**Maitland's Vertebral
Manipulation**

This book is dedicated to the memory of Geoff and Anne Maitland and the legacy they have left for us to nurture and evolve

Content Strategist: *Rita Demetriou-Swanwick*
Content Development Specialist: *Sheila Black*
Project Manager: *Anne Collett*
Designer: *Christian Bilbow*
Illustration Manager: *Jennifer Rose*

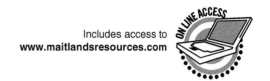
Includes access to
www.maitlandsresources.com

Maitland's Vertebral Manipulation

Management of Neuromusculoskeletal Disorders
Volume 1

EIGHTH EDITION

Edited by

Elly Hengeveld
MSc BPT OMTsvomp Clin Spec fisioswiss/MSK IMTA Member
Oberentfelden, Switzerland

Kevin Banks BA MMACP MCSP SRP IMTA Member
Chartered Physiotherapist, Rotherham, UK

Consulting Editor

Matthew Newton HPC Reg, MCSP, MMACP, MIMTA
Teacher, International Maitland Teachers' Association
Orthopaedic Physiotherapy Practitioner, Doncaster, UK

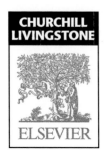

Edinburgh London New York Oxford Philadelphia St Louis Sydney Toronto 2014

CHURCHILL LIVINGSTONE
ELSEVIER

First edition 1964
Second edition 1968
Third edition 1973
Fourth edition 1977
Fifth edition 1986
Sixth edition 2001
Seventh edition 2005
Eighth edition 2014

ISBN 978-0-7020-4066-5

British Library Cataloguing in Publication Data
A catalogue record for this book is available from the British Library

Library of Congress Cataloging in Publication Data
A catalog record for this book is available from the Library of Congress

Notices

Knowledge and best practice in this field are constantly changing. As new research and experience broaden our understanding, changes in research methods, professional practices, or medical treatment may become necessary.

Practitioners and researchers must always rely on their own experience and knowledge in evaluating and using any information, methods, compounds, or experiments described herein. In using such information or methods they should be mindful of their own safety and the safety of others, including parties for whom they have a professional responsibility.

With respect to any drug or pharmaceutical products identified, readers are advised to check the most current information provided (i) on procedures featured or (ii) by the manufacturer of each product to be administered, to verify the recommended dose or formula, the method and duration of administration, and contraindications. It is the responsibility of practitioners, relying on their own experience and knowledge of their patients, to make diagnoses, to determine dosages and the best treatment for each individual patient, and to take all appropriate safety precautions.

To the fullest extent of the law, neither the Publisher nor the authors, contributors, or editors, assume any liability for any injury and/or damage to persons or property as a matter of products liability, negligence or otherwise, or from any use or operation of any methods, products, instructions, or ideas contained in the material herein.

 your source for books, journals and multimedia in the health sciences

www.elsevierhealth.com

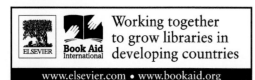 Working together to grow libraries in developing countries

www.elsevier.com • www.bookaid.org

The publisher's policy is to use paper manufactured from sustainable forests

Printed in Great Britain

Last digit is the print number: 10

Contents

Contributors vi

Biography – Geoffrey Douglas Maitland vii

Preface xi

Acknowledgements. xiii

In Memoriam: Kevin Banks (1959-2012). xiv

Glossary xv

1 The Maitland Concept: Assessment, examination and treatment of movement
impairments by passive movement 1
Geoffrey D. Maitland

2 Clinical reasoning: From the Maitland Concept and beyond. 14
Mark A. Jones

3 Communication and the therapeutic relationship. 83
Elly Hengeveld and Geoffrey D. Maitland

4 Management of cervical spine disorders: A neuro-orthopaedic perspective. 116
Robin Blake and Tim Beames

5 Management of thoracic spine disorders 174
Peter Wells and Kevin Banks

6 Management of lumbar spine disorders 228
Elly Hengeveld and Kevin Banks

7 Management of sacroiliac and pelvic disorders. 330
Elaine Maheu and Elly Hengeveld

8 Sustaining functional capacity and performance 380
Elly Hengeveld

Appendix 1 Movement diagram theory and compiling a movement diagram. 404

Appendix 2 Clinical examples of movement diagrams 423

Appendix 3 Examination refinements and movement diagrams 428

Appendix 4 Recording 433

Index. 444

Contributors

Kevin Banks BA MMACP MCSP SRP IMTA Member
Chartered Physiotherapist, Rotherham, UK

Tim Beames MSc BSc(Hons) MCSP
Chartered Physiotherapist; Instructor Neuro Orthopaedic
Institute, London, UK

Robin Blake MCSP DipTP
Chartered Physiotherapist in Private Practice, Kirkby
Malzeard, UK

Elly Hengeveld MSc BPT OMTsvomp Clin Spec fisioswiss/MSK
IMTA Member
Senior teacher IMTA, Oberentfelden, Switzerland

Mark A. Jones BSc(Psych) PT MAppSc
Program Director, Master of Musculoskeletal and Sports
Physiotherapy,
School of Health Sciences, University of South Australia,
Australia

Elaine Maheu BSc PT Grad Dip Manip Ther(SA) FCAMPT
IMTA CGIMS
Manipulative Physiotherapist (Clinical Practice), Montreal;
Instructor and Chief Examiner for the Orthopaedic
Division of the Canadian Physiotherapy Association,
St Laurent, Quebec, Canada

The late Geoffrey D. Maitland MBE AUA FCSP FACP
Specialist Manipulative Physiotherapist, MAppSc
[Physiotherapy], Adelaide, Australia

Peter Wells BA DipTP FCSP FMACP
Senior Teacher, International Maitland Teachers
Association (IMTA); Formerly Physiotherapy Clinician and
Teacher, London, UK

Geoffrey Douglas Maitland MBE AUA FCSP FACP (Monograph), FACP (Specialist Manipulative Physiotherapist) MAppSc (Physiotherapy)

Geoff Maitland worked initially at the Royal Adelaide Hospital and the Adelaide Children's Hospital, with a main interest in the treatment of orthopaedic and neurological disorders. Later he became a part-time private practitioner and part-time clinical tutor at the School of Physiotherapy at the University of South Australia. He continuously studied and spent half a day each week in the Barr–Smith Library and the excellent library at the Medical School of the University of Adelaide.

He immediately showed an interest in careful clinical examination and assessment of patients with neuromusculoskeletal disorders. In those days assessment and treatment by specific passive movements were under-represented in physiotherapy practice. G.D. Maitland learned techniques from osteopathic, chiropractic and bonesetter books as well as from medical books such as those of Marlin, Jostes, James B. Mennell, John McMillan Mennell, Alan Stoddard, Robert Maigne, Edgar Cyriax, James Cyriax and many others. He maintained an extensive correspondence with numerous authors worldwide, who published work on passive mobilizations, manipulation and related topics as for example MacNab from Canada and Alf Breig from Sweden.

As a lecturer, he emphasized clinical examination and assessment. He stimulated students to write treatment records from the very beginning, as he felt that 'one needed to commit oneself to paper to analyze what one is doing'. In 1954 he started with manipulative therapy teaching sessions.

In 1961 he received an award from a special studies fund, which enabled him and his wife Anne to go overseas for a study tour. They visited osteopaths, chiropractors, medical doctors and physiotherapy colleagues whom they had heard and read about and corresponded with in the preceding years. In London, Geoff had interesting lunchtime clinical sessions and discussions with James Cyriax and his staff. From this tour G.D. Maitland established a

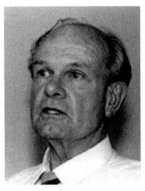

G.D. Maitland (1924–2010), who was born in Adelaide, Australia, trained as a physiotherapist from 1946 to 1949 after serving in the RAAF during the Second World War in Great Britain.

friendship with Gregory P Grieve from the UK. They had extensive correspondence about their clinical experiences and this continued for many years.

Maitland delivered a paper, in 1962, to the Physiotherapy Society of Australia entitled 'The Problems of Teaching Vertebral Manipulation', in which he presented a clear differentiation between manipulation and mobilization and became a strong advocate of the use of gentle passive movement in the treatment of pain, in addition to the more traditional forceful techniques used to increase range of motion. In this context it may be suitable to quote James Cyriax, a founder of orthopaedic medicine and of major influence on the development of manipulative therapy provided by physiotherapists:

> ...more recently Maitland, a physiotherapist from Australia, has been employing repetitive thrusts of lesser frequency but with more strength behind them. They are not identical with the mobilizing techniques that osteopaths misname 'articulation', nor are they as jerky as chiropractors' pressures. The great virtue

of Maitland's work is its moderation. He has not expanded his manipulative techniques into a cult; he claims neither autonomic effects nor that they are a panacea. Indeed, he goes out of his way to avoid theoretical arguments and insists on the practical effect of manipulation… The patient is examined at frequent intervals during the session, to enable the manipulator to assess the result of his treatment so far. He continues or alters his technique in accordance with the change, or absence of change, detected. These mobilizations clearly provide the physiotherapist with a useful addition to those of orthopaedic medicine and, better still, with an introduction to them. She gains confidence from using gentle manoeuvres and, if the case responds well… need seek no further.

Cyriax J 1984 Textbook of Orthopaedic Medicine. Part II – Treatment by Manipulation, Massage and Injection, 11th edition. Ballière-Tindall, London. pp 40–41.

G.D. Maitland became a substantial contributor to the *Australian Journal of Physiotherapy* as well as to other medical and physiotherapy journals worldwide. On the instigation of Monica Martin-Jones, OBE, a leader of the Chartered Society of Physiotherapy in Great Britain, Maitland was asked to publish his work, which resulted in the first edition of *Vertebral Manipulation* in 1964, which was followed by a second edition in 1968. The first edition of *Peripheral Manipulation* was published in 1970, in which the famous 'movement diagram' was introduced, an earlier co-production with Ms Jennifer Hickling in 1965.

Over all the years of lecturing and publishing, Maitland kept treating patients as the clinical work remained his main source of learning and adapting ideas. Geoff treated patients in his private practice for over 40 years and although he closed his practice in 1988, he remained active in treating patients until 1995.

In 1965, one of Maitland's wishes came true; with the help of Ms Elma Caseley, Head of the Physiotherapy School, South Australian Institute of Technology and the South Australian Branch of the Australian Physiotherapy Association, the first three months course on Manipulation of the spine was held in Adelaide. In 1974 this course developed into the one-year postgraduate education 'postgraduate diploma in manipulative physiotherapy' at the South Australian Institute of Technology, now a master's degree course at the University of South Australia.

He was one of the co-founders, in 1974, of the International Federation of Orthopaedic Manipulative Physical Therapy (IFOMPT), a branch of the World Confederation of Physiotherapy (WCPT).

Only in 1978, while teaching one of his first courses in continental Europe in Bad Ragaz, Switzerland, did he recognize, through discussion with Dr Zinn, Director of the Medical Clinic and the Postgraduate Study Centre in Bad Ragaz, that in fact his work and ideas were a specific concept of thought and action rather than a method of applying manipulative techniques. The Maitland Concept of Manipulative Physiotherapy, as it became known, emphasizes a specific way of thinking, continuous evaluation and assessment and the art of manipulative physiotherapy ('know when, how and which techniques to perform, and adapt these to the individual situation of the patient') and a total commitment to the patient.

Maitland has held a long and extensive commitment to various professional associations:

- Australian Physiotherapy Association (APA) where he was on the State branch committee for 28 years in various capacities and a State Delegate to Federal Council for 11 years. In conjunction with others, he was responsible for the revision of the constitution of APA in 1964–1965. In 1977, he put forward a submission regarding Specialization in Manipulative Physiotherapy, a concept which was subsequently accepted in modified form.
- Inaugural President of the Australian College of Physiotherapists for six years and a member of the council for a further six years.
- Member of the Physiotherapy Registration Board of South Australia for 22 years.
- Chairman of the Expert Panel for Physiotherapy for Australian Examining Council for Overseas Physiotherapists (AECOP) for 11 years.
- Australian delegate to IFOMPT for five years and a member of its academic standards committee for another five years.

For his work he was honoured with several awards:

- Member of the Order of the British Empire in 1981.
- Fellowship of the Australian College of Physiotherapists by Monograph in 1970, with a further Fellowship by specialization in 1984.
- Honorary Degree of Master of Applied Science in Physiotherapy from the University of South Australia in 1986.
- Honorary Fellow of the Chartered Society of Physiotherapy (GB).

- Honorary life memberships of the South African Society of Physiotherapy, including the Group of Manipulative Physiotherapy, Manipulative Physiotherapy Association of Australia (MPAA), Swiss Association of Manipulative Physiotherapy (svomp), German Association of Manual Therapy (DVMT), the American Physical Therapy Association (APTA) and the International Maitland Teachers' Association (IMTA).

- He received an award from IFOMPT in appreciation of his service and leadership from its foundation.

- Mildred Elson Award by the World Confederation of Physical Therapy (WCPT) for his life's work in 1995.

In 1992 in Zurzach, Switzerland, the International Maitland Teachers' Association (IMTA) was founded, of which G.D. Maitland was a founding member and inaugural President.

All this work would not have been possible without the loving support of his wife Anne, the mother of their two children, John and Wendy. Anne did most of the graphic arts in Maitland's publications, kept notes, made manuscripts and videotaped many of his courses. Their continuous feedback discipline has been one of the very strengths of the Maitlands, who have been practically inseparable since they met in England during the Second World War. Anne was awarded the protectoress of the Dutch Association of Orthopaedic Manipulative Therapy (NVOMT).

Maitland's work, especially through the mode of thinking and the process of continuous assessment, has laid the foundation for the development of contemporary definitions and descriptions of the physiotherapy process. His life's work has been acknowledged by numerous authors in obituaries at the time of his passing in 2010:

> ...Geoff will be remembered by countless physiotherapists in Australia and overseas. We acknowledge the passing of a truly great clinician, teacher and mentor.
>
> P. Trott, R Grant, 2010, Manual Therapy 15:297

> ...Geoff Maitland's contribution to the physiotherapy profession, and in particular to musculoskeletal physiotherapy, cannot be underestimated. His inspiration and collaboration with our own UK pioneers led to the development of the MACP and really set the foundations for all the extended scope roles and postgraduate physiotherapy education that we enjoy today.
>
> MACP, 2010, Manual Therapy 15:298–299

> ...Geoff was a great listener and a great communicator. He placed a great emphasis on the art and skill of listening [as opposed to just hearing]. He would hang on every word his patients would say so that he did not miss the subtle hints from the language or its tone that would help him understand, in depth, what the individual was experiencing. He would use every facet of 'the bodies capacity to inform' both verbal and non-verbal. He would spot the almost imperceptible nuances of the patient's responses to his treatment. Only he would recognize, in a room full of students, the important meaning of a patient drumming his fingers on the couch. Geoff was a visionary and an innovator. In the preface to the first edition of Vertebral Manipulation [1964] he recognizes 'The practical approach to the use of manipulation is to relate treatment to the patient's symptoms and signs rather than to diagnosis' and that 'it is often impossible to know what the true pathology is ...symptoms and signs [of a disc lesion] may vary widely and require different treatments'
>
> His vision was instrumental in giving us what are now established competencies, including, 'Patient-centred Care', the use of mobilization for pain modulation, and an awareness of 'the nature of the person' and 1st impact on treatment. He highlighted the need for deep and broad theoretical knowledge to support and inform clinical practice. He advocated the discipline of evaluating everything we do to prove our worth and with this came the use of patient reported and orientated outcome measures [subjective and functional asterisks] and the demand for accurate recording of treatment and its effects. Geoff was also at the forefront of research by Physiotherapists for Physiotherapist at a time when it was seen as the role of the Doctor to report on Physiotherapy and decide which Physiotherapy modalities should be prescribed. In summary, G.D. Maitland supported by Anne and his close family and colleagues has established his place in our Profession's History. He is the Donald Bradman of Physiotherapists. Sir Donald, a fellow Australian, had a career Test Match batting average of 99.94 and, as with Geoff, many have aspired to reach such a standard but none, to date, have come anywhere near.
>
> Chairman and members of the International Maitland Teachers' Association, IMTA, 2010, Manual Therapy 15:300–301

Within this context it seems suitable to conclude with a quote from Professor Lance Twomey, Vice Chancellor, Professor of Physiotherapy, Curtin University of Technology, Perth, Australia:

...Maitland's emphasis on very careful and comprehensive examination leading to the precise application of treatment by movement and followed in turn by the assessment of the effects of that movement on the patient, form the basis for the modern clinical approach. This is probably as close to the scientific method as is possible within the clinical practice of physical therapy and serves as a model for other special areas of the profession.

Foreword in Refshauge K & Gass E, 1995, Musculoskeletal physiotherapy. Butterworth-Heinemann, Oxford. p IX

Kevin Banks, Elly Hengeveld

This is the first major revision of *Vertebral Manipulation* since 1986. The editors, in tribute to the legacy of Geoff Maitland, have brought together a team of physiotherapists from all over the world with an expertise in the clinical application of the principles and practice of the 'Maitland Concept'.

A key feature of the revised text is a move away from Geoff Maitland's narrative style of writing to a more evidence-based and analytical view of the role of mobilization and manipulation in clinical practice.

In the 26 years since Geoff Maitland comprehensively updated this text there have been many advances in knowledge in physiotherapy practice. The role of the Maitland Concept in the management of movement-related vertebral disorders needs to be placed in the context of such advances. Contemporary physiotherapy practice is marked by an era of evidence-based practice with the development of guidelines as a decision-making protocol, validity and reliability of clinical assessment instruments, clinical prediction rules, person-centred questionnaires, numeric rating scales, outcome studies and so on.

Nevertheless, the basic principles of this concept of musculoskeletal physiotherapy are as valid as in the origins of their development:

> ...open minded, self-critical thinking, judiciously applying theories into practice, with the primacy of clinical proof. The application of the art of passive movement within the overall concept of movement rehabilitation based on clinical information, progression of treatment and a client-centred attitude.

This concept deals with making decisions collaboratively with a person who seeks the help of a physiotherapist. It emphasizes the art and science of observation, listening, palpation and movement skills. Numeric rating scales may reduce the richness of an individual illness experience to a single number, but careful listening and observation skills may give cues to the world of the individual's thoughts and feelings, which may become determining factors in clinical decision regarding movement rehabilitation. It appears that mixed approaches of active and passive movements lead to better clinical outcomes than either treatment approach alone. Therefore, the art and science of physiotherapy practice encompass the art of passive movement, with the selection and progression of treatment techniques based on clinical information. They also involve teaching active movement and the motivation of patients to change their movement behaviour.

In this process the clinical physiotherapists are encouraged to make use of the best of their personal, theoretical and experiential knowledge bases, the best evidence, and the best of themselves and the patient in order to develop an individualized treatment programme which suits the patient's needs and preferences.

The keynote chapters by GD Maitland from 1987 (*The Maitland Concept: assessment, examination and treatment by passive movement*) and by Mark Jones (*Clinical reasoning: from the Maitland Concept and beyond*) compare and contrast how clinical decision making has developed, to a point whereby an attention to detail in analyzing patient information, forming hypotheses, testing hypotheses in an orderly and structured way, and then evaluating the effectiveness of the decisions made, is underpinned by a deep knowledge of the theoretical basis of clinical reasoning.

The chapter *Communication and the therapeutic relationship* builds on the earlier chapter written by Geoff Maitland in 1986. Several verbatim examples stem directly from the original version. This chapter deals with aspects of person-centredness and individualized communication, as a basis for information exchange and the development of a therapeutic relationship. The individual illness experience of a person has become an important aspect within a bio-psychosocial paradigm of practice, which can be touched by attentive listening and observing as well as conscious communication skills.

The specific vertebral chapters are written from a clinical perspective and review the evidence informing and underpinning how we, as manual therapists, deal with and manage spinal and pelvic pain as they present to us.

Each vertebral region (cervical, thoracic, lumbar, sacroiliac/pelvic) is considered from the point of view of best practice in analyzing and hypothesizing about subjective data, examination, treatment and management of spinal pain conditions.

Robin Blake and Tim Beames, in the chapter *Management of cervical spine disorders: a neuro-orthopaedic perspective*, apply the principles of the Maitland Concept to neck pain. In particular they give us a clearer understanding of how the different mechanisms of pain present in the neck and how, for example, our knowledge of central sensitization has helped us to make sense of patient responses. As a result we learn how to apply manual therapy techniques more effectively with this knowledge in mind. In this chapter there is also an emphasis on managing neurogenic pain and how manual therapy advances in 'neurodynamics' can be integrated with mobilization techniques.

In the chapter, *Management of thoracic spine disorders*, Peter Wells shares his years of expertise in understanding and dealing with a range of complex painful conditions emanating from the vertebral and associated structures in the thoracic spine. This is backed up by a raft of clinical studies which show an association between thoracic manual therapy techniques and relief from shoulder, neck, elbow, groin and thoracic pain.

Kevin Banks and Elly Hengeveld review the *Management of lumbar spine disorders* from the perspective of the role of mobilization and manipulation in helping to de-medicalize low back pain. The evidence reviewed and improved knowledge about motor control and neurodynamic impairments and low back pain has led to a novel way of progressing treatment techniques to include and integrate the three key movement components of non-specific low back pain (arthrogenic, myogenic and neurogenic).

In *Management of sacroiliac and pelvic disorders*, Elaine Maheu and Elly Hengeveld make us realize how often we miss sacroiliac disorders in clinical practice and how, through an attention to detail in examination, we can establish physical impairments in this region. In this chapter there is an emphasis

on how, by thoroughly assessing the sacroiliac joints and pelvis from joint, motor control and neural perspectives, we can show how this region impacts on a whole variety of clinical conditions from the foot to the neck.

The final chapter, on *Sustaining functional capacity and performance*, by Elly Hengeveld explores contemporary paradigms of physical health and wellbeing and the role we have to play as manual therapist and physiotherapists in ensuring patients maintain a productive level of healthy living for themselves. Dependence on medical care and social welfare has become a burden to society when we look at the epidemiology and cost implications of vertebral conditions. The way forward is to use manual therapy as a means to an end in ensuring patients are advised and signposted effectively into sustainable healthy living and maximization of their functional capabilities. The International Classification of Functioning [ICF] is used as the ideal framework for supporting such a desire.

Not all techniques of mobilization and manipulation that are presented in previous editions of *Vertebral Manipulation* are described in these chapters and not all the principles of the concept are detailed. The reason for this is that the authors of each chapter have written in a way that reflects their application of the Maitland Concept to clinical practice and how they have integrated techniques in the light of advancement in professional knowledge.

Additional principles, techniques of examinations and treatment, however, will be made available on the companion website.

As co-editors we hope you enjoy dipping into this text and accessing the companion website (www.maitlandsresources.com) to support the construction of your knowledge and understanding of manipulative physiotherapy and the Maitland Concept. We hope this will give you plenty of deep and contextual learning opportunities to develop your own practice and personal learning goals.

Kevin Banks, Elly Hengeveld 2012

Acknowledgements

Kevin Banks and Elly Hengeveld would like to thank all contributors for sharing their expertise and perspective on the Maitland Concept. They would like to thank Sheila Black and Rita Demetriou-Swanwick from Elsevier for their support, advice and patience. Kevin would also like to thank Rich and Sarah, Will and Rachel for their help with Paintbrush™, Stefan for his photography, Steve and Abi for modelling and all those whose photographs are presented and who have modelled for the figures. Elly expresses her gratitude to Kevin: it has been a privilege for 20 years to work with you in these writing endeavours, as well as in teaching. It is always an enriching experience. Thanks to Hugo Stam for his commitment and to Harry von Piekartz for his support of the work in the Netherlands. Elly also expresses her gratitude to Matthew Newton for his invaluable help at the completion of the electronic version of this publication.

Last, but not least, Kevin and Elly would like to say 'Geoff and Anne, we are sure you are looking down on us and we hope you are happy with what we have done with your lifetimes' work'.

In Memoriam: Kevin Banks (1959–2012)

It is with great sadness that we learned of the death of Kevin Banks. Kevin passed away on 14 November 2012 aged 53 after a short illness.

Kevin has been involved as a co-editor with Elsevier's *Maitland's Peripheral Manipulation*, *Maitland's Vertebral Manipulation* and *Maitland's Clinical Companion*. He passed away as we were completing the manuscripts for the new editions of *Maitland's Peripheral Manipulation* and *Maitland's Vertebral Manipulation*, which he will sadly not be able to see in their final versions.

Kevin was a senior teacher and founding member of the International Maitland Teachers' Association (IMTA). His enquiring thoroughness and critical input played a decisive role in IMTA's further development as an educational institute.

We have lost a friend and colleague dedicated to the teaching and further development of the principles of manipulative or neuromusculoskeletal physiotherapy as initiated by GD Maitland. Kevin saw himself as a practising Clinician and Clinical Educator. His belief that a structured yet flexible clinical practice framework, along with a detailed grounding in clinical reasoning, communication and wise action decision making, is essential for best practice was at the heart of his teaching. Kevin really was a visionary. He knew where his professional area of specialism needed to develop and how to get it there, in a way that many did not. He stated of himself: 'I am driven by the need to enhance learning in a broad and deep range of skills, knowledge and attributes within physiotherapy to ensure that patients have as good a deal as possible.' The patient and their needs were indeed the centre of all he did and strived for in his professional life.

We knew Kevin as a gentle and dedicated person. Many of us have enjoyed his often subtle and unexpected humour and most of all his friendship and kind-heartedness. Kevin has been suddenly taken from us in the prime of his life. We are proud to have been associated with him and will miss him. Our sympathy and thoughts are with his wife, Nancy, and his children Richard, William and Helen.

Elly Hengeveld
Sheila Black and Rita Demetriou-Swanwick (Elsevier)

Chapter 1 The Maitland Concept: assessment, examination and treatment of movement impairments by passive movement

Assessment – Numerous types are practised to monitor the varying stages of the therapeutic process:

1. Analytical assessment in the initial phase
2. Reassessment procedures before and after the application of therapeutic interventions, as well as at the beginning on consecutive sessions
3. Assessment during the application of therapeutic interventions
4. Retrospective assessment, final analytical assessment at the end phase of the therapeutic process.

Maitland Concept, core requirements – Requires open-mindedness, mental agility and mental discipline linked with a logical and methodical process of assessing cause and effect. The central theme demands a positive personal commitment (empathy) to understand what the person (patient) is enduring.

Maitland Concept, key issues – Personal commitment, mode of thinking, techniques, examination, and assessment.

Mode of thinking – The 'science' of physiotherapy enables physiotherapists to make diagnoses and apply the appropriate 'art' of their physical skills; however, the accepted theoretical basis of the profession is continually developing and changing. It is essential that therapists remain open to new knowledge and open-minded in areas of uncertainty. Even with properly attested science applied in its right context, only with precise information concerning the patient's symptoms and signs (of the movement capacity), is development of the physiotherapeutic diagnosis and meaningful treatment possible. Matching the clinical findings to particular theories of anatomical, biomechanical and pathological knowledge, so as to attach a particular 'label' to the patient's condition, may not always be appropriate. Therapists must remain open-minded so that as treatment progresses, the patient is reassessed in relation to the evolution of the condition and the responses to treatment. Clinical evidence should remain the primacy of the clinical work with patients at all times.

Personal commitment to the patient – The necessity of making a conscious effort (particularly during the first consultation) to gain the patient's confidence, trust and relaxed comfort in what may be, at first, an anxious experience. The achievement of this trusting relationship requires many skills, but it is essential if proper *care* is to be provided.

Symbolic permeable brickwall of clinical reasoning – Approach which separates theoretical knowledge from clinical information in clinical decision-making processes, i.e. information from one side can filter through to the other. Thus, theoretical concepts influence examination and treatment, while examination and treatment lead one back to a reconsideration of theoretical premises. It is essential that theoretical knowledge as well as information from 'evidence-based practice' informs clinical work with patients; however, it should not lead to a narrow outlook or prevent innovative practice where required.

Chapter 2 Clinical reasoning: from the Maitland Concept and beyond

Bio-psychosocial model – A framework or approach originally put forward by psychiatrist George L. Engel, University of Rochester. This model proposes that biological, psychological (incorporating thoughts, emotions and behaviours) and social factors all contribute to human functioning, health and disease or illness. This is in contrast to the reductionist biomedical model that previously dominated medicine and physiotherapy where disease and illness were solely attributed to pathogens, genetic or developmental abnormalities or injury.

Clinical reasoning strategies – Various foci of reasoning used by physiotherapists, e.g. diagnostic reasoning, narrative reasoning, reasoning about procedure, interactive reasoning, collaborative reasoning, reasoning about teaching, predictive reasoning and ethical reasoning.

Contributing factors – Predisposing or associated factors (e.g. environmental, psychosocial, behavioural, physical/biomechanical, hereditary) involved in the development or maintenance of the patient's problem.

Deductive reasoning – Backward reasoning from a general premise toward a specific conclusion (associated with hypothesis testing).

Diagnostic reasoning – The reasoning associated with the formation of a physiotherapy 'diagnosis' related to functional limitation(s) and associated physical impairments with consideration of pain mechanisms, tissue pathology and the broad scope of potential contributing factors.

Hypothesis categories – Categories of decisions physiotherapists propose to make through their patient examination and management.

Illness schemata – Individuals' implicit theories of illness that they use to interpret and respond to health threats incorporating the symptoms they associate with the health problem, their beliefs about the immediate and long-term consequences of the problem and its temporal course, and their attributions concerning the cause of the problem and the means by which a cure may be affected.

Inductive reasoning – Forward reasoning from specific cues toward a general judgement (associated with pattern recognition).

Metacognition – Reflective self-awareness and self-monitoring of thinking, knowledge and performance.

Mind map – Pictorial representation of a person's knowledge and organization of knowledge on a specified topic.

Narrative reasoning – Understanding patients' pain, illness and/or disability experiences, or their 'story' incorporating their understanding of their problem and the effect it is having on their life, their expectations regarding management, their feelings and ability to cope and the effects these personal perspectives have on their clinical presentation, particularly whether they are facilitating or obstructing their recovery.

Non-propositional knowledge – Knowledge generated primarily through practice experience.

Pain mechanisms – The input, processing and output mechanisms underlying the patients' activity/

participation restrictions, unhelpful perspectives and physical impairments.

Patient perspectives – Patient's thoughts/beliefs, motivations, feelings, goals, expectations and self-efficacy regarding their pain and disability experience (i.e. psychosocial status).

Propositional knowledge – Knowledge generated formally through research and scholarship.

Socratic questioning – The art of asking questions and pursuing answers originated by Socrates, based on the notion that thinking (e.g. interpretations, opinions, analyses, conclusions) has an underpinning logic or structure which typically is not evident in the initial expression. The purpose of Socratic questioning is to clarify and understand the logic of someone's thoughts (including your own through critical reflection).

Screening questions – Questions (asked by interview or questionnaire) which aim to identify potentially important information from the patient that may not have been volunteered.

Chapter 3 Communication and the therapeutic relationship

Collaborative goal setting – The process in which the physiotherapist defines desired outcomes of treatment *with* the patient, rather than *for* the patient. This is an ongoing process throughout all sessions. It includes goals of treatment, selection of interventions and parameters to assess treatment results.

Communication – Verbal and non-verbal. Can be considered to be a process of the exchange of messages that need to be decoded. A message may contain various aspects: the content of the message, an appeal, an indication of the relationship to the person to whom the message is addressed, and revealing something about the sender of the message (Schulz von Thun 1981).

Watzlawick et al.'s axiom (1969) – 'non-communication does not exist' – indicates that non-verbal communication as well as the absence of words can be a strong message.

Critical phases of the therapeutic process – Throughout the overall physiotherapy process there are some specific 'critical' phases in which particular information needs to be sought or given. Skipping some of the critical phases may result in the physiotherapist missing relevant information regarding diagnosis or assessment. Furthermore, skipping phases may impede the therapeutic relationship as the patient may not understand the purpose of certain procedures.

Immediate-response questions – In various phases of the process of information-gathering (initial sessions, reassessment procedures), the physiotherapist may need to gently interrupt the patient with an interceding 'immediate-response' question to seek clarification of the information given by the patient. This is particularly essential during the subjective examination in the initial session and in reassessment procedures where 'statements of fact' need to be converted into comparisons.

Key phrases, key words, key gestures – These need attention throughout the whole physiotherapy process. If picked up and reacted upon, the physiotherapist may receive important information in assessment and reassessment procedures. Furthermore, they may be indicative clues to the patient's world of thoughts, feelings and emotions, which may be contributing factors to ongoing disability due to pain.

Listening skills – The physiotherapist needs to develop passive and active listening skills to allow the development of a climate in which the patient feels free to reveal any information which seems relevant.

Mirroring – Communication technique which may be employed by the physiotherapist to guide the patient to an increased awareness with regard to use of the body, posture or elements of the individual illness experience. Often starts off with, 'I see you doing…' or 'I hear you saying…'.

Paralleling – An important communication technique, in which the physiotherapist follows the patient's line of thought rather than letting the physiotherapeutic procedures of subjective examination prevail.

Therapeutic relationship – Distinct from a personal relationship. Communication and the conscious development of a therapeutic relationship are considered important elements to enhance a climate in which the patient can learn, develop trust and recover full function.

Yellow flags – Psychosocial risk factors, which may hinder the process to full recovery of function.

Chapter 4 Management of cervical spine disorders: a neuro-orthopaedic perspective

Allodynia – Pain due to a stimulus that does not normally provoke pain.

Bio-psychosocial – Describes the personal construct of attitudes and beliefs related to injury and pain and how these interact with social, cultural, linguistic and workplace influences (Butler 2000). For bio-psychosocial model, see Chapter 2 definition above.

Central sensitization – Increased responsiveness of nociceptive neurons in the central nervous system to their normal or subthreshold afferent input.

Dysaesthesia – An unpleasant abnormal sensation, whether spontaneous or evoked.

Hyperalgesia – Increased pain sensation from a stimulus that normally provokes pain.

Hypoalgesia – Diminished pain in response to a normally painful stimulus.

Mature organism model (Gifford 1998) – The mature organism model is a conceptual model for incorporating pain mechanisms into the science of stress biology and the bio-psychosocial model of pain. This model is also referred to the as the circular model (Butler 2000).

Neuralgia – Pain in the distribution of a nerve or nerves.

Neuromatrix – Can be considered as a vast interconnecting, highly flexible, plastic network of groups of neurons in the brain activated and sculptured by any and every lifetime activity and experience (Melzack 1990), which integrates multiple inputs to produce the output pattern that evokes pain (Melzack 1999).

Neuropathic pain – Pain caused by a lesion or disease of the somatosensory nervous system.

Neuropathy – A disturbance of function or pathological change in a nerve: in one nerve, mononeuropathy; in several nerves, mononeuropathy multiplex; if diffuse and bilateral, polyneuropathy.

Neurosignatures/neurotags – Outputs of the neuromatrix (Melzack 1999) and the pattern of activity that creates the perception of any sensory stimulation in the brain. The perception of pain can be considered a 'neurotag' for pain (Butler & Moseley 2003) and determines the particular qualities and other properties of the pain experience and behaviour.

Nociception – The neural process of encoding noxious stimuli.

Nociceptive neuron – A central or peripheral neuron of the somatosensory nervous system that is capable of encoding noxious stimuli.

Nociceptive pain – Pain that arises from actual or threatened damage to non-neural tissue and is due to the activation of nociceptors.

Nociceptive stimulus – An actually or potentially tissue-damaging event transduced and encoded by nociceptors.

Nociceptor – A high-threshold sensory receptor of the peripheral somatosensory nervous system that is capable of transducing and encoding noxious stimuli.

Noxious stimulus – A stimulus that is damaging or threatens damage to normal tissues.

Paraesthesia – An abnormal sensation, whether spontaneous or evoked.

Peripheral neuropathic pain – Pain caused by a lesion or disease of the peripheral somatosensory nervous system.

Peripheral sensitization – Increased responsiveness and reduced threshold of nociceptive neurons in the periphery to the stimulation of their receptive fields.

Radicular pain – Pain found in the distribution of a known dermatome or nerve tract possibly due to inflammation or other irritation of the nerve root.

Radiculopathy – Not a specific condition, but rather a description of a problem in which one or more nerves are affected and do not work properly (a neuropathy).

Representation – The central nervous system is the ultimate representational device. It has the ability to represent the whole body embracing anatomy, physiology, movement, pain, emotion and disease (Melzack 1990).

Sensitization – Increased responsiveness of nociceptive neurons to their normal input, and/or recruitment of a response to normally subthreshold inputs.

Virtual body – The representation of the real body in the brain. The identification of pain and related symptoms are always expressed in the virtual body in the brain.

WAD – Whiplash-associated disorders.

Chapter 5 Management of thoracic spine disorders

Bio-psychosocial – A framework or approach originally put forward by the psychiatrist George L. Engel, University of Rochester. See Chapter 2 definition of bio-psychosocial model, above.

Multi-area, multi-symptomatic – Patients with complex and chronic problems often present with many areas of symptoms affecting them in many ways. Therapists, in such instances, should regard them each as a part of one problem, with separate and discrete structural and neurological inputs.

Somatic simulating visceral, visceral simulating somatic – Knowledge of: anatomy; innervations of body tissue; referred pain; clinical studies; and clinical experience ensure that therapists should always be aware that a painful stimulus of somatic tissue (e.g. the thoracic intervertebral joints) can simulate pain from a visceral organ (e.g. the gall bladder) and vice versa. In some instances the two simulating situations may co-exist.

Red flags – Signs and symptoms which indicate the presence of serious pathology, and the requirement for urgent medical attention.

'Make the features fit' – One of the most important part of assessment of a patient. The manipulative physiotherapist will tell the patient that his problem is like a jigsaw puzzle, and it is her job to 'make all the pieces fit'. She needs his help and collaboration to do this. As a result of this partnership all the clinical information, therapist's knowledge and patient and therapist's experience can be analyzed and linked together in order to enhance effective therapeutic decisions.

Passive mobilization techniques – Manual therapy treatment techniques performed, usually, by a therapist on a patient. The techniques are performed in such a manner (oscillatory/sustained stretch, position in range, amplitude, speed, rhythm and duration) that they are always under the control of the patient.

Chapter 6 Management of lumbar spine disorders

Demedicalization of low back pain – The need for such a condition to be managed in the community rather than in a hospital.

Low back pain – Characterized by pain and discomfort localized below the costal margin and above the inferior gluteal fold, with or without leg pain.

'Make features fit' – See Chapter 5 definition, above.

Prognosis – A forecast of the future history of a patient's disorder based on the probability of physical, psychological and functional recovery of the patient and the disorder.

Chapter 7 Management of sacroiliac and pelvic disorders

Form closure, force closure – Biomechanical properties contributing to the stability of the pelvic girdle. *Form closure* refers to a stable situation with closely fitting joint surfaces, in which no extra forces are needed to maintain the state of the system, once it is under a certain load. *Force closure* is achieved by the local and global stabilizing muscle systems of the pelvis, lumbar spine and legs.

Pelvic girdle pain – Generally arises in relation to pregnancy, trauma, arthritis and osteoarthritis. Pain is experienced between the posterior iliac crest and the gluteal fold, particularly in the vicinity of the sacroiliac joint (SIJ). The pain may radiate in the posterior thigh and can also occur in conjunction with/or separately in the symphysis. The endurance capacity for standing, walking and sitting is diminished. The diagnosis of pelvic girdle pain (PGP) can be reached after exclusion of lumbar causes. The pain or functional disturbances in relation to PGP must be reproducible by specific clinical tests (Vleeming et al. 2008).

Chapter 8 Sustaining movement capacity and performance

Cognitive behavioural principles – Key cognitive behavioural aspects, which may need to be integrated into physiotherapeutic approaches, include:

- Recognition of potential barriers to full functional recovery
- The process of collaborative goal setting
- Phases of behavioural change
- Compliance enhancement
- Patient-education.

Collaborative goal setting – The process of defining treatment objectives, parameters to monitor treatment results and selection of treatment intervention with the patient rather than for the patient. It is essential to consider collaborative goal-setting as a process throughout all treatment sessions rather than a single moment at the beginning of the treatment series. In fact, ongoing information and goal-setting may be considered essential elements of the process of individualized treatment.

Functional restoration and movement capacity – From the profession-specific perspective of physiotherapists, functional restoration aims at sustaining optimum movement capacity of an individual. Treatment objectives encompass enhancement of movement functions, overall well-being and purposeful actions in daily life, in order to allow patients to participate in their chosen activities of life (in their roles as spouse, family member, friend; in sports, leisure activities and work).

Movement continuum theory

– This theory describes human movement from micro level to macro level. It serves as a basis for the development of the body-of-knowledge of physiotherapists and encompasses all concepts and methods in physiotherapy practice.

Phases of functional restoration towards full movement capacity

– In functional restoration programmes, physiotherapists need to adapt the treatment to the various stages of functional capacity: acute and subacute stages, phase of functional restoration and supporting a healthy lifestyle with regard to activity and rest. Passive mobilizations may play an important role during the acute and subacute phases; however, all passive movements should be considered as a kick-start to active movement as well as an enhancement of bodily perception to movement. Therapists should learn to recognize which patients might develop ongoing pain and disability and to adapt their treatment approach. In all phases it is recommended to follow a cognitive-behavioural attitude towards clinical practice.

Appendix 4 Recording

POMR – Problem oriented medical records, containing soap acronym.

SOAP notes – Recording of therapy sessions must include detailed information, yet must be brief and provide a simple overview. Within this concept use has been made of the so-called 'SOAP' notes (Weed 1964, Kirk 1988). The acronym SOAP refers to the various parts of the assessment process:

1. Collection of subjective information
2. Collection of objective information
3. Performing an assessment
4. Develop and formulate a plan.

References

Butler DS: *The sensitive nervous system*. Adelaide, 2000, NOI Publications.

Butler DS, Moseley GL: *Explain pain*. Adelaide, 2003, NOI Publications.

Gifford L: Pain, the tissues and the nervous system: a conceptual model, *Physiotherapy* 84:27–33, 1998.

Kirk D: *Problem orientated medical records: guidelines for therapists*. London, 1988, Kings Fund Centre.

Melzack R: Phantom limbs and the concept of a neuromatrix. *Trends in Neuroscience* 13:88–92, 1990.

Melzack R: From the gate to the neuromatrix. *Pain Supplement* 6:S121–S126, 1999.

Schulz von Thun F: *Miteinander Reden – Störungen und Klärungen. Allgemeine Psychologie der Kommunikation*. Reinbek bei Hamburg, 1981, Rowohlt Taschenbuch Verlag.

Vleeming A, Albert HB, Östgaard HC, et al: European Guidelines for the diagnosis and treatment of pelvic girdle pain. *European Spine Journal* 17:794–819, 2008.

Watzlawick P, Beavin J, Jackson DJ: *Menschliche Kommunikation*. Bern, 1969, Huber Verlag.

Weed L: Medical records, medical education and patient care. *Irish Journal of Medical Science* 6:271–282, 1964.

The Maitland Concept: Assessment, examination and treatment of movement impairments by passive movement

Geoffrey D. Maitland

CHAPTER CONTENTS

Introduction 1
Commitment to patient 2
Primacy of clinical evidence 2
Techniques 5
Examination 6
Assessment 7

Primacy of clinical evidence, commitment to the patient, communication skills, passive movement, mobilization, manipulation

It would be difficult for me as an individual who has been involved in the practice of manipulative physical therapy in Australia for the past three decades to objectively assess my particular contribution to the discipline. I therefore begin this chapter, by way of explanation and justification, with a relevant and pertinent quotation from Lance Twomey:

> In my view, the Maitland approach to treatment differs from others, not in the mechanics of the technique, but rather in its approach to the patient and his particular problem. Your attention to detail in examination, treatment and response is unique in

Physical Therapy, and I believe is worth spelling out in some detail:

- The development of your concepts of assessment and treatment
- Your insistence on sound foundations of basic biological knowledge
- The necessity for high levels of skill
- The evolution of the concepts. It did not 'come' to you fully developed, but is a living thing, developing and extending
- The necessity for detailed examination and for the examination/treatment/re-examination approach.

This area is well worth very considerable attention because, to me, it is the essence of 'Maitland'.

Although the text of this chapter deals with 'passive movement,' it must be very clearly understood that the author does not believe that passive movement is the only form of treatment that will alleviate musculoskeletal disorders. What the chapter *does* set out to do is to provide a conceptual framework for treatment, which is considered by many to be unique. Thus, for want of a better expression, the particular approach to assessment, examination and treatment outlined in this chapter is described as 'the Maitland Concept,' and referred to hereafter as 'the Concept.'

To portray all aspects of 'the Concept' by the written word alone is difficult since so much of it depends upon a particular clinical pattern of reasoning. The approach is not only methodical, but

This chapter is a reprint from Twomey LT, Taylor JR (1987) Physical Therapy of the Low Back. Churchill Livingstone, New York. With permission from Elsevier.

also involved and therefore difficult to describe adequately without clinical demonstration. *The Maitland Concept requires open-mindedness, mental agility, and mental discipline linked with a logical and methodical process of assessing cause and effect. The central theme demands a positive personal commitment (empathy) to understand what the person (patient) is enduring.* The key issues of 'the Concept' that require explanation are personal commitment, mode of thinking, techniques, examination, and assessment.

A personal commitment to the patient

All clinicians would claim that they have a high level of personal commitment to every patient. True as that may be, many areas of physical therapy require that a deeper commitment to certain therapeutic concepts be developed than is usual. Thus, the therapist must have a personal commitment to care, reassure, communicate, listen and inspire confidence.

All therapists must make a conscious effort (particularly during the first consultation) to gain the patient's confidence, trust and relaxed comfort in what may be at first an anxious experience. The achievement of this trusting relationship requires many skills, but it is essential if proper *care* is to be provided.

Within the first few minutes, the clinician must make the patient believe that he wants to know what the patient feels; not what his doctor or anyone else feels, but what the patient himself feels is the main issue. This approach immediately puts the patient at ease by showing that we are concerned about his symptoms and the effect they are having.

We must use the patient's terminology in our discussions: we must adapt our language (and jargon) to fit his; we must make our *concern* for his symptoms show in a way that matches the patient's feelings about the symptoms. In other words, we should adapt our approach to match the patient's mode of expression, not make or expect the patient to adapt to our personality and our knowledge. The patient also needs to be *reassured* of the belief and understanding of the therapist.

Communication is another skill that clinicians must learn to use effectively and appropriately. As far as personal commitment is concerned, this involves understanding the non-verbal as well as the verbal aspects of communication so that use can be made of it to further enhance the relationship between patient and clinician. Some people find that this is a very difficult skill to acquire, but however much effort is required to learn it, it must be learned and used.

Listening to the patient must be done in an open-minded and non-judgmental manner.

It is most important to accept the story the patient weaves, while at the same time being prepared to question him closely about it. Accepting and listening are very demanding skills, requiring a high level of objectivity.

It is a very sad thing to hear patients say that their doctor or physical therapist does not listen to them carefully enough or with enough sympathy, sensitivity, or attention to detail. The following quotation from *The Age* (1982), an Australian daily newspaper, sets out the demands of 'listening' very clearly:

> Listening is itself, of course, an art: that is where it differs from merely hearing. Hearing is passive; listening is active. Hearing is involuntary; listening demands attention. Hearing is natural; listening is an acquired discipline.

Acceptance of the patient and his story is essential if trust between patient and clinician is to be established. We must accept and note the subtleties of his comments about his disorder even if they may sound peculiar. Expressed in another way, he and his symptoms are 'innocent until proven guilty' (that is, his report is true and reliable until found to be unreliable, biased or false). In this context, he needs to be guided to understand that his body can tell him things about his disorder and its behaviour that we (the clinicians) cannot know unless he expresses them. This relationship should *inspire confidence* and build trust between both parties.

This central core of the concept of total commitment must begin at the outset of the first consultation and carry through to the end of the total treatment period.

Other important aspects of communication will be discussed later under Examination and Assessment (and Chapter 3).

A mode of thinking: the primacy of clinical evidence

As qualified physical therapists, we have absorbed much scientific information and gained a great deal of clinical experience, both of which are essential for providing effective treatment. The 'science' of our discipline enables us to make diagnoses and apply the appropriate 'art' of our physical skill. However, the accepted theoretical basis of our profession is continually developing and changing. The gospel of yesterday becomes the heresy of tomorrow. It is essential that we remain open to new knowledge and open-minded in areas of uncertainty, so that inflexibility and tunnel vision do not result in a misapplication of our 'art.' Even with properly attested science applied in its right context, with precise information concerning the patient's symptoms and signs, a correct diagnosis is often difficult. Matching of the clinical findings to particular theories of anatomic, biomechanical, and pathologic knowledge, so as to attach a particular 'label' to the patient's condition, may not always be appropriate. Therapists must remain open-minded so that as treatment progresses, the patient is reassessed in relation to the evolution of the condition and the responses to treatment.

In summary, the scientific basis underlying the current range of diagnoses of disorders of the spine is incompletely understood. It is also changing rapidly with advances in knowledge and will continue to do so. In this context, the therapist may be sure of the clinical evidence from the patient's history and clinical signs, but should beware of the temptation to 'fit the diagnosis' to the inflexible and incomplete list of options currently available. The physical therapist must remain open-minded, not only at the initial consultation, but also as noting the changing responses of the patient during assessment and treatment. When the therapist is working in a relatively 'uncharted area' like human spinal disorders, one should not be influenced too much by the unreliable mass of inadequately understood biomechanics, symptomatology and pathology.

As a consequence of the above, a list of practical steps to follow has been drawn up. In the early era of its evolution, 'the Maitland Concept' had as its basis the following stages within a treatment:

1. Having assessed the effect of a patient's disorder, to perform a single treatment technique
2. To take careful note of what happens during the performance of the technique
3. Having completed the technique, to assess the effect of the technique on the patient's symptoms including movements

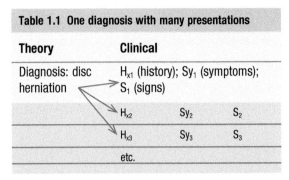

Table 1.1 One diagnosis with many presentations

Theory	Clinical		
Diagnosis: disc herniation	H_{x1} (history); Sy_1 (symptoms); S_1 (signs)		
	H_{x2}	Sy_2	S_2
	H_{x3}	Sy_3	S_3
	etc.		

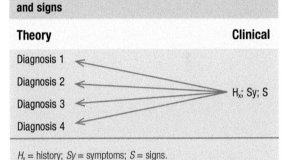

Table 1.2 Different diagnoses for one set of symptoms and signs

Theory	Clinical
Diagnosis 1	
Diagnosis 2	
Diagnosis 3	H_x; Sy; S
Diagnosis 4	

H_x = history; Sy = symptoms; S = signs.

4. Having assessed steps 2 and 3, and taken into account the available theoretical knowledge, to plan the next treatment approach and repeat the cycle from step 1.

It becomes obvious that this sequence can only be useful and informative if both the clinical history taking and physical examinations have been accurate.

The actual pattern of the concept requires us to keep our thoughts in two separate but interdependent compartments: the *theoretical* framework; and the *clinical* assessment. An example may help to clarify these concepts. We know that a lumbar intervertebral disc can herniate and cause pain, which can be referred into the leg. However, there are many presentations that can result from such a herniation (Table 1.1).

The reverse is also true – a patient may have one set of symptoms for which more than one diagnostic title can be applied (MacNab 1971; Table 1.2).

Because of the circumstances shown in Tables 1.1 and 1.2, it is obvious that it is not always possible to have a precise (biomedical) diagnosis for every patient treated. The more accurate and complete our theoretical framework, the more appropriate will be our treatment. If the theoretical framework

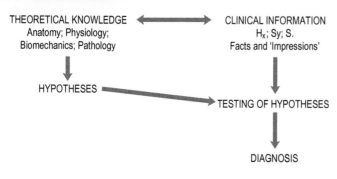

THEORETICAL KNOWLEDGE
Anatomy; Physiology;
Biomechanics; Pathology

CLINICAL INFORMATION
H_x; Sy; S.
Facts and 'Impressions'

HYPOTHESES

TESTING OF HYPOTHESES

DIAGNOSIS

Figure 1.1 • Flowchart demonstrating relationships and contexts for theoretical and clinical knowledge with related hypotheses. (H_x = history; Sy = symptoms; S = signs.) Reproduced from Twomey LT, Taylor JR, eds (1988) *Physical therapy of the low back*, p. 140, Churchill Livingstone with permission from Elsevier.

Table 1.3 Symbolic, permeable brick wall

Theory	B			Clinical
	R		W	
	I		A	
	C		L	
Diagnosis	K		L	H_x; Sy; S

H_x = history; Sy = symptoms; S = signs.

is faulty or deficient (as most are admitted to be), a full and accurate understanding of the patient's disorder may be impossible. The therapist's humility and open-mindedness are therefore essential, and inappropriate diagnostic labels must not be attached to a patient prematurely. The theoretical and clinical components must, however, influence one another. With this in mind, I have developed an approach separating theoretical knowledge from clinical information by what I have called the *symbolic, permeable brick wall* (Table 1.3). This serves to separate theory and practice, and to allow each to occupy (although not exclusively) its own compartment. That is, information from one side is able to filter through to the other side. In this way, theoretical concepts influence examination and treatment, while examination and treatment lead one back to a reconsideration of theoretical premises.

Using this mode of thinking, the brick-wall concept frees the clinician's mind from prejudice, allowing the therapist to ponder the possible reasons for a patient's disorder; to speculate, consider a hypothesis and discuss with others the possibilities regarding other diagnoses without anyone really knowing all the answers, yet all having a clear understanding of the patient's symptoms and related signs (Fig. 1.1).

This mode of thinking requires the use of accurate language, whereas inaccurate use of words betrays faulty logic. The way in which an individual makes a statement provides the listener with an idea both of the way that person is thinking and of the frame of reference for the statement.

A simple example may help to make this point clear. Imagine a clinician presenting a patient at a clinical seminar, and on request the patient demonstrates his area of pain. During the ensuing discussion, the clinician may refer to the patient's pain as 'sacroiliac pain.' This is a wrong choice of words. To be true to 'the Concept' we have outlined, of keeping clinical information and theoretical interpretations separate, one should describe the pain simply as a 'pain in the sacroiliac area.' It would be an unjustified assumption to suggest that pathology in the sacroiliac joint was the source of pain, but the former description above could be interpreted in this way. On the other hand, describing the pain as 'in the sacroiliac area' indicates that we are considering other possible sites of origin for the pain besides the sacroiliac joints, thereby keeping our diagnostic options open until we have more evidence. This is an essential element to 'the Concept.' Some readers may believe that attention to this kind of detail is unnecessary and pedantic. Quite the opposite is true. The correct and careful choice of words indicates a discipline of mind and an absence of prejudice, which influence all our diagnostic procedures including the whole process of examination, treatment and interpretation of the patient's response.

A clinician's written record of a patient's examination and treatment findings also show clearly whether the therapist's thinking processes are right or wrong. A genuine scientific approach involves logical thinking, vertical and lateral thinking, and inductive and deductive reasoning. It requires a mind that is uncluttered by confused and unproven theory, which is at the same time able to use proven facts, and has the critical ability to distinguish between well-attested facts and unsubstantiated opinions. It requires a mind that is honest, methodical, and self-critical. It also requires a mind that has the widest possible scope in the areas of improvisation and innovation.

Techniques

Many physical therapy clinicians are continually seeking new techniques of joint mobilization. When they hear a new name or when a new author has written a book on manipulation, they attempt to acquire the 'new' technical skills, and immediately apply them. In reality, the techniques are of secondary importance. Of course, if they are poorly performed or misapplied, treatment may fail and the therapist may lose confidence in the techniques. However, in my view there are many acceptable techniques each of which can be modified to suit a patient's disorder and the clinician's style and physique. Accordingly, I consider that there is no absolute set of techniques that can belong or be attributed to any one person. There should be no limit to the selection of technique: the biomechanically based techniques of Kaltenborn; the 'shift' techniques of McKenzie; the combined-movements technique of Edwards; the osteopathic and chiropractic technique; the Cyriax techniques; the Stoddard technique; the bonesetters' techniques; the Maigne techniques; and the Mennell techniques. All of these techniques are of the present era. Every experienced practitioner must feel totally free to make use of any of them. The most important consideration is that the technique chosen be appropriate to the particular patient or situation and that its effect should be carefully and continually assessed.

Techniques of management

Within the broad concept of this chapter, there are certain techniques of management that are continually used, but are not described by other authors. These techniques are as follows.

When treating very painful disorders passive-treatment movements can be used in an oscillatory fashion ('surface stirring' as described by Maitland 1985) but with two important provisos:

1. The oscillatory movement is performed without the patient experiencing any pain whatsoever, nor even any discomfort

2. The movement is performed only in that part of the range of movement where there is no resistance, i.e. where there is no stiffness or muscle spasm restricting the oscillations.

One may question how a pain-free oscillatory movement, which avoids every attempt to stretch structures, can produce any improvement in a patient's symptoms. A scientific answer to this question has been suggested (Maitland 1985) but there is a far more important clinical conclusion. It has been repeatedly shown clinically that such a technique does consistently produce a measurable improvement in range of movement with reduction in pain and disability and no demonstrable harmful effects. This demonstrates that the treatment is clinically and therefore 'scientifically,' correct even though an adequate theoretical explanation for its effectiveness may not yet be available. Reliable and repeated demonstration of effectiveness must validate a treatment method. To know how the method achieves the result is a theoretical problem for science to solve. The 'scientific' examination must match the primary clinical observation, the latter being the aspect of which we can be sure.

This example demonstrates once more how this mode of thinking so essential to 'the Concept' is so necessary for the further development of treatment methods. Without this mode of thinking we would never have found that passive-movement treatment procedures can successfully promote union in non-uniting fractures (McNair & Maitland 1983, McNair 1985).

Oscillatory movements as an important component of passive movement are referred to above in relation to the treatment of pain. There is another treatment procedure that requires oscillatory movement to be effective. This is related to the intermittent stretching of ligamentous and capsular structures. There are clearly defined areas of application for this treatment, which are described elsewhere (Maitland 1985).

There are occasions when a passive treatment movement needs to be performed with the opposing joint surfaces compressed together (Maitland 1980). Without the compression component, the technique would fail to produce any improvement in the patient's symptoms.

Utilizing the movements and positions by which a patient is able to reproduce his symptoms as an initial mandatory test is essential to 'the Concept.' This tactic, like the formalized examination of combined movements (the original contribution in cooperation with Edwards 1979) is very special to 'the Concept.'

Although it is frequently recognized that straight-leg raising can be used as a treatment technique for low lumbar disorders, it is not widely appreciated that the technique may be made more effective by using straight-leg raising in the 'Slump test' position (Maitland 1979). In the same slumped position, the neck flexion component of the position may be effectively utilized when such movement reproduces a patient's low back pain.

'Accessory' movements produced by applying alternating pressure on palpable parts of the vertebrae are also very important in terms of techniques and 'the Maitland Concept.' Any treatment concept that does not include such techniques is missing a critical link essential to a full understanding of the effects of manipulation on patients with low lumbar disorders.

It is important to remember that there is no dogma or clear set of rules that can be applied to the selection and use of passive-movement techniques; the choice is open ended. A technique is the brainchild of ingenuity. 'The achievements are limited to the extent of one's lateral and logical thinking' (Hunkin 1985).

Examination

The care, precision and scope of examination required by those using this 'concept' are greater and more demanding than other clinical methods I have observed. 'The Concept's' demands differ from those of other methods in many respects.

The history taking and examination demand a total commitment to understanding what the patient is suffering and the effects of the pain and disability on the patient. Naturally, one is also continually attempting to understand the cause of the disorder (the theoretical compartment of 'the Concept').

Examination must include a sensitive elucidation of the person's symptoms in relation to:

1. Precise area(s) indicated on the surface of the body
2. The depth at which symptoms are experienced
3. Whether there is more than one site of pain, or whether multiple sites overlap or are separate

4. Changes in the symptoms in response to movements or differences in joint positions in different regions of the body.

The next important and unique part of the examination is for the patient to reenact the movement that best reveals his disorder or, if applicable, to reenact the movement that produced the injury. The function or movement is then analyzed by breaking it into components in order to make clinical sense of particular joint-movement pain responses, which are applicable to his complaint.

The routine examination of physiologic movements performed with a degree of precision rarely utilized by other practitioners. If the person's disorder is an 'end-of-range' type of problem, the details of the movement examination required are:

1. At what point in the range are the symptoms first experienced; how do they vary with continuation of the movement; and in what manner do the symptoms behave during the symptomatic range?
2. In the same way and with the same degree of precision, how does muscle spasm or resistance vary during the symptomatic range?
3. Finally, what is the relationship of the symptoms (a) to the resistance or spasm (motor responses); and (b) during that same movement? There may be no relationship whatsoever, in which case, for example, the stiffness is relatively unimportant. However, if the behaviour of the symptoms matches the behaviour of the stiffness, both should improve in parallel during treatment.

An effective method of recording the findings of all components of a movement disorder is to depict them in a 'movement diagram.' These also are an innovative part of 'the Concept.' The use of movement diagrams facilitates demonstration of changes in the patient's condition in a more precise and objective manner. They are discussed at length in the Appendix 4.

If the patient's disorder is a 'pain through range' type of problem, the details of the movement examination required are:

1. At what point in the range does discomfort or pain first increase?
2. How do the symptoms behave if movement is taken a short distance beyond the onset of discomfort? Does intensity markedly increase or is the area of referred pain extended?

3. Is the movement a normal physiological movement in the available range or is it protected by muscle spasm or stiffness? Opposing the abnormal movement and noting any change in the symptomatic response compared with entry 2 is performed to assess its relevance to the course of treatment.

Palpatory techniques

The accessory movements are tested by palpation techniques and seek the same amount and type of information as described above. They are tested in a variety of different joint positions. The three main positions are:

1. The neutral mid-range position for each available movement i.e. midway between flexion/extension, rotation left and right, lateral flexion left and right and distraction/compression

2. The joint is in a 'loose-packed position' (MacConaill & Basmajian 1969) at the particular position where the person's symptoms begin, or begin to increase

3. Position is at the limits of the available range.

These palpatory techniques of examination and treatment have been peculiar to this 'concept' from its beginnings. As well as seeking symptomatic responses to the movement as described above, the palpation is also used to assess positional anomalies and soft-tissue abnormalities, which are at least as critical to 'the Concept' as the movement tests.

The testing of physiologic and accessory movement can be combined in a variety of ways in an endeavour to find the comparable movement sign most closely related to the person's disorder. Edwards (1983) originally described a formal method of investigating symptomatic responses and treating appropriate patients using 'combined movement' techniques. In addition, joint surfaces may be compressed, both as a prolonged, sustained firm pressure and as an adjunct to physiologic and accessory movement. These are two further examples of examination developed as part of 'the Maitland Concept.'

Differentiation tests are perfect examples of physical examination procedures that demonstrate the mode of thinking so basic to 'the Maitland Concept.' When any group of movements reproduces symptoms, 'the Concept' requires a logical and thoughtful analysis to establish which movement of which joint is affected. The simplest example of this is passive supination of the hand and forearm, which when held in a stretched position reproduces the patient's symptoms. The stages of this test are as follows:

1. Hold the fully supinated hand/forearm in the position that is known to reproduce the pain

2. Hold the hand stationary and pronate the distal radio-ulnar joint 2° or 3°

3. If the pain arises from the wrist, the pain will increase because in pronating the distal radio-ulnar joint, added supination stress is applied at the radiocarpal and midcarpal joints

4. While in the position listed in entry 1, again hold the hand stationary, but this time increase supination of the distal radio-ulnar joint. This decreases the supination stretch at the wrist joints and will reduce any pain arising from the wrist. However, if the distal radio-ulnar joint is the source of pain, the increased supination stretch will cause the pain to increase.

All types of differentiation tests require the same logically ordered procedure. These functional tests follow the same logic as the subjective modes of assessment described at the beginning of this chapter and provide additional evidence leading to accurate diagnosis.

Assessment

In the last few years it would appear that physical therapists have discovered a new 'skill,' with the lofty title of 'problem solving.' This is, and always should be, the key part of all physical therapy treatment. Being able to solve the diagnostic and therapeutic problems and thus relieve the patient of his complaint is just what physical therapists are trained to do. For many years, manipulative physical therapy has been rightly classed as empirical treatment. However, since manipulative physical therapists began to be more strongly involved in problem-solving skills, treatment has become less empirical and more logical. On the basis that the pathology remains unknown in the majority of cases and the effects of the treatment on the tissues (as opposed to symptoms) are unknown, the treatment remains empirical in form. This is true with almost all of the medical science. Nevertheless, the approach to the patient and to physical treatment has become more logical and scientific within 'the Maitland Concept.'

Minds existed before computers were developed and manipulative therapists are trained to sort out and access 'input' so that appropriate and logical 'output' can be produced. Appropriate problem-solving logic will relate clinical findings to pathology and mechanical disorders. This process of 'sorting out' we have called *assessment* and assessment is the key to successful, appropriate, manipulative treatment, which, because of the reliability of its careful and logical approach, should lead to better and better treatment for our patients.

Assessment is used in six different situations:

1. Analytical assessment at a first consultation
2. Pretreatment assessment
3. Reassessment during every treatment session proving the efficacy of a technique at a particular stage of treatment
4. Progressive assessment
5. Retrospective assessment
6. Final analytical assessment.

Analytical assessment

A first consultation requires skills in many areas, but the goals require decisions and judgments from the following five areas:

1. The diagnosis
2. The phase of the disorder
3. The degree of stability of the disorder at the time of treatment
4. The presenting symptoms and signs
5. The characteristics of the person.

Without communication and an atmosphere of trust, the answers to the different assessment procedures (1–5) cannot be reliably determined. By using one's own frame of reference and endeavouring to understand the patient's frame of reference, the characteristics of the patient can be judged. By making use of non-verbal skills, picking out key words or phrases, knowing what type of information to listen for and recognizing and using 'immediate-automatic-response' questions (all described later), accurate information can be gained at this first consultation. The physical examination is discussed under the heading, Examination.

Pretreatment assessment

Each treatment session begins with a specific kind of assessment of the effect of the previous session on the patient's disorder (its symptoms and changes in movement). Since the first consultation includes both examination and treatment of movements, the assessment at the second treatment session will not be as useful for therapy as it will be at the following treatment sessions.

When the patient attends subsequent treatment sessions, it is necessary to make both subjective and physical assessments, i.e. subjective in terms of how they feel; objective in terms of what changes can be found in quality and range of movement and in related pain response. When dealing with the subjective side of assessment, it is important to seek spontaneous comments. It is wrong to ask, 'How did it feel this morning when you got out of bed, compared with how it used to feel?' The start should be 'How have you been?' or some such general question, allowing the patient to provide some information that seems most important to him. This information may be more valuable because of its spontaneous nature.

Another important aspect of the subjective assessment is that statements of fact made by a patient must always be converted to comparisons to previous statements. Having made the subjective assessment, the comparative statement should be the first item recorded on the patient's case notes. And it must be recorded as a *comparison-quotation* of his opinion of the effect of treatment. (The second record in the case notes is the comparative changes determined by the objective movement tests.) To attain this subjective assessment, communication skills are of paramount importance. There are many components that make up the skill, but two are of particular importance:

1. *Key words or key phrases*. Having asked the question, 'How has it been?' a patient may respond in a very general and uninformative way. However, during his statements he may include, for example, the word 'Monday.' Latch on to Monday, because Monday meant something to him. Find out what it was and use it. 'What is it that happened on Monday? Why did you say Monday?'
2. A patient frequently says things that demand an immediate-automatic-response question. As a response to the opening question given above,

the patient may respond by saying, 'I'm feeling better.' The immediate-automatic-response to that statement, even before he has had a chance to take breath and say anything else, is, 'better than what?' or 'better than when?' It may be that after treatment he was worse and that he is better than he was then, but that he is not better than he was before the treatment.

One aspect of the previous treatment is that it (often intentionally) provokes a degree of discomfort. This will produce soreness, but if the patient says he has more pain, the clinician needs to determine if it is treatment-soreness or disorder-soreness. For example, a patient may have pain radiating across his lower back and treatment involves pushing on his lumbar spine. He is asked to stand up and is asked, 'How do you feel now compared with before I was pushing on your back?' He may say, 'it feels pretty sore.' He is then asked, 'Where does it feel sore?' If he answers, 'It's sore in the center', the clinician may consider that it is likely to be treatment pain. But if he answers, 'It's sore across my back' then the clinician may conclude that it is disorder pain. If it were treatment soreness it would only be felt where the pressure had been applied. If the soreness spreads across his back, the treatment technique must have disturbed the disorder.

In making subjective assessments, a process is included of educating the patient in how to reflect. If a patient is a very good witness, the answers to questions are very clear, but if the patient is not a good witness, then subjective assessment becomes difficult. Patients should learn to understand what the clinician needs to know. At the end of the first consultation, patients need to be instructed in how important it is for them to take notice of any changes in their symptoms. They should report all changes; even ones they believe are trivial. The clinician should explain, 'Nothing is too trivial. You can't tell me too much; if you leave out observations, which you believe to be unimportant, this may cause me to make wrong treatment judgments.' People need to be reassured that they are not complaining, they are informing. Under circumstances when a patient will not be seen for some days or if full and apparently trivial detail is needed, they should be asked to write down the details. There has been criticism that asking patients to write things down makes them become hypochondriacs. This is a wrong assessment in my experience, as the exercise

provides information that might otherwise never be obtained.

There are four specific times when changes in the patient's symptoms can indicate the effect of treatment. They are as follows:

1. *Immediately after treatment*. The question can be asked, 'How did you feel when you walked out of here last time compared with when you walked in?' A patient can feel much improved immediately after treatment yet experience exacerbation of symptoms one or two hours later. Any improvement that does not last longer than one hour indicates that the effect of the treatment was only palliative. Improvement that lasts more than four hours indicates a change related to treatment.

2. *Four hours after treatment*. The time interval of four hours is an arbitrary time and could be any time from three to six hours. It is a 'threshold' time interval beyond which any improvement or examination can be taken to indicate the success or failure of the treatment. Similarly, if a patient's syndrome is exacerbated by treatment, the patient will be aware of it at about this time.

3. *The evening of the treatment*. The evening of the day of treatment provides information in regard to how well any improvement from treatment has been sustained. Similarly, an exacerbation immediately following treatment may have further increased by evening. This is unfavourable. Conversely, if the exacerbation has decreased, it is then necessary to know whether it decreased to its pretreatment level or decreased to a level that was better than before that day's treatment. This would be a very favourable response, clearly showing that the treatment had alleviated the original disorder.

4. *On rising the next morning*. This is probably the most informative time of all for signalling a general improvement. A patient may have no noticeable change in his symptoms on the day or night of the treatment session, but may notice that on getting out of bed the next morning his usual lower back stiffness and pain are less, or that they may pass off more quickly than usual. Even at this time span, any changes can be attributed to treatment. However, changes that are noticed *during* the day after treatment, or on getting out of bed the second morning after treatment, are far less likely to

be as a result of treatment. Nevertheless, the patient should be questioned in depth to ascertain what reasons exist, other than treatment, to which the changes might be attributed.

Because accurate assessment is so vitally and closely related to treatment response, each treatment session must be organized in such a way that the assessments are not confused by changes in the treatment. For example, if a patient has a disorder that is proving very difficult to help and at the eighth treatment session he reports that he feels there may have been some slight favourable change from the last treatment, the clinician has no alternative in planning the eighth treatment session. In the eighth treatment, that which was done at the seventh must be repeated in exactly the same manner in every respect. To do otherwise could render the assessment at the ninth treatment confusing. If the seventh treatment is repeated at the eighth session, there is nothing that the patient can say or demonstrate that can confuse the effect attributable to that treatment. If there was an improvement between the seventh and the eighth treatment (and the eighth treatment was an identical repetition of the seventh treatment), yet no improvement between the eighth treatment and the ninth treatment time, the improvement between treatments seven and eight could not have been due to treatment.

There is another instance when the clinician must recognize that there can be no choice as to what the eighth treatment must be. If there had been no improvement with the first six treatments and at the seventh treatment session a totally new technique was used, the patient may report at the eighth session that there had been a surprisingly marked improvement in symptoms. It may be that this unexpected improvement was due to treatment or it may have been due to some other unknown reason. There is only one way that the answer can be found – the treatment session should consist of no treatment techniques at all. Objective assessment may be made but no treatment techniques should be performed. At the ninth session, if the patient's symptoms have worsened considerably, the treatment cannot be implicated in the cause because none had been administered. The clinician can then repeat the seventh treatment and see if the dramatic improvement is achieved again. If it is, then the improvement is highly likely to have been due to that treatment.

Whatever is done at one treatment session is done in such a way that when the patient comes back the next time, the assessment cannot be confusing.

Another example of a different kind is that a patient may say at each treatment session that he is 'the same,' yet assessment of his movement signs indicates that they are improving in a satisfactory manner and therefore that one would expect an improvement in his symptoms. To clarify this discrepancy, specific questions must be asked. It may be that he considers he is 'the same' because his back is still just as stiff and painful on first getting out of bed in the morning as it was at the outset of treatment. The specific questioning may divulge that he now has no problems with sitting and that he can now walk up and down the stairs at work without pain. Although his sitting, climbing and descending stairs have improved, his symptoms on getting out of bed are the same and this explains his statement of being 'the same.' The objective movement tests will have improved in parallel with his sitting and stair-climbing improvements.

Assessment during every treatment session

Proving the value or failure of a technique applied through a treatment session is imperative. Assessment (problem solving) should be part of all aspects of physical therapy. In this chapter it is related to passive movement. There are four kinds of assessment and probably the one that most people think of first is the one in which the clinician is trying to prove the value of a technique that is being performed on a patient.

Proving the value of a technique

Before even choosing which technique to use, it is necessary to know what symptoms the patient has and how his movements are affected in terms of both range and the pain response during the movement. Selection of a treatment technique depends partly on knowing what that technique should achieve while it is being performed. In other words, is it the aim to provoke discomfort and, if so, how much 'hurt' is permissible? It is also necessary to have an expectation of what the technique should achieve after it has been performed.

With these considerations in mind, it is necessary to keep modifying the treatment technique until it achieves the expected goal during its performance. Assuming that this is achieved and that the technique has been performed for the necessary length of time, the patient is then asked to stand, during which time he is watched to see if there are any nuances that may provide a clue as to how his back is feeling. The first thing is to then ask him is, 'How do you feel now compared with when you were standing there before the technique?' It is then necessary to clarify any doubts concerning the interpretation of what he says he is feeling. It is important to understand what the patient means to say if the subjective effect of the technique is to be determined usefully.

Having subjectively assessed the effect of the technique, it is then necessary to reexamine the major movements that were faulty, to compare them with their state before the technique. An important aspect of checking and rechecking the movements is that there may be more than one component to the patient's problem. For example, a man may have back pain, hip pain and vertebral-canal pain. Each of these may contribute to the symptoms in his lower leg. On reassessing him after a technique, it is necessary to assess at least *one* separate movement for *each* of the components, so it can be determined what the technique has achieved for each component. It is still necessary to check all of the components even if it is expected that a change will only be effected in one of the components. Having completed all of these comparison assessments, the effect of that technique at that particular stage of the disorder is now recorded in detail.

Progressive assessment

At each treatment session the symptoms and signs are assessed for changes for their relation to the previous treatment session and to 'extracurricular' activities. At about each fourth treatment session a subjective assessment is made, comparing how the patient feels today with how he felt four treatments previously. The purpose of this progressive assessment is to clarify and confirm the treatment by assessment of the treatment response. One is often surprised by the patient's reply to a question, 'How do you feel now compared with 10 days (i.e. four treatments) ago?' The goal is to keep the

treatment-by-treatments assessment in the right perspective in relation to the patient's original disorder.

Retrospective assessment

The first kind of retrospective assessment is that made routinely at each group of three or four treatment sessions when the patient's symptoms and signs are compared with before treatment began, as described above.

A second kind of retrospective assessment is made toward the end of treatment when the considerations relate to a final assessment. This means that the clinician is determining:

1. Whether treatment should be continued

2. Whether spontaneous recovery is occurring

3. Whether other medical treatments or investigations are required

4. Whether medical components of the disorder are preventing full recovery

5. What the patient's future in terms of prognosis is likely to be?

A third kind of retrospective assessment is made when the patient's disorder has not continued to improve over the last few treatment sessions. Under these circumstances, it is the subjective assessment that requires the greatest skill and its findings are far more important than the assessment of the objective-movement tests. The clinician needs to know what specific information to look for. This is not a facetious remark, since it is the most common area where mistakes are made, thereby ruining any value in the assessment. The kinds of question the clinician should ask are as follows:

'During the whole time of treatment, is there anything I have done that has made you worse?'

'Of the things I have done to you, is there any one particular thing (or more) that you feel has helped you?'

'Does your body tell you anything about what it would like to have done to it to make it start improving?'

'Does your body tell you anything about what it would like to have done to it to make it start improving the treatment's effect?'

'Do your symptoms tell you that it might be a good plan to stop treatment for, say, two weeks after which a further assessment and decision could be made?'

And so the probing interrogation continues until two or three positive answers emerge, which will guide the further measures that should be taken. The questions are the kind that involve the patient in making decisions and that guide the clinician in making a final decision regarding treatment.

There is a fourth kind of retrospective assessment. If treatment is still producing improvement but its rate is less than anticipated, a good plan is to stop treatment for two weeks and to then reassess the situation. If the patient has improved over the two-week period, it is necessary to know whether the improvement has been a day-by-day affair thus indicating a degree of spontaneous improvement. If the improvement only occurred for the first two days after the last treatment, then it would seem that the last treatment session was of value and that a further three or four treatments should be given followed by another 2-week break and reassessment.

Final analytical assessment

When treatment has achieved all it can, the clinician needs to make an assessment in relation to the possibility of recurrence, the effectiveness of any prophylactic measures, the suggestion of any medical measures that can be carried out and, finally, an assessment of the percentage of remaining disability. The answers to these matters are to be found by analyzing all the information derived from:

1. The initial examination
2. The behaviour of the disorder throughout treatment
3. The details derived from retrospective assessments
4. The state of affairs at the end of treatment, taking into account the subjective and objective changes.

This final analytical assessment is made easier as each year a clinician's work builds up experience. It is necessary for this experience to be based on a self-critical approach and on analysis of the results, with the reasons for these results.

Conclusion

The question has often been asked, 'How did this method of treatment evolve?' The attributes necessary to succeed in this treatment method are an analytical, self-critical mind and a talent for improvisation.

With this as a basis, the next step is to learn to understand how a patient's disorder affects him. Coupled with this is the need to have sound reasons for trying a particular technique and then the patience to assess its effect. In 'the Maitland Concept,' over the years this has developed into a complex interrelated series of assessments as described in the body of this text.

Q Why are painless techniques used to relieve pain?

A Experience with patients who have had manipulative treatment elsewhere allows us to inquire as to which kind of technique was used and to observe its effect. When patients emphasize the extreme gentleness of some successful clinicians, one is forced to the conclusion that there must be ways of moving a joint extremely gently and thus improving patients' symptoms. Having accepted this fact (and that is not always easy) the obvious next step is to reproduce these techniques. For example, a technique one patient may describe can then be used on other patients who fit into the same kind of category. The clinician can learn what its possibilities are via the assessment process.

Q Why conversely, are some of the techniques quite vigorous and painful?

A When treatment reaches a stage when nothing seems to help, a useful axiom is, 'Find the thing that hurts them and hurt them.' This should not be interpreted as being cruel to a patient, or that one is 'out to hurt them', come what may. The hurting is a controlled progressive process with a strong emphasis on assessment. From using this kind of treatment on appropriate patients, it has become obvious how firmly some disorders need to be pushed to the point of eliciting pain in order to aid recovery. This approach may be seriously questioned by some practitioners, but it can be a most useful technique in appropriate circumstances.

Q How did treating joints using strong compression of the joint surfaces come about?

A If, for example, a patient has shoulder symptoms only when lying on it and if normal examination methods reveal very little, then the thought processes go something like this:

'I believe him when he says he has a shoulder problem.'
'There is nothing to indicate any serious or sinister disorder.'
'He hasn't responded to other treatments.'
'So it must be possible to find something on examination that relates to his problem.'
'How can I find that something? What lead is there?'

'He says, 'I can't lie on it.''

'So I will ask him to lie on it and then move it around and see what happens.'

By thus experimenting with techniques (improvisation) until the patient's pain can be reproduced, having found the thing that hurts him, treatment should then aim to hurt him in this *controlled* manner, as stated above.

A quandary then arises:

'As the patient doesn't move his shoulder around when he's asleep and lying on it, why is my examination using compression only, without movement, not painful?'

One would expect it to be painful!

'However, he has to lie on it for half an hour before pain forces him to change his position, so try compression again but make it stronger and sustain it longer.'

After half a minute or so of sustained maximum compression without movement his pain will certainly appear.

Q How about the Slump test and treatment, how did this evolve?

A Some patients who have low back pain complain about difficulty getting into a car. By reenacting the action and analyzing it, it is found that it was not the flexing of the lumbar spine that made getting into the car difficult; i.e. it was the head/neck flexion that provoked the low back symptoms. Examination using standard movement tests for structures between the head and the sacrum do not reveal anything; so reenact the particular movements and remember that the only structure connecting both areas must be in the vertebral column, most likely within the vertebral canal. To put these structures on stretch was the only method that reproduced the complaint. The maximum stretch position is the position now referred to as the 'slump position'.

Q We now read of using mobilizing techniques to make a non-uniting fracture unite. How did this come about?

A In the past, traditional methods used to stimulate union have been:

1. Remove all support for the fracture site and allow the patient to take weight through the fracture; and

2. Surgically explore the area and make both ends of the fracture site bleed and then splint them in apposition again. If such things can promote union then why not try passively moving the fracture site? Based on this reasoning and linking it with our axiom 'find the thing that hurts and hurt them,' it was found that it was possible to cause 'fracture-site pain.' This characteristic pain was found to have two other characteristics:

◆ Pain stopped *immediately* when the treating movement was stopped; and

◆ No side-effects were provoked. This then meant that the treatment could be repeated and in fact pain became harder to provoke: union took place.

References

The Age: 1982. 21 August

Edwards BC: Combined movements of the lumbar spine: examination and clinical significance, *Aust J Physiother* 25:147, 1979.

Edwards BC: Movement patterns, International Conference on Manipulative Therapy, Manipulative Therapists' Association of Australia, Perth, 1983.

Hunkin K: 1985. Unpublished publication.

MacConaill MA, Basmajian SV: *Muscles and movements*, Baltimore, 1969, Waverley Press.

MacNab I: Negative disc exploration: an analysis of the causes of nerve root involvement in 68 patients, *J Bone Joint Surg* 53A:891, 1971.

McNair JFS, Maitland GD: The role of passive mobilization in the treatment of a non-uniting fracture site – a case study, International Conference on Manipulative Therapy, Perth, 1983.

McNair JFS: Non-uniting fractures management by manual passive mobilization. Proceedings Manipulative Therapists' Association of Australia, Brisbane, 1985, pp 88.

Maitland GD: Negative disc exploration: positive canal signs, *Aust J Physiother* 25:6, 1979.

Maitland GD: The hypothesis of adding compression when examining and treating synovial joints, *J Orthop Sports Phys Ther* 2:7, 1980.

Maitland GD: Passive movement techniques for intra-articular and periarticular disorders, *Aust J Physiother* 31:3, 1985.

Clinical reasoning: From the Maitland Concept and beyond

2

Mark A. Jones

CHAPTER CONTENTS

Introduction 14

Clinical reasoning and evidence-based practice 15

Critical thinking and clinical reasoning 16

Importance of skilled clinical reasoning to expert practice 17

Clinical reasoning and the bio-psychosocial model of health and disability 18

Clinical reasoning as a hypothesis-oriented and collaborative process 19

Clinical reasoning and knowledge 25

Clinical reasoning and cognition/metacognition 26

Skilled questioning important to critical thinking and learning 27

Skilled questioning important to clinical practice 27

Facilitating application of bio-psychosocial practice: clinical reasoning strategies and hypothesis categories 31

Pattern recognition 43

Complexity of clinical reasoning 44

Errors of clinical reasoning 44

Improving clinical reasoning: learning through clinical reasoning 46

Clinical reasoning reflection forms 53

Key words

Clinical reasoning, critical thinking, bio-psychosocial, patient perspectives, diagnostic reasoning, narrative reasoning, hypothesis categories, pattern recognition

Introduction

Geoff Maitland always insisted on a systematic and comprehensive patient examination that in his words 'enables you to live the patient's symptoms over 24 hours'. All patient information regarding their problem, its effects on their life and the associated physical impairments found on physical examination had to be analysed with the aim of 'making features fit'. Patient treatments were never recipes or protocols, rather specific treatments were based on thorough analysis of the subjective (i.e. patient interview) and physical findings combined with knowledge of research, clinical patterns, treatment strategies that had been successful for similar presentations and systematic reassessment of all interventions. While Geoff did not refer to this process of information gathering, analysis, decision making, intervention and reassessment as clinical reasoning, it clearly was a structured and logical approach in line with contemporary clinical reasoning theory. Consistent with the aim of contemporary evidence-based practice, his 'Brick Wall' concept emphasized consideration of both research and experienced-based evidence with the research providing a general guide and the patient's unique presentation determining how that research was applied and ultimately the specific interventions to trial. The open-minded yet critically reflective bio-psychosocial philosophy of practice that Geoff promoted is evident in the following quote:

> The Maitland concept requires open-mindedness, mental agility and mental discipline linked with a logical and methodical process of assessing cause and effect. The central theme demands a positive personal commitment (empathy) to understand what the person (patient) is enduring. The key issues of 'the concept' that require explanation are personal commitment, mode of thinking, techniques, examination and assessment.
>
> (Maitland 1987, p. 136)

In this chapter the clinical reasoning implicit in 'The Maitland Concept' is made explicit. The importance of skilled clinical reasoning to expert practice and to evidence-based practice is noted. The components of critical thinking inherent in skilled clinical reasoning are highlighted. The role clinical reasoning plays in assisting application of bio-psychosocial models of health and disability, such as the World Health Organization International Classification of Functioning, Disability and Health (ICF) (WHO 2001), is discussed along with frameworks for directing and organizing the different foci of thinking and categories of decision making needed to understand both the person and their problem(s) and to guide a collaborative approach to management. Lastly, common errors of reasoning are considered and the value of skilled reflective reasoning to learning and to the continual evolution of physiotherapy practice is stressed.

Clinical reasoning defined

> Clinical reasoning is a reflective process of inquiry and analysis carried out by a health professional in collaboration with the patient with the aim of understanding the patient, their context and their clinical problem(s) in order to guide evidence-based practice.
>
> (Brooker 2013)

More simply it is the thinking and decision making associated with clinical practice that enables therapists to take the best-judged action for individual patients. In this sense, clinical reasoning is the means to 'wise' action (Cervero 1988, Harris 1993).

Clinical reasoning and evidence-based practice

Evidence-based practice (EBP), defined as 'the integration of best research evidence with clinical expertise and patient values' (Sackett et al. 2000, p. 1), is critical to minimize misconceptions in clinical theory and practice and to understand how best to work with patients in their health management. Clinical practice is subject to unrecognized bias, taken-for-granted assumptions and errors of reasoning that necessitate audits of practice as encouraged by the evidence-based movement. In fact, Thomas Kuhn, a science historian, highlights how the majority of misconceptions through the history of science, including such things as the function of the heart as the organ of thought, can almost universally be attributed to a lack of critical appraisal of contemporary theory (Kuhn 1970). However, EBP was never intended to be prescriptive. Our current body of research is either incomplete or incomplete in its reporting to adequately guide therapists in their recognition and management of the multitude of patient problems we face (Jones et al. 2006). Common limitations with physiotherapy effectiveness studies include high drop-out rates or loss to follow-up, lack of blinding (patient, therapist, measurer), lack of random and concealed allocation to treatment arms, lack of adequate identification of population subgroups, artificial isolation of treatment interventions in determining their effect and lack of evidence of sustainable outcomes. As such, practicing clinicians face the daunting challenge of maintaining best practice based on best evidence when the evidence is still largely not available or is incomplete. Even when primary research studies (or systematic reviews) testing therapeutic interventions for the condition of interest are available, numerous issues must be considered for the clinician to have confidence in the applicability of the findings including whether their patient matches the population studied (often made difficult by lack of homogeneity of subjects and insufficient consideration of psychosocial variables) and whether the intervention tested can be replicated. Very few studies provide sufficient detail and justification of the assessments and treatments (e.g. what precisely was done including details of positions, dosage, sequence and progression; who treated the patients including level of procedural competence; what was the therapeutic environment including associated explanations, instructions, verbal cues and advice) to enable clinicians to replicate the assessments and management (educatively, behaviourally and humanistically) with confidence. Application of evidence to practice requires skilled clinical reasoning. Skilled clinical reasoning is underpinned by skilled critical thinking.

Critical thinking and clinical reasoning

While generic thinking skills are themselves insufficient for expertise in clinical practice (Boshuizen and Schmidt 2008, Elstein et al. 1978), skilled clinical reasoning incorporates the fundamentals of critical thinking. Critical thinking is a field of study on its own (e.g. see Baron & Sternberg 1987, Brookfield 1987, de Bono 1994, Forneris 2004, Mezirow 1990, 1991, 2000, Nickerson et al. 1985, Schön 1983, 1987). Paul and Elder (2007) provide a clear and simple overview of critical thinking which they propose has three dimensions: the analytic, the evaluative and the creative. Critical thinking generally involves analyzing and assessing information, issues, situations, problems, perspectives and thinking processes. It enables the judging of information regarding its accuracy, precision, completeness and relevance to facilitate understanding and identification of solutions. It enables creation of new insights and knowledge. While everyone is already capable of thinking, and as Nickerson (1985, p. 28) points out, 'All of us compare, classify, order, estimate, extrapolate, interpolate, form hypotheses, weigh evidence, draw conclusions, devise arguments, judge relevance, use analogies and engage in numerous activities that are typically classified as thinking', this is not to say that we do these things well in all circumstances, or that we couldn't learn to do them better. Steven Brookfield (1987, p. ix), a prominent researcher and writer in the field of adult learning and critical thinking, summarizes the value of critical thinking and reasoning as follows:

- When we become critical thinkers we develop an awareness of the assumptions under which we, and others, think and act
- We learn to pay attention to the context in which our ideas and actions are generated
- We become sceptical of quick fix solutions, of single answers to problems, and of claims of universal truth

- We also become open to alternative ways of looking at and behaving in the world
- Critical thinking influences all aspects of our lives. For example, in our personal relationships we can learn to see our own actions through the eyes of others
- At our workplace we seek democracy and take initiative in forming new directions
- We become aware of the potential for distortion and bias in media depictions
- We value political freedom, we practice democracy, we encourage a tolerance of diversity, and we hold in check the demagogic tendencies of politicians.

In addition to Brookfield's list, critical thinking and reasoning are also important to:

- Improve lifelong learning
- Avoid misdirection in beliefs
- Discover alternative understandings and solutions and generate new ideas
- Optimize health care outcomes
- Improve social interactions
- Analyze arguments of others thereby making you less susceptible to manipulation by others
- Increase earning power; and
- Enrich your life aesthetically by becoming more observant.

For some therapists who already possess good critical thinking skills, developing skilled clinical reasoning mostly requires acquiring the necessary research and practice knowledge with which to apply those skills. However, others either lack those fundamental critical thinking skills or they fail to use them, instead falling into the trap of uncritically following routines and protocols. Even skilled therapists are vulnerable to habits of practice and over allegiance to particular approaches or paradigms of practice. It can be difficult to critically examine your own perspective when you consider as Brookfield (2008, p. 68) notes:

No matter how much we may think we have an accurate sense of our practice, we are stymied by the fact that we are using our own interpretive filters to become aware of our own interpretive filters! ... To some extent we are all prisoners trapped within the perceptual frameworks that determine how we view our experiences. A self-confirming cycle often develops whereby our uncritically accepted assumptions shape clinical actions which then serve only to confirm the truth of those assumptions. It is very difficult to stand outside ourselves and see how some of our most deeply held values and beliefs lead us into distorted and constrained ways of thinking and practicing.

Suggestions for improving critical thinking in general through 'Socratic questions' along with skilled clinical questioning to optimize the quality of patient information obtained are discussed later in the chapter.

> **Key message**
>
> A challenge of evidence-based practice is to critically appraise both research-based and experience-based sources of evidence and to use critical thinking and reasoning skills to apply that evidence to practice.

Importance of skilled clinical reasoning to expert practice

Research into expertise in a number of fields (e.g. physics, mathematics, medicine, chess) has identified the following generic characteristics (Glaser & Chi 1988):

- Experts excel in their own domains
- Experts possess large repertoire of well-developed profession specific patterns they recognize
- Experts solve problems fast with less error
- Experts see problems at a deeper level, spending more time analyzing problems qualitatively (i.e. more aware of contextual cues in the presentation)
- Experts have strong self-monitoring skills
- Experts possess the affective dispositions necessary to learn from their experiences including:
  - inquisitiveness
  - open-mindedness
  - honesty
  - diligence
  - self-confidence
  - flexibility
  - empathy
  - humility.

Clinical expertise, of which clinical reasoning is a component, can be viewed as a continuum along multiple dimensions including clinical outcomes and personal attributes such as knowledge, technical skills, communication and interpersonal skills, cognitive/metacognitive proficiency, professional judgment and empathy (Higgs & Jones 2000). Health professions' research into clinical expertise (e.g. Beeston & Simons 1996, Benner 1984, Elstein et al. 1978, Edwards et al. 2004a, Embrey et al. 1996, Jensen et al. 2007, Jensen et al. 2008, Mattingly & Fleming 1994, May & Dennis 1991, Patel & Groen 1986, Payton 1985, Thomas-Edding 1987) has identified the following characteristics and expectations of expert clinicians:

- Experts value participation of others (patients, family, other health professionals)
- Experts value different forms of knowledge in their reasoning (research and experienced based)
- Experts' theory, practice, reasoning and intuition are intertwined through practical experience
- Experts are patient-centred, collaborative with superior practice based knowledge. For example patients are viewed as active participants in therapy
- Primary goal of care is empowerment of patients through collaboration between patient and therapist
- Expert has a strong moral commitment to beneficence or doing what is in the patient's best interest
- Expert is willing to serve as a patient advocate or moral agent in helping them become successful
- Experts have good communication skills
- Experts use collaborative problem-solving to help patients learn how to resolve their problems on their own, fostering self-efficacy and empowering them to take responsibility
- Experts share their expertise to assist others; and
- Experts communicate their reasoning well at an appropriate level depending on who they are speaking to.

Many of the generic and health professions' specific characteristics of expertise above are also associated with skilled clinical reasoning. Physiotherapy specific research investigating expert practice (e.g. Edwards et al. 2004a, Embrey et al. 1996, Jensen et al. 1990, Jensen et al. 1992, Resnik & Jensen 2003) has contributed significantly to our evolving understanding of clinical reasoning, much of which is reported in the text *Expertise in physical therapy practice* (Jensen et al. 2007). Key dimensions of skilled clinical reasoning emanating from this research include:

- Clinical reasoning is situated within a bio-psychosocial model of health
- Clinical reasoning is complex, non-linear and cyclical in nature involving both inductive and deductive reasoning
- Clinical reasoning is patient-centred involving a collaborative exchange to achieve a mutual understanding of the problem and to negotiate an agreed-upon plan for addressing that problem
- Clinical reasoning requires different foci of thinking, or 'reasoning strategies' within which expert physiotherapists make judgments
- Clinical reasoning plays a critical role in reflective learning from practice experiences and in the development of clinical expertise.

Clinical reasoning and the bio-psychosocial model of health and disability

Contemporary understanding of health and disability recognizes disability is not simply the cumulative effects of physical impairments, rather disability is also socially constructed (e.g. Borrell-Carrió et al. 2004, Imrie 2004, Johnson 1993, Werner 1998). This broader view of disability is consistent with

the holistic bio-psychosocial philosophy of practice as depicted in the World Health Organization ICF framework (World Health Organization 2001) (Fig. 2.1). The bio-psychosocial model initially put forward by Engel:

> …dispenses with the scientifically archaic principles of dualism and reductionism and replaces the simple cause-and-effect explanations of linear causality with reciprocal causal models.
>
> (Engel 1978, p. 175)

However, despite overwhelming evidence for the bio-psychosocial philosophy of practice, many therapists still practice in a predominantly biomedical mode. Some argue it's not their role (i.e. 'I'm a physiotherapist not a psychologist'); some agree it is important but see psychosocial factors as only relevant to chronic pain; some have a dualistic conception of bio-psychosocial rather than understanding it as a genuine integration of mind and body (Borrell-Carrió et al. 2004, Duncan 2000, Engel 1978, Pincus 2004); some claim to be bio-psychosocial but their actual practice does not reflect this approach (Argyris & Schön 1978, Jorgensen 2000, Mattingly & Fleming 1994); and some do practice bio-psychosocially but due to a lack of formal training they tend to be informal and superficial with an over focus on behavioural over cognitive and social factors (Sharp 2001, Sim & Smith 2004).

The ICF framework depicted in Figure 2.1 portrays the patient's clinical presentation through the boxes across the middle of the diagram incorporating impairments of body functions and

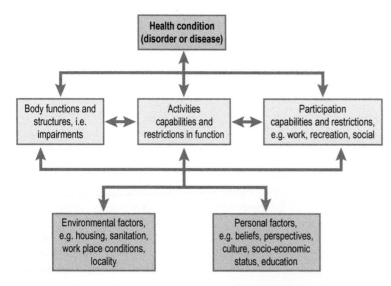

Figure 2.1 • Adaptation of World Health Organization International Classification of Functioning, Disability and Heath Framework (World Health Organization 2001, p. 18).

structures, restrictions and capabilities in functional activities and restrictions and capabilities in their ability to participate in life situations (e.g. work, family, sport, leisure). This clinical presentation of impairments, activity and participation restrictions (i.e. the patient's 'disability') is represented as an outcome of interactions between the biomedical health condition (i.e. disorder, disease, illness) and contextual environmental and personal factors. Environmental factors include architectural characteristics, social attitudes, legal and social structures, climate, terrain, etc. Personal factors include gender, age and psychological features such as thoughts/ beliefs, feelings, coping styles, health and illness behaviours, social circumstances, education, past and current experiences. Environmental and personal factors can positively or negatively influence the clinical presentation. Bidirectional arrows are used between the different factors to reflect the reciprocal relationship between components. Understanding a patient's clinical presentation therefore necessitates attention to their physical health, environmental and personal factors. While physiotherapists are generally well prepared to assess and manage the physical dimensions of the patient's health condition, formal education and experience assessing, analyzing and managing environmental and personal factors is often less developed and less structured. The ICF framework provides an excellent overarching profile of the scope of areas in which physiotherapists must be competent to holistically understand and manage their patients with a growing body of physiotherapy literature now available relating the ICF to categorization of clinical problems and to clinical reasoning (e.g. Childs et al. 2008, Cibulka et al. 2009, Edwards & Jones 2007a, Escorpizo et al. 2010, Jette 2006, Logerstedt et al. 2010, McPoil et al. 2008, Steiner et al. 2002). The scope of clinical reasoning required to practice within this biopsychosocial framework is discussed next.

Key message

Research into expertise and clinical reasoning reveals that many of the attributes of experts are also associated with skilled clinical reasoning. Expert physiotherapists reason and practice within a holistic bio-psychosocial model of health and disability consistent with the World Health Organization ICF framework and contemporary health care.

Clinical reasoning as a hypothesis-oriented and collaborative process

Understanding the clinical reasoning underlying a physiotherapist's assessment and management of a patient requires consideration of the thinking process of the therapist, the thinking process of the patient and the shared decision making between therapist and patient. Figure 2.2 presents a biopsychosocial framework of clinical reasoning as a collaborative process between physiotherapist and patient (Edwards & Jones 1996). The left-hand side of Figure 2.2 depicts the therapist's thinking while the right represents the patient's. The arrows linking the two sides reflect the collaborative nature of the process.

The physiotherapist's thinking

The therapist's reasoning is an ongoing hypothesisoriented process of perception, interpretation and synthesis of information. Information about or from the patient must first be perceived as relevant and then interpreted. Both perception and interpretation are directly related to the therapist's knowledge base (e.g. novices often miss relevant information, struggle to identify and give weight to the most relevant information, and may interpret information incorrectly or superficially). Once identified and interpreted, information must then be synthesized with other information obtained. This is a higher order thinking skill, again directly related to the clinician's organization of knowledge. It is useful to conceptualize the working interpretations made throughout the patient examination and ongoing management as hypotheses as this discourages premature conclusions. Instead, further information obtained is interpreted and considered against existing hypotheses (i.e. tested) as either supporting or not-supporting. This process of hypothesis generation involves a combination of specific data interpretations or inductions (generalizing from the specific) and the synthesis of multiple clues or deductions (instancing from generalizations) that, taken together, has been characterized as hypotheticodeductive or 'backward reasoning' (Arocha et al. 1993, Patel & Groen 1991). In this sense clinical reasoning is a cyclic process of information perception and interpretation (i.e. hypothesis generation)

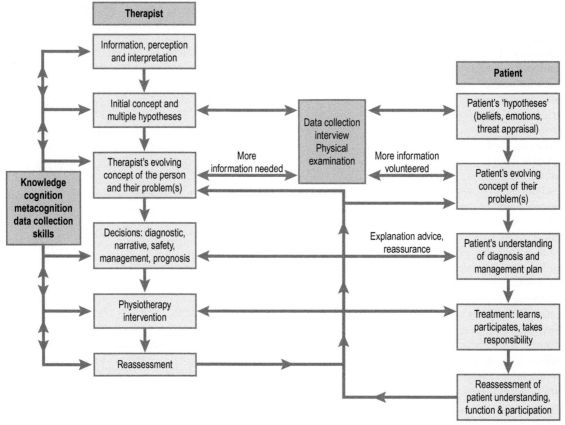

Figure 2.2 • Collaborative reasoning model (Edwards & Jones 1996, Jones & Rivett 2004).

followed by further information collection, interpretation and synthesis (i.e. hypothesis testing, modification and additional hypothesis generation). The reassessments following treatment interventions represent another example of hypothesis testing as reflected in the arrow in Figure 2.2 which runs from reassessment back up to the therapist's evolving understanding of the problem and person. It is important for student physiotherapists to learn to think on their feet. While examination routines are helpful to ensure a thorough and systematic assessment of the neuro-musculoskeletal system, examination by rote (i.e. simply following a protocol without reasoning) is inefficient and likely to lead to recipe treatments that are not tailored to the individual patient and so are less effective.

The hypothetico-deductive reasoning process portrayed in the left side of Figure 2.2 underpins the diagnostic process used in medicine and physiotherapy. While experts with extensive experience and superior knowledge are often able to use pattern recognition (discussed later) to circumvent

extensive generation and testing of competing hypotheses when confronting familiar presentations (Elstein & Schwarz 2002, Kaufman et al. 2008, Patel & Groen 1986, Patel et al. 1986), the process of differential diagnosis still exists as typically the two or three most likely patterns are considered. However, where medical diagnosis normally has a disease or pathology focus, physiotherapy physical diagnostic reasoning tends to incorporate a broader analysis of the patient's functional capabilities and physical impairments along with their established or hypothesized pathology as they relate to the presenting activity and participation restrictions (APTA 2003, Jensen et al. 2007, Jones & Rivett 2004).

The patient's thinking

Understanding the patient as a person rather than simply their biomedical physical problems requires understanding their perspectives or their thoughts, feelings, self-efficacy and coping strategies as reflected in the boxes on the right side of Figure 2.2. Patients' beliefs and feelings which are counterproductive to their management and recovery can contribute to their lack of involvement in the management process, poor self-efficacy and ultimately a poor outcome. Patients acquire their own ideas and associated feelings regarding their health problems from their personal experiences including advice from medical practitioners, family and friends. While typically not thought of as such, these can be equated to their 'hypotheses' regarding what is going on with their body, how serious it is and what can and should be done about it. A brief summary of research findings demonstrating the potential influences of patients' perspectives on their clinical presentation, expectations and willingness to self-manage follows.

Patients' perspectives of their problem have been shown to impact on their levels of pain tolerance, attempts to adjust or cope, their mood and pain related disability and eventual outcome (Craig 2006, Flor & Turk 2006, Gottlieb et al. 2001, Jensen et al. 2003, King et al. 2002, Williams & Keefe 1991, Wilson et al. 1993). Levels of anxiety have been shown to influence pain severity, complications following surgery and days of hospitalization (DeGroot et al. 1997, Pavlin et al. 1998, Salkovskis 1996). Anxiety is most common when symptoms are unexplained, the future is uncertain and the patient is concerned about the perception of others. A reciprocal relationship exists so that negative thoughts elicit negative moods and negative feelings in turn adversely influence patients' appraisals of their problem. Reduction in pain-related anxiety has been demonstrated to predict improvement in functioning, affective distress, pain and activity levels (McCracken & Gross 1998). Patients' preoccupation with negative thoughts and self-statements about their circumstances and future prospects (i.e. 'catastrophizing') is a risk factor for pain-related fear and long-term disability (Pincus 2004, Vlaeyen & Linton 2000). Greater worry about pain is also associated with hypervigilance, or over-attention and misinterpretation of body sensations. Negative, unhelpful thoughts tend to relate to the meaning patients attribute to their problem or pain. Patients with low self-efficacy (i.e. low perception and confidence in ability to cope and make a change) tend to be convinced their own efforts will not be successful and tend to use less constructive coping strategies. This perceived helplessness has been related to pain level and disability (Gatchel et al. 2007).

Assessment, management and reassessment of patients' thoughts and feelings contribute to both the patient's and the therapist's evolving understanding of the significance these factors have to the clinical presentation. When unhelpful thoughts and feelings are successfully addressed patients gain a deeper understanding of their problem that includes recognition of the extent to which their incorrect and often excessively negative perspectives have been contributing to it. This new more constructive understanding enhances their self-efficacy and self-management. Assessing a patient's perspectives requires an understanding of what makes up a health perspective.

Health perspectives (pain, illness, self)

Research into patient's health and disability perspectives highlights important components that make up a patient's understanding/beliefs and concerns about their problem. The experience of pain is integrally associated with personal perceptions and social influences such that patients' pain perceptions, experiences and coping combine into a pain or disability experience lived as a whole (Kleinman et al. 1992, Sim & Smith 2004). As such, the various elements can never truly be isolated. However, greater understanding of the components of the pain experience and their interrelationships is important to guiding what information the physiotherapist listens for and seeks out (either through questionnaire or interview) when attempting to understand the person and any psychosocially related factors that may be contributing to their presentation. Research in medical anthropology, medical sociology and cognitive psychology has all contributed to the understanding of illness representations or schemas (e.g. Bishop 1991, Pincus & Morley 2001, Skelton & Croyle 1991, Sim & Smith 2004, Turk & Rudy 1992). Leventhal et al. (1980) put forward the notion that patients' mental representations of health threats determine how they respond to those threats. Illness schemata are defined as individuals' 'implicit theories of illness' that they use in order to interpret and respond to health threats. These illness (or pain) schemas are like imprints, or patterns of interconnected features, learned (consciously or unconsciously) through social and personal experiences. Skelton and Croyle (1991, p. 4) report on illness cognition research that demonstrates illness schemas comprise the following elements:

1. Concrete symptoms and a label (e.g. a common cold vs pneumonia) that facilitate identification of the health problem
2. Beliefs about the immediate and long-term consequences of the problem, and
3. Its temporal course, and attributions concerning the cause of the problem and the means by which a cure may be affected.

Research has also identified a number of dimensions that people use in evaluating their health problem including their perception of its seriousness, social desirability, personal responsibility, controllability and changeability (Bishop 1991). Therefore it is not only the person's existing beliefs and assumptions that make up their illness schema and contribute to determining their coping but also their appraisal of the threat their medical condition poses. This highlights the importance of assessing, and if necessary addressing through education, the patient's threat appraisal (Jones & Edwards 2006, Moseley 2004).

A person's understanding, expectations and concerns about different types of pain (e.g. needle injection pain, toothache pain, back pain, etc.) would make up their pain schema which Pincus and Morley (2001) suggest comprises beliefs regarding the immediate sensory-intensity, spatial and temporal features of pain along with the initial affective responses and self-protective behaviours that ensue. The pain schema would also likely include a similar appraisal as the illness schema regarding its seriousness and controllability/changeability.

Lastly, Pincus and Morley (2001) discuss a 'self' schema as a complex multifaceted construct that relates to who you are with reference to who you used to be (prior to your perceived change in self) and who you would like to be in the future. It includes an evaluative dimension that contributes to an individual's sense of self-worth. Pain and disability have the potential to disrupt aspects of the self, such that repeated failures to function 'normally' and the negative emotions that result can lead to changes in a person's self-image (Osborn & Smith 1998, Sim & Smith 2004, Steen & Haugli 2000).

Pincus and Morley (2001) also propose that these different schemas can be enmeshed so that a pain schema for example may enmesh with an illness schema and elicit interpretations of the pain as a marker or part of a larger illness or health problem. Similarly, perceptions of the threat a pain condition

or illness may create can be enmeshed with the patient's self-worth as with the chronic back pain patient whose pain has not been adequately explained by the medical system who develops perceptions (real or imagined) that his family, employer and/or co-workers don't believe him, causing him to feel he is not a good work-mate, spouse, parent, etc.

The value of this concept of different pain, illness and self schemas to patients' presentations is not for physiotherapists to attempt to classify a patient's schemas or their theoretical schema enmeshment, instead the value is to our clinical reasoning and the scope of patient perspectives we listen for and seek out when attempting to assess psychosocial factors. Patients are clearly not homogeneous when you consider the different pathologies that can cause pain and disability, the continuum of any particular pathology (minor to extensive), the physical impairments that can predispose to the problem or be created by the problem, and the different perspectives (understandings, beliefs, fears, coping mechanisms, self-image, etc.) that exists in varying combinations. This is important to our clinical reasoning as it highlights theory we must understand (e.g. pain and disability associations with psychosocial factors), skills we must acquire in order to assess (e.g. questioning about psychosocial factors, questionnaires to use) and manage (e.g. education and cognitive-behavioural strategies, referral pathways) this dimension of our patients' presentations. Understanding patients' perspectives is also important as their understanding, attributions, feelings, etc., will influence other perspectives. For example, expectations of management such as the perspective 'my disc is out' causing the expectation that nothing can be done or perhaps physical/passive treatment is required; expectations regarding personal responsibility and self-management, such as the perspective/belief that 'the problem is my degenerative spine', without appreciating the physical (e.g. relative flexibility, motor control, fitness), lifestyle and environmental factors that may have predisposed the degenerative spine to become symptomatic and require a significant contribution of self-management; and expectations regarding the future as with the perspective 'my back-knee-shoulder, etc. is stuffed and I will never be able to work-exercise-etc. again'. Understanding patients' problems diagnostically and understanding patients' perspectives require considerable bio-psychosocial research and practice knowledge.

The level of education physiotherapists receive in psychosocial assessment and management varies considerably. Jones and Edwards (2006) have suggested the following categories of information are screened when assessing patients' perspectives (i.e. psychosocial status):

- What are patient's perspectives of their experience?
  - their understanding of their pain/condition?
  - their coping strategies?
  - their management expectations and goals?
  - their threat appraisal with regard to its seriousness, social desirability, personal responsibility, controllability and changeability?
  - their level of stress and distress?
    - stress: over-attention to sensory information and fear-avoidance or more extensive over-attention to overall health with catastrophizing cognitions and overt symptoms of stress?
    - distress: natural, harmless feelings of frustration to more significant and higher levels of distress (e.g. depression) affecting their 'self'?
- How does patient think they are perceived by others and how does this affect how they feel about themselves?
  - attention seeking or response to society's expectations? Some will feel they need to justify their pain as real and not just in their head
- How does the patient compare themself with others?
  - what they can and can't do?
  - their self-worth?
  - their perception of their contributions? For example:
    - positive comparisons where self-esteem is strengthened: 'I could be worse off, I could be stuck in a wheelchair'
    - negative comparisons that reinforce their despair and threat of rejection
- Does patient avoid activities/withdraw from others due to pain/disability/social stigma?
- What is the patient's 'motivation' for change? For example:
  - how ready they are for change?
  - how important do they feel change is?

- how confident do they feel they are in their own abilities to make changes?

As a measure of their 'motivation' the patient can then be asked: 'On a scale of 0 to 100, how ready are you to make these changes? How important are these changes to you? How confident/ able are you to make these changes?'

There is now also a wide range of questionnaires available for screening patients' psychosocial related issues (see Table 2.1 for an example). While these questionnaires provide a helpful resource, on their own they are insufficient to guide the physiotherapist's management. They provide useful insight to a patient's thoughts, beliefs and feelings but they generally do not provide the basis of those thoughts and feelings. As such, physiotherapists need to review the completed questionnaire with the patient to explore further the patient's answers. That is, questionnaires such as these should not be seen as a replacement for the interview questions suggested above, rather they should be used as an adjunct and an objective means of documenting and scoring patients' psychosocial status.

It is beyond the scope of this chapter to extend this discussion to the physical and cognitive-behavioural management strategies needed to address patient perspectives judged as contributing to their disability and/or presenting as obstacles to their recovery. However, there is now very helpful physiotherapy literature providing suggestions on assessment and management strategies specifically targeting patients' unhelpful thoughts, feelings and behaviours (e.g. Harding 1998, Johnson & Moores 2006, Keefe, Scipio & Perri 2006, Kendall & Watson 2000, Main & Watson 2002, Main et al. 2008, Muncey 2002, Strong & Unruh 2002).

Clinical reasoning as collaboration between therapist and patient

Thinking of clinical reasoning through examination and management as a therapeutic alliance where collaboration, rather than simply compliance, is sought is important to encourage students and therapists to involve their patients in the decision making process (Edwards et al. 2004b, Higgs & Hunt 1999, Jensen et al. 2002, Payton et al. 1998, Trede & Higgs 2008). While obviously the patient has come to the physiotherapist seeking their expertise, treatment and advice, patients who have been given an opportunity to share in the decision making have

Table 2.1 Examples of psychosocial screening questionnaires

Questionnaire	Purpose	Source
Fear-avoidance Beliefs Questionnaire	To measure patients' beliefs about how physical activity and work affect their low back pain. It can help identify patients for whom psychosocial interventions may be beneficial	Waddell et al. (1993)
Tampa Scale of Kinesiophobia	To measure patients' fear of movement/re-injury in persistent pain. The Tampa Scale Kinesiophobia-11 (TSK-11) uses 11 out of the 17 items from the original version of the Tampa Scale of Kinesiophobia	Woby et al. (2005)
Örebro Musculoskeletal Pain Screening Questionnaire	To identify how likely it is that workers with soft tissue injury will develop long-term problems (screening for yellow flags). This screening questionnaire, when completed 4–12 weeks after musculoskeletal injury, predicts long-term disability and failure to return to work	Linton and Hallden (1998)
Centre for Epidemiologic Studies-Depression Scale	To measure anxiety, depression and depressed mood symptoms	Radloff (1977)
Kessler Physiological Distress Scale	To measure non-specific psychological distress (primarily intended as a measure of mood, anxiety and depression)	Kessler et al. (2002)
Chronic Disease Self-efficacy Scales	To measure patients' beliefs that they can manage their chronic condition (e.g. symptom control, role function, emotional functioning and communicating with physicians).	Lorig et al. (1996)
Self-Efficacy for Managing Chronic Disease 6 Item Scale	To measure patients' symptom control, role function, emotional functioning and communicating with physicians	Lorig et al. (2001)
Perceived Health Confidence Scale	To measure patients' views of their competence in taking care of their health. It is a domain-specific measure of the degree to which an individual feels capable of effectively managing their health outcomes.	Smiths, Wallston and Smith (1995)
Perceived Stress Scale	To measure patients' perception of stress. It is a measure of the degree to which situations in one's life are appraised as stressful. The scale also includes a number of direct queries about current levels of experienced stress	Cohen, Kamarck and Mermelstein (1983)
Pain Self-efficacy Questionnaire	To measure chronic pain patients' self-rated confidence in performing activities despite the presence of pain	Nicholas (2007)
Modified Somatic Perceptions Questionnaire	To measure clinically significant psychological distress in patients with persistent back pain (a measure of heightened somatic and autonomic awareness related to anxiety and depression)	Main (1983)
PHQ9 and PHQ2	PHQ-9: To assist diagnosis and guide management of depression. PHQ-2: To identify patients who may have depression and require referral for further diagnostic assessment.	Arroll et al. (2010)

been shown to take greater responsibility for their own management, are more satisfied with their health care (reducing risk of formal complaints) and have a greater likelihood of achieving better outcomes (Arnetz et al. 2004, Edwards et al. 2004b, Trede & Higgs 2008). Despite acknowledging the importance of being collaborative with their patients many physiotherapists do not respond to patients' life and treatment priorities or work with patients in collaboratively setting goals (Edwards et al. 2004b). Patient learning (i.e. altered understanding and improved health behaviour), improved self-efficacy and shared responsibility in management are primary outcomes sought in a collaborative reasoning approach.

Therapist learning also occurs through collaboration. That is, when patients are given the opportunity to tell their story rather than simply answer questions, reflective therapists, who attend to individual patient presentations noting features that appear to be linked (such as increased stress affecting one patient's symptoms but not another's), will learn the variety of ways in which patients' health, cognition, behaviour, movement and pain can interact. Specific strategies for involving patients in their health care, including when differences in opinion exist, are addressed by Edwards et al. (2004b) and Trede and Higgs (2008).

The box on the far left-hand side of Figure 2.2 highlights important variables influencing the therapist's clinical reasoning including their knowledge base, their cognitive, metacognitive (including critical thinking), and their data collection skills.

 Key message

Clinical reasoning is a collaborative process between therapist and patient. The therapist must continually think on their feet through a cyclic process of information perception and interpretation, hypothesis generation, further data collection, synthesis of working interpretations and hypothesis modification that occurs throughout the initial assessment and ongoing management and reassessments. Simultaneously with their 'diagnostic' assessment and reasoning the therapist must assess and evaluate, through interview and questionnaire, the patient as a person including their pain or disability experiences as reflected through their thoughts, feelings, self-efficacy and coping strategies regarding their perceived health threats.

Clinical reasoning and knowledge

The importance of knowledge to physiotherapists' clinical reasoning is highlighted in Jensen's expertise research where expert physiotherapists were seen to possess a broad, multidimensional knowledge base acquired through professional education and reflective practice where both patients and other health professionals were valued as sources for learning (Jensen et al. 2007). All forms of knowledge are important including physiotherapists' broader worldview, their philosophy of practice and their medical and physiotherapy specific knowledge (Cusick 2001, Higgs and Hunt 1999, Hooper 1997, Jensen et al. 2007, Unsworth 2004). However, it is not simply how much an individual knows, rather it is their organization of knowledge that is most

important (Chi et al. 1988, Ericsson & Smith 1991, Hayes & Adams 2000, Rumelhart & Ortony 1977). Glaser (1984, p. 99) states that 'effective thinking is the result of conditionalized knowledge – the knowledge that becomes associated with the conditions and constraints of its use'. In other words, for knowledge to be accessible in a clinical setting it must be organized or linked to its clinical significance. While not addressed here, this has important implications to physiotherapy educators to ensure that the basic sciences underpinning physiotherapy practice are taught in a manner that facilitates this clinical link (e.g. Problem based/experiential learning) and that practical and clinical subjects also strategically link their content to the relevant basic sciences (e.g. biomechanics, pain science, etc.).

Knowledge emerges from what we believe or hold to be true (Higgs et al. 2008). Physiotherapists utilize a combination of propositional knowledge ('knowing that') generated formally through research and scholarship and non-propositional knowledge ('knowing how') generated primarily through practice experience. Higgs and Titchen (1995) divide non-propositional knowledge further into professional craft knowledge and personal knowledge. Craft knowledge comprises professional knowledge such as procedural and communication knowledge and skills, based on academic propositional knowledge that has been refined and contextualized through clinical experience. Personal knowledge includes that knowledge acquired through personal life experiences (including community and cultural) that contribute to shaping a person's beliefs, values and attitudes, or what Mezirow (1990, 1991) has called their 'meaning perspective' (also synonymous with Maitland's 'Frame of reference'). As already discussed, a person's perspectives (therapist and patient) significantly influence their interpersonal interactions and their expectations. Therapists who are alert to both community and their own attitudes (i.e. personal knowledge) regarding for example different population subgroups (e.g. ethnic, workers compensation, substance abuse) are better able to safeguard against their own assumptions, biases/prejudices leading to premature or incorrect judgments.

Understanding and successfully managing patients' problems requires a rich organization of all three types of knowledge. Propositional knowledge provides us with theory and research substantiation on which to base our practice while non-propositional professional craft knowledge provides us with the means to use that theory and research evidence in the clinic.

The importance of craft knowledge cannot be overstated. Maitland placed enormous emphasis on clinical skills (subjective questioning and examination/treatment procedures). While these were initially taught as propositional knowledge of subjective and physical examination routines and correct execution of examination and treatment techniques, they were then refined through clinical supervision to be tailored to patients' particular presentations with continual clarification of patient answers and adjustment of examination and treatment procedures. It was not uncommon for Maitland to demonstrate on a patient a treatment procedure he had never used in exactly the way it was being demonstrated, as he had adapted the procedure to the patient's particular presentation. That nicely illustrates the use of craft knowledge and the importance of using propositional knowledge as a guide, not a prescription, for how to practise.

Clinical reasoning and cognition/metacognition

In addition to the therapist's organization of knowledge, their cognitive skills (e.g. data synthesis/analysis and purposeful inquiry strategies) and their metacognitive skills (self-awareness and critical reflection) are key factors influencing their clinical reasoning proficiency. Cognition in clinical reasoning commences with the perception of what is relevant. Closely related to knowledge, perception includes recognizing potentially relevant cues available from medical records/reports and patient information (verbal and non-verbal) obtained directly through interview and from the physical examination. A student's reasoning may be limited simply due to their inability to recognize important information.

Physiotherapists' decisions regarding physical assessment (e.g. extent of assessment that can be safely carried out and which assessments to prioritize at the first appointment), physical diagnosis, influence of environmental and psychosocial factors, treatment and prognosis relate to their ability to synthesize and analyze the mass of information obtained about a patient's presentation and the weighting they have given (consciously or unconsciously) to the various findings. Synthesis (e.g. for consistency of information) and analysis (i.e. for meaning and recognition of patterns) are higher

order forms of cognition. A challenging aspect of analysis is that one cue can alter the interpretation of another. For example, patients with significant central sensitization in their clinical presentation may have provocative physical examination tests that on their own would implicate pathology/impairment of a particular structure/tissue. However, when the pain provoked is considered in light of an apparent dominant central pain state it may actually be a false positive, painful due to the sensitization rather than actual local pathology (Meyer et al. 2006, Nijs et al. 2010, Wolf 2011).

Metacognition is a form of self-awareness that incorporates monitoring of yourself (e.g. your performance, your thinking, your knowledge) as though you are outside yourself observing and critiquing your practice. There is an integral link between cognition, metacognition and knowledge acquisition or learning from clinical practice experience (Eraut 1994, Higgs et al. 2004, Higgs et al. 2004, Schön 1987). For example, following protocol assessments without reasoning requires little cognition beyond remembering a routine that was memorized. In contrast, questions and physical assessments used with a specific purpose in mind provide a more complete picture of the patient's presentation while enabling working hypotheses to be 'tested' and clinical patterns recognized. While hopefully all therapists think, not all therapists think about their thinking. It is this self-awareness and self-critique that prompts the metacognitive therapist to reconsider their hypotheses, plans and management.

This self-awareness is not limited to formal hypotheses considered and treatments selected as metacognitive awareness of performance is also important. This for example underpins the experienced therapist's immediate recognition that a particular phrasing of a question or explanation was not clear. Similarly metacognitive awareness of the effectiveness of a physical procedure enables immediate recognition that the procedure needs to be adjusted or perhaps should be abandoned as for example when cues such an increase in muscle tone or the patient's expression signal the procedure was not achieving its desired effect.

Lastly metacognition is important to recognizing limitations in knowledge. The student or therapist who lacks awareness of their own knowledge limitations will learn less. Experts not only know a lot in their area of practice, they also know what they don't know. That is, the expert is typically very quick to recognize a limitation in their knowledge (e.g. a patient's medication they are unfamiliar with, a medical condition, a peripheral nerve sensory and motor distribution) and act on it by consulting a colleague or appropriate resource. In short metacognition and critical reflection are important means to continued professional career-long learning.

Motivation to acquire knowledge through entry level physiotherapy education emanates from internal interests enhanced by formal assessment requirements to pass a subject/program. Knowledge acquisition in clinical practice is driven largely by personal desire to understand more and achieve better outcomes. Inherent in the learning through formal academia and through clinical practice is the critical thinking and reasoning ability to ask skilled questions of yourself (i.e. critical reflection) and of others (educators, colleagues, patients). What follows is a brief discussion of skilled questioning important to critical thinking in general (e.g. self-reflection and discussions/debates with students, classmates, work colleagues and educators) and skilled questioning specific to clinical practice.

Skilled questioning important to critical thinking and learning

Socratic questioning

Thinking is driven by questions in that questions define or clarify issues being discussed. An open and questioning mind is a prerequisite to skilled critical thinking and reasoning which in turn cultivates deep learning. The art of asking questions and pursuing answers originated by Socrates (Athens, c. 469–399 BC), called 'Socratic questioning', is based on the notion that thinking (e.g. interpretations, opinions, analyses, conclusions) has a logic or structure that underpins it that typically is not evident in the initial expression (Paul & Elder 2007). The purpose of Socratic questioning is to clarify and understand the logic of someone's thought (including your own through critical reflection). Paul and Elder (2006, pp. 54–55) note that:

> All thinking has assumptions; makes claims or creates meaning; has implications; focuses on some things and throws others into the background; uses some concepts or ideas and not others; is defined by purposes, issues, or problems; uses or explains some facts and not others; is relatively clear or unclear; is relatively deep or superficial; is relatively critical or uncritical; is

relatively elaborated or underdeveloped; is relatively mono-logical or multi-logical.

Through disciplined questioning complex ideas and concepts can be explored, truth can be sought, unrecognized issues and problems can be revealed, assumptions can be made apparent, what is known and not known can be made evident and the logical implications of thought can be highlighted. From an educator's perspective Paul and Elder (2006, p. 55) highlight the value of successful Socratic questioning discussions to:

> …take student thought from the unclear to the clear, from the unreasoned to the reasoned, from the implicit to the explicit, from the unexamined to the examined, from the inconsistent to the consistent, from the unarticulated to the articulated.

Edited examples of different types of Socratic questions related to critical thinking in general (but also relevant to critical thinking in the clinic) as suggested by Paul and Elder (2006, pp. 5–7, 20–23) are highlighted in Box 2.1.

Skilled questioning important to clinical practice

The accuracy and effectiveness of our clinical judgments is influenced by the quality of information (e.g. patient interview and physical examination) on which those judgments are based. The manner in which an examination and therapy is provided with respect to patient rapport and the level of therapist interest, empathy and confidence conveyed influences patients' information volunteered, motivation for change, willingness to participate in self-management and their outcome in general (Klaber et al. 1997). While the specific questions and sequence of questions asked will vary according to education and personal experience, the aim should be the same, that is to understand the patient's problem and their individual pain/disability experience in order to inform effective, collaborative management.

Many of the generic critical thinking questions outlined above are equally relevant to skilled patient questioning. Maitland offered excellent examples of questioning strategies to optimize the quality of information obtained (Maitland 1986). Perhaps the one he emphasized most was to never assume and therefore to always clarify the patient's meaning.

| Box 2.1

Edited examples of 'Socratic questions'

Questions that target the parts of thinking

Questions that probe purpose:

(All thought reflects an agenda or purpose. Assume that you do not fully understand someone's thought (including your own) until you understand the agenda behind it.)

- What is the purpose of ___?
- What was your purpose when you said___?

Questions that probe assumptions:

(All thought rests upon assumptions. Assume that you do not fully understand a thought until you understand what that thought takes for granted.)

- What are you assuming? How would you justify taking this for granted here?
- You seem to be assuming ___. Do I understand you correctly?
- All of your reasoning depends on the idea that ___. Why have you based your reasoning on ___ rather than ___?
- Is your assumption always the case? Why do you think the assumption holds here?

Questions that probe information, reasons, evidence, and causes:

(All thoughts presuppose an information base. Assume that you do not fully understand the thought until you understand the background information (facts, data, experiences) that supports or informs it.)

- On what information are you basing that comment?
- What are your reasons for saying that?
- How do we know this information is accurate? How could we verify it?
- Why do you think that is true?
- Is there an alternative interpretation/conclusion?
- What experience convinced you of this? Could your experience be distorted?
- Could you explain your reasons to us?
- What led you to that belief?
- Do you have any evidence to support your assertion?
- How does that information apply to this case?

Questions about viewpoints or perspectives:

(All thought takes place within a point of view or frame of reference. Assume that you do not fully understand a thought until you understand the point of view or frame of reference that places it on an intellectual map.)

- From what point of view are you looking at this? Are there other perspectives?

- You seem to be approaching this issue from ___ perspective. Why have you chosen that perspective?
- How would other groups/types of people respond? Why? What would influence them?
- Does anyone else see this another way?

Questions that probe implications and consequences:

(All thought is headed in a direction. It not only begins somewhere (resting on assumptions), it also goes somewhere (has implications and consequences). Assume that you do not fully understand a thought unless you know the most important implications and consequences that follow from it.)

- What are you implying by that?
- When you say ___, are you implying ___?
- What effect would that have?
- Would that necessarily happen or only probably happen?
- Have you considered the implications of that?

Questions about the question:

(All thought is responsive to a question. Assume that you do not fully understand a thought until you understand the question that gives rise to it.)

- I am not sure exactly what question you are raising. Could you explain it?
- The question in my mind is this ___. Do you agree or do you see another question at issue?
- Is this the same issue as ___?
- Can we break this question down at all?
- Is the question clear? Do we understand it?
- What does this question assume?
- To answer this question, what other questions would we have to answer first?

Questions that probe concepts and ideas:

(All thought involves the application of concepts. Assume that you do not fully understand a thought until you understand the concepts that define and shape it.)

- What is the main idea you are using in your reasoning? Could you explain that idea?
- Why/how is this idea important?
- What was the main idea guiding our thinking as we try to reason through this issue? Is this idea causing us problems?
- What main theories do we need to consider in figuring out ___?
- What idea is this author using in her or his thinking?

Box 2.1—cont'd

Questions that probe inferences and interpretations:

(All thought requires the making of inferences, the drawing of conclusions, the creation of meaning. Assume that you do not fully understand a thought until you understand the inferences that have shaped it.)

- What conclusions are we coming to about ___?
- How did you reach that conclusion?
- Is there a more logical inference we might make in this situation?
- Could you explain your reasoning?
- Given all the facts, what is the best possible conclusion?

Questions that target the quality of reasoning

The quality of thinking can be evaluated by its clarity, precision, accuracy, relevance, depth, breadth, logicalness and fairness.

Questioning clarity:

(Assume that you do not fully understand a thought except to the extent you can elaborate, illustrate and exemplify it.)

- What do you mean by____?
- What is your main point?
- Could you put that another way?
- Could you give me an example?
- Could you explain that further?
- Why do you say that?
- Let me see if I understand you; do you mean ___ or ___?
- How does this relate to our discussion/problem/issue?

Questioning precision:

(Assume that you do not fully understand a thought except to the extent that you can specify it in detail.)

- Could you give me more details about that?
- Could you be more specific?

Questioning accuracy:

(Assume that you have not fully assessed a thought except to the extent that you have checked to determine whether it represents things as they really are.)

- How could we verify that?
- Can we trust the accuracy of these data given the questionable source from which they come?

Questioning relevance:

(Thinking is always capable of straying from the task, question, problem, or issue under consideration. Assume that you have not fully assessed thinking except to the extent that you have ensured that all considerations used in addressing it are genuinely relevant to it.)

- How does that relate to the issue?
- Could you explain the connection between your point and the issue?

Questioning depth:

(Thinking can either function at the surface of things or probe beneath that surface to deeper matters and issues. Assume that you have not fully assessed a line of thinking except to the extent that you have determined the depth required for the task at hand.)

- Is this issue/question simple or complex? Is it easy or difficult to understand/evaluate/answer?
- What makes this a complex issue/question?
- How are we dealing with the complexities inherent in the issue/question?

Questioning breadth:

(Thinking can be more or less broad or narrow-minded and that breadth of thinking requires the thinker to think insightfully within more than one point of view or frame of reference. Assume that you have not fully assessed a line of thinking except to the extent that you have determined how much breadth of thinking is required.)

- What points of view are relevant to this issue?
- Do we need to look at this from another perspective?

Data from Paul and Elder 2006, pp. 5–7, 20–23.

There are numerous examples of where this is helpful including the following:

Clarification for precision

There are many situations where the patient makes a general statement that requires clarification to understand precisely their meaning. Examples include such things as constancy of symptoms (where clarification of 'constant' reveals daily symptoms but not every moment of the day); area of symptoms (where for example patient's perception of their 'shoulder' is clarified to actually be their supraspinous fossa); and aggravating factors (where for example 'walking' requires clarification regarding what aspect of the walking is a problem – time, speed, distance, surface, phase of gait, etc.?).

Clarification for accuracy

Patient responses are often generalizations where the lack of accuracy can lead to misinterpretations. Examples here include reassessments of previous treatment sessions (where the patient reports no benefit but clarification reveals symptoms significantly improved for a period of time before returning); and patient reports of what others have said or the attitude/support of others (e.g. doctors, employers, family) that reflect the patient's perspective but not always reality.

Clarification for relevance

While it is important to always give patients a voice and an opportunity to tell their story, it is also necessary to control the interview for time management. This requires considerable communication skills to establish the relevance of a particular tangent the patient seems to be taking and diplomacy to bring them back on track while still conveying interest.

Clarification for completeness

Completeness (thoroughness) of examination and reassessments is necessary to ensure nothing important is missed. This relates to another clinical reasoning tactic referred to as 'screening questions'.

Screening questions

Patients will typically volunteer the information they feel is important and related to their main problem. However, they will often not appreciate the potential importance of other information they may feel is unrelated. Without thorough screening, information may be missed and as a result reasoning compromised. Important areas to use screening questions for completeness include mapping out the patient's symptoms, establishing their behaviour of symptoms and medical screening for precautions and contraindications to examination and treatment.

While the patient will obviously describe their main complaint they may not feel other symptoms and problems in other body areas are relevant. Clearing other body areas, as emphasized by Maitland, ensures the main complaint is considered in the context of the patient's broader health presentation. For example, when clarified a recent peripheral joint pain may turn out to be part of a broader systemic disorder, only recognized when further screening reveals involvement of other joints. Similarly, patients will report their main symptom(s) but may not consider other symptoms as relevant or may not even recognize other feelings as symptoms until questioned. Examples of common neuromusculoskeletal symptoms that should be screened for include:

- Neuropathic symptoms (numbness, paraesthesias, etc.)
- Vascular and autonomic symptoms (swelling, skin colour, skin dryness/perspiration)
- Weakness
- Stiffness
- Clicks, clunks, giving way, locking
- Vertebrobasilar insufficiency (VBI)/ cervical arterial dysfunction (CAD) symptoms (related to cervical problems), spinal cord symptoms (related to spinal problems), cauda equina symptoms (related to lumbar problems).

As with mapping out the patient's symptoms, when questioning in order to determine aggravating factors, patients will often only mention what they remember or consider most significant. However, if the therapist is reasoning through the examination they should, based on the patient's area of symptoms, consider different structures that may be involved and with that knowledge direct further questions to 'test' those hypotheses. For example, a posterior buttock pain may be emanating from the hip, the sacroiliac joint, the buttock muscles/soft tissues, a neural source (e.g. sciatic or nerve root), or be referred from the lumbar spine. While no aggravating activity will affect a single joint or structure in isolation, questions about other potential aggravating factors that tend to affect one area more than another can assist the evolving picture. For example, if the buttock pain is worsened by crossing the legs and/or squatting, the hip and/or sacroiliac joint-associated tissues are incriminated. This can then be considered against other aggravating factors explicitly screened for which relate to spinal movements and neurodynamics; it may also highlight movements and structures that must be examined and differentiated. The third main area where it is important to screen for completeness, medical screening for precautions, and contraindications to examination and treatment will be discussed later within the section on Hypothesis Categories.

Effects of therapist's questioning/ manner on the patient

While the patient interview is largely about gaining information to understand the patient and their problem, the nature and manner (i.e. tone, non-verbal behaviours) of the therapist's questions and responses to patient answers will influence the interest the patient perceives the therapist has in them, the confidence they have in the therapist and the success of the therapeutic relationship in general (Klaber et al. 1997). Maitland emphasized the importance of establishing patient rapport through the interest and belief conveyed in what they say and through the thoroughness of examination you demonstrate. Our questions and responses (verbal and non-verbal) are interpreted by patients as conveying our thoughts. Many patients report negative experiences with medical and other health professionals who they felt didn't listen or believe them. Without good rapport the patient is less likely to collaborate in providing the necessary information or participate in the management jeopardizing the eventual outcome.

Skilled questioning should be open but specific. The therapist should seek understanding of the person and their problem(s), be efficient while giving the patient a voice, and constantly clarify responses for precision, accuracy, relevance and completeness. The therapeutic relationship, reasoning and outcome are all enhanced when the therapist's listening and responding conveys interest, acknowledgement/empathy, respect, and collaboration while reserving judgment. While patients may need to be challenged at some stage regarding their beliefs, attitudes and health behaviours, argumentation should be avoided and where possible opportunities should be sought to support patient self-efficacy. Patients are unlikely to make the necessary lifestyle changes unless they believe they have the capacity to do so. Brief summaries of your understanding of the patient's story, including your assessment of their perspectives, are important to validate the patient's meaning. While physical impairments such as range of movement and strength are quantitative measures that can be judged against established normative data, patient perspectives represent qualitative data that does not lend itself

to absolute interpretations of normality (i.e. adaptive versus maladaptive/unhelpful perspectives) and hence require validation with the patient (Edwards et al. 2004b, Stewart et al. 2011).

Key message

Metacognitive awareness of your own thinking, performance and knowledge is essential to self-critique and learning. Socratic questioning is a critical thinking tactic helpful to clarifying and understanding the logic of someone else's and your own thoughts. A key Socratic question particularly important to skilled questioning in clinical practice is clarification of meaning for precision, accuracy and relevance. Clarification for completeness can be achieved through the use of 'Screening Questions' for other types of symptoms, other aggravating/easing factors and medical screening for safety. Attention also must be given to the nature and manner of our questions and responses to patients as the interest, belief and empathy we convey will influence the confidence they have in us and the success of the therapeutic relationship and outcome.

Facilitating application of bio-psychosocial practice: clinical reasoning strategies and hypothesis categories

Being able to practice within a bio-psychosocial framework requires different sets of knowledge and clinical skills to be able to understand both the biomedical problem (disease, disorder, illness) and the environmental and personal factors that may predispose or contribute to the problem. As such a distinction can be made between understanding and managing the physical problem to effect change versus understanding and interacting with the person to effect change. To assist physiotherapists' application of bio-psychosocial practice, we have promoted the evolution of our understanding and recommended use of two frameworks for guiding the focus of decision making required (clinical reasoning strategies) and the types of decisions required (hypothesis categories) (American Physical Therapy Association 2003, Christensen et al. 2011, Edwards et al. 2004a, Jones 1987, 1992, 1995, 1997a, 1997b, Jones et al. 2002, Jones and Rivett 2004, Jones et al. 2008).

Clinical reasoning strategies

While clinical reasoning is often equated with diagnostic decision making, in reality that represents only a small portion of the reasoning that actually occurs in clinical practice. In a qualitative research study of clinical reasoning in physiotherapy, Edwards and colleagues (Edwards 2000, Edwards et al. 2004a) identified patterns in the focus of expert physiotherapists' clinical reasoning in three different fields of physiotherapy (musculoskeletal, neurological and domiciliary care). Individual expert therapists in all three fields employed a range of 'clinical reasoning strategies', despite the differing emphases of their examinations and management. The clinical reasoning strategies identified were each associated with a range of diverse clinical actions. While this was the first physiotherapy study to elucidate expert physiotherapists use of this full range of strategies, they have been identified previously either by research, by theoretical proposition or by an exposition of the relevant skills in the literature of medicine, nursing, occupational therapy and physiotherapy under the following names: diagnostic or procedural reasoning (Elstein et al. 1978, Fleming 1991); interactive reasoning (Fleming 1991); conditional or predictive reasoning (Fleming 1991, Hagedorn 1996); narrative reasoning (Benner et al. 1992, Mattingly 1991); ethical reasoning (Barnitt & Partridge 1997, Gordon et al. 1994, Neuhaus 1988); teaching as reasoning (Sluijs 1991); and collaborative decision making (Beeston and Simons 1996, Jensen et al. 2007, Mattingly & Fleming 1994). The clinical reasoning strategies identified by Edwards and colleagues (Edwards 2000, Edwards et al. 2004a) can be grouped broadly under a classification of 'Diagnosis' and 'Management' as follows:

Diagnosis

1. *Diagnostic reasoning* is the formation of a diagnosis related to functional limitation(s) and associated physical impairments with consideration of pain mechanisms, tissue pathology and the broad scope of potential contributing factors.
2. *Narrative reasoning* involves understanding patients' pain, illness and/or disability experiences, or their 'story'. This incorporates their understanding of their problem and the effect it is having on their life, their

expectations regarding management, their feelings and ability to cope and the effects these personal perspectives have on their clinical presentation, particularly whether they are facilitating or obstructing their recovery.

Management

3. *Reasoning about procedure* is the decision making behind the selection, implementation and progression of treatment procedures.
4. *Interactive reasoning* is the purposeful establishment and ongoing management of therapist-patient rapport.
5. *Collaborative reasoning* is the nurturing of a therapeutic alliance towards the interpretation of examination findings, the setting of goals and priorities and the implementation and progression of treatment.
6. *Reasoning about teaching* is the planning, execution and evaluation of individualized and context sensitive teaching, including education for conceptual understanding and education for physical performance (e.g. exercise, posture, sport technique correction).
7. *Predictive reasoning* is the therapist's judgment regarding prognosis and their interaction with the patient to envision future scenarios with collaborative exploration of the different paths identified and the implications each holds.
8. *Ethical reasoning* involves the recognition and resolution of ethical dilemmas which impinge upon the patient's ability to make decisions concerning their health and upon the conduct of treatment and its desired goals.

The reasoning and judgments made within these different reasoning strategies span a continuum from biomedically focused diagnostic reasoning to psychosocially focused 'narrative' reasoning. The diagnostic reasoning focus and the associated procedural management of physical impairments are aligned more with the experimental quantitative research paradigm with its underlying assumptions that reality, truth and/or knowledge are best understood in an objective, measurable, generalizable and predictable framework (Edwards et al. 2004a, Jones et al. 2008). In contrast patients' pain and disability experiences (i.e. their perspectives) are less amenable to objective measurement against normative standards. As such narrative reasoning is more aligned with the interpretive qualitative research paradigm with its underlying assumptions that truth, reality and/or knowledge are context dependent, socially constructed with multiple realities. The 'normality' versus 'abnormality' language of diagnostic reasoning is too absolute and therefore less appropriate to understanding patient's pain and disability experiences through narrative reasoning (Mattingly 1991, Stewart et al. 2011) and to understanding the effects patients thoughts and feelings can have on biological phenomena such as movement (Edwards et al. 2006).

When examining and treating a patient the therapist's thinking and actions should incorporate a combination of both diagnostic and narrative oriented assessments, interventions (e.g. procedural and educative) and re-assessments. Edwards (Edwards 2000, Edwards et al. 2004a, Edwards & Jones 2007b) demonstrated that these occur dialectically, meaning the therapist will move back and forth in attending (assessing and responding) to these different dimensions of the patient's presentation as dictated by the immediate circumstances. For example, the therapist may be performing a procedure to a physical impairment that elicits a patient response relevant to understanding their perspective, necessitating a fluidity of reasoning and action that explores the patient meaning and possibly even its relationship to the procedure being performed. That is, diagnostic and narrative reasoning are not carried out separately, rather they are intertwined with the key being the therapist's knowledge and ability to listen for and question patient perspectives both in a structured manner and as opportunities arise. While physical/biomedical and psychosocial factors represent different dimensions of a patient's presentation, in reality they are closely related such that each can influence the other (Borrell-Carrió et al. 2004, Duncan 2000, Engel 1978, Leventhal 1993, Pincus 2004). Further, it is not possible to fully understand a patient's pain and disability experience without a comprehensive physical examination that reveals the extent of physical impairment and disability they have to cope with. Similarly, understanding patient's perspectives provides the therapist with valuable insight that will assist their interpretation of movement and pain responses that may not fit typical patterns of pathology and nociception.

Hypothesis categories

While the clinical reasoning strategies provide a framework to assist students and practising therapists recognize the different focus of thinking required, it is also helpful to recognize the different types of clinical decisions required in the application of these different reasoning strategies. It is not necessary or even appropriate to stipulate a definitive list of decisions all physiotherapists in all areas of physiotherapy practice must consider, as this would only stifle the independent and creative thinking important to the evolution of our profession. However, a minimum list of categories of decisions that can/should be considered is helpful to those learning clinical reasoning as it provides them with initial guidance to understand the purpose of their questions and physical assessments, encourages holistic reasoning and breadth of thought, and creates a framework in which to organize their clinical knowledge as it relates to decisions that must be made (i.e. diagnosing, understanding patients' perspectives, determining therapeutic interventions, establishing rapport/therapeutic alliance, collaborating, teaching, prognosis and managing ethical dilemmas). Any group (profession, area of practice, physiotherapy educators, and physiotherapy departments/practices) can critically reflect on the categories of decisions important for optimal biopsychosocial practice and patient care. What follows is a list of 'hypothesis categories' initially proposed by Jones (1987) that has continued to evolve through professional discussion to this current format (see Box 2.2). Some evidence is available to support these categories by demonstrating that physiotherapists generate and test diagnostic and management hypotheses throughout their encounters with patients (Doody & McAteer 2002, Rivett & Higgs 1997). Anecdotal evidence from experienced physiotherapists and clinical educators also has supported the relevance and use of these particular hypothesis categories across all areas of physiotherapy practice with some variation in emphasis between therapists working in neurological, paediatric, cardiopulmonary care settings compared to outpatient musculoskeletal and sports physiotherapy. Nevertheless, these particular hypothesis categories are not being recommended for uncritical use by all therapists and whatever categories of decisions are adopted should continually be reviewed to ensure

Box 2.2

Hypothesis categories

- Activity capability/restriction
- Participation capability/restriction
- Patient's perspectives on their experience
- Pathobiological mechanisms
- Physical impairments and associated body structures/tissue sources of symptoms
- Contributing factors to the development and maintenance of the problem
- Precautions and contraindications to physical examination and treatment
- Management/treatment selection
- Prognosis

From Jones and Rivett 2004, Jones et al. 2008.

they reflect contemporary health care and physiotherapy practice.

Activity capability/restriction

Patients' activity capabilities and restrictions directly relate to the ICF framework of health and disability presented in Figure 2.1 and refer to the patient's functional abilities and restrictions (e.g. walking, lifting, sitting, etc.) that are volunteered and for which they are further screened. To gain a complete picture it is important the therapist identifies those activities the patient is capable of alongside those that are restricted.

Participation capability/restriction

Patients' participation capabilities and restrictions refer to the patient's abilities and restrictions to participate in life situations (e.g. work, recreation/sport, family, etc.). Again, determining participation capabilities, including modified participation (e.g. modified work duties) is important as this will contribute to other decisions such as prognosis and management. It is particularly important to pay attention to the proportionality of activity and participation restrictions and the physical pathology/impairments identified through examination. When activity and participation restrictions are out of proportion to identified pathology and physical impairments then it is likely the patient's perspectives on their experience (i.e. psychosocial

factors) will be negatively contributing to their disability.

Patient perspectives on their experience

Patient perspectives on their experience relates to the patient's psychosocial status which the therapist tries to understand through their narrative reasoning (as discussed earlier in this chapter under 'The patient's thinking'). It incorporates such things as the patient's understanding of their problem (including attributions about the cause and beliefs about pain), their goals and expectations for management, the stressors in their life and any relationship these have with their clinical presentation, as well as the effects the problem and any stressors appear to have on their thoughts, feelings, motivations, their coping and self-efficacy.

Pathobiological mechanisms

The pathobiological mechanisms category incorporates hypotheses about pathology or tissue mechanisms and hypotheses about pain mechanisms. While neither of these can be validated on the basis of a clinical examination alone, biomedical knowledge of pathology and pain combined with clinical and research supported knowledge of typical clinical patterns enables therapists to hypothesize with reasonable confidence about the likely pathology and dominant pain mechanism, both of which have implications to other categories of decisions including precautions/contraindications, management and prognosis.

Pathology within the neuromusculoskeletal system can be considered at both the process and structure levels. For example, in some presentations the process (e.g. inflammatory, degenerative, ischaemic, infection, etc.) or syndrome (e.g. stenosis, impingement, instability) underpinning a person's pain and disability can be identified even when the exact structures or tissues cannot be confirmed. In other presentations the pathology can be confirmed through a combination of clinical and medical investigations (e.g. spondylolisthesis, muscle tears/tendinopathy, disc disease, etc.). Since pathology can be asymptomatic and clinical presentations within a symptomatic pathology will vary according to the extent of pathology and influence of both physical and psychological factors, skilled clinical reasoning necessitates that the therapist avoid simply administering prescribed pathology focused treatments. Rather, therapists must consider the safety and management implications of a hypothesized pathology and then strike a balance between treating the associated physical impairments and unhelpful patient perspectives while also utilizing research evidence and theory supporting pathology directed treatments (e.g. tendinopathy – Cook & Purdam 2009; intervertebral disc – Adams et al. 2010, exercise for tissue repair – Khan & Scott 2009; Van Wingerden 1995, etc.).

Pain mechanisms refer to the different input, processing and output mechanisms underlying the patients' activity/participation restrictions, unhelpful perspectives and physical impairments. These are explained more comprehensively elsewhere (e.g. Butler 2000, Fields et al. 2006, Gifford 1998a, 1998b, 1998c, Gifford et al. 2006, Meyer et al. 2006) but briefly the input mechanisms include the sensory and circulatory systems that inform the brain about the internal and external environment. Two input pain mechanisms relevant to physiotherapists are nociceptive mechanisms and peripheral neuropathic mechanisms (Butler 2000, Galea 2002, Gifford 1998a, Gifford 1998d, Meyer et al. 2006, Wright 2002). Technically all pain perception is an output from our central nervous system as nociceptive activity following a noxious stimuli will always be subjected to central modulation and it is this modulation that ultimately determines whether pain is perceived or not. However, clinically it is useful to recognize patterns of pain perception associated with nociceptive activity triggered by a peripheral stimulus such as tissue injury or overload. That is, nociceptive pain involving chemical and mechanical activation of nociceptors in somatic or visceral tissues such as joints, muscles, bone, meninges, peripheral nerve sheaths and the various viscera has a recognizable clinical pattern (Butler 2000, Smart et al. 2012a, Wolf 2011). While clinical patterns for different pain mechanisms are not fully validated, broadly nociceptive pain includes local symptoms plus or minus referral to areas of common segmental innervation (Bielefeldt & Gebhart 2006, Bogduk 1993, Schaible 2006, Smart et al. 2012a, Vicenzino et al. 2002) (chronic nociceptive pain may only present with referred symptoms), a predictable stimulus-response relationship with aggravating and easing factors (Butler 2000, Nijs, Van Houdenhove & Oostendorp 2010, Smart et al. 2012a), a history of either trauma or specific predisposing factors (e.g. overload, new activity, etc.), physical impairments that are proportional to the symptoms, activity and participation restrictions and a predictable response to treatment.

Peripheral neuropathic pain refers to symptoms with contributions from neural tissue outside the dorsal horn or cervicotrigeminal nucleus as occurs with spinal nerve root or peripheral nerve irritation/ compression. Peripheral neuropathic pain can be less clear in its presentation (Butler 2000, Devor 2006, Gifford 1998d). Common features include: the type of symptoms (e.g. numbness, pins and needles, weakness, burning, itching, etc.); quality of symptoms (severe, shooting if acute); area of symptoms (distribution according to nerve although nerve root pain is typically not in classic dermatomes while paraesthesias are more dermatomal; Smart et al. 2012b); symptoms often worse at night; symptoms aggravated by movements and positions that compress or stretch the involved nerve (Smart et al. 2012b) or by situations that elicit stress or anxiety (possibly reflecting a component of central sensitization); symptoms eased by movements and positions that unload the nerve; physical impairments in neural conduction (i.e. positive neurological findings), neural mechansensitivity (i.e. positive neurodynamic and neural palpation findings) and in interfacing tissues that can compress or irritate neural tissue (e.g. structures forming borders of intervertebral foramina, adjacent muscles and fascia).

Central processing refers to the neural modulation of both input and output that occurs throughout the central nervous system/neuromatrix (e.g. Fields et al. 2006, Gatchel et al. 2007, Melzack 2005, Moseley 2003, Nijs et al. 2010, Wolf 2011) in response to internal and external sensory inputs including physical (e.g. overloaded tissues), cognitive and emotional input (e.g. thoughts, fears, anxiety, frustrations, self-efficacy, etc.). While the central nervous system is always processing input and generating output, maladaptive central processing is known to underpin some pain states causing increased responsiveness to a range of stimuli including emotional stressors, mechanical pressure, chemical substances, light, sound, cold and heat (Nijs et al. 2010). The increased sensitivity (or decreased load tolerance) can co-exist with somatic or visceral noxious stimulus nociception but can also be evoked or maintained without a peripheral noxious stimulus. Symptom provocation therefore occurs out of proportion to existing pathology and can even exist when overt pathology no longer exists. Wolf (2011) reports evidence that central sensitization has been demonstrated in a wide range of conditions commonly treated by physiotherapists including rheumatoid arthritis, osteoarthritis, temporomandibular disorders, fibromyalgia, chronic musculoskeletal disorders, headache, neuropathic pain, complex regional pain syndrome, post-surgical pain and visceral pain hypersensitivity syndromes. With central sensitization normally non-noxious stimuli and loads become provocative often creating false positive findings in the physical examination (i.e. physical testing is provocative despite the lack of overt pathology) leading to ineffective management when pain mechanisms are not understood (Butler 2000, Gifford 1998c).

Currently diagnostic criteria and biomarkers for central sensitization are lacking (Wolf 2011). However, contemporary thinking extrapolated from a broad range of research supports the observation that maladaptive central symptoms no longer follow the predictable pattern of pain with nociceptive and peripheral neuropathic contributions (Butler 2000, Nijs et al. 2010, Smart et al. 2012c, Wolf 2011). Instead, activity and participation restrictions and symptoms are typically out of proportion to the physical impairments and the symptom behaviour is less predictable with spontaneous pains, latent pains, inconsistent stimulus-response relationships to aggravating and easing factors and more pronounced associations with psychosocial stressors. Pain may be disproportionate to the nature and extent of injury or pathology with strong association to psychosocial factors and diffuse, non-anatomical areas of pain or tenderness to palpation (Smart et al. 2012c). Traditional nociceptively oriented therapies may produce short-term gains but are themselves ineffective in making lasting changes.

Melzack (2005) describes the neuroscience of patients' thoughts, feelings and pain as neurosignatures of a widely distributed neural network involving diverse areas of the brain he calls the 'body-self neuromatrix'. Since these neurosignatures are related in part to our own subjective experiences or perceptions (e.g. pain and what it means, interpretation of what others' think, etc.) they are like our own 'virtual reality' of our experienced existence (Revonsuo 1995, 2006). That is our conscious experience is a construction of our brain. In this sense the chronic pain patient with significant central sensitization is trapped in their own representations/ neurosignatures of their internal and external world.

This is what cognitive-behavioural therapy attempts to change by firstly identifying unhelpful perspectives and then by assisting the patient to construct more adaptive perspectives, feelings and behaviours through a combination of providing convincing alternative understandings and through behavioural strategies that facilitate controlled reactivation (e.g. graded exposure, pacing, relaxation, flare-up management; e.g. Donaghy et al. 2008, Gatchel et al. 2007, Harding & Williams 1995, Keefe et al. 2006, Linton & Nordin 2006, Main et al. 2008, Muncey 2002, Strong & Unruh 2002, Turk & Flor 2006). There is now a convincing body of literature supporting the efficacy of neuroscience based pain education and cognitive-behavioural interventions for chronic low back pain patients and for preventing progression from acute to chronic pain. For example, Moseley (2004) demonstrated that individualized pain education to moderately disabled chronic low back pain patients successfully changed patients' pain cognitions (i.e. understanding) and physical performance (e.g. straight leg raise and forward bending). Vlaeyen et al. (2002) demonstrated an exposure in vivo (individually tailored practice tasks developed on the basis of graded hierarchy of fear-eliciting situations) intervention resulted in reductions in chronic low back pain patients' pain-related fear, pain catastrophizing, pain disability, pain vigilance while increasing their physical activity levels. Linton and Nordin (2006) reported on a 5-year follow-up of a randomized clinical trial investigating the efficacy of a cognitive-behavioural intervention for prevention of chronic back pain. The effects of six (2-hour) cognitive-behavioural sessions promoting patients' individualized problem solving, risk analysis, activity scheduling and other coping strategies were compared with an information comparison group who received standardized pamphlets emphasizing self-help, remaining active and ergonomic, 'back school' based information. The cognitive-behavioural group improvements demonstrated at an initial 1-year follow-up (Linton & Andersson 2000) were maintained at this 5-year follow-up including significantly less pain, greater activity levels, better quality of life, better general health and significantly fewer days off work due to illness.

Lastly the output mechanisms refer to the effects of central nervous system/neuromatrix modulation that produce, for example, our cognitions, emotions, learning, sleep and language as well as our motor, autonomic, endocrine and immune system functions, all of which can be adversely affected in some acute, and particularly chronic, pain conditions. In fact pain itself is an output in that it is a perception of our brain in response to the internal and external influences discussed above. While it is beyond the scope of this chapter to cover the neurophysiology and clinical presentations of these different systems, the reader is referred to a variety of resources that provide clinically relevant overviews with reference to the underlying basic science research (Butler 2000, Gifford 1998c, Jänig & Levine 2006, Mackinnon 1999, Martin 1997, Sapolsky 1998).

At present, contemporary thinking holds that if a patient presents with a 'normal' adaptive pain mechanism, wherein symptoms are the result of pathology or abnormal load to specific structures/ tissues, it is appropriate to identify and treat relevant physical impairments while also addressing physical, environmental and psychosocial contributing factors. However, when 'abnormal' maladaptive central pain mechanisms are hypothesized to be present, management requires attention to stressors (physical and non-physical) thought to be sensitizing the nervous system and use of cognitive-behavioural strategies to promote increased activities, participation and general fitness. Making these judgments is not simple as often clinical features of several pain mechanisms will be present along with clear physical impairments that may or may not prove relevant. This is where skilled clinical reasoning to recognize the overlapping patterns combined with short-term treatments and re-assessments to identified relevant physical impairments will assist in establishing how much an apparent central sensitization is being driven by the symptomatic physical impairments or other co-existing cognitions, emotions and life stressors. In some cases physical impairments and disability will underpin the stress, frustrations, etc. that a patient is experiencing with resolution of the pain and the negative psyche following thorough assessment and skilled physical and environmental management. Here it is important to recognize that symptomatic physical pathology/impairment is also a source of stress that can affect neuromodulation and the neuromatrix (Melzack 2001) in order to avoid the erroneous assumption that all stress is necessary psychosocial in origin, requiring hands off therapy. In other cases sensitization is driven by both physical and cognitive/affective factors necessitating management of both. In contrast, extreme central sensitization driven primarily by psychosocial factors requires cognitive-behavioural management (Donaghy et al. 2008, Harding & Williams 1995,

Muncy 2002, Strong & Unruh 2002, Turk & Flor 2006) and is unlikely to be helped by tissue-based approaches.

Physical impairments and associated structures/ tissue sources

Clinical decisions identifying and judging the relevance of the patient's physical impairments combined with hypotheses regarding structures involved and potential sources of any symptoms provoked are based on findings obtained throughout the subjective and physical examination combined with re-assessments following targeted interventions to different impairments. The physical impairments are the specific regional neuromusculoskeletal abnormalities found through physical examination including impairments in posture, active and passive movement, soft tissue, neurodynamics and motor control/strength/etc. Physical impairments may be symptomatic and directly associated with the source of the patient's symptoms or asymptomatic but still contributing by altering stress/load elsewhere causing other structures to be symptomatic. Asymptomatic physical impairments must be analysed with regard to the structures responsible (e.g. restricted passive hip extension due to hip joint hypomobility, hip flexor tightness/tone or both) and whether the impairment is truly contributing to other structures being symptomatic. Again, this requires specific treatments, re-assessments and skilled reasoning to determine. Symptomatic physical impairments also have to be analysed as to the structures (and pathology) implicated and for their particular clinical presentation with respect to pain (e.g. minor to severe, non-irritable to irritable), mobility (e.g. stiff to hypermobile), dynamic control (e.g. weakness/ inadequate stabilization to over-activity), and the relationship of pain provocation to passive movement (i.e. Maitland's passive movement diagram), all of which represent non-propositional craft knowledge that assists selection and progression of treatment. While clinical examination generally cannot confirm the actual source of a patient's symptoms, clues from the area and behaviour of symptoms, history, physical examination and treatments/ re-assessments, combined with knowledge of common clinical patterns, will enable the therapist to hypothesize with confidence the likely structures at fault and possibly their pathology.

Table 2.2 Body chart depicting an example of symptom location and the potential sources that should be considered for that symptom area

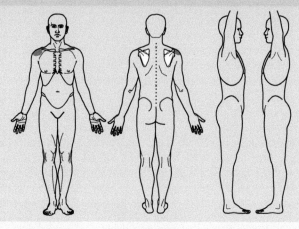

Potential local somatic sources	Potential local neural sources	Potential sources of somatic referral	Potential nerve root sources	Potential sources of visceral referral
Glenohumeral periarticular (rotator interval structures, capsule and ligaments) Glenohumeral intrarticular (glenoid labrum, biceps attachment, joint surface) Subacromial space (rotator cuff, biceps, bursa, coraco-acromial ligament, acromion) Acromioclavicular joint	Axillary nerve Suprascapular nerve	Any C5/6 motion segment structures (muscle, posterior intervertebral joint) Any somatic structure sharing the C5-6 innervation	C3-7 Nerve roots	Visceral structures with common innervation to shoulder (e.g. phrenic nerve C3-5 innervates diaphragm, pericardium, gallbladder, pancreas) Visceral structures capable of irritating diaphragm (heart, spleen (L), kidneys, pancreas, gall bladder (R), liver (R)

As an example of generating hypotheses regarding possible sources of the patient's symptoms based on the area of symptoms, consider the body chart in Table 2.2 depicting a common area of shoulder pain and the potential sources of that pain that should be considered.

Considering potential structures involved within the suggested columns assist a though generation of hypotheses that can then be tested with further questioning through the behaviour of symptoms (aggravating and easing factors), history, medical screening and physical examination–treatment–re-assessment. As alluded to earlier, hypotheses about specific sources of the patient's symptoms must be made with consideration of the dominant pain mechanisms hypothesized. Symptomatic local tissue impairment is likely an accurate reflection of structures involved in nociceptive dominant patterns where maladaptive central processing can create false positives causing 'healthy' structures/tissues to be symptomatic.

Contributing factors

Hypotheses regarding potential contributing factors represent the predisposing or associated factors involved in the development or maintenance of the patient's problem. These include environmental, psychosocial, behavioural, physical/biomechanical and hereditary factors.

The potential physical contributing factors that can create excessive strain causing another structure to be symptomatic are quite varied. Examples here include hip extension stiffness causing increased lumbar spine strain during walking and weakness of the scapular upward rotators causing increase subacromial strain during shoulder elevation. Just as physical impairments commonly exist without becoming symptomatic (i.e. sources of pain), physical impairments can also cause increased strain without those tissues becoming symptomatic. While these impairments still represent risk factors for musculoskeletal symptoms later (analogous to dietary risk factors for heart disease), establishing their relevance in a patient's current pain presentation requires systematic intervention to alter the impairment and reassessment of the effect. Often this can be established relatively quickly with procedures that immediately address the impairment (e.g. manual assistance or taping of the scapula) or brief trial treatments to assess their benefit.

Even with the same pathology different patients can have different physical, environmental and psychosocial contributing factors necessitating quite different management. For example, three patients can present with similar subacromial bursitis pathology causing subacromial pain but quite different predisposing contributing factors necessitating quite different management. Patient 1, for example, may present with a tight posterior glenohumeral joint capsule causing increased anterosuperior humeral head translation during overhead activities that result in bursal irritation. Patient 2 has good posterior capsule mobility, as reflected in their good range of humeral internal rotation and horizontal flexion, but this patient has poor control/strength of their scapular force couples which are required to upwardly rotate the scapula, resulting in inadequate rotation, a narrowed subacromial outlet during overhead activities and bursal irritation. Patient 3 also has a motor control/strength problem but not of the scapula, instead the rotator cuff force couples responsible for maintaining humeral head depression during elevation are ineffective resulting in increased superior translation and, again, bursal irritation. Knowledge of common contributing factors to different clinical problems combined with skilled reasoning to establish their relevance is essential. While treatment directed to the hypothesized source of the patient's symptoms is often effective in relieving symptoms, contributing factors must be addressed in order to minimize reoccurrence.

The scenario above of one pathology (subacromial bursitis) having three different clinical presentations requiring three different approaches to management is one example of the philosophical principle contained within the 'Brick wall' concept put forward by Maitland (Maitland 1986; also see Chapter 1). While research evidence provides some guidance to management of different pathologies/problems, variation in clinical presentations necessitates that the therapist's management decisions are based on consideration of the patient's unique clinical presentation combined with contemporary knowledge from the current body of research evidence.

Precautions and contraindications to physical examination and treatment

Patient safety is paramount and there are a range of decisions within this hypothesis category that therapists must consider including: whether a physical examination should be carried out at all (versus immediate referral for further medical consultation/investigation) and if so the extent of examination that can be safely performed that will minimize the risk of aggravating the patient's symptoms; whether specific safety tests are indicated (e.g. vertebrabasilar insufficiency testing, neurological, blood pressure/heart rate, instability tests); whether any treatment should be undertaken (versus referral for further consultation/investigation); and the appropriate dose/strength of any physical interventions planned. A number of factors will contribute to determining the extent of physical examination and treatment that is safe to perform, including the following:

- Dominant pain mechanism (peripheral neuropathic and maladaptive central processing typically require more caution)
- Patient's perspectives (anxious, fearful, angry patients, particularly with negative past medical/physiotherapy experiences require more caution)
- Severity and irritability of symptoms (Maitland 1986)
- Nature of the pathology (e.g. rheumatoid arthritis or osteoporosis require caution due to weakened tissues)
- Progression of the presentation (e.g. worsening problems require more caution)
- Presence of other medical conditions that may masquerade as a musculoskeletal problem or co-exist and require consideration and monitoring so that musculoskeletal interventions do not compromise the patient's other health

problems (e.g. cardiac and respiratory conditions).

Medical screening for other health problems requires knowledge of the body systems and common features of medical conditions, particularly those that overlap with neuromusculoskeletal problems. This form of screening is not for the purpose of assigning a medical diagnosis; rather medical screening by physiotherapists is for the purpose of identifying patients who may have medical conditions that require further investigation and medical consultation. It is particularly important to first contact practitioners who see patients that have not previously been evaluated by a medical practitioner but is it also important to physiotherapists practising under referral as non-musculoskeletal conditions may have been missed or developed since the patient last saw their doctor. Physiotherapists should be familiar with recognized 'red flags' which are signs and symptoms that may indicate the presence of more serious pathology and systemic or viscerogenic pathology/disease which should elicit consideration of referral for further consultation/investigation. There are different lists of 'red flags' available in the literature but two excellent resources written for physiotherapists are Boissonnault (2011) and Goodman and Snyder (2013). As an example of important medical screening to guide clinical reasoning regarding precautions and contraindications to physical examination and treatment, Goodman and Snyder (2013) provide the lists of 'Guidelines for medical referral' and 'Precautions and contraindications to therapy':

Readers are referred to Goodman and Snyder (2013) for additional lists of 'red flags' and 'Guidelines for immediate medical attention'.

Physiotherapists need to develop a through yet efficient system of medical screening. The texts by Boissonnault (2011) and Goodman and Snyder (2013) provide a comprehensive Review of Systems that assist therapists to recognize combinations of symptoms and signs that may reflect non-musculoskeletal conditions requiring further medical consultation. Both texts also provide examples of information to include in a medical screening questionnaire which is an excellent way to thoroughly and efficiently screen a patient's medical health. Having completed the questionnaire the physiotherapist must then review the patient's responses and clarify conditions or symptoms/signs ticked to establish their history, medical management and relationship with the patient's current problem.

Management and treatment

Management in this context refers to the overall health management of the patient, including consultation and referral to other health professionals, health promotion interventions (e.g. fitness assessment and management) and patient advocacy as required (e.g. with insurers or employers). Treatment refers to the specific therapeutic interventions (physical and educational) carried out during an appointment and the underlying reasoning required to determine which impairments to address, which to address first, the strategy/procedure and dosage to use, the outcome measures to reassess and the self-management appropriate for optimizing change (in understanding, impairment, activity and participation).

Most important to skilled reasoning is that there are no recipes! Health care in general and physiotherapy care in particular are not an exact science. While clinical trials and theory extrapolated from basic science provide helpful guides to management for different problems, these should not be taken as prescriptions. Instead, therapists must judge how their patient matches the population in the research reported and then tailor their management to the individual patient's unique lifestyle, goals, activity and participation restrictions, perspectives, pathobiological mechanisms and physical impairments. Since research supported management efficacy is still lacking for most clinical problems, skilled reasoning is the therapist's best tool to minimize the risk of mismanagement and over servicing.

The bio-psychosocial model highlights the need for management to be holistic (i.e. addressing physical, environmental, psychosocial as required) with systematic and thorough re-assessments to determine inter-relationships between different physical impairments (e.g. presence of a neurodynamic impairment secondary to a soft tissue interface impairment) and between physical impairments and cognitive/affective factors (e.g. education to improve understanding leading to a decrease in patient fear and concurrent improvement in movement impairments). Management of contributing factors is essential to minimize risk of reoccurrence and patient understanding and active involvement is critical to promoting self-efficacy, self-management and long-term success.

As discussed earlier, much of the reasoning and practice knowledge associated with selection, delivery and progression of treatment falls within the area of professional craft knowledge. Since such knowledge typically lacks direct research validation therapists must be diligent in their personal reflection and critique to minimize the trap of falling into habits of practice. As discussed later, a good strategy to avoid this is to subject your reasoning and practice to critical appraisal from your peers through patient reviews and case study discussions.

Prognosis

Prognosis refers to the therapist's judgment regarding their ability to help their patient and an estimate of how long this will take. Broadly a patient's prognosis is determined by the nature and extent of patient's problem(s) and their ability and willingness to make the necessary changes (e.g. lifestyle, psychosocial contributing factors, physical contributing factors) to facilitate recovery or improved quality of life within a permanent disability. Clues will be available throughout the subjective and physical examination and the ongoing management including the:

- Patient's perspectives and expectations
- Extent of activity/participation restrictions
- Nature of problem (e.g. systemic disorder such as rheumatoid arthritis versus local ligamentous such as ankle sprain)
- Extent of 'pathology' and physical impairments
- Social, occupational and economic status
- Dominant pain mechanisms present
- Stage of tissue healing
- Irritability of the disorder

- Length of history and progression of disorder
- Patient's general health, age and pre-existing disorders.

While prognostic decisions also are not an exact science (Jeffreys 1991) it is helpful to consider a patient's prognosis by reflecting on the positives and negatives from the list above.

The decisions required in clinical practice will determine the information sought (e.g. safety information considered important necessitates safety oriented questions and physical tests). However, the hypothesis category framework is not intended to direct the order in which information is obtained or the precise inquiries and physical tests utilized to obtain that information. For example, musculoskeletal physiotherapists will typically follow a systematic subjective and physical examination as depicted in Table 2.3.

Clinical reasoning within the hypothesis category framework involves consideration of the different categories of decisions as information unfolds. While it is not possible or desirable to stipulate what hypothesis categories a therapist should be considering at any given point in time (e.g. it is not realistic or cognitively efficient to consider every hypothesis category after every new piece of information is obtained), equally the therapist should not simply be obtaining information without thinking. Mostly during the examination the therapist will be trying to understand the patient and their problem(s) in order to plan their management including judging how much physical examination can be safely performed and which physical examination procedures are most important to prioritize at the first appointment. For this focus the therapist would need to

Table 2.3 Typical components of the subjective and physical examinations used by musculoskeletal physiotherapists

Subjective examination	Physical examination
1. Personal profile (e.g. work, activity level, sport, recreation, living/social circumstances)	1. Functional assessment
	2. Posture
	3. Active movements
2. Patient's understanding/beliefs, feelings, coping, expectations and goals	4. Passive physiological and passive accessory movements
3. Area and description of symptoms/disability	5. Neurodynamics, neurological
4. Behaviour of symptoms/disability	6. Soft tissue assessment
5. Questions to identify precautions and contraindications to physical examination and treatment	7. Muscle length
	8. Motor awareness, control and proprioception
	9. Muscle strength, endurance, etc.
6. History and past history	10. Vascular assessment
	11. Specific safety tests as required (e.g. cardiorespiratory, VBI, instability, etc.)

consider the patient's activity and participation capabilities and restrictions, the patient's perspectives, the pathobiological mechanisms, the structures/sources and contributing factors implicated from the subjective examination (hence requiring priority in examination), the precautions to physical examination and treatment, physical impairments found on physical testing and the structures/sources implicated, and management clues (emanating from both the subjective and physical examination). It is the therapist's ability to think on their feet through the examination and ongoing management that leads to their qualification of patient responses and the variations in examination routines. That is, all tests are not performed on every patient.

Interpreting information across different hypothesis categories

Patient information will inform several hypothesis categories at the same time. Just as the therapist may be asking a pathology/impairment oriented question but receive a patient answer that sheds light on their perspectives (i.e. psychosocial status), a question directed at understanding their activity capability and restrictions will often provide clues to other hypothesis categories at the same time. Consider for example a 72-year-old patient's response to a question regarding what aggravates their back and bilateral leg pains?

> Walking. I'm afraid to even try anymore. Even short 5–10 minute walks make the back and legs worse and then I have to sit down to ease it off. Sitting is good but I can't sit all day! I can't even help out around the house anymore or get over to see the grandchildren. I'm really worried it might be something serious.

This one answer provides the following hypothesis categories information:

- Activity restriction: walking
- Activity capability: sitting
- Participation restrictions: helping around house and seeing grandchildren
- Patient perspectives: afraid to try walking, worried it may be serious
- Pathobiological: clues to nociceptive, neuropathic, vascular claudication, stenosis (neuropathic claudication)

- Physical impairments/sources: back and leg symptoms related; lumbar joints and nerve roots implicated
- Contributing factors: age
- Precautions: age, easily aggravated, bilateral leg pain, patient's fears/worry
- Prognosis: (−) age, disability, extent of symptoms, neuropathic, perspectives; (+) easing factor.

In the end the therapist gains clues to the different hypothesis categories throughout the whole examination and ongoing management that must be interpreted, weighed for significance and analyzed with other supporting and negating information. The knowledge that underpins the different clinical decisions comes from a broad range of both propositional and craft knowledge. Learning theory suggests that for knowledge to be clinically accessible it needs to be acquired within the conditions and constraints for which it will be used (Glaser 1984, Greeno 1998, Lave & Wenger 1991). This is typically achieved in physiotherapy education through the use of experiential/problem based teaching strategies. With the same aim, the hypothesis categories provide a bio-psychosocially oriented organizing framework to link academic knowledge to the clinical reasoning through the patient examination–treatment–re-assessment process facilitating the learning of clinical patterns.

Key message

Understanding the patient's problem and their pain or disability experience and making the necessary decisions regarding management requires different foci of thinking, or 'Reasoning Strategies'. Where diagnostic reasoning and the associated procedural management of physical impairments can be linked with the experimental quantitative research paradigm that emphasizes objective measurement against normative standards, narrative reasoning is more aligned with interpretive qualitative research where objective independent measurement of normality is less appropriate requiring therapists validate their interpretations of patients' perspectives with the patient themselves. Hypothesis categories represent different types of clinical decisions therapists consider throughout the patient examination and ongoing management. They also provide a useful bio-psychosocially oriented framework for organizing clinically relevant information.

Pattern recognition

Pattern recognition is characteristic of all mature thought (Nickerson et al. 1985). Experts across a wide range of professions have been shown to possess a large repertoire of profession specific patterns that enable them to more quickly recognize familiar problems and associated solutions (Chi et al. 1988, Higgs & Jones 2008, Jensen et al. 2007, Schön 1983). Pattern recognition relates to memory storage where knowledge has been shown to be stored in chunks or patterns that facilitate more efficient communication and thinking (Anderson 1990, Ericsson & Smith 1991, Hayes & Adams 2000, Newell & Simon 1972, Rumelhart & Ortony 1977). These patterns form categories or prototypes of frequently experienced situations (e.g. symptoms, signs, predisposing factors) that individuals use to recognize and interpret other situations, a process referred to in the medical literature as 'forward reasoning' (Elstein & Schwarz 2002, Patel & Groen 1986, Boshuizen & Schmidt 2008, Higgs & Jones 2008). Clinical patterns can be either generic prototypes, as found in textbooks, or they may be memories of particular patient presentations (Brooks et al. 1991, Schmidt et al. 1990) where the clinical pattern becomes meaningful through its instantiation with a real patient (Boshuizen & Schmidt 2008).

The information contained in a clinical pattern is quite varied. Boshuizen and Schmidt (2008) review the research on the development of expertise in medicine and suggest that medical clinical patterns, called 'illness scripts' (originally proposed by Feltovich & Barrows, 1984), typically include the 'enabling conditions', that is the conditions or constraints under which a disease occurs (e.g. personal, social, medical, hereditary, environmental); the 'fault', that is the pathophysiological process taking place; and the 'consequences of the fault', that is the signs and symptoms. Illness scripts are consistent with the clinical patterns physiotherapists learn and look for within their diagnostic reasoning, although the pathophysiological process will not always be confirmed.

Clinical patterns also exist when interpreting patients' perspectives through narrative reasoning and should incorporate at a deeper level: not simply the patient's perspective but also the basis of the perspective and its relationship with the behaviour and history of their symptoms/disability. Similarly clinical patterns exist within the hypothesis categories of precautions/contraindications (i.e. recognizing typical clinical features that signal the need for caution ± referral) and prognosis (i.e. recognizing typical features that support a positive or negative outcome and whether change is likely to be quick or slow).

Forward reasoning or pattern recognition enables efficiency in examination with familiar presentations. Pattern recognition is required to generate hypotheses while hypothesis testing (i.e. backward reasoning) provides the means by which those patterns are refined, proved reliable and new patterns such as recognition of common features in a particular subgroup of patients are learned (Barrows & Feltovich 1987). Where experts are able to function largely via pattern recognition with familiar problems, novices who lack sufficient knowledge and experience to recognize clinical patterns will rely on the slower hypothesis testing approach to work through a problem. However, when confronted with a complex, unfamiliar problem, the expert, like the novice, will rely more on the hypothesis-oriented method of clinical reasoning (Barrows & Feltovich 1987, Patel & Groen 1991).

The advantage of pattern recognition is its efficiency and ability to reduce cognitive load. The disadvantage of pattern recognition is the risk of missing or misinterpreting important features or differential diagnoses. If clinical patterns become the focus of your attention where you examine patients only to determine which pattern their problem fits into, then the accuracy of your reasoning will depend on whether their presentation fits a clinical pattern you know. That is, when patterns become the focus of your attention it can be difficult to see outside the

> ### Key message
>
> Experts in all professions, including physiotherapy, acquire a large repertoire of profession-specific patterns that enable them to quickly recognize problems and their solutions (e.g. common clinical presentations and the appropriate management). Clinical patterns exist and can be learned within all hypothesis categories. However, as useful as clinical patterns are to efficient clinical practice, they are also one of the greatest sources of errors in reasoning as even experienced therapists can fall into habits of practice where they over focus on their favourite clinical patterns causing them to miss or misinterpret important information to competing hypotheses.

patterns you know resulting in over-emphasis on those features that most closely match a pattern you recognize. This will be discussed further later under common errors in clinical reasoning.

Complexity of clinical reasoning

The similarity of the clinical reasoning process to common logic where both involve information collection, perception/interpretation/analysis, hypothesis generation/modification makes it easy to understand. However, in reality clinical reasoning is complex, challenging to execute and subject to error. The complexity of clinical reasoning relates to a number of factors including: the complexity of many patients' problems, particularly when the physical (biomedical) is considered alongside the environmental and personal (psychosocial) factors; the subjective nature of much of the information that must be interpreted (e.g. patient reports, therapist observations and feel); the lack of absolute or research validated interpretations for much of the patient information obtained (i.e. patient reports and therapists' physical tests used); and the necessity for therapists to reason across different categories of clinical judgments at the same time, while obtaining information, qualifying responses and working through a systematic examination–treatment–re-assessment process that is tailored to the patient's unique presentation.

Christensen reviews the literature of complexity theory as it relates to health care and physiotherapy and relates this to the complexity inherent in many patient presentations (Christensen 2009, Christensen et al. 2008a). She utilizes a model of organizational management approaches to problem solving originally proposed by Stacey (1996) and adapted by Zimmerman et al. (2001, p. 141) to illustrate the continuum of patient presentations from the simple to the complex (see Fig. 2.3). Clinical decisions made in conditions of high certainty tend to be associated with more linear cause and effect relationships as opposed to decisions where cause and effect are less clear and consequently decisions less certain. Here, the greater the clinician's knowledge (research and experience-based) the greater their certainty. The agreement axis relates to the extent of consensus within a group, team or organization (e.g. physiotherapy and medical professions). Decisions made in conditions of high certainty and high

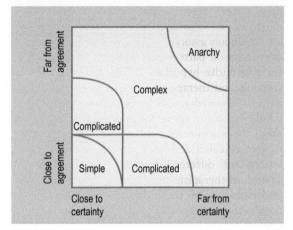

Figure 2.3 • Adaptation of Stacey agreement and certainty matrix, with kind permission of Brenda Zimmerman (Zimmerman et al. 2001, p. 141).

agreement are characterized as falling into the simple zone where the problem and its management are clear and supported by evidence. In contrast, decisions made in conditions of little certainty and high levels of disagreement fall within the zone of anarchy often leading to either poor decisions or avoidance of decisions all together. The largest zone between simple and anarchy is the zone of complexity where much of physiotherapy practice and reasoning occurs. Again this can be related to the complexity of clinical presentations combined with the lack of sufficient evidence and/or agreement regarding diagnosis (pathology and impairment) and management. Most patient problems are multifactorial, often with more than one source of pain or impairment and typically with their own unique mix of environmental, psychosocial, cultural and physical contributing factors requiring a mixture of management interventions. As such, while clinical reasoning is relatively easy to understand, skilled reasoning is difficult to do.

Errors of clinical reasoning

Errors in clinical reasoning are frequently linked to errors in cognition (Kempainen et al. 2003, Rivett & Jones 2004, Scott 2000). Examples of these include overemphasis on findings which support an existing hypothesis, misinterpretation of non-contributory information as confirming an existing hypothesis, rejection of findings which do not support a favoured hypothesis, and incorrect interpretation related to limitations in knowledge and inappropriately applied inductive and deductive logic. Errors such as these are commonly associated with habits of thinking and over-focus on pattern recognition resulting in bias for a favourite hypothesis. The challenge here for students and therapists is to learn and use clinical pattern knowledge while not relying solely on it. Clinical pattern knowledge, particularly in musculo-skeletal physiotherapy, is typically unproven due to lack of research and variability in clinical presentations for different problems and pathologies. Therefore therapists must obtain a comprehensive understanding of the patient's presentation that enables them to consider what 'diagnostic' pattern(s) (pathology and impairment based) are implicated so that any research supported management is considered while at the same time not limiting themselves to classification according to textbook patterns or treatment according to set protocols. While many musculoskeletal problems will fit into clear clinical patterns (e.g. muscle strains, ligament sprains) many problems also do not fit, either because there is more than one symptomatic pathology/impairment or simply because there are considerable variations in physical, environmental and personal (i.e. psycho-social) factors that contribute to patients' clinical presentations. Thorough examination and a systematic process of treatment and re-assessment will often enable therapists to gradually determine the key factors responsible for the patient's pain and disability eventually allowing identification of the most likely clinical pattern. However, even when a specific clinical syndrome cannot be established, as long as appropriate medical screening has been conducted for potential systemic or visceral problems, treatment of presenting symptoms and impairments with emphasis on restoring function will usually be effective.

Associated with over-focusing on clinical patterns is reaching a premature conclusion regarding the patient's presentation. Initial impressions will sometimes bias interpretations of other information. This error typically occurs when the therapist is biased by a dominant cue and does not adequately consider or rule out (through further questioning and physical assessment) alternative explanations/hypotheses. A good example here is of the patient who arrives with a medical diagnosis. While that is clearly important to consider, it does not obviate the need for thorough examination as the diagnosis may be wrong or there may be other problems not detected by the referring doctor. Even with a correct diagnosis (structures involved ± pathology) the therapist must still establish how that diagnosis manifests with respect to specific symptoms and impairments and the stage of the disorder (e.g. acute/inflammatory versus subacute/mechanical versus chronic). By thinking of these early impressions as 'working hypotheses', and ensuring competing diagnostic and narrative hypotheses are entertained, premature conclusions can be avoided.

While efficiency is important, many errors stem from a general lack of thoroughness in information obtained and hypotheses generated and tested. The use of 'screening questions' (related to other types of symptoms, other aggravating/easing factors, and medical screening for safety) will minimize the risk of missing relevant information. Thoroughness of the physical examination for musculoskeletal problems requires good knowledge of the potential sources (i.e. tissue or structure) of the patient's symptoms and knowledge of structures or mechanisms (e.g. motor control, biomechanics, ergonomics) that may be contributing directly or indirectly to increased load (i.e. strain) on the symptomatic area.

Errors in reasoning can also be precipitated by lack of skilled questioning, as discussed earlier. Here the most common example is making assumptions without explicitly clarifying the patient's meaning (e.g. patient's 'shoulder pain' actually occurring in the supraspinous fossa; back pain aggravated by walking down hills rather than just any walking; patient's fear of aggravating their pain being an adaptive concern causing avoidance of overdoing activities and not a more maladaptive total avoidance). This last example touches on an error within the narrative reasoning focus. Other common narrative reasoning related errors include the following:

- Therapist views biomedical and psychosocial as separate, assuming that their role as a physiotherapist is to manage only the biomedical, with the psychosocial exclusively the responsibility of psychologists and counsellors
- Therapist does not attempt to understand biomedical diagnosis in the context of patient's personal circumstances
- Therapist does not screen psychosocial factors or their psychosocial assessment is too superficial, leading to judgments based on insufficient assessment. Common examples here include:
  - patient does not volunteer personal problems so therapist assumes none exist

○ therapist relies on psychosocial screening questionnaires without giving the patient an opportunity to qualify their responses, including the basis of those responses

○ therapist does not explore effects of problem on patient's self, understanding/beliefs, symptoms, expectations and future prospects

○ patient alludes to stress at work/home but therapist does not clarify or establish history and relationship of stress to clinical presentation

○ therapist does not clarify if patient is coping with their problem or what coping strategies they use or have tried

○ therapist approaches narrative reasoning judgements in same way as diagnostic reasoning judgements, assuming patient perspectives can be understood/measured as maladaptive by a standard normative interpretation (such as range of movement).

Reasoning errors related to management are often the result of reasoning errors made through the examination (e.g. lack of thoroughness, not considering competing hypotheses, poor questioning and manual skills resulting in inaccurate information, etc.). Also common is inadequate re-assessment of appropriate management outcomes (e.g. pain, physical impairments, function, quality of life, disability measures) to determine the value of any intervention but also to establish the significance and relationship between different impairments. For example, systematic re-assessment of several impairments (active and passive movement, soft tissue, neurodynamics, motor control) following spinal mobilization for pain and stiffness may reveal improvement in neurodynamics and motor control supporting their relationship to the spinal stiffness. While most therapists recognize the importance of re-assessment of function and physical impairments, re-assessment of patient understanding following explanation/education is less appreciated and practiced.

Lastly a lack of self-awareness (i.e. metacognition) is a reasoning error that limits the therapist's ability to recognize other errors and limits their learning from reflections on their experiences.

Improving clinical reasoning: learning through clinical reasoning

Physiotherapists must be competent in the examination, reasoning and management of a wide range of patient problems, many of which are complex and multifactorial. In addition they must be capable of effectively managing unfamiliar, ambiguous presentations outside their current knowledge and skill base. So how can therapists and students improve their critical thinking and reasoning to minimize errors of reasoning and assist their management of the diverse variety of familiar to difficult and unfamiliar presentations they encounter? Christensen et al. (2008a, p. 102) review the 'capability' literature and offer the following definition of capability as it relates to clinical reasoning:

> Capability in clinical reasoning involves integration and effective application of thinking and learning skills to make sense of, learn collaboratively from and generate knowledge within familiar and unfamiliar clinical experiences.

Acquisition of clinical reasoning capability should be facilitated throughout the physiotherapy professional entry education. This does not always occur with some schools having no overt academic content covering clinical reasoning theory and/or no explicit framework or strategies for ensuring clinical educators facilitate application of clinical reasoning to practice consistent with contemporary theory (Christensen 2009, Christensen et al. 2008b). Students in those programs tend to develop their clinical reasoning capability through self-directed learning with the individual views/knowledge of their clinical educators often having a significant influence (positive and negative).

Key message

All therapists are vulnerable to reasoning errors in both their diagnostic and their narrative-oriented reasoning. Inadequate knowledge, poor data collection skills (i.e. communication, observational and manual), lack of thoroughness (i.e. examination and re-assessments), habits of thinking (e.g. over-focus on clinical patterns) and lack of reflection/metacognition are common underlying causes. Being less familiar, narrative reasoning errors appear to relate to poor understanding of the bio-psychosocial model, superficial assessments of patients' perspectives and premature or unfounded judgments, all likely related to less explicit education in psychosocial assessment and management.

Christensen (2009) provides a comprehensive report of students' development of clinical reasoning capability across four physiotherapy programs in the USA. It is beyond the scope of this chapter to cover this topic in detail. Instead, key findings and implications of her research are briefly mentioned here and interested readers can refer to the references (Christensen 2009, Christensen et al. 2008a, 2008b) for further details. Christensen discusses four dimensions of clinical reasoning capability in the context of her research including reflective thinking, critical thinking, dialectical thinking and complexity thinking, each of which have been briefly addressed in this chapter. She discusses the role of professional socialization in shaping students' approach to clinical reasoning and proposes educators incorporate learning activities that assist students to see their own clinical reasoning as a reflection of their professional identity as a physiotherapist where the profession's espoused philosophy of practice, professional values, ethics and behavioural expectations are apparent in their practice and their reasoning. She discusses the need to strengthen connections between academic classroom learning of clinical reasoning and clinical application/learning of clinical reasoning. She proposes that this can be enhanced through classroom clinical reasoning focused learning activities that utilize existing models and frameworks within the literature to give form to clinical reasoning concepts and their clinical application (an educational process called reification, Wenger 1998) in order to assist students' understanding of clinical reasoning. Examples of frameworks that can be used in classroom theoretical discussions and case studies include models of clinical reasoning (e.g. Fig. 2.2), models of health and disability (e.g. Fig. 2.1) and the clinical reasoning strategies and hypothesis categories presented in this chapter. Lastly she emphasizes the importance of students having supervised clinical experiences that include overt attention to their developing clinical reasoning from clinical educators who are themselves familiar with clinical reasoning theory, skilled in their own clinical reasoning and skilled in facilitating students' clinical reasoning.

Maitland advocated open-mindedness (e.g. not being limited by current knowledge), analytical thinking (e.g. making features fit by attending to all aspects of the patient's story including features that do not immediately make sense) and use of advanced inquiry skills (i.e. questioning and physical assessments) to maximize the quality of information obtained. Inherent in Maitland's approach and unanimously promoted throughout the critical thinking, clinical reasoning, and education literature in general is continual reflection to note, critique, discuss and revise our research and experience based knowledge and actions (e.g. Brookfield 1987, Clouder 2000, Cranton 1994, Forneris 2004, Higgs& Jones 2008, Mezirow 2000, Rodgers 2002, Schön 1983, 1987). Reflection in clinical reasoning is the basis for experiential learning from practice (Christensen et al. 2008b; Eraut 1994; Schön 1987). In addition to the obvious reflection on a patient's problem, students and therapists should also reflect on their own thinking and the factors that limit it (e.g. knowledge).

Brookfield (2008) discusses critical appraisal as a process of recognizing and researching the assumptions that underpin clinical practice. EBP necessitates critical appraisal of available evidence with formal appraisal tools available according to the type of research. Critical appraisal applied to clinical reasoning requires reflection on existing knowledge, the basis of that knowledge and the assumptions underpinning or associated with that knowledge. This sort of critical reflection should improve clinical reasoning itself while also fostering learning through clinical reasoning.

Assumptions are taken-for-granted beliefs acquired through life and through formal education that are often tacit and hence typically not considered or challenged. Uncritically accepted assumptions often emerge from professional philosophies or approaches to practice or from personal experiences that have shaped one's views. Without scrutiny such assumptions place us at risk of thinking (in everyday life) and reasoning (in practice) on the basis of inaccurate and biased 'knowledge' (i.e. views/opinions) making us vulnerable to misinterpretations, inaccurate judgments and ultimately less effective health care.

Brookfield (2008) categorizes assumptions as paradigmatic, prescriptive and causal. Paradigmatic assumptions are the broad structuring assumptions we use to order the world into fundamental categories. They are typically the most difficult assumptions to recognize and change as they are supported by our personal experiences. A classic example of a paradigmatic assumption in medicine and physiotherapy is the traditional biomedical paradigm that equates pathology with symptom presentation and disability. The more contemporary bio-psychosocial model requires a broader consideration of environmental and personal or psychosocial factors alongside pathology in the assessment, analysis and management of patients' health problems.

Prescriptive assumptions relate to what we think should happen in a particular situation. Clinically related examples, including assumptions about clinical syndromes (e.g. chronic pain, shoulder impingement) or assumptions about patients themselves (e.g. different ethnic groups, workers compensation cases) can lead to inaccurate generalizations regarding their presentation, their attitude/motivation and the appropriate management. It is these sorts of prescriptive assumptions that commonly underpin failure to recognize the uniqueness of patients' individual clinical presentations and uncritical application of research findings and protocols of treatment. Prescriptive assumptions are inevitably related to our paradigmatic assumptions. For example, if you are biomedically (as opposed to bio-psychosocially) biased you are more likely to treat patients with a particular pathology or clinical syndrome the same rather than modifying your treatment to the patient's individual presentation.

Causal assumptions are assumptions about how different parts of the world (or human body) work (or do not work as with health) and what is required to create change (e.g. promote improved health). Physiotherapy and medicine in general are replete with causal assumptions typically based on unproven clinical management extrapolations from basic research or bias from personal experience not supported by adequate follow-up or critical comparison to other approaches.

What follows are some specific suggestions for facilitating students' and practising therapists' clinical reasoning drawn from research and personal experiences of educators across the health professions (Christensen et al. 2002, Higgs & Jones 2008, Rivett & Jones 2004, Scott 2000, Watts 1995). It is important that learning activities are well planned to target specific aspects of clinical reasoning (e.g. hypothesis generation, hypothesis testing, diagnostic versus narrative reasoning, etc.) while linking core biomedical and psychosocial theory to examination and management principles applied to simulated and real patient presentations. Students should have opportunity to reflect on their existing knowledge/ understandings and to question new information covered (concepts, principles, clinical patterns, management strategies) in order to promote construction of new knowledge/understandings that are acquired through critical consideration (as opposed to rote memory) in the context of clinical scenarios. There is a wealth of educational and clinical reasoning specific literature available to guide educators' development of learning activities. While it is beyond the scope of this chapter to review that literature, publications by Shepard and Jensen (2002), Higgs (1990, 1992, 1993, 2008), Higgs and Edwards (1999), Higgs and Hunt (1999), Higgs et al. (2008) and Rivett and Jones (2008) are helpful resources.

Understanding clinical reasoning theory

Just as students are expected to learn basic and applied science theory from presentations and review of literature, they should also be presented with contemporary theory and research of clinical reasoning. Ideally they should read selected clinical reasoning literature with activities or assignments that require them to demonstrate their understanding and application of that theory to practice. Reading literature from medicine, physiotherapy and the other allied health professions (e.g. Higgs et al. 2008) provides students with a comprehensive overview that will assist construction of their own understanding while at the same time giving them insight to the reasoning of their colleagues in other health professions.

Facilitated clinical reasoning through case studies and real patients

Real or hypothetical clinical problems can be used in clinical reasoning learning activities presented as paper-based, computer-based, filmed or through the use of simulated patients (trained actors). The text *Clinical reasoning for manual therapists* (Jones & Rivett 2004) provides theory chapters on clinical reasoning, learning theory and improving clinical reasoning as well as 23 case study contributions from recognized musculoskeletal clinical experts around the world. Through their cases the experts are questioned about their evolving reasoning, with the case providing valuable resources for educators and practicing therapists to use in clinical reasoning learning activities. A recent monograph entitled *Clinical reasoning and evidence-based practice,* available as an independent study course through the American Physical Therapy Association (Christensen et al. 2011) also provides a good overview of clinical reasoning theory linked to three patient cases. Newer books also now commonly include case studies and associated clinical reasoning (e.g. see Lee 2011, Vicenzino et al. 2011). When using case studies drawn from published resources or your own clinical experiences it is important that the cases are selected with an appropriate level of complexity for the student group with strategically planned discussions around aspects of clinical reasoning, basic science and physiotherapy examination, clinical pattern and management theory all linked to EBP (including experience and research-based evidence). Clinical reasoning activities with real patients are essential for students to develop their clinical reasoning capability within the variability of clinical presentations (problems and people), variability of practice environments and variability of time constraints inherent in real life practice. It is often useful to bridge the learning between case studies/simulated patients and students' reasoning through real patients they examine and treat with opportunities for students to observe patient demonstrations (and discuss associated reasoning) by their educators.

Whether using case studies, simulated or real patients it is essential that educators access students' thoughts in order to understand the reasoning and knowledge on which they base their reasoning. Students' reflections on their reasoning can be encouraged before, during and after the patient case/encounter. While stopping part way through an examination or treatment of a real patient is time consuming, it is also invaluable in exploring the student's immediate perceptions, interpretations and synthesis of patient information. The educator clearly must provide feedback and share their own interpretations but at the same time allow students the opportunity to explore (within reason and without risk to patient safety) their own reasoning even if it proves to be less efficient/effective than that of the educator. A balance is required to shape the student's knowledge, skills and reasoning without necessarily forcing them to only think and do the same as you. Peer coaching involving demonstration, observation, collaborative practice, feedback and reasoning discussions between students has also been demonstrated to be effective in facilitating student reasoning (Ladyshewsky & Jones 2008).

Self-reflection worksheets and clinical pattern diaries

Often educator / student ratios and time constraints prohibit one-on-one discussion with all students on every case. Here, use of self-reflection worksheets completed by students following their patient encounter is effective in accessing students' reasoning and promoting their self-awareness. Two examples of clinical reasoning self-reflection forms (long and short versions) are provided in Appendix 2.1. These have evolved to their present form from Maitland's original 'planning sheet' and readers are invited to use or modify them according to your own teaching and learning needs. Students commonly find the forced reflection these forms require is itself illuminating in highlighting information they failed to obtain or areas of knowledge and reasoning where they need further work. This, combined with feedback from the clinical educator, makes them a useful teaching, self-reflection and assessment tool.

Requiring students to compile a diary of clinical patterns facilitates their knowledge organization around common clinical patterns for use in their clinical reasoning. While there are a variety of ways clinical patterns can be presented, two examples of templates for constructing a clinical pattern used in the Master of Musculoskeletal and Sports Physiotherapy program, University of South Australia (single pattern versus comparative pattern) are available in Appendix 2.2. The content for constructing the patterns will come from the literature, ideally with acknowledgment of the level of supporting evidence used. Importantly for these patterns to become meaningful, educators should encourage students to include summaries of real patients they have seen who fit a particular pattern as this instantiation promotes deeper learning and highlights that clinical presentations typically do not match textbook patterns perfectly, enabling students to learn common variations and recognition of overlap between different patterns.

Mind maps

Mind maps (Buzan 2009) (also called concept and cognitive maps, although some differences exist) are another teaching and assessment strategy useful for facilitating metacognition, knowledge organization and clinical reasoning. A mind map is a pictorial representation of a person's knowledge and organization of knowledge on a specified topic. As such, it externalizes for the learner and the assessor the breadth and depth of the learner's understanding with potential to reveal preconceptions, assumptions, misunderstandings and biases. Cahill and Fonteyn (2008) review the literature on mind mapping and attribute its theoretical basis to the learning theory espoused by Ausubel (1963) who is credited with identifying the importance of relationships between concepts to a person's understanding and thinking. Meaningful (i.e. deep as opposed to superficial or rote) learning occurs when new learning is related to existing concepts or knowledge structures resulting in some change in understanding. This may be revision of a previous concept and/or new insight to relationships with other concepts previously not appreciated. Buzan and Buzan (1996) draw parallels between the mind map and the associative nature of brain pathways and argue for the importance of learning associations to improving understanding and memory. A growing body of education research is now available supporting the efficacy of mind mapping for promoting meaningful learning (see Cahill & Fonteyn 2008).

There are different processes for creating mind maps described in the literature. In natural science education students are often given a group of related concepts accompanied by a lecture after which the students are asked to create a mind map depicting their understanding of the concepts and any relationships between concepts. Arrows are generally used to illustrate relationships and words may be written along the arrows to qualify the nature of the particular relationship (e.g. 'leads to', 'causes', etc.). Cahill and Fonteyn (2008) describe how they had student nurses complete mind maps representing their 'thinking about a patient case' including patient problems, assessments, interpretations and management. At the University of South Australia, Master of Musculoskeletal and Sports Physiotherapy programme we have used mind maps as both a teaching and assessment tool. We start by having the students brainstorm on a sheet of paper everything they know about a specified topic prior to reading or receiving a lecture on the topic (e.g. inflammation, subacromial impingement). The students are then asked to number the items they brainstormed by grouping related items (i.e. giving every item that they feel should be categorized together the same number, for example for a common clinical presentation such as 'groin pain' all symptoms might be given a '1', signs

a '2', possible pathologies a '3' and so on). After completing the categorization of items the students then transfer those category headings and items within categories to another paper. Lastly students are asked to illustrate the relationships between categories (or concepts) by their placement on the paper (e.g. predisposing factors may be above pathology and signs and symptoms) and by arrows between categories with words along the arrows to qualify the relationship. The process of constructing a mind map itself is often illuminating to the student highlighting gaps in their knowledge. When time allows for students to complete maps prior to another learning activity (reading, lecture, demonstration) the pre-mind map promotes self-awareness (i.e. metacognition) of what they know and do not know about the nominated topic. This alone is valuable as students are then more likely to engage in the learning activity with greater interest and interaction as they listen for and ask about the gaps in their knowledge. Ideally a post-mind map is completed after the learning activity which enables the student to review new information and revise previous understandings. The second map will almost always have greater breadth and depth of information and relationships represented reflecting the learning and knowledge reorganization that has occurred. We have used this formatively to facilitate deeper learning and we have used it as a summative assessment for a whole course on 'Ethics and communication' where students are required to complete pre-course and post-course mind maps illustrating their understanding of the constructs and relationships between clinical reasoning and ethical reasoning (Jones et al. 2013). In this case students also wrote a brief essay explaining their second map which provided further insight to their understanding and learning through the course.

Lateral/creative thinking

Logical (also called vertical) thinking is essential to inductively recognize clinical patterns and to deductively substantiate those patterns through hypothesis oriented questioning and physical assessment (i.e. differential diagnosis). While this hypothetico-deductive process is clearly important to diagnostic reasoning and to advances in knowledge through quantitative research, lateral thinking is also important to the generation of new insights and discoveries that enable the individual therapist and the profession to advance their knowledge and practice. In fact, Kuhn (1970), in his text *The structure of scientific revolutions*, points out that many of the major breakthroughs in science did not occur due to carefully controlled scientific research, rather they often emerged from accidents or the lone insight of an individual. As long as a student's or therapist's clinical reasoning is logical and safe, lateral thinking should be encouraged. If we only encourage logical thinking and practice within the realm of what is 'known' or substantiated by research evidence we limit the variability and creativity of thinking that is important to the generation of new ideas.

Logical and its associated scientific thinking typically discourage individual intuition (i.e. gut feelings). However, in reality both the frontal cortex (cognition) and limbic system (emotions) are involved in most decisions to varying degrees. Research investigating the effects of over analyzing (too much logic) versus insufficient analysis (relying too much on emotions/gut feelings) suggests both can lead to poor decisions (Lehrer 2009). That decision-making research was primarily conducted in the realm of day to day decisions (e.g. which wine or food product you prefer, which house to buy, on field sports decisions, etc.) rather than clinical decision making. However, given the reality that health and disability are not an absolute science where judgments are black and white, correct or incorrect, intuition and emotions will also be involved in clinical reasoning. It is easy to imagine the errors of clinical reasoning that might occur with relying completely on gut feelings but could being too analytical and resistant to intuition also lead to clinical judgment errors? This has not been investigated but at the very least personal intuition should be reflected on and even pursued (i.e. line of questioning, physical assessment, treatment intervention) as it may lead to a fruitful outcome (e.g. useful information, positive response to intervention) that would not have been discovered if obvious logical avenues are the only things pursued. That is, new ideas and new approaches can emerge from intuition as well as logic.

Teaching lateral thinking centres on helping students recognize their current thinking processes (e.g. interpretations of patient information, diagnostic and management decisions) and encouraging them to think more widely, outside what may seem obvious and logical to them (de Bono 1970, 1994). Lateral thinking is relative to each individual's perspectives. That is, what is logical to one person

is not necessarily logical to another. De Bono characterizes vertical thinking as logical, sequential, predictable thinking where the thinker aims to systematically make sense of all information. In contrast lateral thinking involves restructuring and escape from old patterns, looking at things in different ways and avoidance of premature conclusions. The logical thinker attends only to what is obviously relevant where the lateral thinker recognizes that sometimes seemingly irrelevant information assists in viewing the problem from a different perspective. As a practical example of encouraging lateral thinking a student could be encouraged to conduct a review of patient progress and their reasoning (i.e. Maitland's 'retrospective assessment') where the student is explicitly asked to identify their dominant interpretation of the patient's diagnosis (e.g. pathology vs impairment, physical vs psychosocial, etc.) and the dominant approach they have been taking in their management to date (e.g. passive or dynamic bias, bias to treating source versus contributing factors, bias to physical impairments vs psychosocial factors, etc.). It is difficult to think laterally/creatively if you cannot first recognize how you have been thinking or approaching the problem thus

Key message

For student physiotherapists to develop their clinical reasoning capabilities, reasoning theory and supervised clinical application need to be explicit in the professional entry education. Frameworks such as the WHO ICF, models of clinical reasoning, clinical reasoning strategies and hypothesis categories all have the potential to assist. Reflection in the form of self-critique of knowledge, reasoning and performance will promote learning through clinical reasoning, particularly when assumptions underpinning clinical practice are critically examined. Many learning activities are available to facilitate improved clinical reasoning capability including: understanding clinical reasoning theory (e.g. review of literature); supervised reasoning through case studies and real patients; clinical reasoning self-reflection worksheets; clinical pattern diaries; and mind mapping. While logical thinking/reasoning is essential to safe effective practice, lateral/creative thinking is important to the generation of new ideas and discoveries. Little is known about the use and value of intuition or gut feelings in clinical reasoning, but research in non-clinical decision making suggests intuition should not be discarded and therapists should listen to and explore their gut feelings.

far. Once recognized, the student can then be encouraged to think more laterally about alternative interpretations of the patient's presentation and alternative management approaches. Maitland's way of emphasizing this process was to physically turn around in a circle, take a deep breath and start again. If students and therapists always follow the same interpretations and always manage problems the same way they never learn the place for alternative interpretations or that other approaches may be equally or even more effective.

We are all imposters

Every student and therapist will have experienced the uncomfortable situation of having to treat a patient who is not responding to treatment and whose presentation is not fully understood. Confirmation of pathology is often not possible from medical investigations or clinical assessment. Symptoms and physical impairments also commonly exist without overt pathology and many physical impairments exist without symptoms making it challenging to be clear which factors in the patient's life and clinical presentation are genuinely contributing to their symptoms and disability. Fortunately treatment of impairments is often effective in more straightforward nociceptive dominant presentations even when pathology is unclear. But as discussed earlier, many patient presentations are complex and multifactorial. Physical impairments are present alongside psychosocial issues and it is not always clear how much each is driving or contributing to the patient's disability. Systematic treatment addressing the different components hypothesized as being potentially relevant is not always effective causing some to conclude the problem is centrally mediated and the patient lacks understanding, acceptance, motivation and/or self-efficacy to actively participate in the rehabilitation recommended and to make the necessary lifestyle changes. While these factors may well underpin a patient's failed management they are difficult to assess/measure (Stewart et al. 2011) and challenging to manage. When a patient is not responding to treatment the therapist will inevitably go through a period of inner torment as they question whether they lack adequate knowledge of the latest research or missed something in the presentation. Many

therapists in this situation are hesitant to acknowledge their lack of understanding to the patient. They may similarly hesitate to request assistance from a colleague in fear that their examination and management will be judged incompetent. In short, they feel like an imposter who does not know enough, isn't skilled enough and are afraid they will be found out (Brookfield 2008). I chose to finish on this note as I see it as an unspoken reality that restricts some students' and therapists' learning and makes their practice less enjoyable. So what is the solution to minimize the struggle against 'impostership'? Brookfield (2008) discusses this phenomenon and suggests the answer is to go public. That is, to acknowledge to both patient and colleagues when you are not clear and would like a second opinion. Earlier I indicated that expert clinicians not only know a lot, they also know what they don't know. The student has the impression that the expert solves all patient problems and never needs assistance. All experienced clinicians will know how false that assumption is. The expert has become an expert precisely because they recognize their limitations and they act on them, often consulting other colleagues. When teachers and senior therapists acknowledge their difficult cases, their 'failures', it can be enormously reassuring to those less experienced making them more comfortable to ask for help. A second opinion may uncover missed information important to management or errors in reasoning but may also support the management trialled in which case other referral pathways should be considered. Creating an environment in the classroom or clinic where students/therapists feel comfortable discussing theory, research and clinical principles they don't understand is important. This can be facilitated through clinical discussion groups where patient cases are presented. Here it is important to not focus only on everyone's success, rather cases should be included that were not understood or where, in hindsight, errors were recognized. Health, disability and physiotherapy assessment and management are not exact sciences. Skilled clinical reasoning is important to work through the myriad of factors in a patient's presentation and critical reflection (metacognition) is important to recognizing limitations in knowledge, communication, procedural skills, and reasoning. When reflection leads to action (e.g. change in practice, request for assistance) the result is life-long learning.

Master of Musculoskeletal and Sports Physiotherapy
School of Health Sciences
UNIVERSITY OF SOUTH AUSTRALIA
CLINICAL REASONING REFLECTION FORM

NAME .... DATE .... PATIENT'S NAME...............................
Please provide a de-identified copy of the patient's bodychart with the form

PERCEPTIONS / INTERPRETATIONS
ON COMPLETION OF THE SUBJECTIVE EXAMINATION

It is important to recognise that the patient's presentation and factors affecting it (eg physical, environmental, psychosocial and health management via physiotherapy or other means) can be characterised in pain language/mechanisms by the dominant Input, Processing or Output pain mechanisms that appear to be affected. This should be considered when forming judgements regarding the other hypothesis categories as interpretations of the patient's symptoms, psychosocial status and signs will vary with the dominance of pain mechanisms present.

1. ACTIVITY CAPABILITY/RESTRICTION
Identify the key abilities and restrictions the patient has in executing activities:
- **Abilities** _____
- **Restrictions** _____

2. PARTICIPATION CAPABILITY/RESTRICTION
Identify the key abilities and restrictions the patient has with involvement in life situations
(work, family, sport, leisure):
- **Abilities** _____
- **Restrictions** _____

3. PATIENT'S PERSPECTIVES ON THEIR EXPERIENCE

3.1 What is your assessment of the patient's understanding of their problem? Specifically consider their threat appraisal with respect to severity, social desirability / self-concept, personal responsibility, controllability and changeability (positive, negative, neutral – explain). Does the patient's understanding and threat appraisal present a potential barrier to their recovery?

_____
_____
_____

3.2 What is your assessment of the patient's feelings (positive and negative) about their problem, its effect on their life and how it has been managed to date? Do any expressed negative feelings present a potential barrier to their recovery?

_____
_____
_____

3.3 Does the patient have any **explicit coping strategies** (for pain, stress, unhelpful thoughts/emotions) and if so do they appear to be adaptive or maladaptive? Does the patient convey **any avoidance behaviours** (to activities or participation) and if so does this appear reasonable for their disability or is it potentially maladaptive?

_____
_____
_____

3.4 What effect do you anticipate the patient's attitude to: 1) physical exercise, and 2) self-management will have on your management?

_____

_____

_____

3.5 Identify one experience from the patient's story that appears representative for them and provide your assessment of what that experience means to the patient

_____

_____

_____

3.6 What is your assessment of the patient's expectations from Physiotherapy? Specifically comment whether you feel they are appropriate or whether they may reflect maladaptive understanding and emotions that together will need to be addressed in your management.

_____

_____

What are the patient's goals related to their problem(s), their general health management and your specific physiotherapy management? What is your assessment of their goals (e.g. appropriate, if not,why not)?

_____

_____

_____

4.   PATHOBIOLOGICAL MECHANISMS

4.1   Tissue Mechanisms

What is your hypothesis regarding tissue health? Is there a clinical pattern of a specific process (e.g. Degenerative? Ischaemic? Over strain? Inflammatory?) Explain.

_____

_____

_____

Is there a clinical pattern of a specific pathology? Explain.

_____

_____

_____

If there has been overt tissue injury, at what stage of the inflammatory/healing process would you judge the injury to be? (e.g. acute inflammatory phase 0 – 72 hours, proliferation phase 72 hours – 6 weeks, remodelling & maturation phase 6 weeks – several months).

_____

_____

_____

4.2 Pain Mechanisms

List the subjective evidence which supports each specific mechanism of symptoms. Remember that all mechanisms are operating in every presentation. The aim of this table is to identify patient cues that support involvement of that mechanism.

Input Mechanisms		Processing Mechanisms	Output Mechanisms
Nociceptive Symptoms	Neuropathic Symptoms	Central Sensitisation	Behaviour (health & illness), Motor function, Thoughts/beliefs and cognitive function, Emotions, Autonomic nervous system, Neuroendocrine system, Immune system

4.3

Draw a "pie chart" on the diagram below that reflects the proportional involvement of the pain mechanisms (Nociceptive, Neuropathic, Central Sensitisation, Output specifying which output system(s)) apparent after completing the subjective examination.

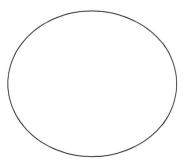

5.   THE POTENTIAL NOCICEPTIVE SOURCE(S) OF THE SYMPTOMS

5.1 **If** a "nociceptive" dominant pain mechanism is hypothesised, list in order of likelihood all possible structures that might contribute to a nociceptive mechanism for each area/component of symptoms.

Source	Area 1:	Area 2:	Area 3:	Area 4:
Somatic local				
Somatic referred				
Neurogenic				
Vascular				
Visceral				

6.   CONTRIBUTING FACTORS

6.1 Based on the subjective examination, are there any contributing factors hypothesised as associated with the development or maintenance of the patient's symptoms, activity and participation restrictions?

- **Hypothesised Physical factors based on knowledge of patient's activity levels/fitness, work and lifestyle, sport, medical and neuro-musculoskeletal history** (e.g.biomechanical, muscle length/strength/control, joint mobility, neural mobility, posture, etc.):

  _____

  _____

- **Environmental/ergonomic factors** (work place set up etc.):

  _____

  _____

- **Psychosocial factors** (e.g. patient's perspectives/understanding of problem & requirements for recovery/management, feelings regarding problem & its management, attributions, health beliefs and behaviours):

  _____

  _____

- **Health related factors** (e.g. health related issues that will affect the symptoms and development of the symptoms):

  _____

  _____

  _____

7. THE BEHAVIOUR OF THE SYMPTOMS

7.1 Give your interpretation of each of the following:

- **Severity:** _____
  (Symptom 1)   Low   High

- **Severity:** _____
  (Symptom 2)   Low   High

- **Irritability:** _____
  (Symptom 1)   Non-irritable   Very irritable

- **Irritability:** _____
  (Symptom 2)   Non-irritable   Very irritable

Give an example of irritability

_____
_____
_____

7.2 What is the relationship of the patient's activity/participation restrictions &/or symptoms to each other? *(this question is only relevant if more than one activity or participation restriction and/or more than set of symptoms)*

- **Behavioural:** Does the current pattern of activity and participation restrictions have a common theme such as flexion, extension, load, posture, stress related?

_____
_____

- **Behavioural:** Are the different symptoms related in their behaviour (e.g. respond together to aggravating and easing factors)? If so, in what way?

_____
_____

- **Historical (**e.g. Are the symptoms, activity and participation restrictions related historically? If so, in what way?)

_____
_____

7.3 Provide your interpretation of the contribution of mechanical &/or inflammatory features to the nociceptive component:

- Inflammatory: _____
                   0   10

- Mechanical: _____
                   0   10

- List those factors that support your decision

Inflammatory	Mechanical

8.   HISTORY OF THE SYMPTOMS

8.1 Give your *interpretation* of the history (present & past) for each of the following:

- **Nature of the onset** (e.g.is it consistent with a particular process, pathology or clinical syndrome and does it suggest a dominant pain mechanism?)

_____

_____

_____

- **What is the extent of physical impairment & associated tissue damage/change** hypothesised to be present? (e.g. mild versus severe &supporting evidence. Also, does this fit with a predominantly peripherally evoked or centrally mediated process?)

_____

_____

_____

- **What are the implications for the physical examination?** (specifically, how do your priorities change for day 1 physical examination?)

_____

_____

_____

- **What is the progression of the presentation since onset?** (better, worse, same, variability/stability)

_____

_____

_____

- **Is the patient's symptom presentation consistent with the history?** (Explain your answer)

_____

_____

_____

9.   HEALTH CONSIDERATIONS, PRECAUTIONS AND CONTRAINDICATIONS TO PHYSICAL EXAMINATION AND MANAGEMENT

9.1 Is there anything specific in the patient's answers to the "Medical Screening Questionnaire"(or your abbreviated initial screening) that represents a potential or clear caution/contraindication to your physical examination and management? Specify.

_____

_____

_____

Is there anything in your subjective examination questioning that indicates the need for caution in your physical examination or management? (e.g.highly irritable/inflammatory condition, rapidly worsening, progressive neurologically, red flag issues not identified in questionnaire, potential cervical arterial dysfunction, spinal cord or cauda equina compression/ischaemia, weight loss, medications, investigations etc.)? Specify.

_____

_____

_____

9.2 IF precautions are identified above, identify what action is indicated (e.g.Medical consultation, specific safety screening such as instability tests, cervical artery tests,etc.).

_____

_____

_____

9.3 Does the patient's general health or level of physical fitness indicate the need for consideration of health screening &/or fitness testing? **YES/NO**

- If yes, what health screening questionnaire(s) would you consider using?

_____

_____

_____

- What cardiovascular fitness testing would be appropriate?

_____

_____

- What other specific fitness screening tests would be appropriate?

_____

_____

- Is this testing a Day 1 priority? Explain your answer. **YES/NO**

_____

_____

9.4 At which points under the following headings will you limit your physical examination?

- Circle the relevant description.

Local symptoms (consider each component)	Referred symptoms (consider each component)	Dysthesias	Symptoms of CAD	Visceral or other system symptoms
	Short of P1	Short of Production		
Point of onset/ increase in resting symptoms	Point of onset/ increase in resting symptoms	Point of onset/ increase in resting symptoms	Point of onset/ increase in resting symptoms	Point of onset/ increase in resting symptoms
Partial reproduction	Partial reproduction	Partial reproduction		Partial reproduction
Total reproduction	Total reproduction	Total reproduction		Total reproduction

9.5 Is there any health, red flag or precaution-related reason to limit your examination(separate from your symptom provocation decision above)? Consider your responses to question 9.1 and 9.3 in making your decision.

- Circle the relevant description

Active examination

- Active movement short of limit
- Active limit
- Active limit + overpressure
- Additional tests

Passive examination

- Passive movement short of R1
- Passive movement into moderate resistance
- Passive movement into full overpressure

IF you hypothesise a dominant central sensitisation in the patient's presentation (e.g.as per pie chart on 4.3), indicate how you will attend to this in your physical examination.

_____

_____

_____

- If your hypothesis is a dominant central sensitisation, what would be your priorities for Day 1?

_____

_____

_____

_____

9.6   **Is a neurological examination necessary?**   **YES/NO**

•   **If so, indicate which neurological structures should be included** (e.g. nerve root, peripheral nerve, spinal cord, cauda equina, cranial nerves).

_____

_____

•   Is this examination a Day 1 priority? Explain your answer   **YES/NO**

_____

_____

9.7   **If relevant, do you expect a comparable sign(s) to be easy/hard to find?** (e.g. are the patient's symptoms easy to provoke so likely to be easy to reproduce in the clinic?)

•   Explain your answer   **EASY/HARD**

_____

_____

_____

_____

9.8   **What are the clues (if any) in the subjective examination to any specific treatment techniques or approach to treatment that may be appropriate?** (e.g. a particular movement or position that is pain relieving might form the basis of a mobilising technique, postural symptoms might indicate need for an endurance program, indications of chronic pain might indicate the need for an educational bias to your management)

•   Explain your answer   **YES/NO**

_____

_____

_____

_____

10. WRITE OUT YOUR PLAN FOR YOUR PHYSICAL EXAMINATION
- Highlight with an * those procedures to be included on Day 1

Functional tests:	
Functional outcome measure:	
Posture:	
Fitness related tests • **CV tests** • **Strength/endurance**	
Active movements:	
Passive movements: • **Physiological** • **Accessory**	
Resistive tests:	
Neurological examination:	
Neurodynamic:	
Soft tissue:	
Motor control:	
Other:	

PERCEPTIONS, INTERPRETATIONS, IMPLICATIONS
FOLLOWING THE PHYSICAL EXAMINATION AND FIRST TREATMENT

11. **Identify the key PHYSICAL IMPAIRMENTS from your physical examination that may require management/reassessment** (e.g. posture, movement pattern impairments, motor control impairments, soft tissue/joint/muscle/neural mobility/sensitivity, fitness levels, strength/power/endurance)

1.	
2.	
3.	
4.	
5.	
6.	
7.	
8.	
9.	
10.	
11.	
	List any assessments not completed Day 1:

12. THE SOURCES AND PATHOBIOLOGICAL MECHANSIMS OF THE PATIENT'S SYMPTOMS

12.1 List the components of symptoms and pathobiological mechanisms identified in Sections 4 & 5 and number in order of likelihood the possible structure(s) at fault for each apparent component. Then identify the supporting & negativing evidence from the *PHYSICAL EXAMINATION* for each structure and pathobiological mechanism (you may need to attach an additional page to complete the list)

Component	Possible structure(s) at fault	Physical Examination Supporting Evidence	Physical Examination Negating Evidence
e.g. Left mid cervical pain	Left PIV joints C2-5	• Thickened soft tissue over laminae C2-5 • Tenderness C2-5 • Active LF & rotation left limited range	• PPIVMs LF & rotation left C2/3 –5/6 normal ROM • Stiffness unilateral PA C2/3-5/6

12.2 List the supporting and negating evidence from the PHYSICAL EXAMINATION for the Pain and Tissue Mechanisms listed below:

Pain Mechanisms	Supporting Evidence	Negating Evidence
Input Mechanisms: • Nociceptive • Neuropathic		
Processing Mechanism: • Central Sensitisation • Potentially maladaptive cognitive and/or affective cues apparent during the physical examination		
Motor & Other Output Mechanisms: • Motor • Other		

Tissue Healing Mechanisms	Supporting Evidence	Negating Evidence

If an overt (macro or micro) tissue injury has occurred (e.g. muscle/tendon/ligament/etc) such that the tissues will go through the understood healing process, identify the features from the Physical Examination that support the phase of healing:

Acute inflammatory phase		
Proliferation phase		
Remodelling and maturation phase		

12.3 What does P/E suggest regarding tissue health (process, specific pathology, clinical syndrome) and how does that fit with previous tissue health hypothesis from S/E?

• Explain your answer   **YES/NO**

_____

_____

_____

_____

12.4 Based on your full S/E and P/E assessment and analysis list the favourable and unfavourable prognostic indicators (consider for example: pain and tissue mechanisms, patient perspectives, inflammatory versus mechanical presentation, degree of irritability, nature of onset and progression, effects of previous interventions, medical screening findings, extent of physical impairments and possible contributing factors):

Favourable	Unfavourable

12.5 Based on your assessment of favourable and unfavourable prognostic indicators, indicate whether you feel you/physiotherapy can assist this patient and state as specifically as you can (e.g. days, weeks, months) how much time or number of treatments are likely to be required.

• Able to help?

• How much time is required?

• Percentage improvement anticipated?

IMPLICATIONS OF PERCEPTIONS AND INTERPRETATIONS ON ONGOING MANAGEMENT

13. MANAGEMENT

13.1 Is there anything about your physical examination findings which would indicate the need for caution in your management? Explain YES/NO

13.2 Does your interpretation of the physical examination findings change the anticipated emphasis of treatment? Explain YES/NO

13.3 What was your management on Day 1 (e.g. explanation/advice, exercise, passive mobilisation, general exercise, referral for further investigation etc.)

• Why was this chosen over other options?

• **If passive treatment was used, what was your principal treatment technique(s)?** (indicate technique, position in which it was performed, grade, dosage)

- **What physical examination findings support your choice?** (include in your answer a movement diagram of the most comparable passive movement sign *[most positive passive movement]*)

_____
_____
_____
_____

MOVEMENT DIAGRAM

13.4 • **If dynamic management was used, what was your principal focus/starting point?** (indicate exercise, position in which it was performed/taught, dosage)

_____
_____

13.5 • **If education was your starting point, what was your principal focus?** (indicate key messages targeted)

_____
_____

13.6 What was the effect of your Day 1 intervention?

- Subjective response:

_____
_____

- Physical response:

_____
_____

What is your expectation of the patient's response over the next 24 hours?

_____
_____

13.7 What is your plan and justification of management for this patient?

- Overall management plan (e.g. general components of clinical presentation requiring attention)

_____
_____

- Type of treatment

_____
_____

- Priorities with treatment

_____
_____

- Attention to components other than the primary presentation

_____
_____

- Rate of progress etc.

_____
_____

13.8 **Is attention to the general fitness/cardiovascular health of the patient a priority in your management? Explain**   **YES/NO**

_____

_____

- If so, how do you plan to incorporate this in your overall management?

_____

_____

13.9 **Do you envisage a need to refer the patient to another health provider** (e.g. physician, orthopaedic surgeon, neurologist/neurosurgeon, vascular surgeon, endocrinologist, psychologist/psychiatrist, anaesthetist, dietician, Feldencrais practitioner, Pilates practitioner, gym instructor etc.)

- Explain:

_____

_____

14. **REFLECTION ON PAIN MECHANISMS, SOURCE(S), CONTRIBUTING FACTOR(S) AND PROGNOSIS**

AFTER THIRD VISIT

14.1 **How has your understanding of the patient and the patient's problem(s) changed from your interpretations made following the first session?**

_____

- How have the patient's perceptions of his/her problem and management changed since the first session?

_____

- Are the patient's needs being met?

_____

_____

14.2 **On reflection, what clues (if any) can you now recognise that you initially missed, misinterpreted, under or over-weighted?**

_____

- What would you do differently next time?

_____

- Have you been able to address all components as indicated in your management plan or advance your treatment at the rate planned? Explain

                                                                                                         YES/NO

_____

- If not, what barriers have prevented you advancing your treatment as you planned?

_____

_____

AFTER SIXTH VISIT

14.3 **How has your understanding of the patient and the patient's problem changed from your interpretation made following the third session?**

_____
_____

- How have the patient's perceptions of his/her problem and management changed since the third session?

_____
_____

- Have the patient's expectations been met?

_____
_____

14.4 **On reflection, what clues (if any) can you now recognise that you initially missed, misinterpreted, under or over-weighted?**

_____
_____

- What would you do differently next time?

_____
_____

- Have you been able to address all components as indicated in your management plan or advance your treatment at the rate planned? Explain

                                                                    YES/NO

_____
_____

- If not, what barriers have prevented you advancing your treatment as you planned?

_____
_____

14.5 **If the outcome is to be short of 100% (i.e. "cured") at what point will you cease management and why?**

_____
_____

AFTER DISCHARGE

14.6 **How has your understanding of the patient and the patient's problem changed from your interpretations made following the sixth session?**

_____
_____

- How has the patient's perceptions of his/her problem and management changed since the third session?

_____
_____

- How much have you been able to address the patient's concept of self-efficacy, responsibility for self-management and perceptions of the importance of healthy lifestyle in management of his/her problem?

_____
_____

14.7 **In hindsight, what were the principal source(s) and pathobiological mechanisms of the patient's symptoms?**

_____
_____
_____
_____

• What were the patient's principal health/fitness related issues?

_____
_____

• How successful have you been in addressing all components of the patient's problem? Explain

_____
_____
_____
_____

14.8 **Identify the key subjective and physical features (i.e. clinical pattern) that would help you recognise this presentation in the future**

Subjective	Physical

Master of Musculoskeletal and Sports Physiotherapy
School of Health Sciences
UNIVERSITY OF SOUTH AUSTRALIA
CLINICAL REASONING REFLECTION FORM

STUDENT.........................DATE.............PATIENT'S NAME.............................

PERCEPTIONS / INTERPRETATIONS
ON COMPLETION OF THE SUBJECTIVE EXAMINATION

1. **ACTIVITY & PARTICIPATION CAPABILITY/RESTRICTION**
   Abilities ....
   Restrictions ....

2. **PATHOBIOLOGICAL MECHANISMS**
   Identify the DOMINANT Pain Mechanism and supporting evidence:
   ....
   ....
   If relevant, specify the stage of Tissue Healing: ....
   ....

3. **PATTERN OF AGGRAVATION**
   Indicate the dominant pattern of aggravation (e.g. flexion, extension, sustained
   positions, movement, load, stress, etc.):..
   ....

4. **SOURCE OF THE SYMPTOMS**
   Identify the possible tissue sources for each symptom:
   Symptom 1..
   Symptom 2..
   Symptom 3..

5. **CONTRIBUTING FACTORS**
   List any potential contributing factors identified in the subjective examination:
   ....
   ....

6. **DAY 1 PRIOITIES**
   Specify your priorities for physical examination on Day 1:...................................
   ....
   ....

7. **PRECAUTIONS & CONTRAINDICATIONS**
   List any features suggesting caution or contraindication to P/E or treatment:.............
   ....

8. **YELLOW FLAGS**
   Identify any Yellow Flags and how you plan to attend to them in your P/E and
   treatment:..
   ....

9. **EXPECTATIONS AND GOALS**
   Specify the patient's expectations/goals, whether you consider them realistic and how
   you may suggest breaking them down into short versus longer term goals:
   ....
   ....
   ....

PERCEPTIONS / INTERPRETATIONS
ON COMPLETION OF THE PHYSICAL EXAMINATION

10. PHYSICAL IMPAIRMENTS
Identify physical impairments found on the physical examination:...........................
....
....

11. PATHOBIOLOGICAL MECHANISMS
Specify the findings from the P/E supporting or not-supporting the dominant pain
mechanisms and tissue mechanisms hypothesised in the S/E:.............................
....
....

12. SOURCE OF THE SYMPTOMS / PHYSICAL IMPAIRMENTS
Indicate the tissue sources (general or specific as appropriate) of the symptoms and/or
physical impairments supported by the physical examination:.................................
....
....

13. BROAD MANAGEMENT AND SPECIFIC TREATMENTS
Specify and justify your broad management plan at this stage and the specific
treatment(s) you plan for Day 1:...
....
....

14. REASSESSMENT / OUTCOME MEASURES
Identify the key S/E and P/E reassessments you plan to monitor:...........................
....

15. EXPLANATION
Highlight the focus of the explanation you gave to the patient:...............................
....

PERCEPTIONS / INTERPRETATIONS
ON COMPLETION OF DAY 1 TREATMENT

16. REASSESSMENT
What are your thoughts following reassessment of today's treatment?....................
....

17. PLANS FOR FURTHER ASSESSMENT
Identify any further assessments (S/E or P/E) you plan to do:...............................
....
....

18. TREATMENT PROGRESSION AND SELF-MANAGMENT
What are your immediate plans for progression of today's treatment?......................
....
What self-management do you plan to suggest and when will you do so?................
....

19. PROGNOSIS
Indicate how long you think the problem will take to resolve and list the positive and
negative prognostic indicators from the S/E, P/E and response to treatment Day 1:....
Positives..
Negatives...

Sample of a comparative clinical pattern

Title of the pattern:

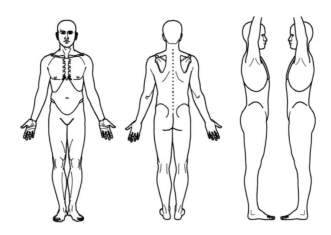

References:			
	Comparative Pattern 1	**Comparative Pattern 2**	**Comparative Pattern 3**
Typical epidemiological features • *Age, gender, activity, work, sport typically associated with the condition*	•	•	•
Area of symptoms	•	•	•
Characteristics of symptoms	•	•	•
Typical activity capability/restriction	•	•	•
Behaviour of symptoms • *24 hour pattern* • *Typical aggravating/easing factors*	•	•	•
Typical history of condition	•	•	•

Pathobiological mechanisms • *Primary mechanisms operating with the initial presentation*	•	•	•
Proposed pathology	•	•	•
Physical impairments & associated structure/tissue sources (ie P/E findings) • *Incorporated into this section should be an indication of the evidence available on the diagnostic accuracy of any particular test as reported in the textbook (Cleland 2007) or elsewhere as appropriate*	•	•	•
Typical contributing factors • *These may be physical, biomechanical, psychosocial, medical etc*	•	•	•
Precautions/contraindications to P/E and treatment • *Only those specific to this condition*	•	•	•
Diagnostic imaging useful for the condition • *Expected positive findings*	•	•	•
Typical prognosis	•	•	•
Management/treatment selection • *Emphasis on musculoskeletal &/or sports physiotherapy* • *Include management options reported in literature (with indication of level of evidence)* • *Options provided for you in class and on placement*	•	•	•
Differential diagnosis • *Include key differentiating characteristics*	•	•	•

Sample of a clinical pattern

Title of the pattern

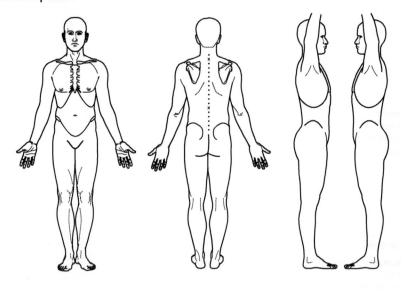

References:	
Typical epidemiological features • *Age, gender, activity, work, sport typically associated with the condition*	•
Area of symptoms	•
Characteristics of symptoms	•
Typical activity capability/restriction	•
Behaviour of symptoms • *24 hour pattern* • *Typical aggravating/easing factors*	•
Typical history of condition	•

Pathobiological mechanisms • *Primary mechanisms operating with the initial presentation*	•
Proposed pathology	•
Physical impairments & associated structure/tissue sources(ie P/E findings) • *Incorporated into this section should be an indication of the evidence available on the diagnostic accuracy of any particular test as reported in the textbook (Cleland 2007) or elsewhere as appropriate*	•
Typical contributing factors • *These may be physical, biomechanical, psychosocial, medical etc*	•
Precautions/contrain dications to P/E and treatment • *Only those specific to this condition*	•
Diagnostic imaging useful for the condition • *Expected positive findings*	•
Typical prognosis	•
Management/treatment selection • *Emphasis on musculoskeletal &/or sports physiotherapy* • *Include management options reported in literature (with indication of level of evidence)* • *Options provided for you in class and on placement*	•
Differential diagnosis • *Include key differentiating characteristics*	•

References

Adams MA, Stefanakis M, Dolan P: Healing of a painful intervertebral disc should not be confused with reversing disc degeneration: implications for physical therapies of discogenic back pain, *Clin Biomechan* 25:961–971, 2010.

American Physical Therapy Association: *Guide to physical therapist practice* (Revised ed 2), Alexandria, 2003, American Physical Therapy Association.

Anderson JR: *Cognitive psychology and its implications*, ed 3, New York, 1990, Freeman.

Argyris C, Schön D: *Organizational learning: a theory in action perspective*, Reading, 1978, Addison-Wesley.

Arnetz JE, Almin I, Bergström K, et al: Active patient involvement in the establishment of physical therapy goals: Effects on treatment outcome and quality of care, *Adv Physiother* 6:50–69, 2004.

Arocha JF, Patel VL, Patel YC: Hypothesis generation and the coordination of theory and evidence in novice diagnostic reasoning, *Med Decis Making* 13:198–211, 1993.

Arroll B, Goodyear-Smith F, Crengle S, et al: Validation of PHQ-2 and PHQ-9 to Screen for Major Depression in the Primary Care Population, *Ann Fam Med* 8:348–353, 2010.

Ausubel DP: *The psychology of meaningful verbal learning*, New York, 1963, Grune and Stratton.

Barnitt R, Partridge C: Ethical reasoning in physical therapy and occupational therapy, *Physiother Res Int* 2:178–192, 1997.

Baron JB, Sternberg RJ: *Teaching thinking skills: Theory and practice*, New York, 1987, WH Freeman and Company.

Barrows H, Feltovich P: The clinical reasoning process, *Med Educ* 21:86–91, 1987.

Beeston S, Simons H: 'Physiotherapy practice: Practitioners' perspectives, *Physiother Theory Pract* 12:231–242, 1996.

Benner P: *From novice to expert: Excellence and power in clinical nursing practice*, Menlo Park, 1984, Addison-Wesley.

Benner P, Tanner C, Chesla C: From beginner to expert: Gaining a differentiated clinical world in critical care nursing, *Adv Nurs Sci* 14(3):13–28, 1992.

Bielefeldt K, Gebhart GF: Visceral pain: basic mechanisms. In McMahon SB, Koltzenburg M, editors: *Wall and Melzack's textbook of pain*, ed 5, Edinburgh, 2006, Elsevier, pp 721–736.

Bishop GD: Understanding the understanding of illness: lay disease representations. In Skelton JA, Croyle RT, editors: *Mental Representation in Health and Illness*, New York, 1991, Springer-Verlag, pp 32–59.

Bogduk N: The anatomy and physiology of nociception. In Crosbie J, McConnell J, editors: *Physiotherapy foundations for practice – key issues in musculoskeletal physiotherapy*, Oxford, 1993, Butterworth-Heinemann, pp 48–87.

Borrell-Carrió F, Suchman AL, Epstein RM: The bio-psychosocial model 25 years later: Principles, practice, and scientific inquiry, *Ann Fam Med* 2(6):576–582, 2004.

Boshuizen HPA, Schmidt HG: The development of clinical reasoning expertise. In Higgs J, Jones MA, Loftus S, Christensen N, editors: *Clinical reasoning in the health professions*, ed 3, Amsterdam, 2008, Butterworth Heinemann Elsevier, pp 113–121.

Boissonnault WG: *Primary care for the physical therapist. Examination and triage*, ed 2, St Louis, 2011, Elsevier.

Brooker C: *Mosby's 2013 Dictionary of Medicine, nursing and health professions*, ed 9, Edinburgh, 2013, Elsevier.

Brookfield SD: *Developing critical thinkers. Challenging adults to expore alternative ways of thinking and acting*, San Francisco, 1987, Jossey-Bass.

Brookfield S: Clinical reasoning and generic thinking skills. In Higgs J, Jones MA, Loftus S, Christensen N, editors: *Clinical reasoning in the health professions*, ed 3, Amsterdam, 2008, Butterworth Heinemann Elsevier, pp 65–75.

Brooks L, Norman GR, Allen S: Role of specific similarity in a medical diagnostic task, *J Exp Psychol Learn Mem Cogn* 120:278–287, 1991.

Butler DS: *The sensitive nervous system*, Adelaide, 2000, Noigroup Publications.

Buzan T: *The mind map book*, Harlow, 2009, Pearson Education Limited.

Buzan T, Buzan B: *The mind map book*, New York, 1996, Plume/Penguin.

Cahill M, Fonteyn M: Using mind mapping to improve students' metacognition. In Higgs J, Jones MA, Loftus S, Christensen N, editors: *Clinical Reasoning in the Health Professions*, ed 3, Amsterdam, 2008, Butterworth-Heinemann Elsevier, pp 485–491.

Cervero RM: *Effective continuing education for professionals*, San Francisco, 1988, Jossey-Bass.

Chi TH, Glaser R, Farr MJ, editors: *The Nature of Expertise*, Hillsdale, 1988, Lawrence Erlbaum Associates.

Childs JD, Cleland JA, Elliott JM, et al: Neck pain: clinical practice guidelines linked to the International Classification of Functioning, Disability, and Health from the Orthopaedic Section of the American Physical Therapy Association, *J Orthop Sports Phys Ther* 38(9):A1–A34, 2008.

Christensen N: 'Development of clinical reasoning capability in student physical therapists', *Unpublished PhD thesis*, 2009, University of South Australia.

Christensen N, Jones M, Carr J: Clinical reasoning in orthopaedic manual therapy. In Grant R, editor: *Physical therapy of the cervical and thoracic spine*, ed 3, Edinburgh, 2002, Churchill Livingstone.

Christensen N, Jones MA, Higgs J, Edwards I: Dimensions of clinical reasoning capability. In Higgs J, Jones MA, Loftus S, Christensen N, editors: *Clinical Reasoning in the Health Professions*, ed 3, Amsterdam, 2008a, Butterworth-Heinemann Elsevier, pp 101–110.

Christensen N, Jones MA, Edwards I, Higgs J: Helping physiotherapy students develop clinical reasoning capability, In Higgs J, Jones MA, Loftus S, Christensen N, editors: *Clinical Reasoning in the Health Professions*, ed 3, Amsterdam, 2008b, Butterworth-Heinemann Elsevier, pp 389–396.

Christensen N, Jones M, Edwards I: Clinical Reasoning and Evidence-based Practice. Independent Study

Course 21.2.2: *Current Concepts of Orthopaedic Physical Therapy*, ed 3, La Crosse, 2011, Orthopaedic Section, APTA, Inc.

Cibulka MT, White DM, Woehrle J, et al: Hip pain and mobility deficits – hip osteoarthritis: clinical practice guidelines linked to the International Classification of Functioning, Disability, and Health from the Orthopaedic Section of the American Physical Therapy Association, *J Orthop Sports Phys Ther* 39(4):A1–A25, 2009.

Clouder L: Reflective practice in physiotherapy education: A critical conversation, *Stud Higher Ed* 25(2):211–223, 2000.

Cohen S, Kamarck T, Mermelstein R: A global measure of perceived stress, *J Health Soc Behav* 24: 386–396, 1983.

Cook JL, Purdam CR: Is tendon pathology a continuum? A pathology model to explain the clinical presentation of load-induced tendinopathy, *Br J Sports Med* 43:409–416, 2009.

Craig KD: Emotions and psychobiology. In McMahon S, Koltzenburg M, editors: *Wall and Melzack's textbook of pain*, ed 5, 2006, Elsevier, pp 231–240.

Cranton P: *Understanding and promoting transformative learning: A guide for educators of adults*, San Francisco, 1994, Jossey-Bass.

Cusick A: Personal frames of reference in professional practice. In Higgs J, Titchen A, editors: *Practice knowledge and expertise in the health professions*, Oxford, 2001, Butterworth Heinemann, pp 91–95.

de Bono E: *Lateral thinking. Creativity step by step*, New York, 1970, Harper and Row.

de Bono E: *De Bono's thinking course*, New York, 1994, MICA Management Resources.

DeGroot KI, Boeke S, van den Berge HJ, et al: Assessing short- and long-term recovery from lumbar surgery with pre-operative biographical, medical and psychological variables, *Br J Health Psychol* 2:229–243, 1997.

Devor M: Response of nerves to injury in relation to neuropathic pain. In McMahon SB, Koltzenburg M, editors: *Wall and Melzack's Textbook of pain*, ed 5, Edinburgh, 2006, Elsevier Churchill Livingstone, pp 905–927.

Donaghy M, Nicol M, Davidson K: *Cognitive-behavioural interventions in physical and occupational therapy*, Edinburgh, 2008, Butterworth-Heinemann Elsevier.

Doody C, McAteer M: Clinical reasoning of expert and novice physiotherapists in an outpatient orthopaedic setting, *Physiotherapy* 88(5):258–268, 2002.

Duncan G: Mind-body dualism and the bio-psychosocial model of pain: what did Descartes really say? *J Med Philos* 25:485–513, 2000.

Edwards IC: Clinical reasoning in three different fields of physiotherapy – a qualitative case study approach. Vols. I and II, *Unpublished thesis submitted in partial fulfilment of the Doctor of Philosophy in Health Sciences*, University of South Australia, Adelaide, Australia, The Australian Digitized Theses Program, 2001, 2000, Available at: http://www.library.unisa.edu.au/adt-root/public/adt-SUSA-20030603-090552/index.html.

Edwards IC, Jones MA: Collaborative reasoning, *Unpublished paper submitted in partial fulfillment of the Graduate Diploma in Orthopaedics*, Adelaide, Australia, 1996, University of South Australia.

Edwards I, Jones MA: The role of clinical reasoning in understanding and applying the International Classification of Functioning, Disability and Health (ICF), *Kinesitherapie* 71:e1–e9, 2007a.

Edwards I, Jones M: *Clinical reasoning and expertise*. In Jensen GM, Gwyer J, Hack LM, Shepard KF, editors: *Expertise in physical therapy practice*, ed 2, Boston, 2007b, Elsevier, pp 192–213.

Edwards I, Jones M, Carr J, Braunack-Mayer A, Jensen G: Clinical reasoning strategies in physical therapy, *Phys Ther* 84(4):312–335, 2004a.

Edwards I, Jones M, Higgs J, Trede F, Jensen G: What is collaborative reasoning? *Adv Physiother* 6:70–83, 2004b.

Edwards I, Jones MA, Hillier S: The interpretation of experience and its relationship to body movement: a clinical reasoning perspective, *Man Ther* 11:2–10, 2006.

Elstein AS, Schwarz A: Clinical problem solving and diagnostic decision making: Selective review of the cognitive literature, *Br Med J* 324:729–732, 2002.

Elstein AS, Shulman L, Sprafka S: *Medical problem solving: An analysis of clinical reasoning*, Cambridge, 1978, Harvard University Press.

Embrey DG, Guthrie MK, White OR, Dietz J: Clinical decision making by experienced and inexperienced pediatric physical therapists for children with diplegic cerebral palsy, *Phys Ther* 76(1):20–33, 1996.

Engel G: The bio-psychosocial model and the education of health professionals, *Ann NY Acad Sci* 310:535–544, 1978.

Eraut M: *Developing professional knowledge and competence*, London, 1994, Routledge Falmer.

Ericsson A, Smith J, editors: *Toward a general theory of expertise: Prospects and limits*, New York, 1991, Cambridge University Press.

Escorpizo R, Stucki G, Cieza A, et al: Creating an interface between the International Classification of Functioning, Disability and Health and physical therapist practice, *Phys Ther* 90(7):1053–1067, 2010.

Feltovich PJ, Barrows HS: Issues of generality in medical problem solving. In Schmidt HG, de Volder ML, editors: *Tutorials in problem-based learning: A new direction in teaching the health professions*, Assen, 1984, Van Gorcum, pp 128–141.

Fields HL, Basbaum AI, Heinricher MM: Central nervous system mechanisms of pain modulation. In McMahon SB, Koltzenburg M, editors: *Wall and Melzack's textbook of pain*, ed 5, Edinburgh, 2006, Elsevier Churchill Livingstone, pp 125–142.

Fleming MH: The therapist with the three-track mind, *Am J Occup Ther* 45:1007–1014, 1991.

Flor H, Turk DC: Cognitive and learning aspects. In McMahon SB, Koltzenburg M, editors: *Wall and Melzack's Textbook of pain*, ed 5, Edinburgh, 2006, Elsevier Churchill Livingstone, pp 241–258.

Forneris SG: Exploring the attributes of critical thinking: A conceptual basis, *IJNES* 1(1), Article 9, 2004.

Galea MP: Neuroanatomy of the nociceptive system. In Strong J, Unrush AM, Wright A, Baxter GD, editors: *Pain: a textbook for therapists*, Edinburgh, 2002, Churchill Livingstone, pp 13–41.

Gatchel RJ, Bo Peng Y, Peters ML, Fuchs PN, Turk DC: The

bio-psychosocial approach to chronic pain: scientific advances and future directions, *Psychol Bull* 133(4): 581–624, 2007.

Gifford L: Tissue and input related mechanisms. In Gifford L, editor: *Topical issues in pain: Whiplash – science and management. Fear-avoidance beliefs and behaviour*, Falmouth, 1998a, CNS Press, pp 57–65.

Gifford L: Central mechanisms. In Gifford L, editor: *Topical issues in pain: Whiplash – science and management. Fear-avoidance beliefs and behaviour*, Falmouth, 1998b, CNS Press, pp 67–80.

Gifford L: Output mechanisms. In Gifford L, editor: *Topical issues in pain: Whiplash – science and management. Fear-avoidance beliefs and behaviour*, Falmouth, 1998c, CNS Press, pp 81–91.

Gifford L: Acute low cervical nerve root conditions: symptoms, symptom behaviour and physical screening, *In Touch* 85(Winter):4–19, 1998d.

Gifford L, Thacker M, Jones MA: Physiotherapy and pain. In McMahon SB, Koltzenburg M, editors: *Wall and Melzack's Textbook of pain*, ed 5, Edinburgh, 2006, Elsevier Churchill Livingstone, pp 603–617.

Glaser R: Education and thinking: the role of knowledge, *Am Psychol* 39:93–104, 1984.

Glaser R, Chi MTH: Overview. In Chi MTH, Glaser R, Farr MJ, editors: *The nature of expertise*, Hillsdale, 1988, Lawrence Erlbaum.

Gottlieb A, Golander H, Bar-Tal Y: The influence of social support and perceived control on handicap and quality of life after stroke, *Aging Clin Exp Res* 13:11–15, 2001b.

Goodman CC, Snyder TEK: *Differential diagnosis for physical therapists. Screening for referral*, ed 5, St Louis, 2013, Elsevier.

Gordon M, Murphy CP, Candee D, Hiltunen E: Clinical judgement: an integrated model, *Adv Nurs Sci* 16:55–70, 1994.

Greeno JG: The situativity of knowing, learning, and research, *Am Psychol* 53(1):5–26, 1998.

Hagedorn R: Clinical decision-making in familiar cases: a model of the process and implications for practice, *Br J Occup Ther* 59: 217–222, 1996.

Harding V: Application of the cognitive-behavioural approach. In Pitt-Brooke J, Reid H, Lockwood J, Kerr K, editors: *Rehabilitation of movement: Theoretical bases of clinical practice*, London, 1998, WB Saunders, pp 539–583.

Harding V, de C Williams A: Extending physiotherapy skills using a psychological approach: Cognitive-behavioural management of chronic pain, *Physiotherapy* 81(11):681–688, 1995.

Harris IB: New expectations for professional competene. In Curry L, Wergin J, editors: *Educating professionals: Responding to new expectations for competence and accountability*, San Francisco, 1993, Jossey-Bass, pp 17–52.

Hayes B, Adams R: Parallels between clinical reasoning and categorization. In Higgs J, Jones MA, editors: *Clinical reasoning in the health professions*, ed 2, Oxford, 2000, Butterworth Heinemann, pp 45–53.

Higgs J: Fostering the acquisition of clinical reasoning skills, *NZ J Physio* 18:13–17, 1990.

Higgs J: Developing clinical reasoning competencies, *Physiotherapy* 78(8):575–581, 1992.

Higgs J: A programme for developing clinical reasoning skills in graduate physiotherapists, *Med Teach* 15(2):195–205, 1993.

Higgs J: Educational theory and principles related to learning clinical reasoning. In MA Jones, DA Rivett, editors: *Clinical reasoning for manual therapists*, Edinburgh, 2008, Butterworth Heinemann, pp 379–402.

Higgs J, Titchen A: The nature, generation and verification of knowledge, *Physiotherapy* 81(9):521–530, 1995.

Higgs, J, Edwards, H, editors: *Educating beginning practitioners*, Oxford, 1999, Butterworth Heinemann.

Higgs J, Hunt A: Rethinking the beginning practitioner: introducing the 'Interactional Professional. In Higgs J, Edwards H, editors: *Educating beginning practitioners*, Oxford, 1999, Butterworth-Heinemann, pp 10–18.

Higgs J, Jones MA: Clinical reasoning in the health professions. In Higgs J, Jones MA, editors: *Clinical reasoning in the health professions*, ed 2, Oxford, 2000, Butterworth Heinemann, pp 3–14.

Higgs J, Jones MA: Clinical decision making and multiple problem spaces. In Higgs J, Jones MA, Loftus S, Christensen N, editors: *Clinical reasoning in the health professions*, ed 3, Amsterdam, 2008, Butterworth Heinemann Elsevier, pp 3–18.

Higgs J, Andresen L, Fish D: Practice knowledge – its nature, sources and contexts. In Higgs J, Richardson B, Dahlgren MA, editors: *Developing practice knowledge for health professionals*, Edinburgh, 2004, Butterworth Heinemann, pp 51–69.

Higgs J, Jones M, Edwards I, Beeston S: Clinical reasoning and practice knowledge. In Higgs J, Richardson B, Dahlgren MA, editors: *Developing practice knowledge for health professionals*, Edinburgh, 2004, Butterworth Heinemann, pp 181–199.

Higgs J, Jones MA, Titchen A: Knowledge, reasoning and evidence for practice. In Higgs J, MA Jones, S Loftus, N Christensen, editors: *Clinical reasoning in the health professions*, ed 3, Amsterdam, 2008, Butterworth Heinemann Elsevier, pp 151–161.

Higgs J, Jones MA, Loftus S, Christensen N, editors: *Clinical reasoning in the health professions*, ed 3, Amsterdam, 2008, Butterworth Heinemann Elsevier.

Hooper B: The relationship between pretheoretical assumptions and clinical reasoning, *Am J Occup Ther* 51(5):328–337, 1997.

Imrie R: Demystifying disability: a review of the International Classification of Functioning, Disability and Health, *Sociol Health Illn* 26(3):287–305, 2004.

Jänig W, Levine JD: Autonomic-endocrine-immune interactions in acute and chronic pain. In McMahon SB, Koltzenburg M, editors: *Wall and Melzack's textbook of pain*, ed 5, Edinburgh, 2006, Elsevier Churchill Livingstone, pp 205–218.

Jeffreys E: *Prognosis in musculoskeletal injury. A handbook for doctors and lawyers*, Oxford, 1991, Butterworth-Heinemann.

Jensen GM, Shepard KF, Hack LM: The novice versus the experienced clinician: Insights into the work of the physical therapist, *Phys Ther* 70(5):314–323, 1990.

Jensen GM, Shepard KF, Gwyer J, Hack LM: Attribute dimensions that distinguish master and novice physical therapy clinicians in orthopedic settings, *Phys Ther* 72(10):711–722, 1992.

Jensen GM, Lorish CD, Shepard KF: Understanding and influencing patient receptivity to change: The patient-practitioner collaborative model. In Shepard KF, Jensen GM, editors: *Handbook of teaching for physical therapists*, ed 2, Boston, 2002, Butterworth-Heinemann, pp 323–350.

Jensen MP, Nielson WR, Turner JA, et al: Readiness to self-manage pain is associated with coping and with psychological and physical functioning among patients with chronic pain, *Pain* 104: 529–537, 2003.

Jensen GM, Gwyer J, Hack LM, Shepard KF: *Expertise in physical therapy practice*, ed 2, St Louis, 2007, Saunders Elsevier.

Jensen GM, Resnik L, Haddad A: Expertise and clinical reasoning. In Higgs J, Jones MA, Loftus S, Christensen N, editors: *Clinical Reasoning in the Health Professions*, ed 3, Amsterdam, 2008, Butterworth-Heinemann Elsevier, pp 123–135.

Jette AM: Toward a common language for function, disability, and health, *Phys Ther* 86(5):726–734, 2006.

Johnson R: 'Attitudes just don't hang in the air...' disabled people's perceptions of physiotherapists, *Physiotherapy* 79:619–626, 1993.

Johnson R, Moores L: Pain management: integrating physiotherapy and clinical psychology. In Gifford L, editor: *Topical issues in pain 5, Treatment, Communication, Return to Work, Cognitive Behavioural, Pathophysiology*, Falmouth, 2006, CNS Press, pp 311–319.

Jones MA: The clinical reasoning process in manipulative therapy. In Dalziel BA, Snowsill JC, editors: *Proceedings of the fifth biennial conference of the manipulative therapists association of Australia*, Melbourne, 1987, Manipulative Therapists Association of Australia, pp 62–69.

Jones MA: Clinical reasoning in manual therapy, *Phys Ther* 72(12):875–884, 1992.

Jones MA: Clinical reasoning and pain, *Man Ther* 1:17–24, 1995.

Jones MA: Clinical reasoning: The foundation of clinical practice. Part 1, *AJP* 43(3):167–170, 1997a.

Jones MA: Clinical reasoning: The foundation of clinical practice.

Part 2, *AJP* 43(3):213–217, 1997b.

Jones MA, Edwards I: Learning to facilitate change in cognition and behaviour. In Gifford L, editor: *Topical issues in pain 5*, Falmouth, 2006, CNS Press, pp 273–310.

Jones MA, Rivett DA: Introduction to clinical reasoning. In Jones MA, Rivett DADA, editors: *Clinical reasoning for manual therapists*, Edinburgh, 2004, Butterworth Heinemann, pp 3–24.

Jones MA, Edwards I, Gifford L: Conceptual models for implementing bio-psychosocial theory in clinical practice, *Man Ther* 7:2–9, 2002.

Jones MA, Grimmer K, Edwards I, et al: Challenges in applying best evidence to physiotherapy, *Internet J All Health Sci Prac* 4(3), 2006, Online, http://ijahsp.nova.edu/articles/vol4num3/jones.htm. [Accessed February 10, 2011].

Jones MA, Jensen G, Edwards I: Clinical reasoning in physiotherapy. In Higgs J, Jones MA, Loftus SS, Christensen N, editors: *Clinical reasoning in the health professions*, ed 3, Amsterdam, 2008, Butterworth Heinemann Elsevier, pp 245–256.

Jones M, van Kessel G, Swisher L, et al: Cognitive maps and the structure of observed learning outcome assessment of physiotherapy students' ethical reasoning knowledge, *Assess Eval High Educ* 2013. DOI:10.1080/02602938.2013.772951

Jorgensen P: Concepts of body and health in physiotherapy: the meaning of the social/cultural aspects of life, *Physiother Theory Pract* 16(2): 105–115. 2000.

Kaufman DR, Yoskowitz NA, Patel VL: Clinical reasoning and biomedical knowledge: implications for teaching. In Higgs J, Jones MA, Loftus S, Christensen N, editors: *Clinical Reasoning in the Health Professions*, ed 3, Amsterdam, 2008, Butterworth-Heinemann Elsevier, pp 137–149.

Keefe F, Scipio C, Perri L: Psychosocial approaches to managing pain: current status and future directions. In Gifford L, editor: *Topical issues in pain 5: Treatment, communication, return to work, cognitive behavioural, pathophysiology*, Falmouth, 2006, CNS Press, pp 241–256.

Kempainen RR, Migeon MB, Wolf FM: Understanding our mistakes: a primer on errors in clinical reasoning, *Med Teach* 25(2): 177–181, 2003.

Kendall N, Watson P: Identifying psychosocial yellow flags and modifying management. In Gifford L, editor: *Topical Issues of Pain 2, Bio-psychosocial assessment and management, Relationships and pain*, Falmouth, 2000, CNS Press, pp 131–139.

Kessler RC, Andrews G, Colpe LJ, et al: Short screening scales to monitor population prevalences and trends in non-specific psychological distress, *Psychol Med* 32(6): 959–976, 2002.

Khan KM, Scott A: Mechanotherapy: how physical therapists' prescription of exercise promotes tissue repair, *Br J Sports Med* 43:247–251, 2009.

King G, Tucker MA, Baldwin P, et al: A life needs model of pediatric service delivery: services to support community participation and quality of life for children and youth with disabilities, *Phys Occup Ther Pediatr* 22(2):53–77, 2002.

Klaber Moffett JA, Richardson PH: The influence of the physiotherapist-patient relationship on pain and disability, *Physiother Theory Pract* 13:89–96, 1997.

Kleinman A, Brodwin PE, Good BJ, Good MJD: Pain as human experience, an introduction. In Good MJD, Brodwin PE, Good BJ, Kleinman A, editors: *Pain as human experience: An anthropological perspective*, Berkeley, 1992, University of California Press, pp 1–28.

Kuhn TS: *The Structure of Scientific Revolutions*, ed 2, Chicago, 1970, University of Chicago Press.

Ladyshewsky R, Jones MA: Peer coaching to generate clinical reasoning skills. In Higgs J, Jones MA, Loftus S, Christensen N, editors: *Clinical Reasoning in the Health Professions*, ed 3, Amsterdam, 2008, Butterworth-Heinemann Elsevier, pp 433–440.

Lave J, Wenger E: *Situated learning: Legitimate peripheral participation*, Cambridge, 1991, Cambridge University Press.

Lee D: *The pelvic girdle. An integration of clinical expertise and research*, Edinburgh, 2011, Churchill Livingstone Elsevier.

Lehrer J: *How we decide*, Boston, 2009, Mariner Books.

Leventhal H: The pain system: a multilevel model for the study of motivation and emotion, *Motiv Emot* 17:139–146, 1993.

Leventhal H, Meyer D, Nerenz D: The common sense representation of illness danger. In Rachman S, editor: *Contributions to Medical Psychology*, vol 2, New York, 1980, Pergamon Press, pp 7–30.

Linton SJ, Andersson T: Can chronic disability be prevented? A randomized trial of a cognitive-behavior intervention and two forms of information for patients with spinal pain, *Spine* 25:2825–2831, 2000.

Linton SJ, Hallden K: Can we screen for problematic back pain? A screening questionnaire for predicting outcome in acute and subacute back pain, *Clin J Pain* 14(3):209–215, 1998.

Linton SJ, Nordin E: A 5-year follow-up evaluation of the health and economic consequences of an early cognitive behavioural intervention for back pain: A randomised controlled trial, *Spine* 31(8):853–858, 2006.

Logerstedt D, Snyder-Mackler L, Ritter R, et al: Knee stability and movement coordination impairments: knee ligament sprain, *J Orthop Sports Phys Ther* 40(4): A1–A37, 2010.

Lorig K, Stewart A, Ritter P, et al: *Outcome Measures for Health Education and other Health Care Interventions*, Thousand Oaks, 1996, Sage Publications, pp 24–25, 41–45.

Lorig KR, Sobel DS, Ritter PL, et al: Effect of a self-management program for patients with chronic disease, *Eff Clin Pract* 4:256–262, 2001.

McCracken LM, Gross RT: The role of pain-related anxiety reduction in the outcome of multidisciplinary treatment for low back pain: Preliminary results, *J Occup Rehabil* 8:179–189, 1998.

McPoil T, Martin R, Cornwall M, et al: Heel pain–plantar fasciitis: clinical practice guidelines linked to the International Classification of Function, Disability, and Health from the Orthopedic Section of the American Physical Therapy Association, *J Orthop Sports Phys Ther* 38(4):A1–A18, 2008.

Mackinnon LT: *Advances in exercise immunology*, Champaign, 1999, Human Kinetics.

Main CJ: The Modified Somatic Perception Questionnaire (MSPQ), *J Psychosom Res* 27(6):503–514, 1983.

Main C, Watson P: The distressed and angry low back pain patient. In Gifford L, editor: *Topical Issues in Pain 3*, Falmouth, 2002, CNS Press, pp 175–192.

Main C, Sullivan M, Watson P: *Pain management: Practical applications of the bio-psychosocial perspective in clinical and occupational settings*, Edinburgh, 2008, Churchill Livingstone.

Maitland GD: *Vertebral Manipulation*, ed 5, London, 1986, Butterworth-Heinemann.

Maitland GD: The Maitland concept: assessment, examination, and treatment by passive movement. In Twomey LT, Taylor JR, editors: *Clinics in physical therapy. Physical therapy for the low back*, New York, 1987, Churchill Livingstone, pp 135–155.

Martin P: *The sickening mind: brain, behaviour, immunity and disease*, London, 1997, Harper Collins.

Mattingly C: The narrative nature of clinical reasoning, *Am J Occup Ther* 45:998–1005, 1991.

Mattingly C, Fleming MH: *Clinical reasoning: forms of inquiry in a therapeutic practice*, Philadelphia, 1994, F.A. Davis.

May BJ, Dennis JK: Expert decision making in physical therapy-a survey of practitioners, *Phys Ther* 71(3):190–206, 1991.

Melzack R: Pain and the neuromatrix in the brain, *J Dent Educ* 65(12):1378–1382, 2001.

Melzack R: Evolution of the neuromatrix theory of pain, *Pain Pract* 5:85–94. 2005.

Meyer RA, Ringkamp M, Campbell JN, Raja SN: Peripheral mechanisms of cutaneous nociception. In McMahon SB, Koltzenburg M, editors: *Wall and Melzack's textbook of pain*, ed 5, 2006, Elsevier, pp 3–34.

Mezirow J: *Fostering critical reflection in adulthood: A guide to transformative and emancipatory learning*, San Francisco, 1990, Jossey-Bass.

Mezirow J: *Transformative dimensions of adult learning*, San Francisco, 1991, Jossey-Bass.

Mezirow J: Learning to think like an adult: Core concepts of transformation theory. In Mezirow J, editor: *Learning as transformation: Critical perspectives on a theory in progress*, San Francisco, 2000, Jossey-Bass, pp 3–33.

Moseley GL: A pain neuromatrix approach to patients with chronic pain, *Man Ther* 8:1–11, 2003.

Moseley GL: Evidence for a direct relationship between cognitive and physical change during an education intervention in people with chronic low back pain, *Eur J Pain* 8:39–45, 2004.

Muncey H: Explaining pain to patients. In Gifford L, editor: *Topical issues in Pain 4 – Placebo and nocebo, pain management, muscles and pain*, Falmouth, 2002, CNS Press, pp 157–166.

Neuhaus BE: Ethical considerations in clinical reasoning: the impact of technology and cost containment, *Am J Occup Ther* 42:288–294, 1988.

Newell A, Simon HA: *Human problem solving*, Englewood Cliffs, 1972, Prentice-Hall.

Nicholas MK: The pain self-efficacy questionnaire: taking pain into account, *Eur J Pain* 11:153–163, 2007.

Nickerson RS, Perkins DN, Smith EE: *The teaching of thinking*, Hillsdale, 1985, Lawrence Erlbaum Associates.

Nijs J, Van Houdenhove B, Oostendorp RAB: Recognition of central sensitization in patients with musculoskeletal pain: Application of pain neurophysiology in manual therapy practice, *Man Ther* 15:135–141, 2010.

Osborn M, Smith JA: The personal experience of chronic benign lower back pain: An interpretative phenomenological analysis, *Br J Health Psychol* 3:65–83, 1998.

Patel VL, Groen G: Knowledge-based solution strategies in medical reasoning, *Cogn Sci* 10:91–116, 1986.

Patel VL, Groen GJ: The general and specific nature of medical expertise: A critical look. In Ericsson A, Smith JJ, editors: *Toward a general theory of expertise: prospects and limits*, New York, 1991, Cambridge University Press, pp 93–125.

Patel VL, Groen G, Frederiksen C: Differences between medical students and doctors in memory for clinical cases, *Med Educ* 20:3–9, 1986.

Paul R, Elder L: *The thinker's guide to: the art of Socratic questioning*, Dillon Beach, 2006, Foundation for Critical Thinking.

Paul R, Elder L: *A guide for educators to: Critical thinking competency standards*, Dillon Beach, 2007, Foundation for Critical Thinking.

Pavlin DJ, Rapp SE, Pollisar N: Factors affecting discharge time in adult outpatients, *Anesth Analg* 87: 816–826, 1998.

Payton OD: Clinical reasoning process in physical therapy, *Phys Ther* 65(6):924–928, 1985.

Payton OD, Nelson CE, Hobbs MSC: Physical therapy patients' perceptions of their relationships with health care professionals, *Physiother Theory Pract* 14:211–221, 1998.

Pincus T: The psychology of pain. In French SS, Sim J, editors: *Physiotherapy a Psychosocial Approach*, Edinburgh, 2004, Elsevier, pp 95–115.

Pincus T, Morley S: Cognitive-processing bias in chronic pain: a review and integration, *Psychol Bull* 127:599–617, 2001.

Radloff LS: The CES-D scale: a self depression scale for research in the general population, *Appl Psychol Measures* 1:385–401, 1977.

Resnik L, Jensen GM: Using clinical outcomes to explore the theory of expert practice in physical therapy, *Phys Ther* 83(12):1090–1106, 2003.

Revonsuo A: Consciousness, dreams and virtual realities, *Phil Psychol* 8(1):35–54, 1995.

Revonsuo A: *Inner presence. Consciousness as a biological phenomenon*, Cambridge, 2006, The MIT Press.

Rivett DA, Higgs J: Hypothesis generation in the clinical reasoning behavior of manual therapists, *J Phys Ther Educ* 11(1):40–45, 1997.

Rivett DA, Jones MA: Improving clinical reasoning in manual therapy. In MA Jones, DA Rivett, editors: *Clinical reasoning for manual therapists*, Edinburgh, 2004, Butterworth Heinemann, pp 3–24.

Rivett DA, Jones MA: Using case reports to teach clinical reasoning. In Higgs J, Jones MA, Loftus S, Christensen N, editors: *Clinical reasoning in the health professions*, ed 3, Amsterdam, 2008, Butterworth Heinemann Elsevier, pp 477–484.

Rodgers C: Defining reflection: Another look at John Dewey and reflective thinking, *Teach Coll Rec* 104(4):842–866, 2002.

Rumelhart DE, Ortony E: The representation of knowledge in memory. In Anderson RC, Spiro RJ, Montague WE, editors: *Schooling and the Acquisition of Knowledge*, Hillsdale, 1977, Lawrence Erlbaum, pp 99–135.

Sackett D, Straus S, Richardson W, et al: *Evidence-based medicine: How to practice and teach EBM*, ed 2, Edinburgh, 2000, Churchill Livingstone.

Salkovskis P: The cognitive approach to anxiety: threat beliefs, safety seeking behaviour, and the special case of health anxiety and obsessions. In Salkovskis P, editor: *Frontiers of Cognitive Therapy*, London, 1996, The Guilford Press, pp 48–74.

Sapolsky RM: *Why zebras don't get ulcers. An updated guide to stress, stress-related diseases, and coping*, New York, 1998, Freeman.

Schaible H-G: Basic mechanisms of deep somatic pain. In McMahon SB, Koltzenburg M, editors: *Wall and Melzack's textbook of pain*, ed 5, 2006, Elsevier, pp 621–633.

Schön DA: *The reflective practitioner*, New York, 1983, Basic Books.

Schön DA: *Educating the reflective practitioner: Toward a new design for teaching and learning in the professions*, San Francisco, 1987, Jossey-Bass.

Schmidt H, Norman G, Boshuizen H: A cognitive perspective on medical expertise: Theory and implications, *Acad Med* 65(10):611–620, 1990.

Scott I: Teaching clinical reasoning: a case-based approach. In Higgs J, Jones MA, editors: *Clinical reasoning in the health professions*, ed 2, Oxford, 2000, Butterworth Heinemann, pp 290–297.

Sharp TJ: The "safety seeking behaviours" construct and its application to chronic pain, *Behav Cogn Psychother* 29:241–244, 2001.

Shepard KF, Jensen GM: *Handbook of teaching for physical therapists*, ed 2, Oxford, 2002, Butterworth-Heinemann.

Sim J, Smith MV: The sociology of pain. In French S, Sim J, editors: *Physiotherapy a Psychosocial Approach*, Edinburgh, 2004, Elsevier, pp 117–139.

Skelton JA, Croyle RT: Mental representation, health, and illness: an Introduction. In Skelton JA, Croyle RT, editors: *Mental Representation in Health and Illness*, New York, 1991, Springer-Verlag, pp 1–9.

Sluijs EM: Patient education in physiotherapy: towards a planned approach, *Physiotherapy* 77:503–508, 1991.

Smart KM, Blake C, Staines A, et al: Mechanisms-based clasificaitons of musculoskeletal pain: Part 3 of 3: Symptoms and signs of nociceptive pain in patients with low back (+/– leg) pain, *Man Ther* 17(4):352–357, 2012a.

Smart KM, Blake C, Staines A, et al: Mechanisms-based classifications of musculoskeletal pain: Part 2 of 3: Symptoms and signs of peripheral neuropathic pain in patients with low back (+/– leg) pain, *Man Ther* 17(4):345–351, 2012b.

Smart KM, Blake C, Staines A, et al: Mechanisms-based classifications of musculoskeletal pain: Part 1 of 3: Symptoms and signs of central sensitisation in patients with low back (+/– leg) pain, *Man Ther* 17(4):336–344, 2012c.

Smiths MS, Wallston KA, Smith CA: Development and validation of the perceived health competence scale, *Health Educ Res* 10(1):51–64, 1995.

Stacey RD: *Strategic management and organizational dynamics*, London, 1996, Pitman Publishing.

Steen E, Haugli L: Generalised chronic musculoskeletal pain as a rational reaction to a life situation? *Theor Med* 21:581–599, 2000.

Steiner WA, Ryser L, Huber E, et al: Use of the ICF model as a clinical problem-solving tool in physical therapy and rehabilitation medicine, *Phys Ther* 82(11): 1098–1107, 2002.

Stewart J, Kempenaar L, Lauchalan D: Rethinking yellow flags, *Man Ther* 16:196–198, 2011.

Strong J, Unruh AM: Psychologically based pain management strategies. In Strong J, Unruh AM, Wright A, Baxter GDGD, editors: *Pain. A textbook for therapists*, Edinburgh, 2002, Churchill Livingstone, pp 169–185.

Thomas-Edding D: 'Clinical problem solving in physical therapy and its implications for curriculum development', Paper presented at the Tenth International Congress of the World Confederation of Physical Therapy, Sydney, Australia, 1987, May 17–22.

Trede F, Higgs J: Collaborative decision making. In Higgs J, Jones MA, Loftus S, Christensen N, editors: *Clinical reasoning in the health professions*, ed 3. Amsterdam, 2008, Butterworth Heinemann Elsevier, pp 31–41.

Turk DC, Flor H: The cognitive-behavioural approach to pain management. In McMahon SB, Koltzenburg M, editors: *Wall and Melzack's textbook of pain*, ed 5. Edinburgh, 2006, Elsevier Churchill Livingstone, pp 339–348.

Turk DC, Rudy TE: Cognitive factors and persistent pain: a glimpse into Pandora's box, *Cognit Ther Res* 16:99–122, 1992.

Unsworth CA: Clinical reasoning: how do pragmatic reasoning, worldview and client-centredness fit? *Br J Occup Ther* 67(1):10–19, 2004.

Van Wingerden BAM: *Connective tissue in rehabilitation*, Vaduz, 1995, Scipro Verlag.

Vicenzino B, Souvlis T, Wright A: Musculoskeletal pain. In Strong J, Unrush AM, Wright A, Baxter GD, editors: *Pain: A textbook for therapists*, Edinburgh, 2002, Churchill Livingstone, pp 327–349.

Vicenzino B, Hing W, Rivett D, Hall T: *Mobilisation with Movement, The art and the science*. Edinburgh, 2011, Churchill Livingstone.

Vlaeyen JWS, Linton SJ: Fear-avoidance and its consequences in chronic musculoskeletal pain: a state of the art, *Pain* 85:317–332, 2000.

Vlaeyen JWS, de Jong J, Geilen M, et al: The treatment of fear of movement/(Re)injury in chronic low back pain: Further evidence on the effectiveness of exposure in vivo, *Clin J Pain* 18:251–261, 2002.

Waddell G, Newton M, Henderson I, et al: A fear-avoidance belief's questionnaire (FABQ) and the role of fear-avoidance beliefs in chronic low back pain and disability, *Pain* 52:157–168, 1993.

Watts NT: Teaching the components of clinical decision analysis in the classroom and clinic. In Higgs J, Jones M, editors: *Clinical reasoning in the health professions*, Oxford, 1995, Butterworth-Heinemann, pp 204–212.

Wenger E: *Communities of practice: Learning, meaning, and identity*, Cambridge, 1998, Cambridge University Press.

Werner D: Disabled persons as leaders in the problem solving process. In *Nothing about us without us: Developing innovative technologies for, by and with disabled persons*, Palo Alto, 1998, Health Wrights.

Woby SR, Roach NK, Urmston M, Watson PJ: Psychometric properties of the TSK-11: a shortened version of the Tampa Scale for Kinesiophobia, *Pain* 117(1–2): 137–144, 2005.

World Health Organization: *International classification of functioning, disability and health*, Geneva, 2001, World Health Organization.

Williams DA, Keefe FJ: Pain beliefs and the use of cognitive-behavioral coping strategies, *Pain* 46:185–190, 1991.

Wilson P, Henry J, Nicholas M: Cognitive methods in the management of chronic pain and tinnitus, *Aust Psychol* 28:172–180, 1993.

Wolf CJ: Central sensitization: Implication for diagnosis and treatment of pain, *Pain* 152:s2–215, 2011.

Wright A: Neurophysiology of pain and pain modulation. In Strong J, Unrush AM, Wright A, Baxter GD, editors: *Pain: A textbook for therapists*, Edinburgh, 2002, Churchill Livingstone, pp 43–64.

Zimmerman BJ, Lindberg C, Plsek PE: *Edgeware: Insights from complexity science for health care leaders*, ed 2, Irving, 2001, VHA Inc.

Communication and the therapeutic relationship

3

Elly Hengeveld   Geoffrey D. Maitland

CHAPTER CONTENTS

A review of the relevance of the
therapeutic relationship in physiotherapy
literature 83

Aspects of communication and
interaction. 86

Shaping of interactions 89

Communication techniques. 90

Process of collaborative goal setting. 94

Critical phases in the therapeutic
process. 95

Verbatim examples of various phases in
the therapeutic process. 98

 Key words

Verbal communication, non-verbal communication,
interaction, therapeutic relationship, critical phases of
the therapeutic process

Introduction

As described in former editions of Maitland's work
(Maitland 1986, 1991), well-developed communication skills are essential elements of the physiotherapy process. They serve several purposes:

- To aid the process of information-gathering
  with regard to physiotherapy diagnosis,

treatment planning and reassessment
of results
- To possibly help develop a deeper understanding
  of the patient's thoughts, beliefs and feelings
  with regard to the problem. This information
  assists in the assessment of psychosocial aspects
  which may hinder or enhance full recovery of
  movement functions
- Empathic communication with the above-
  mentioned objectives also enhances the
  development of a therapeutic relationship.

Therapeutic relationship

Based on changing insights on pain as a multidimensional experience, the therapeutic relationship is
considered to have increasing relevance in physiotherapy literature. It is debated that interpersonal
communication, next to academic knowledge and
technical expertise, constitutes one of the cornerstones of the art of health professions (Gartland
1984a). Furthermore, it is considered that the physiotherapy process depends strongly on the interaction between the physiotherapist and the patient, in
which the relationship may be therapeutic in itself
(Stone 1991). The World Confederation of Physical
Therapy (WCPT 1999) describes the interaction
between patient and physiotherapist as an integral
part of physiotherapy, which aims to achieve a
mutual understanding. Interaction is seen as a 'prerequisite for a positive change in body awareness and
movement behaviours that may promote health and

wellbeing' (WCPT 1999, p. 9). The physiotherapist may be seen as a treatment modality next to the physical agents applied (Charmann 1989), in which all the physiotherapist's mental, social, emotional, spiritual and physical resources need to be used to establish the best possible helping relationship (Pratt 1989). It is recommended that every health professional establishes a therapeutic relationship with a client-centred approach, with empathy, unconditional regard and genuineness (Rogers 1980). In particular, empathy and forms of self-disclosure by the therapist are seen as important elements of a healing environment (Schwartzberg 1992) in which markedly empathic understanding may support patients to disclose their feelings and thoughts regarding the problem for which they are seeking the help of a clinician (Merry & Lusty 1993).

The physiotherapist's role in the therapeutic relationship

It is recognized that within the therapeutic process a physiotherapist may take on a number of different roles:

- Curative
- Prophylactic
- Palliative (KNGF 1998)
- Educational (French et al. 1994, KNGF 1998)
- Counselling (Lawler 1988).

In relation to counselling it is argued that physiotherapists may often be involved in counselling situations, without being fully aware of it (Lawler 1988). The use of counselling skills may be considered as distinct from acting as a counsellor, the latter being a function of psychologists, social workers or psychiatrists (Burnard 1994). However, it is recommended that every clinician learns to use counselling skills within their framework of clinical practice (Horton & Bayne 1998).

It appears that over the years of clinical experience physiotherapists view their roles with regard to patients differently. As junior physiotherapists they may consider themselves more in an expert, curative role, providing treatment from the perspective of their professional expertise, while more senior physiotherapists seem to endeavour to meet patients' preferences of therapy (Mead 2000) and engage more in social interactions with the patients (Jensen et al. 1990), thus considering themselves more in the role of a guide or counsellor.

The positive effects of a therapeutic relationship are seen in:

- Actively integrating a patient in the rehabilitation process (Mattingly & Gillette 1991)
- Patient empowerment (Klaber Moffet & Richardson 1997)
- Compliance with advice, instructions and exercises (Sluys et al. 1993)
- Outcomes of treatment, such as increased self-efficacy beliefs (Klaber Moffet & Richardson 1997)
- Building up trust to reveal information which the patient may consider as discrediting (French 1988)
- Trust to try certain fearful activities again or re-establishing self-confidence and wellbeing (Gartland 1984b).

Notwithstanding this, the therapeutic relationship is often seen as a non-specific effect of treatment, meeting prejudice in research and being labelled as a placebo effect, which needs to be avoided (Van der Linden 1998). However, it is argued that each form of treatment in medicine knows placebo responses, which need to be investigated more deeply and used positively in therapeutic settings (Wall 1994). These placebo effects seem to be determined more by characteristics of the clinician than by features of the patients, such as friendliness, reassurance, trustworthiness, showing concern, demonstrating expertise and the ability to establish a therapeutic relationship (Grant 1994).

Research and the therapeutic relationship

In spite of an increasing number of publications, relatively few physiotherapy texts seem to deal explicitly with the therapeutic relationship when compared with occupational therapy or nursing literature. A CINAHL database search over the period 1989–2012 under the key words 'patient–therapist relationship AND physical therapy' and 'therapeutic relationship AND physical therapy' was performed: 14 entries (from a total of 1021 entries dealing with 'patient–therapist relationship'), and seven entries (compared with 150 entries under the heading 'therapeutic relationship') respectively, were published in physiotherapy-related journals. This notion is confirmed by Roberts and Bucksey (2007). In an observational study they investigated the content and prevalence of communication between therapists and patients with back pain. They identified verbal and non-verbal behaviours as observable tools for observation and video analysis, but they conclude that communication is an extremely important element of the therapeutic relationship, but underexplored in scientific research. Nevertheless, the World Confederation of Physical Therapy in the *Description of Physical Therapy* (1999) declared the interaction with the patient as an integral part of physiotherapy practice, and the Chartered Society of Physiotherapy in Great Britain, in the third edition of its *Standards of Physiotherapy Practice*, emphasizes the relevance of a therapeutic relationship and communication as key components of the therapeutic process (Mead 2000). These viewpoints seem to be shared by the majority of physiotherapists in Sweden. In a study with primary qualitative research and consequently a questionnaire with Likert-type answers, it was concluded that the majority of physiotherapists attributed many effects of the treatment to the therapeutic relationship and the patient's own resources rather than to the effects of treatment techniques alone (Stenmar & Nordholm 1997).

It is recommended that within a therapeutic relationship patients need to be treated as equals and experts in their own right, and that their reports on pain need to be believed and acted upon. Opportunities need to be provided to communicate, to talk with and listen to the patients about their problems, needs and experiences. In addition, independence needs to be encouraged in choosing personal treatment goals and interventions within a process of setting goals *with* rather than *for* a patient (Mead 2000).

Various studies have been undertaken with elements of the therapeutic relationship among patients and physiotherapists. In various surveys of patients it was concluded that patients appreciated positive regard and willingness to give information next to professional skills and expertise (Kerssens et al. 1995), communication skills and explanations on their level of thinking about their problem, and treatment goals and effects as well as confidentiality with the information given (de Haan et al. 1995). In a qualitative study on elements of quality of physiotherapy practice, patient groups regarded the ability to motivate people and educational capacities as essential aspects (Sim 1996).

Besley et al. (2011) identified in a literature study key features of a therapeutic relationship, which included: patient expectations with regard to the therapeutic process and outcomes; personalized therapy regarding acceptance in spite of cultural differences and holistic practice; partnership, relating to trust, mutual respect, knowledge exchange, power balance and active involvement of the patient; physiotherapist roles and responsibilities, including the activation of patients' own resources, being a motivator and educator and the professional manner of the therapist; congruence between the therapist and patient, relating to goals, problem identification and treatment; communication, in particular non-verbal communication, active listening and visual aids; relationship/relational aspects, encompassing friendliness, empathy, caring, warmth and faith that the therapist believes the patient; and influencing factors, as waiting time, quick access to the therapist, having enough time allocated to the sessions, knowledge and skills of therapist.

Hall et al. (2010), in another review on the influence of the therapeutic relationship on treatment outcomes, concluded that particularly beneficial effects could be found in treatment compliance, depressive symptoms, treatment satisfaction and physical function.

The therapeutic relationship and physiotherapy education and practice

Indications exist that various dimensions of the therapeutic relationship are neglected in physiotherapy education and practice. In a qualitative study in Great Britain among eight physiotherapists offering low back pain education it was concluded that only one participant followed a patient-centred approach, with active listening to the needs of the patients, while the remaining physiotherapists followed a therapist-centred approach (Trede 2000). In a survey among physiotherapists in The Netherlands it was concluded that almost all physiotherapists felt that insufficient communication skills training had been given during their undergraduate education (Chin et al. 1993). Furthermore, in a qualitative study the participants felt that aspects of dealing with intimacy during daily clinical encounters between patients and physiotherapists have been neglected (Wiegant 1993). In a qualitative study among clinical instructors of undergraduate physiotherapy students it was noted that the clinical supervisors preferred to give feedback to the students on technical skills rather than on social skills (Hayes et al. 1999). This may have the consequence that some students will never learn about the relevance of the therapeutic relationship in the physiotherapy process and later will not make the elements of this relationship explicit in their clinical reasoning processes.

Often physiotherapists consider communication as a by-product in therapy and don't consider this as 'work' (Hengeveld 2000); for example, 'every time the patient attended she had so many questions that it cost 10 minutes of my treatment time and I could not start working with her'.

A study with interviews of 34 recipients of physiotherapy treatment showed that patients not only appreciate the outcomes of care but also the process in which therapy has been delivered. The following elements were identified as key dimensions that contribute to patient satisfaction with physiotherapeutic treatment:

- *Professional and personal manner* of the therapist (friendly, sympathetic, listening, respectful, skilled, thorough, inspiring confidence)
- *Explaining and teaching* during each treatment (identifying the problem, guidance to self-management, process of treatment, prognosis)
- How the *treatment was consultative* (patient involvement in the treatment process, responses to questions, responsiveness to self-help needs)
- The *structure* and time with the therapist (e.g. short waiting time, open access and enough time)
- The *outcome* (treatment effectiveness and gaining self-help strategies).

It is concluded that it is essential to establish expectations, values and beliefs with regard to physiotherapy treatment in order to optimize patient satisfaction with the delivered treatment (May 2001).

In order to develop a fruitful therapeutic relationship, well-developed communication skills and an awareness of some critical phases of the therapeutic process are essential.

Communication and interaction

Most people consider that communication between two people who speak the same language is simple, routine, automatic and uncomplicated. However, even in normal day-to-day communications there are many instances in which misunderstandings occur. Even if the same words are being used, they may have different meanings to the individuals involved in the communication.

Communication may be seen as a process of sending messages, which have to be decoded by the receiver of these messages. A message may contain various aspects: the content of the message, an appeal, an indication of the relationship to the person to whom the message is addressed, and revealing something about the sender of the message (Schulz von Thun 1981). This follows some of the axioms on communication as defined by Watzlawick in which it is discussed that 'non-communication does not exist' – in other words, communication always takes place, whether the participants are aware of it or not. Every communication bears aspects of content and relationship, and human communication follows digital and analogue modalities, the latter referring to verbal and non-verbal communication, which ideally should occur congruently (Watzlawick et al. 1969).

Many errors in communication occur as a result of different understanding and interpretation as well as to the selection of words. The cartoon depicted in Figure 3.1 highlights some of the difficulties which may occur during verbal communication. The last three lines in the cartoon bear greatest significance. This could be saying, 'What I said was so badly worded that it did not express the thought that was in my mind', or it is possible that the receiver tuned in, or listened closely only to those parts of the message that fitted their own way of thinking, and ignored other parts that did not. It is also possible that the receiver's expectations or frame of mind altered their perception.

The feedback loop of Figure 3.2 indicates some of the coding errors which may occur during a communication between a 'sender' and a 'receiver' of a message.

Communication, as any other skill in clinical work, is an ability which can be learned and refined by continuous practice. Attention to one level of communication (e.g. content and meaning of words) can be practised step by step, until a high level of skill in uncovering meanings is developed. A good way of discovering more about an individual style of interviewing and communication is to record it on video or audiotape. Play it back to yourself and to constructive peers and supervisors.

I know that you believe you understand what you think I said, but, I am not sure you realize that what you heard is not what I meant!

Figure 3.1 • One of the problems of communication.

The skill must be developed to a high level if a patient's problem is to be understood without any detail being missed. The learning of this skill requires patience, humility, clarity and constructive self-criticism. Words, phrases and intonation need to be chosen carefully when asking questions to avoid being misunderstood, and patients must be listened to carefully so that the meanings of the words they use are not misinterpreted (Maitland 1986). Attention needs to be given not only to *what* is said, but also to *how* it is said (Main 2004), including a careful observation of the body language of the patient.

The physiotherapist should not be critical of the way a patient presents. The very presentation *itself* is a message, needing to be decoded in the same way as the many other findings that the subjective and physical examinations reveal. Various elements may lead to misinterpretation of the severity of the patient's symptoms and/or disability.

The various ways that a person may experience pain or limitation of activities may lead to different expressions of pain behaviour. Some may seem stoic and do not appear to experience much distress, while others seem to suffer strongly and have high anxiety levels. The way people express pain, distress or suffering may be due to learning factors, including

the family and the culture in which the person has been brought up. If patients are not fluent in the language of the examiner, their non-verbal expression to explain what is being experienced may be more exaggerated from the perspective of the examiner. Some patients will comment only on the symptoms that remain and do not comment on other aspects of the symptoms or activity levels that may have improved. The skilled physiotherapist can seek the positive side of the symptomatic changes rather than accepting the more negative approach of the patient. Overall, it is essential for the physiotherapist to develop an attitude of unconditional regard towards the patient and the situation, as suggested by Rogers (1980), even if the physiotherapist does not fully understand the patient's behaviour and manners with regard to pain and disability.

Aspects of communication

Communication consists of various components:

- Verbal components
- Non-verbal components, such as tone of voice, body posture and movements and so on.

It is important that the physiotherapist creates a setting in which a free flow of communication is possible, allowing an uncomplicated exchange of information. Attention to the physical distance to the patient, not too far and not too close, often enhances the process of information gathering. At times a gentle touch will allow a quicker exchange of information, for example when the physiotherapist would like to know which areas of the body are free of symptoms. The physiotherapist may gently touch, for example, the knee of a patient in order to interrupt their somewhat garrulous dialogue, so they can highlight an important aspect of the information given or seek further clarification.

Congruence of verbal and non-verbal communication is essential. Eye contact is important, as is a safe environment in which not too many outside disturbances hinder the establishing of an atmosphere in which patients can develop trust to disclose information which they think might be compromising.

It is important that the physiotherapist pays attention not only to *what* is said, but also to *how* it is said. Often the body posture or the intonation of the voice or certain key words and phrases give indications of the individual illness experience, especially if certain words are used which may have a

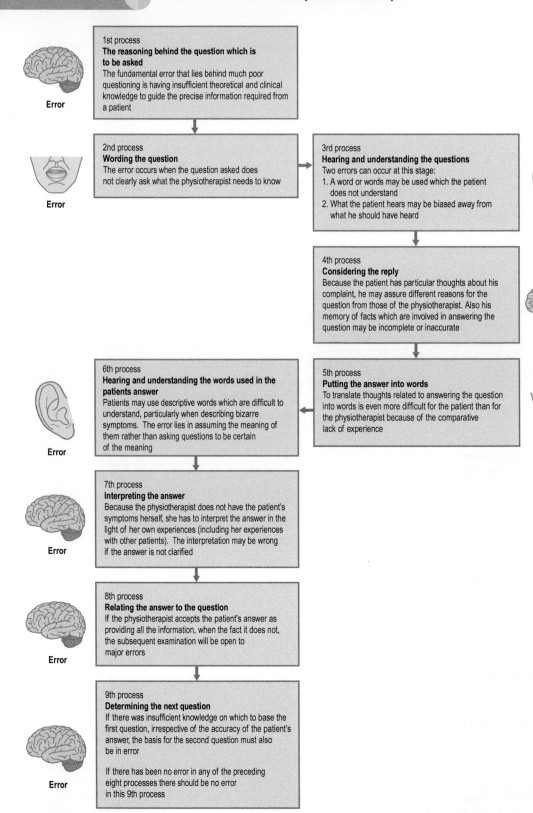

Error

1st process
The reasoning behind the question which is to be asked
The fundamental error that lies behind much poor questioning is having insufficient theoretical and clinical knowledge to guide the precise information required from a patient

Error

2nd process
Wording the question
The error occurs when the question asked does not clearly ask what the physiotherapist needs to know

3rd process
Hearing and understanding the questions
Two errors can occur at this stage:
1. A word or words may be used which the patient does not understand
2. What the patient hears may be biased away from what he should have heard

Error

4th process
Considering the reply
Because the patient has particular thoughts about his complaint, he may assure different reasons for the question from those of the physiotherapist. Also his memory of facts which are involved in answering the question may be incomplete or inaccurate

Error

6th process
Hearing and understanding the words used in the patients answer
Patients may use descriptive words which are difficult to understand, particularly when describing bizarre symptoms. The error lies in assuming the meaning of them rather than asking questions to be certain of the meaning

Error

5th process
Putting the answer into words
To translate thoughts related to answering the question into words is even more difficult for the patient than for the physiotherapist because of the comparative lack of experience

Error

7th process
Interpreting the answer
Because the physiotherapist does not have the patient's symptoms herself, she has to interpret the answer in the light of her own experiences (including her experiences with other patients). The interpretation may be wrong if the answer is not clarified

Error

8th process
Relating the answer to the question
If the physiotherapist accepts the patient's answer as providing all the information, when the fact it does not, the subsequent examination will be open to major errors

Error

9th process
Determining the next question
If there was insufficient knowledge on which to base the first question, irrespective of the accuracy of the patient's answer, the basis for the second question must also be in error

If there has been no error in any of the preceding eight processes there should be no error in this 9th process

Error

Figure 3.2 • Feedback loop.

more emotional content (e.g. 'it is all very terrible'). These may be clues to the patient's world of thoughts, feelings and emotions, which may be contributing factors to ongoing disability due to pain (Kendall et al. 1997). Attention to these aspects often allows the physiotherapist to perform a psychosocial assessment as an integral part of the overall physiotherapy-specific assessment.

As pointed out in various chapters of this edition and in Hengeveld & Banks (2014), many details are asked in order to be able to make a diagnosis of the movement disorder and its impact on the patient's life. Critics may say that the patient will not be able to provide all this information. However, it has long been a principle of the Maitland Concept that the *body has the capacity to inform*. If the physiotherapist carefully shapes the interview, pays attention to details such as selection of words and body language and explains regularly why certain questions or interventions are necessary, the patient will learn what information is of special relevance to the physiotherapist and pay attention to this.

Shaping of interactions

During the overall series of treatment, as well as in each session, it is important that the physiotherapist shapes the interaction deliberately, if a conscious nurturing of the therapeutic relationship seems necessary.

As in other counselling situations, each series of therapy, as well as each treatment session, knows three phases of interaction (Brioschi 1998):

- *Initial phase* – a 'joining' between physiotherapist and patient takes place on a more personal level in order to establish a first contact; personal expectations are established; the patient's questions may be addressed; the specific objectives of physiotherapy or of the session are explained; the specific setting is clarified (e.g. number of sessions, treatment in an open or closed room). The first subjective and physical examinations or the subjective reassessment takes place. It is essential that in this phase the (ongoing) process of collaborative goal setting has started.
- *Middle phase* – working on the treatment objectives and using interventions in a collaborative way; regular reassessment to confirm the positive effects of the selected treatment interventions. It is important that all

aspects of goal setting, selection of interventions and reassessment parameters are defined in a collaborative problem-solving process between the physiotherapist and the patient.

- *End phase* of the session or of the treatment series – summary; attention to the patient's questions; recommendations, instructions or self-management strategies including reassessment; addressing of organizational aspects. Often it is very useful to ask the patient to reflect on what has been particularly useful in the current treatment session or series and what has been learned so far.

Often both the information and the end phase (including the final analytical assessment in the last sessions of the treatment series) seem to be neglected, mostly due to lack of time. However, once the more explicit procedures of the session are finished, towards the end of the session the patient often reveals information on the individual illness experience which may be highly essential for the therapy. The following example highlights this aspect.

A 72-year-old lady presents to the physiotherapist with a hip problem. Joint mobilizations in lying and muscle recruitment exercises in sitting and standing are performed. At the end of the session, when saying goodbye, the lady tells the physiotherapist that she was going to visit her daughter in another town. However, she was not confident in getting on a bus, as the steps were so high and the drivers would move off too quickly before she was even seated. On the levels of disability and activity resources, as defined by the *International Classification of Functioning, Disability and Health* (WHO 2001), it was more relevant to redefine goals of treatment on activity and participation levels and for the patient to practise actually walking to and finding trust on entering the bus, rather than working solely on the functional impairments in the physiotherapy practice. This information was not given in the initial examination session, in spite of deliberate questioning by the physiotherapist.

Shaping of a therapeutic climate: listening and communication

In order to stimulate a safe environment in which a free flow of information can take place, the development of listening skills is essential. Therapists may well hear what they expect to hear rather than listening to the words the patient uses. The following quotation may serve to underline this principle:

> Listening is itself, of course, an art: that is where it differs from merely hearing. Hearing is passive; listening is active. Hearing is voluntary, listening demands attention. Hearing is natural, listening is an acquired discipline.
>
> *(The Age* 1982)

It is essential to develop the skills of active and passive listening:

- *Passive listening* means showing that the therapist is listening, with body posture directed towards the patient, maintaining eye contact, and allowing the patient to finish speaking.
- *Active listening* encourages patients to tell their story and allows the therapist to seek further clarification.

Active listening may include clarifying questions such as 'Could you tell me more about this?', repetition and summary of relevant information such as 'If I have understood you correctly, you would like to be able to play tennis again and find more trust in riding your bicycle?', or asking questions with regard to the personal illness experience, for example, 'How do you feel about your back hurting for so long?'

With active and passive listening skills the therapist can show that they have understood the patient.

In order to shape a therapeutic climate of unconditional regard (Rogers 1980), it is essential that the responses and reactions of the therapist are non-judgemental and neutral. Irony, playing the experience of the patient down, talking too much of oneself, giving maxims, threatening ('if you won't do this then your back will never recuperate') or just lack of time may jeopardize the development of the therapeutic relationship (Keel 1996, cited in Brioschi 1998).

If patients reveal personal information, it is essential that they are given the freedom to talk as much about it as they feel necessary. At all times the physiotherapist should avoid forcing patients to reveal personal information which they would rather have kept to themselves. This may happen if the physiotherapist asks exploratory questions too aggressively. Some excellent publications with regard to 'sensitive practice' have been published, and are recommended for further exploration of this issue (Schachter et al. 1999).

Giving advice too quickly, offering a single solution, talking someone into a decision or even commanding may hinder the process of activating the patient's own resources in the problem-solving process. If possible, it is better to *guide* people by *asking questions* rather than *telling* them what to do. This is particularly essential in the process of collaborative goal setting in which the patient is actively integrated in defining treatment objectives. In this process it is important to define treatment objectives on activity and participation levels (WHO 2001) which are meaningful to the patient. Too frequently it seems that the physiotherapist is directive in the definition of treatment goals and in the selection of interventions (Trede 2000). Ideally the therapist may offer various interventions from the perspective of professional expertise to reach the agreed goals of treatment, and the decision is left to the patient to decide which solution may be best for the problem.

Communication techniques

Communication is both a skill and an art. Various communication techniques may be employed to enhance the flow of information and the development of the therapeutic relationship.

- Style of questions:
  - Open questions (e.g. 'What is the reason for your visit?')
  - Questions with aim (e.g. 'Could you describe your dizziness more?', 'What do you mean by pinched nerves?')
  - Half-open questions – as suggested in the subjective examination. The questions are posed with an aim, but they leave the patient the freedom to answer spontaneously. These questions often start with *how, when, what, where* (e.g. 'How did it start?', 'When do you feel it most?', 'What impact does it have on your daily life?', 'Where do you feel it at night?')
  - Alternative questions – leave the patient a limited choice of responses (e.g. 'Is the pain only in your back or does it also radiate to your leg?')
  - Closed questions – can only be answered with yes or no (e.g. 'Has the pain got any better?')

○ Suggestive questions – leave the patient little possibility for self-expression (e.g. 'But you *are* better, aren't you?')

It may be necessary to employ a mixture of question styles in the process of gathering information. Half-open questions and questions with aim may provide information concerning biomedical and physiotherapy diagnosis; frequently, however, they are too restricting if the physiotherapist wants to get an understanding of the patient's thoughts, feelings and beliefs with regard to the individual illness experience and psychosocial assessment. Such questions may provoke answers of social desirability or the patient may not reveal what is actually being experienced:

- Modulation of the voice and body language – as described before
- Summarizing of information – in the initial phase this technique is often useful during the subjective examination in various stages: after the completion of the main problem and 'body chart', after the establishment of the behaviour of symptoms, after completion of the history and as a summary of the subjective and physical examinations
- Mirroring – in which the physiotherapist neutrally reports what is observed or heard from the patient
- (Short) pauses before asking a question or giving an answer
- Repetition (with a question) of key words or phrases.

Probably the first requirement during interviews with patients is that the physiotherapist should retain control of the interview. Even if the physiotherapist decides to employ forms of 'narrative clinical reasoning' rather than procedural clinical reasoning (Chapter 2), it is necessary that the physiotherapist keeps an overview of the individual story of the patient and the given information which is particularly relevant to establish a diagnosis of a movement disorder and its contributing factors.

It is essential to use the patient's language whenever possible, as this makes things that are said or asked much clearer and easier to understand.

A versatile physiotherapist can develop various ways to stop or interrupt a more garrulous patient, by making statements such as 'I was interested to hear about X, could you tell me more?' Another possibility may be gently touching the patient's knee before stating, 'I would like to know more about

this'. Interposing a question at a volume slightly higher than the patient's or with the use of non-verbal techniques such as raising a hand, making a note, or touching a knee, tends to interrupt the chain of thought and this may be employed if the spontaneous information does not seem to be forthcoming. More reticent patients need to be told kindly that it seems they find it hard to talk about their complaints but that it is necessary for them to do so. They should be reassured that they are not complaining, but *informing*.

The following strategies are important to keep in mind during the interview:

- Speak slowly
- Speak deliberately
- Use the patient's language and wording, if possible
- Keep questions short
- Ask only one question at a time
- Pose the questions in such a manner that as much as possible spontaneous information can be given (see above).

Paralleling

When a patient is talking about an aspect of their problem, their mind is running along a specific line of thought. It is likely that the patient could have more than one point they wish to express. To interrupt the patient may make them lose their place in their story. Therefore, unless the physiotherapist is in danger of getting confused, the patient should not be stopped if at all possible while the therapist follows the patient's line of thought. However, a novice in the field may rather first practice the basic procedures of interviewing, as paralleling is a skill which is learned by experience. Paralleling may be a time-consuming procedure if the patient starts off with a long history of, for example, 20 years. It may then be useful to interrupt and ask the patient what the problem is *now* and why help is being sought from the physiotherapist *now* – and from then on the physiotherapist may use the technique of paralleling.

Paralleling means that, from the procedural point of view the physiotherapist would like to get information (e.g. about the localization of symptoms), whereas the patient is talking about the behaviour of the symptoms. However, using 'paralleling' techniques does not mean that the physiotherapist should let the patient talk on without seeking clarification or using the above-mentioned communication techniques.

Immediate-response questions

At times the employment of immediate-response questions is essential. If during the first consultation a patient gives important information with regard to the planning of physical examination and treatment, immediate-response questions may be needed. Example:

> Patient: 'I feel it mostly with quick movements.'
> Therapist: 'Quick movements of what?'

Follow the patient's answer with: 'In what direction?', or: 'Are you able to show me that quick movement now?' The information on the area of the movement and the direction of the movement may be decisive in the selection of treatment techniques.

During subsequent treatments in the reassessment phases, the physiotherapist is in a process with the patient of *comparing* changes in the symptoms and signs. Frequently, however, the patient may give information which is a 'statement of fact'. The patient may say, 'I had pain in my back while watching football on television'. This is a statement of fact and is of no value as an assessment, unless it is known what would have happened during 'watching television' before starting treatment. This statement demands an immediate-response question: 'How would you *compare* this with, for example, 3 weeks ago, when we first started treatment?' The patient may respond that in fact 3 weeks ago he was not able to watch television at all, as the pain in his back was too limiting. Using immediate-response questions during this phase of reassessment prevents time being wasted and valuable information being lost. If the physiotherapist employs this technique kindly but consistently in the first few treatment sessions, the patient may learn to *compare* changes in his condition rather than to express statements of fact. *At reassessment, convert statements of fact into comparisons!*

Furthermore, immediate-response questions may be needed with non-verbal responses. There are many examples in which the examiner must recognize a non-verbal response either to a question or to an examination movement. The physiotherapist must qualify such expressions. For example, in response to a question the patient may respond simply by a wrinkle of the nose. The

immediate-response question, in combination with a mirroring technique may be: 'I see that you wrinkled your nose – that doesn't look too good. Do you mean that it has been worse?' etc.

Key words and phrases

During patients' discourses they will frequently make a statement or use words that could have great significance – the patient may not realize it, but the therapist must latch onto it while the patient's thoughts are moving along the chosen path. The physiotherapist could use it either immediately by interjecting or by waiting until the patient has finished. For example, the therapist might say:

> Q 'You just mentioned your mother's birthday – what does that relate to?'
>
> A 'Well, I can remember that it was on my mother's birthday that I was first aware of discomfort in my shoulder when I reached across the table to pick up her birthday cake.'

By instantly making use of the patient's train of thought (paralleling) the development of the progressive history of the patient's shoulder pain is easier to determine for both the therapist and the patient, because, in fact, the patient's mind is clearly back at the birthday party.

As another example, having asked the question at subjective reassessment procedures, 'How have you been?', the patient may respond in a general and rather uninformative way. However, during subsequent statements the patient may include, for example, the word 'Monday'. This may mean something to the patient and therefore it is often effective to use it and ask, 'What was it about Monday?', or 'What happened on Monday?'

Bias

It is relatively easy to fall into the trap of asking a question in such a way that the patient is influenced to answer in a particular way. For example, the therapist may wish to know whether the last two sessions have caused any change in the patient's symptoms or activity levels. The question can be asked in various ways:

1. 'Do you feel that the last two treatments have helped you?'
2. 'Has there been any change in your symptoms as a result of the last two treatments?'
3. 'Have the last two treatments made you any worse in any way?'

The first and third questions are posed with aim, nevertheless they are suggestive. The first question, however, is biased in such a way that it may push the patient towards replying with 'yes'. The second and third questions are acceptable, as the second question has no specific bias and the third question biases the patient away from a favourable answer. Both questions allow the patient to give any spontaneous answer, even if the therapist is hoping that there has been some favourable change.

Purpose of the questions and assuming

Purpose of the questions

In efficient information gathering it is essential for the physiotherapist to be aware of the purpose of the questions – no question should be asked without an understanding of the basic information that can be gained (see Chapters 1 and 2 of this volume, and Chapters 1 and 2 of the Peripheral Manipulation volume). For beginners in the field it is essential to know which questions may support the generation of which specific hypotheses.

Before asking a question it is vital for the physiotherapist to be clear about several things:

1. What information is required and why?
2. What is the best possible way to word the question?
3. Which different answers might be forthcoming?
4. How the possible reply to this question might influence planning ahead for the next question.

A mistake that often occurs with trainee manipulative physiotherapists is the accepting of an answer as being adequate when in fact it is only vaguely informative, incomplete or of insufficient depth. The reason for accepting an inadequate answer is usually that trainee physiotherapists do not clearly understand why they are asking the question and therefore do not know the number of separate answers they must hear to meet the requirements of the question. The same reason can lead to another error: allowing a line of thought to be diverted by the patient, usually without realizing it.

Assuming

If a patient says that pain is 'constant', it is wrong to assume that this means constant throughout the day and night. The patient may mean that, when the pain is present, it is constant, but not all day long. It is important to check the more exact meaning: is it 'steady' or 'unchanging in degree', 'constant in location' or 'constant in time'?

Assuming may lead to one of the major errors in clinical reasoning processes: misinterpretation of information, leading to overemphasis or blinding out of certain information. Therefore it is well worth remembering: *never assume anything!*

Pain and activity levels

Sometimes the Maitland Concept is criticized for putting too much focus on the pain experience and some may state that 'talking about pain causes some people to develop more pain'.

If in examination and reassessment procedures the physiotherapist focuses solely on the pain sensation and omits to seek information on the level of activities, bias towards the pain sensation may occur and some patients may be influenced to focus mainly on their pain experience. It may then seem that they develop an increased bodily awareness and become more protective towards movements which may be painful. It is therefore essential that the physiotherapist establishes a balanced image of the pain including the concomitant activity limitations and resources. Sometimes the pain experience does not seem to improve and leaves the patient and physiotherapist with the impression that 'nothing helps'. However, if the level of activity normalizes and the patient may successfully employ some self-management strategies once the pain is experienced again, both the patient and physiotherapist may become aware of positive changes, *if* they look for them.

Some physiotherapists prefer, with some patients, not to talk about pain and to focus only on the level of activity and may even make a verbal contract with the patient to no longer talk about pain and only about function (Hengeveld 2000). However, often this is not of much help, as it denies one of the major complaints for which the patient is seeking therapy, and in fact it denies the most important personal experience of the patient. Nevertheless, in such cases it may be useful to use metaphors for the pain experience, wellbeing and activity levels. For example, rather than asking, 'How is your pain?', the therapist may ask, 'What does your body tell you now in comparison with before?' or, 'If the pain is like a high wave on the ocean in a storm, how is the wave now in comparison with before?'

On the other hand, some patients prefer to focus on their activities rather than on the pain sensation alone. The following statement was once overheard in a clinical situation:

> Patient to physiotherapist: 'You always talk about the pain. However it is like having a filling of a tooth – if I give it attention, I will notice it. However I still am able to eat normally with it.

thus indicating that, to the patient, it is important to be able to function fully and that he will accept some degree of discomfort.

The process of collaborative goal setting

As stated earlier, it is recommended that within a therapeutic relationship patients need to be treated as equals and experts in their own right. Within this practice following a process of collaborative goal setting is recommended (Mead 2000).

There are indications that compliance with the recommendations, instructions and exercises may increase if treatment objectives are defined in a collaborative rather than a directive way (Riolo 1993, Sluys et al. 1993, Bassett & Petrie 1997).

It is essential to consider collaborative goal setting as a *process* throughout all treatment sessions rather than a single moment at the beginning of the treatment series. In fact, ongoing information and goal setting may be considered essential elements of the process of informed consent.

Various agreements between the physiotherapist and patient may be made in the process of collaborative goal setting:

- Initially the physiotherapist and patient need to define treatment objectives collaboratively
- Additionally, the parameters to monitor treatment results may be defined in a collaborative way
- The physiotherapist and patient need to collaborate on the selection of interventions to achieve the desired outcomes
- In situations where 'sensitive practice' seems especially relevant, some patients may need to be given the choice of a male or a female physiotherapist or may express their preference regarding a more open or an enclosed treatment room (Schachter et al. 1999).

Frequently, physiotherapists may ask a patient at the end of the subjective examination what would be the goal of treatment. Often the response will be that the patient would like to have less pain and no further clarification of this objective takes place. In some cases this approach may be too superficial, especially if the prognosis is that diminution of pain intensity and frequency may not be easily achieved. This may be the case in certain chronic pain states or where secondary prevention of chronic disability seems necessary. Patients commonly state that their goal of treatment is 'having less pain'; however, after being asked some clarifying questions it often transpires that they wish to find more control over their wellbeing with regard to pain, in order to be able to perform certain activities again.

In the initial session during subjective examination, various stages occur in which collaborative goal setting may take place by the communication technique of summarizing:

- After the establishment of the main problem and the areas in which the patient may feel the symptoms
- After the establishment of the 24-hour behaviour of symptoms, activity levels and coping strategies
- After establishment of the history
- After completion of the physical examination (at this stage it is essential to establish treatment objectives collaboratively, not only in the reduction of pain, but also to define clear goals on the levels of activity which need to be improved and in which circumstances the patient may need self-management strategies to increase control over wellbeing and pain).

The relatively detailed process of collaborative goal setting needs to be continued during each session in its initial phase. It is essential to clarify if the earlier agreed goals are still to be followed up. If possible, it is useful to explain to the patient the diverse treatment options on how the goals may be achieved and then let the patient make the choice of the interventions.

Another phase of collaborative goal setting takes place in later stages during retrospective assessment procedures. In this phase a reconsideration of treatment objectives is often necessary. Initially the physiotherapist and patient may have agreed to work on improvement of pain, pain control with self-management strategies, educational strategies with regard to pain and movement, and to treat impairments of local functions, such as pain-free joint movement and muscular recruitment. In later stages it is essential to establish goals with regard to activities which are meaningful for the patient. If a patient is able to return to work after a certain period of sick leave, it is important to know about those activities which the patient seems most concerned about and where the patient expects to develop symptoms again. For example, an electrician who needs to kneel down in order to perform a task close to the floor may be afraid that in this case his back may start to hurt again. It may be necessary to include this activity in the training programme in combination with simple self-management strategies which can be employed immediately in the work-place.

This phase of retrospective assessment, including a prospective assessment with redefinition of treatment objectives on activity and participation levels, is considered one of the most important phases of the rehabilitation of patients with movement disorders (Maitland 1986).

To summarize, the process of collaborative goal setting should include the following aspects (Brioschi 1998):

- The reason for referral to physiotherapy
- The patient's definition of the problem, including goals and expectations
- Clarification of questions with regard to setting, frequency and duration of treatment
- Hypotheses and summary of findings of the physiotherapist, and clarification of the possibilities and limitations of the physiotherapist, resulting in agreements, collaborative goal definitions and a verbal or sometimes written treatment contract.

Critical phases of the therapeutic process

In order to shape the therapeutic process optimally, special consideration needs to be given to the information which is given to the patient and sought by the physiotherapist in specific phases of the therapeutic process. In fact, the educational task of the physiotherapist may start at the beginning of the first session in which the expectations of the patient towards physiotherapy need to be clarified.

If some of these critical phases are skipped it is possible that the process of actively integrating the patient into the therapeutic process is impeded. Attention to these phases supports the development of mutual trust and understanding, enhances the therapeutic relationship and aids in the development of a treatment plan. In these various stages regular interventions of collaborative goal setting should take place, clarifying step-by-step:

- The goals of treatment
- What possibilities exist to achieve these goals
- Where certain limitations may be present.

It is essential that the physiotherapist not only points out the possibilities of treatment, but also indicates, carefully and diplomatically, the possible limitations with regard to achievable goals. This is particularly essential in those cases where the patient seems to have almost unrealistic expectations of the physiotherapist, which it may not be possible to fulfil. Particularly with patients with chronic disability due to pain, it is frequently necessary to point out that the physiotherapy interventions may not necessarily be able to reduce the pain, but that the physiotherapist can work with them to find ways to establish more control over their wellbeing and to normalize the level of activities which are meaningful to them.

In general it is useful to pay attention to these critical phases in order to 'keep the patient on board'. It is stated that novices in the field tend to be more mechanical in their interactions with patients in which their own procedures seem to prevail above the direct interactions with the patient (Jensen et al. 1990, 1992, Thomson et al. 1997). However, it is essential that the patient understands the scope and limitations of physiotherapy as a movement science as well as the reason for certain questions and test procedures. At times it can be observed in supervision or examination situations that physiotherapists appear to be preoccupied with their procedures of examination, treatment, recording and reassessment and seem to forget to *explain* to patients what they are doing and why. It may happen in such cases that the patient is not able to distinguish between a reassessment and a treatment procedure. Furthermore, by paying attention to the information of some critical phases, the physiotherapist may address some 'yellow flags', which may hinder the full recovery of movement function. Secondary prevention of chronic disability may start with the welcoming and initial assessment of the patient's problem.

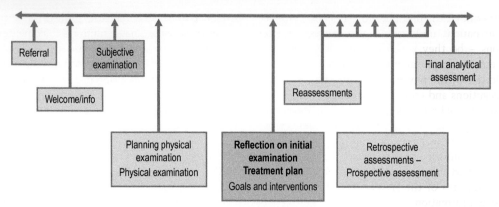

Figure 3.3 • Critical phases in the therapeutic process in which specific consideration is given to the information process.

The critical phases of the therapeutic process (Fig. 3.3) need specific consideration with regard to providing and gathering of information.

Welcoming and information phase

After some 'joining' remarks to help the patient feel at ease as a first step towards development of a therapeutic relationship, it is important to inform the patient in this phase about the specific movement paradigm of the physiotherapy profession – the 'clinical side' of the brick wall analogy of the Maitland Concept. The patient may have different beliefs or paradigms from the physiotherapist as to the causes of the problem and the optimum treatment strategies, which may create an implicit conflict situation if not clarified in time. The physiotherapist may explain this to the patient in the following way:

> I am aware that your doctor has seen you and diagnosed your problem as osteoarthritis of the hip and I have this diagnosis in the back of my head. However, my specific task as a physiotherapist is to examine and treat your movement functions. Maybe you have certain habits in your daily life, or you may have stiff joints or muscles which react too late. I need to ask some questions about this and I would like to look in more detail at your movements. Often when these movements improve, the pain of the osteoarthritis may also normalize. Is this what you yourself expected as a treatment for your problem?

Starting a session in this manner often prevents the patient from feeling irritation that the physiotherapist is starting off with an examination, when this may have already been done by the referring doctor. Furthermore, the patient may learn immediately that the physiotherapist follows a somewhat different perspective to problem-solving processes than a medical doctor. Too often patients do not understand that each member in an interdisciplinary team follows a unique frame of reference which is specific to their profession (Kleinmann 1988).

Some questions with regard to yellow flags may also be addressed with this information (Kendall et al. 1997, Main 2004):

- Is the patient expecting physiotherapy to help?
- Which beliefs does the patient have with regard to movement if something hurts?
- Does the patient feel that the problem has not been examined enough?

It is essential to be aware of certain key remarks indicating these points, for example, 'Well, the doctor did not even bother to make an X-ray…'. If these points are addressed early enough in the treatment series, some patients may start to develop trust and carefully embark on a treatment, which they initially may have approached sceptically, especially if they have already had various encounters with many different health-care practitioners (Main & Spanswick 2000).

Subjective examination

The subjective examination serves several purposes as described in the chapters on assessment and examination (see Chapters 1 and 2 of this volume, and Chapters 1 and 2 of the Peripheral Manipulation volume).

It is essential to pay attention not only to what is said but also to how things are said by the patient. Key words, gestures and phrases may open a window to the world of the individual illness experience, which may be decisive in treatment planning.

Furthermore, the physiotherapist needs to ensure that the patient understands the purpose of the questions – be they a baseline for comparison of treatment results in later reassessment procedures or indicative of the physiotherapy diagnosis, including precautions and contraindications.

Most essential are the various steps in collaborative goal setting, which preferably take place throughout the overall process of subjective examination. With information on the main problem and the 'body chart', the physiotherapist may develop a first general idea of the treatment objectives; with increasing information throughout the whole examination, this image of the various treatment goals should become more and more refined.

Planning of the physical examination

The planning phase between the subjective and the physical examination is crucial from various perspectives. The main objective of this phase is the planning of the physical examination in its sequence and dosage of the examination procedures. However, it is important to summarize the relevant points of the subjective examination first and then to describe the preliminary treatment objectives on which the patient and the physiotherapist have agreed so far. Furthermore, it is essential to explain to the patient the purpose of the physical examination.

Physical examination

In order to integrate the patient actively in this phase of examination, it is recommended that the physiotherapist explains why certain test procedures are performed and teaches the patient to become aware of the various parameters which are relevant from the physiotherapist's perspective – for example, it may be important during active test movements to educate the patient that the physiotherapist is interested not only in any symptom the patient may feel, but also in the range of motion, the quality of the movement and the trust of the patient in the particular movement test. During palpation sessions and the examination of accessory movements, the patient should be encouraged not only to describe any pain but also any sensations of stiffness at one level in the spine in comparison with an adjacent level. This is a procedure which requires highly

developed communication skills; however, it can be an important phase in the training of the perception of the patient.

Furthermore, it is recommended that physiotherapists inform patients not only about those tests which serve as a reassessment parameter, but also about the test movements that have been judged to be normal. Frequently it appears that physiotherapists are more likely to be deficit oriented in their examinations; however, to many patients it is a relief to hear from the therapist which movements and tests are considered to be normal.

Sometimes patients may indicate their anxiousness with certain test procedures (e.g. SLR) based on earlier experiences. In such cases it is essential to negotiate directly with the patient how far the physiotherapist will be allowed to move the limb. In fact, 'trust to move' may become an important measurable and achievable parameter, which may indicate the first beneficial changes in the condition of the patient.

Ending a session

Sufficient time needs to be planned for the ending of a session. On the one hand the physiotherapist may instruct the patient about how to observe and *compare* the possible changes in symptoms and activity levels. Furthermore, the therapist may need to warn the patient of a possible exacerbation of symptoms in certain circumstances. A repetition of the first instructions, recommendations or self-management strategies may be necessary in order to enhance short-term compliance (Hengeveld 2003). As described in 'Shaping of interactions' above, attention needs to be given to unexpected key remarks of the patient as these may be indicative of the individual illness experience and relevant treatment objectives.

Evaluation and reflection of the first session, including treatment planning

This phase includes summarizing relevant subjective and physical examination findings, making hypotheses explicit, outlining the next step in the process of collaborative goal setting for treatment and, if possible, collaboratively defining the subjective and physical reassessment parameters. If the physiotherapist is confronted with a recognizable clinical presentation, this phase may have occurred partially already during the examination process ('reflection in action'). However, in more complicated presentations or in new situations the physiotherapist may need more time to reflect on this phase after the first session ('reflection on action') before explaining the physiotherapy viewpoints to the patient and suggesting a treatment plan (Schön 1983). In particular, trainees and novices in the field need to be given sufficient *time* to reflect before entering the next treatment session in order to develop comprehensive reflective skills (Alsop & Ryan 1996). The completion of a clinical reasoning form may aid the learning process of the students in the various phases of the therapeutic process.

Reassessments

As stated earlier, it is essential that patients are able to recognize reassessment procedures as such and do not confuse them with a whole set of procedures in which they may not be able to distinguish between treatment and evaluation. Education of patients may be required to observe possible changes in terms of comparisons, rather than statements of fact. Cognitive reinforcement at the end of a reassessment procedure may be helpful to support the learning processes of both the patient and the physiotherapist. If the physiotherapist employs educational strategies it may be necessary to perform a reassessment on this cognitive goal as well. Often it is useful to integrate questions with regard to self-management strategies in the opening phase of each session during the subjective reassessments. However, from a cognitive–behavioural perspective, the way a patient is asked if they are capable of doing their exercises and to evaluate the effects of these can be decisive in the development of understanding and compliance.

Retrospective assessment

In an earlier edition of Maitland's work it was stated that retrospective assessments are crucial aspects of the Concept. In retrospective assessment in particular, the physiotherapist evaluates patients' awareness of changes to their symptoms as one of the most important elements of evaluation. The only way to get this information is with skills in communication and awareness of possible changes in symptoms, signs, activity levels and illness behaviour. The physiotherapist evaluates the results of the treatment so far, including the effects of self-management strategies. In this phase it is essential to (re)define collaboratively with the patient the treatment objectives for the next phase of treatment, preferably on levels of activity and participation (WHO 2001) ('prospective assessment') and leading to an optimum state of wellbeing with regard to movement functions.

Final analytical assessment

This phase includes the reflection of the overall therapeutic process, when assessment is made of which interventions have led to which results. Often it is useful to reflect with the patient what has been learned so far. In order to enhance long-term compliance, the physiotherapist may anticipate collaboratively with the patient on possible future difficulties in activities or work and which self-management interventions may be useful if there is any recurrence (Sluys et al. 1993).

Verbatim examples

Although communication with a patient is a two-way affair, the main responsibility for its effectiveness lies with the therapist rather than with the patient. The therapist should be thinking of three things (Maitland 1991):

1. I should make every effort to be as sure as is possible that I understand what the patient is trying to tell me
2. I should be ready to recognize any gaps in the patient's communication, which I should endeavour to fill by asking appropriate questions
3. I should make use of every possible opportunity to utilize my own non-verbal expressions to show my understanding and concern for the patient and his plight.

The following verbatim examples in this text are used to provide some guidelines which will, it is hoped, help the physiotherapist to achieve the depth, accuracy and refinement required for good assessment and treatment.

The guidelines should not be interpreted as preaching to the ignorant – they are given to underline the essence of careful and precise communication as an integral part of overall physiotherapy practice.

Welcoming and information phase

As described above, the welcoming and information phase may be an essential stage to 'get a patient on board' in the physiotherapy process. This phase needs an explanation on the paradigms in physiotherapy, which can be understood easily by the patient. It is essential to find out if the patient can be motivated to physiotherapy and to develop trust in what is lying ahead in the therapy sessions.

In this phase it is also important to find out if a patient has already consulted a number of different specialists in the medical field for the problem. Often the patient may have received various opinions and viewpoints and is left confused, especially if they seem to have a more externalized locus of control with regard to their state of health (Rotter 1966, Härkäpää et al. 1989, Keogh & Cochrane 2002, Roberts et al. 2002). A patient may indicate by certain key phrases the expectation of a single cure according to the biomedical model, whereas the physiotherapist expects to treat the patient according to a movement paradigm in which self-management strategies may play an important role: 'I have seen so many specialists – everybody says something different. Why don't they find out what is wrong with me and then do something about it?'

There are many ways to respond to such a statement but it is crucial that such a key remark is not ignored. The physiotherapist may respond in various ways, for example:

Q 'What would you think that they would need to do about it?'

Q 'Now you have come to me – there is a chance that I might also have a different opinion, like all the others. How would you feel about that?'

Initial assessment: subjective examination

As stated above, in this phase it is vital to concentrate on both the patient's actual words and how they are delivered. Furthermore, during the overall process of subjective examination the process of collaborative goal setting should take place, in which treatment objectives are defined in a balanced approach to symptom control and normalization of activities, thereby enhancing overall wellbeing.

'First question' – establishing main problem

When the physiotherapist starts off the subjective examination, the first thing to be determined is the main problem in the patient's own terms. It is important that patients be given every opportunity to express their reasons for seeking treatment, for example with the first question being: 'As far as *you* are concerned … [Pause …] (the pause helps the patient to realize that the therapist is specifically interested in the patient's *own* opinion) … what do *you* feel … [Pause …] is *your main* problem at this stage?'

The patient may start off by answering, 'The doctor said I've got tennis-elbow', or, 'Well, I've had this problem for 15 years'.

In this case the physiotherapist may gently interrupt with an 'immediate-response' question such as:

Q 'What made you go to the doctor?'

A 'Well, because my shoulder hurts of course.'

Q 'Ah, okay, it's your shoulder hurting' (and then immediately making a note of this answer, which indicates to the patient that this is the information the physiotherapist is seeking).

After this answer the physiotherapist may determine the perceived level of disability. At this stage it is also essential to pay attention not only to what is said, but also to how it is said. The use of more emotionally laden words ('it's all very terrible and annoying, I can't do anything anymore'), the non-verbal behaviour of expressing the main problem (e.g. looking away from the area of the symptoms while indicating this, a deep sigh before answering) or a seeming discrepancy between the level of disability and the expected impairments or areas of symptoms may guide the physiotherapist to the development of hypotheses with regard to 'yellow flags', which may facilitate or hinder full recovery of function.

In the determination of the localization of symptoms, at times it is important to ensure that certain areas are free of symptoms, in a sense if 'not even half of 1%' exists. In this case 'immediate-response' questions need to be asked:

Q 'Do you have any symptoms in your leg?'

A 'Not really.'

Q 'Do you mean, nothing at all?'

The response to the examiner's first question with regard to the patient's main problem will guide the next question in one of two directions:

1. The behaviour of the symptoms and the activities of daily living
2. The history of the problem.

Behaviour of the symptoms

Without experience in the choice of words or phrasing of questions, an enormous amount of time can be taken up in determining the behaviour of a patient's symptoms. Unfortunately, it needs time if the skill is to be learned, for nothing teaches as well as experience. The information required relative to the behaviour of a patient's symptoms is:

- The relationship that the symptoms bear to rest, activities and positions
- The constancy, frequency and duration of the intermittent pain and remission, and any fluctuations of intensity ('irritability')
- The ability of the patient to control these symptoms and promote wellbeing (coping strategies)
- The level of activity in spite of the symptoms
- Definition of first treatment objectives on activity and participation levels, as well as further coping strategies.

The following is one example that provides a guide as to the choice of words and phrases that will save time and help the therapist avoid making mistaken interpretations and incorrect assumptions. The conversation that follows is with a man who has had 3 weeks of buttock pain. The text relates only to the behaviour of the buttock pain (adapted from Maitland 1986):

(ET, Examiner's thoughts; Q, question; A, answer)

ET   Earlier in the interview he said his buttock pain was 'constant'. 'Constant' can mean 'constant for 24 hours of the day' or 'constant when it is present' as compared with the momentary sharp pain. This is borne out by the fact that a surprising number of patients say their pain is constant, yet when you ask them, immediately prior to testing the first movement, 'Do you feel any symptoms in your back at this moment?', they will answer 'No'. The 'constant ache' and 'no symptoms' are incompatible. To avoid misinterpreting his use of 'constant', it is essential that this is clarified. It may be possible to gain a more positive manner by tackling the question from the opposite direction:

Q   'At this stage, are there any moments in which you do *not* feel your backache?'
A   'No, it's there all the time.'
ET   The next question is to ask him is if he has any ache if he awakens during the night, because this is the most likely time for him to be symptom-free.
Q   'How does it feel if you waken during the night?'
A   'All right.'
Q   'Do you mean it is not aching then?'
A   'That's right.'
Q   'Do you mean it is not aching at all?'
A   'That's right.'
Q   'So you do have *some* stages when it is not aching?'
A   'Only at night. It aches all day.'
ET   That's now clear. His thinking processes at the moment relate to 'no symptoms in bed' and 'it aches all day'. I need to know the answers to two associated aspects of the daytime:

1. Does the ache vary during the day? (And if so, how much, why, and how long does it take to subside?)
2. Does he have any stiffness and/or pain on getting out of bed first thing in the morning?

To make use of his current train of thought, the following question should quickly be asked in response to his answer '… it aches all day':

Q   'Does the ache vary at all during the day?'
A   'Yes.'
ET   Well, that doesn't help me much, but it does provide a point from which to work further. There are many ways I can tackle the next few questions. Basically, what I want to know is, does it increase as the day progresses or does it depend on *particular* activities or positions he may adopt? How can I get the answer most quickly? I'll try this first:
Q   'What makes it worse?'
A   'It just gets worse as the day goes on.'
Q   'Do you mean there is nothing you know of which makes it worse – it just gets worse for no obvious reason?'
ET   Assessment and reassessment in particular are easier if there is something he can do to increase or to decrease his ache. I need to ask a more leading question:
Q   'Is there anything you can do, here and now, which you know will hurt your buttock?'
A   'Well, I know that while I have been sitting here it has ached more.'
Q   'Do you mean, sitting normally makes you ache?'
A   'If I sit and watch television it aches.'
ET   Good, this gives me more information with regard to physical examination and reassessment

of treatment. However, I would like to know two things:

1. What can he do by himself to influence the pain? (This will provide me with information with regard to self-management strategies and physical examination.)

2. Are there any *activities* he performs which cause aching? (This information will also be helpful in later reassessment stages.)

I first continue with his current line of thought – sitting and watching TV cause ache.

Q 'Once your back is aching during watching television, is there anything you can do by yourself to influence the ache?'

A 'I just get up and walk around for a while.'

Q 'Do you happen to perform any particular movements?'

A 'I am not aware of this.'

Q 'Are you having any ache right now?'

A 'Yes.'

Q 'What would you like to do right now to reduce it?'

A 'I would like to get up and walk a few steps.' (*Patient gets up and ET observes.*)

Q 'How is it now?'

A 'It's still there, but certainly better than just before.'

Q 'Well, since this improves it a bit, I would suggest that getting up and moving around for a few moments is certainly a good thing to continue, whenever your back is aching more.'

ET Well, I observed him getting up and supporting his back with his hands and he seemed to be having difficulty in straightening his back. This indicates a lumbar movement disorder rather than a hip disorder. In the latter case I would have expected him to have difficulty with walking rather than straightening his back. He could also have moved his leg more to reduce the pain if the hip was a cause of his movement dysfunction.

Now I would like to find out if there are some activities rather than positions which provoke his symptoms. I can combine this with one step of goal setting:

Q 'So, if I understand you correctly, you would like sitting while watching television and getting up after sitting to improve, am I correct?'

A 'Oh sure, that's right.'

Q 'How do you feel when you first get out of bed in the morning?'

A 'I have difficulty putting my socks on, I feel stiff and it aches in my buttock.'

ET The greater value of this answer is the use of the spontaneous key word 'stiffness'. Stiffness in the morning may fit a recognizable clinical pattern of an inflammatory disorder, which can be determined by further questioning.

Q 'How long does the stiffness last?'

A 'Only a few minutes. I'm still aware of it when I lean over the wash-basin to wash my face, but by breakfast it has already gone.'

Some readers may consider the above answers are too good to be true. However, as the physiotherapist learns to ask key questions to elicit spontaneous answers, the responses become more informative and helpful in understanding both the person and his problem, hence the development of a therapeutic relationship and a differentiated baseline for later reassessment procedures.

The behaviour of the patient's symptom of stiffness may also be significant when there is some pathology involved. For example, during the early part of the examination the physiotherapist may develop the hypothesis that ankylosing spondylitis may be the background of the patient's movement disorder. The conversation and thoughts may be something like this:

ET I want to know if his back feels stiff on getting out of bed in the morning. If he has ankylosing spondylitis, his back should be quite stiff and probably painful. Even if it is not very painful, does the stiffness take longer than 2 hours to improve to his normal degree of limited mobility? To gain the maximum value from his answer I must avoid any suggestive questions.

Q 'How does your back feel when you first get out of bed in the morning?'

A 'Not so good.'

Q 'In what way isn't it good?'

A 'It's stiff.'

ET This is a statement, and all statements need to be made factual if they are to be used for prognosis and assessment purposes.

Q 'How stiff?'

A 'Very stiff.'

Q 'How long does it take for this stiffness to wear off?'

A 'Oh, it's fairly good by about midday.'

ET His job may involve shift work, so I must not assume immediately that his stiffness lasts for about 5 hours.

Q 'What time do you get up in the morning?'

A 'About 7 o'clock.'

ET That means that he's stiff for at least 4 hours. That's too long for any ordinary mechanical movement disorder.

History of the problem

History taking is discussed in numerous chapters of this book. The discussion here relates to communication guidelines. Especially in those patients in whom the disorder is of a spontaneous onset, many probing questions are needed to determine the predisposing factors involved in the onset. The following text is but one example of the probing necessary in the history taking of this group of patients:

ET   If I start with open questions, which are vaguely directed, his spontaneous answers may help me considerably to understand those parts of his history that are important to him. Those parts which are important to me I can seek later, if they do not unfold spontaneously.

Q   'How did it begin?'

ET   This may also provide me with information on *when* it began.

A   'I don't know. It just started aching about 3 weeks ago and it isn't getting any better.'

ET   It is necessary to know what precipitated the pain and whether this was mechanical or not. If there was an incident or episode, it was either so trivial that he does not remember, or he doesn't associate it with his symptoms. Before sorting this out, it may save time for me to know if he has had any previous episodes. If he has, they may provide the key to recognizing the historical pattern of a particular movement disorder, as well as the key to this kind of precipitating onset for the present symptoms.

Q   'Have you ever had this, or anything like this before?'

ET   I have to be alert here because he may say 'No' on the basis that previous episodes have been called 'lumbago' and therefore he does not associate them with his present problem, which has been called 'arthritis'.

A 'No.'

ET   I can now direct my questions in several ways, but probably the most informative may be verifying this 'No' answer, as his present thoughts are directed now along 'past history'.

Q   'Do you mean you've never had a day's backache in your life?'

A   'No, not really.'

ET   Ah … 'Not really' means to me that he has had something, so I must clarify this.

Q   'When you say "Not really", it sounds as though you may have had something.'

A   'Well, my back gets a bit stiff if I do a lot of gardening, but then everyone has that, don't they?'

ET   Now it's coming out. What I need to know is whether the degree of stiffness is related to the degree of gardening.

Q   'How long does it take you to recover from a certain amount of gardening?'

A   'It might take 2 or 3 days to get back to normal after a whole weekend in the garden.'

ET   This is very useful information. It helps me to know what his back can tolerate, at least in previous episodes. I don't know yet if his back is about the same in this episode or if it's deteriorating, but to save time I'll go back to the 'here and now' and return to the gardening issue later – provided I do not forget about it! I will need to know the stability of the current disorder as it will guide me in the vigour of treatment and prognosis. The answer may come during other parts of the examination. What I need to know now is how this episode began. His initial vagueness indicates I am going to have to ask some searching questions to find the answers.

There are many ways the questions can be tackled, and the answer to each will take about the same length of time.

Q   'You said that this episode started about 3 weeks ago. Did it come on *suddenly*?'

A   'Yes, fairly quickly.'

ET   Fairly quickly means 'suddenly' to him, but it's not precise enough for me, so I'll need to probe deeper.

Q   'What were you *first* aware of?'

A   'It just started aching.'

Q   'During the morning or the afternoon?'

A   'I don't remember.'

Q   'Do you remember if it came on in one day? In other words, did you have no ache one day and have an ache the next day?'

After a delay, while he ponders the question, the answer comes:

A   'Yes, I think so.'

Q   'Do you happen to remember which day it was?'

ET   To pursue this line of thinking I will guide his memory, which may help him to remember something that might otherwise be lost.

A   'It was a Thursday.'

Q   'Was it aching when you wakened that day or did it come later that day?'

A   'I think I wakened with it, yes. Yes, I'm sure I did because I remember saying to my wife during breakfast that my back was aching.'

Q   'And when you went to bed the night before, was your back aching then?'

A 'No, then I did not feel anything.'

ET That's part of the question solved, or at least as much as I need at the moment. Now to find out what provoked it. The first thing is to make him think about whether there was any trivial incident which occurred during the day before the backache started. If this proves negative, then I'll ask about 'predisposing factors'.

Q 'Did you do anything at all on *Wednesday* that hurt your back even in a minor way, or made you *aware* of your back in any way?'

A 'No, I've been trying to remember if I did anything, but I can't remember any time I could have hurt it.'

ET So now I have to resort to the 'predisposing factors' referred to above. While his mind is orientated towards physical activity, if I continue with questions associated with activities, he will probably be able to answer more quickly. And the answer may be more reliable. To ask him about the non-physical activity 'predisposing factors' (fatigue, disease, etc.) will force him to change his train of thought and it may take more time. I will keep paralleling to his train of thought, as long as I do not lose the overview and don't forget about the other questions.

Q 'Did you do any unusual work on that Wednesday or about that time?'

A 'No.'

Q 'Have you been doing any *heavier* work than usual?'

A 'No.'

Q 'Any work that was *longer* than usual?'

A 'No.'

Q 'Anything changed at work, like new furniture?'

A 'No.'

ET So there isn't any obvious physical activity which has provoked this ache. The next step is to investigate the other 'predisposing factors' – there *must* be a reason for the onset of aching on the Thursday morning.

Q 'At that time, were you unwell, or overtired or under any stress?'

A 'Well, yes I was pretty tired. I'm overdue for holidays and we have had two men off work sick – and now you mention it, we have been working longer hours than usual to meet a deadline – I'd forgotten about that – and I was involved in a lot of lifting and carrying that day.'

ET It often takes quite a long time (which is reasonable) for a person to retrieve pieces of information, so rather than thinking, 'Why didn't you say that when I asked you earlier', I'd be better to think, 'Well at least I didn't miss out on that piece of information'.

Q 'And that is unusual for you, isn't it?'

A 'Well, yes it is. I do have to do quite a bit of lifting, but the pressure was really on at that particular time.'

ET Thank you very much, that's just what I was looking for. Now that it makes sense, the history and the symptoms are compatible.

Now I would like to know, as his train of thought is still '3 weeks ago', if he considered doing any self-management interventions during the day he was lifting so much.

Q 'During that Wednesday when you were lifting so much, did you think of doing any exercises in between to protect your back – or have you learned some things previously?'

A 'Oh no, I was so busy, I did not think of anything other than getting the job done.'

ET Okay, that's something I can understand. It provides me however with hypotheses regarding management – it could be a lumbar movement dysfunction, without prematurely excluding other sources. If it is lumbar, he may need to learn extension movements during the day to compensate for the bending activities. I'll keep that in mind and come back to this later.

As already mentioned, when interviewing more garrulous patients, trying to keep control of the interview is challenging. During history taking these patients tend to go off at tangents and give a lot of detailed information. This may need to be skillfully interposed by gently increasing the volume of your voice and simultaneously touching the patient gently. However, the important thing is that the examiner can retain control of the interview without insulting or upsetting the patient. Nevertheless, every effort should be made to make patients feel that they are not complaining, rather they should be told that they are informing – *'What you don't tell me, I don't know.'*

For example the opening question and answer might be as follows:

Q 'When did it start?'

A 'Well, I was on my way to visit an old aunt of mine, and as I was getting onto…'

This is often a difficult situation – is this the patient's train of thought, which may provide the therapist eventually with valuable spontaneous information, or is it better to interrupt? Some intervening questions to keep control of the interview may be as follows:

Q1 'What happened?'

Q2 'Did you fall?'

Q3 'How long ago was this?'

Initial assessment: physical examination

After a summary of the main findings of the subjective examination and agreed treatment objectives, it is essential that the patient is informed about the purpose of the test movements to allow the patient an active role in the procedures. This may be worded as follows:

> We have agreed that we would try to work on activities like bending over and standing. I've understood that it is important to you that you feel capable of jogging again soon and inviting people to your home. Am I correct? (patient agrees). Now I would like to look more specifically at your movements of your shoulder and neck, in order to see if they all meet the basic requirements to fulfil such tasks.

While performing the test procedures, the purpose of active test movements, as well as the parameters relevant for reassessment procedures can be explained:

Q   'While standing here now, what do you feel in your neck and arm?'

A   'The whole lot.'

Q   'Equally throughout?'

A   'No, the upper arm isn't so bad.'

Q   'Your neck and forearm are more painful, aren't they?'

A   'Yes.'

Q   'Which is worse?'

A   'They're about the same.'

ET   Right, that's clear. Now I would like to test neck flexion.

The patient is asked to bend his head forward and then return to the upright position.

Q   'Did your pain change?'

A   'Yes, the pain in my upper arm increased.'

Q   'Did your forearm change?'

A   'No.'

Q   'And nothing else changed either?'

A   'No.'

Q   'Good. And now, has the upper arm pain subsided back to what it was before?'

A   'Yes.'

Q   'Did that happen immediately you started to come up, or did it take a while to subside?'

A   'It hurt more while I was fully bent forwards.'

ET   That's ideal answering. I now have a complete picture of how the symptoms behave with forward flexion of the neck. I have seen his range and quality of movement – I wonder if he observed this as well.

Q   'I want you to remember this movement – we will use it as a test later on to measure progress. Could you tell me something about how you perceived the way you moved – could you bend as much and as easily as you are used to?'

A   'Can I do it again?'

Q   'Yes.'

A   'It feels much stiffer and I think I normally come further down.'

Q   'I would like you to remember how the pain feels, but also to remember the way you feel able to move. Let's test the next movement now … Could you carefully bend your head backwards?'

Patient does this and makes a grimace.

Q   'Up you go. Where was it?'

A   'In my upper arm again.'

Q   'How is it now?'

A   'Back to normal again.'

Q   'How did you feel about the movement itself?'

A   'I did not feel free; I did not fully trust myself to go further back. I did not go as far as normal.'

Q   'Which movement was more problematic: bending forwards or backwards?'

A   'Backwards; it hurts more and I did not trust myself fully.'

Q   'I would like you to remember this movement also. We will compare this one later on as well.'

ET   Now I would like to perform the other neck movement, if the 'present pain' has not yet increased.

This example demonstrates how much close attention the pain responses to the movement deserve. The physiotherapist usually simultaneously observes the quality and range of movement. However, often it is necessary to guide the patient to this observation in order to teach him all the essential parameters of a test procedure. Furthermore, it is important for the patient to understand that the physiotherapist wants to use these movements in later reassessment procedures to observe if any beneficial changes have occurred. To many patients this is a strange procedure, as they often naturally would want to avoid the painful movements. To omit precision in this area would be a grave mistake. Once the behaviour of the pain is established and the patient understands the purpose of these test procedures, the treatment techniques can be suitably modified and the appropriate care given to treatment and reassessment.

The intonation of the patient's speech can also express much to the physiotherapist. During the consultation every possible advantage should be taken of all avenues of both verbal and non-verbal communication. The more patients one sees, the quicker and more accurate the assessment becomes.

> Q 'Now let me see you bending your head to the left side.'

And so the examination continues. The examples given should show how it is possible to determine very precise, accurate information about the responses to movement without great expenditure of time. Obviously it is not always as straightforward as the example given, but it is nearly always possible to achieve the precision.

Some patients become quickly irritated in subsequent treatment sessions by being asked the same questions in the same detail. The physiotherapist who is tuned into the patient's non-verbal communication will quickly get this message. One way around this, without losing precision, is to vary the question:

'Upper arm again?' or, 'Only upper arm?', or, 'Same?'

Palpation

During palpation sequences and examination of accessory movements it is important to actively integrate the patient in the examination as well. Often the patient will be asked to comment only on any pain. However, if the patient is guided towards giving information on his perception of the tissue quality and comparing the movements of various levels of the spine, he learns that many more subtle parameters may be relevant to reassessment procedures and hence to his wellbeing.

While performing, for example, accessory movement of the cervicothoracic junction the following verbal interactions may take place.

Physiotherapist performs accessory movements of the C5–7 segments:

> Q 'How does it feel when I move on these vertebrae?'
>
> A 'The lower one especially hurts.'
>
> Q (performs central PA movement on C7) 'So this one hurts you the most?'
>
> A 'Yes.'

> Q 'If I move it a little bit less?' (moves less deep into the direction of movement)
>
> 'Now it's less?'
>
> A 'Yes.'
>
> Q 'And if I move so far (goes back to the point where she suspected the pain to start again), then it flares up again?'
>
> A 'Yes.'
>
> Q 'And like this it is less again?'
>
> A 'Yes.'

With this method of questioning the patient may learn several things: first, that the physiotherapist is truly interested not only in finding the painful segments of the spine, but also that the therapist does not want to hurt him unnecessarily. Second, the patient may develop trust in the physiotherapist.

The physiotherapist now examines T1–4, which are not painful but have a very limited range of motion.

> Q 'If I move in this area, how is this?'
>
> A 'Good.'
>
> Q 'Does anything hurt?'
>
> A 'No.'
>
> Q 'Do you notice any difference in elasticity in this area compared with above?' (moves gently in T1–4 area and then back to a more mobile, but pain-free area of the cervical spine)
>
> A 'Well, it's hard to say. It somehow seems much stiffer.'
>
> Q 'That's what I felt as well. I think that this area (C7) may have become so painful because these adjacent areas are stiff. I would like to gently move those painful areas in your neck with these fine movements; however, I would not like to go into the pain (gently shows the movements on the neck of the patient). This area (shows now at T1–4) I would like to treat a bit later, as soon as I know how your neck reacts to these little movements.
>
> Could you sit up again, and we will quickly look at bending forwards and backwards – just to see if your neck has liked these little movements.'

Summarizing the first session: collaborative treatment planning and goal setting

At the completion of the first session, after a subjective and a physical examination as well as a first probationary treatment, including reassessment, it is essential to summarize the main points. This is relevant to train the clinical reasoning processes of the physiotherapist and to inform the patient about the viewpoints of the therapist, to clarify the goals of treatment once more and to define the interventions to achieve these objectives. Furthermore, the parameters which indicate any beneficial treatment effects need to be defined collaboratively with the patient.

The process of collaborative goal setting requires skill in communication as well as in negotiation. At times a patient may simply expect to have 'less pain', although it may seem in the prognosis that reduction in pain intensity and frequency will not be easily achieved. It may even be more challenging if the patient states that 'first the pain has to disappear and then I will think of work and activities'. It is almost always relevant to define goals with control of pain and wellbeing, *including* normalization of activities, as fear avoidance behaviour has been described as one of the major contributing factors to ongoing disability due to pain (Klenermann et al. 1995, Vlaeyen & Linton 2000). However, not only the avoidance of activities but also the avoidance of social contacts and interesting stimuli, e.g. going to the theatre, are important contributing factors (Philips 1987). Furthermore, a lack of relaxation or a lack of bodily awareness during the activities of normal daily life may be relevant contributing factors and may need to be included in the collaborative goal-setting process.

The following interaction could take place:

Q 'What would be your main goal of the treatment with me?'

A 'To have less pain.'

Q 'I understand that. If you had less pain, what would you do again that you are not doing now?'

A 'Well, I would like to work in the garden, I love roses.'

Q 'Are there any other things that you would like to do again?'

A 'I would like to invite people to my house again.'

Q 'What keeps you from doing this now?'

A 'Well, if I invite people to the house and cook for them, then I am afraid that the pain just comes at that time. And I cannot expect much help from my husband in that case.'

Q 'So if I understand you correctly, if you could have a bit more control over your pain, for example with simple movements, you would invite people to your house again and work in the garden with your roses again?'

A 'Oh certainly!'

Q 'When would you be satisfied with your pain? I mean, if your pain was like a wave on the ocean, now it is a very high wave, but does the water need to be totally flat?'

A 'Oh no, I certainly can accept some pain! It just should not get worse than it is right now.'

Q 'Do you mean, that *now* your pain is acceptable, but it should not get worse?'

A 'Yes, that's right!'

Q 'So if I understand you correctly, you would like to perform these activities again, but you do not trust yourself fully to do this?'

A 'Yes, I am afraid to do these things again.'

Q 'What seems more important to you: having more trust in doing these things and controlling the pain a bit, or do you need to be fully pain free?'

A 'Oh no, I don't mind a bit of pain. If possible I would like to be able to cook again, to ride a bicycle and to work in the garden – just those things which make life so much more enjoyable.'

Q 'How about trying to work together on activities like cooking and working in the garden and see if we find ways to control the pain, if this should flare up?'

A 'Well, yes…that would be wonderful of course.'

Q 'I suggest that on the one hand I might perform some movements on your back to loosen it up a bit, as I did before. However, I also think we should find some simple exercises together which you could perform in your daily life, exactly when you may get more pain. Is that something you would be willing to try?'

Initially in this interaction it seems that the patient only seeks 'freedom from pain' in its intensity; however, after a few probing questions it becomes clear that the woman is more probably looking for a *sense of control* over her pain and developing trust in activities that she has avoided so far. The use of a metaphor for the pain (as in this example 'a wave on the ocean') frequently shows that in fact the patient is seeking control rather than simply reduction of pain and improvement in wellbeing. Often it is useful to take the time for this process of clarifying treatment goals as unrealistic expectations may be identified and the patient sometimes learns that there are other worthwhile goals to be achieved in therapy as well. Furthermore, it aids reassessment purposes as both the physiotherapist and patient learn to pay attention to activities which serve as parameters – for example, the trust to move and control over pain rather than sensory aspects of pain alone (e.g. pain intensity, pain localization and so on).

At times physiotherapists think they are involved in a collaborative goal-setting process; however, they may be more directive than they are aware (Chin et al. 1993). In order to enhance compliance with the agreed goals, ideally it is better to guide people by asking questions rather than telling them what to do. The following example may highlight this principle:

The patient is a 34-year-old mother of three young children who takes care of the household and garden, nurses her sick mother-in-law and helps her husband in the bookkeeping of his construction business. She is complaining of shoulder and arm pain. The physiotherapist is treating her successfully with passive movements in the glenohumeral joint. However, the pain is recurrent and the physiotherapist's hypothesis is that lack of relaxation and lack of awareness of tension development in the body and during movements may be very important contributing factors. The physiotherapist would like to begin relaxation strategies which could easily integrate with the patient's daily life and subsequently would like to start work on bodily awareness of relaxed movement during normal daily activities (see also the example of collaborative goal setting discussed below).

Directive interaction

Q 'I think you need more quiet moments during your day. Because you work so much, your shoulder can never recuperate. I suggest that you just take some time off every day for yourself.'

A 'Yes, I think you're right. I should do this.'

This directive way may develop an agreed goal of treatment; however, the patient is not provided with any tools on how to achieve this goal. This may impede short-term compliance (Sluys & Hermans 1990). Furthermore, it has been shown that compliance with suggestions and exercises may increase if goals are defined in a more collaborative way (Bassett & Petrie 1997).

Another approach may be:

Collaborative goal setting by asking questions

Q 'I think you must be quite stress resistant when I see all the things that you are doing in your daily life.'

A 'Oh, well, yes…' (reluctant)

Q 'Yes?' (makes a short pause and looks the patient in the eye)

A 'Oh well, sometimes it is a little bit too much.'

Q 'What are you able to do, when you feel it is becoming a bit too much?'

A 'Well, in 3 months' time my husband and I are going for a long weekend to Paris without the kids.'

Q 'Wow, that's wonderful! Hope you enjoy it! However, Paris is still a long time off. What could you do in the meantime, when things get a bit too much? Have you discovered anything which you could do just during the day?'

A 'I don't know. I don't do anything special. I am not used to doing anything special for such things. Also at home when I was a kid we always worked a lot in our parents' business.'

Q 'I think it would be useful if you could find some moments in the day in which to tank up a bit of energy again, before you continue with all your tasks. I think that your shoulder may benefit a lot from this.' (waits a moment and observes the patient)

A 'I have been thinking about that as well.'

Q 'How would it be if we search for simple things which you could integrate into your daily life in which you can tank up a bit of energy? Maybe you already do very useful things in this regard, but if they're not done consciously, they may not be done frequently enough.'

A 'That's okay.'

Q 'Could you describe a situation where you think it was all a bit too much for you in which your shoulder was hurting as well?'

Beginning of a follow up session: subjective reassessment

Reassessment

In follow-up sessions spontaneous information about reactions to the last treatment is usually sought first, before a comparison to the parameter of the subjective examination is pursued explicitly. If the physiotherapist has suggested some self-management strategies to influence pain, it is also essential to address this somewhere in the subjective reassessment. It is important to remember at all times that statements of fact need to be converted into comparisons. The following communication could take place:

Q 'Well now, how have you been?', or, 'How do you feel now compared with when you came in last time?'

A 'Not too bad.'

ET That tells me nothing, so…

Q 'Any different?'

A   'I don't know if this is usual, but I've been terribly tired.'

ET   *Well, it seems that his symptoms have not been significantly worse. However, I should not just assume that if they had been he would have said so straight away. The tiredness can be related and it can be a favourable sign, so the response to his answer should be:*

Q   'Yes, it's quite common and it can be a good indicator. How have your back and leg been?'

A   'A bit worse.'

ET   *Most responses need qualifying, but for 'worse' clarifying is mandatory: In what way?, Which part?, When?, Why? Spontaneous answers are still important, so I'll keep my questions as non-directive as possible.*

1. In what way?

Q   'In what way is it worse?'

A   'My buttock has been more painful.'

Q   'Sharper or more achy?'

A   'It's more difficult to get comfortable in bed.'

ET   *That's not really answering my question, but it's telling me something about an activity, which I'm going to accept for the moment as being enough of an answer.*

2. Which part?

ET   *Because he may have a nerve root problem I should determine if his calf pain has changed, and it would be better to do this before finding out the 'when' and 'why' of his increased buttock pain. Because I hope his calf hasn't worsened too, I am going to ask the question in a way that will influence him to say 'yes'.*

Q   'Do you mean your calf?'

A   'No, that's about the same.'

ET   *That's makes the answer to what I wanted to know very positive.*

3. When?

Q   'When did you notice your buttock worsening?'

A   'Last night.'

Q   'How about the night before?'

A   'No different from usual.'

Q   'So there was no change from the time you left here after treatment until last night?'

A   'That's right.'

4. Why?

ET   *It is essential to know if this increase was caused by treatment or other causes. I still don't know about his other activities. He may have done much more with his structures that he was not able to do before. Then it may even be a favourable response. At no time should I stop the subjective reassessment in this phase!*

Q   'Do you think it was what I did to you that made it worse?'

A   'Not really, because the night before last was all right. And, actually, when I left here I felt better and I think I even had a better night than usual.'

ET   *That's a good answer – I know treatment did not make him worse, he even felt better. Let me check on that asterisk of sitting.*

Q   'So, you felt better after treatment and the night seemed better. How was sitting compared to before the treatment?'

A   'Actually I think on the first day after treatment I could sit longer at work before it became uncomfortable as usual. However, yesterday I had to sit in an uncomfortable chair for 2.5 hours at a meeting during the evening – my buttock was quite sore during the last hour.'

Q   'So after this sitting you felt the ache in your buttock more?'

A   'Yes.'

Q   'Did you feel anything in your calf then?'

A   'No, only my buttock.'

ET   *Well, the worsening seems related to his sitting, which was already a problem. I have already suggested that he tries out a self-management exercise if his pain increases. I am aware that behaviour does not change overnight, but I am curious to find out if he thought of trying out this exercise last night after the meeting, or if he stuck to his old habits.*

Q   'Were you able, last night, to try out that exercise I showed you last time?'

A   'Exercise? No, I was so busy, I did not even think of it.'

ET   *Okay, that's acceptable in the beginning – I have difficulty in changing my habits as well. But it shows me I have to repeat this exercise today during the session and I want to emphasize particularly the necessity of him trying it out, especially at those times when he has more symptoms. Now I want to know if he has recuperated to his initial state after this episode of sitting.*

Q   'After you went to bed and finally became comfortable, how was your night?'

A   'I slept well, in fact I did not wake up at all last night.'

Q   'Is that unusual?'

A   'Well, it's at least 3 weeks since I could sleep a whole night. This is the first time since my buttock and leg started to hurt.'

Q   'And how were you this morning compared with other mornings?'

A   'I think about the same, back to what it was. A bit stiff for about 10 minutes and some difficulty putting socks on.'

Q 'Thank you. I'd like to summarize what I've heard, but please correct me if I'm wrong. Last night you had more difficulty getting comfortable in bed, but that this may be due to the longer period of sitting?'

A 'Yes I think so.'

Q 'I can imagine that. It would be helpful the next time to try out that exercise of straightening your back to see if you can influence it.'

A 'Okay.'

Q 'So last night you were more uncomfortable in your buttock, but your calf was the same. Immediately after treatment 2 days ago you felt better and you may have slept better. And last night you could sleep the whole night for the first time for 3 weeks?'

A 'Yes that's correct. Overall I think I am a bit better.'

Q 'Okay, now I would like to compare a few of the test movements of last time before we continue with treatment.'

If the physiotherapist had stopped this reassessment procedure relatively early in the conversation, important information would have been lost and in fact the therapist may have ended with the impression that the patient's situation had worsened. Especially in the beginning, it can take much deeper questioning before the patient knows which details to observe and compare. The physiotherapist needs to have a clear picture in mind of all the possible indicators of change, both in the subjective and in the physical examination. Too frequently it can be observed in clinical situations that lack of in-depth questioning leads the physiotherapist to the interpretation that the situation has remained unchanged or worsened, but in fact the disorder has improved somewhat already.

The questioning may also alert the patient to the necessity of trying out the self-management strategies the moment he starts to feel an increase in his symptoms, provided the exercises have been chosen with that objective. It is not unusual for patients to forget these self-management suggestions. However, this should not be interpreted as lack of discipline or motivation; from a cognitive–behavioural perspective the education of self-management strategies deals with change of movement behaviour and habits, which usually do not change overnight.

Effects of self-management strategies

The way the physiotherapist reassesses the self-management strategies may be crucial for the learning process of the patient and the initialization of change in movement behaviour. Random questions will often lead to random answers (Sluys et al. 1993):

Q 'Have you been able to do your exercises?'

A 'Yes.'

Q 'What did they do? Did they help?'

A 'No, not really.'

In comparison with for example:

Q 'Last time I recommended you try out two exercises – have you been able to think of these?'

A 'Yes, I've done them in the morning and in the evening.'

Q 'Very good! You told me that you had symptoms in your shoulder and neck after writing at your computer. Have you thought of doing the exercises then as well?'

A 'No, not at that particular moment. Maybe I should do them then as well.'

Q 'Yes, that's a very good idea. It seems strange, but just at the time that something hurts it might be helpful to try this out. Maybe you can tell me next time what the effects were – are you going to work at your computer again?'

Reassessments of physical examination tests

To determine the effect of a technique both the subjective and the physical parameters need to be assessed. The patient is asked if he feels any different from the treatment intervention. The following conversation shows how this can be done quickly, without sacrificing the depth of information required.

Q 'How do you feel now compared with when you were last in?'

A 'About the same.'

ET *So subjectively he is about the same – now to check the movements.*

Q 'Do you remember a few of the test movements we did before?'

A 'Yes, I lifted my arm, didn't I?'

Q 'Yes – please could you compare that with before? How does your arm feel now?'

ET *I think he has gained about 20° in range before he made a grimace and the quality of the movement looked better.*

A 'It did not make my upper arm worse this time.'

Q 'And now that your arm is down again, is it any worse as a result of lifting it?'

A 'No.'

Q 'Did you notice any difference in the way you moved?'

A 'I think I could lift it a bit higher?'

Q 'Yes, that's what I saw as well. You could move your arm higher before the pain started. How did it feel with regard to the quality of the movement? Did it feel any heavier or more difficult to move up?'

A 'No, I think I could lift my arm a bit more easily.'

Q 'Good. I would now like to summarize: we did these mobilization movements of your arm, which were not painful this time, and now that we have reassessed the lifting of your arm, it seems that your body liked the treatment as you could move the arm higher up and move it with more ease. The pain has not increased, but came on a little bit later in the range of movement. That's a good sign! Could I now check the other movements?

It may be useful, especially if the patient feels that the symptoms have not changed, to ask if he feels that the quantity or quality of the movement has changed. There are at times situations where the patient starts to move more freely with more range, but the pain is still the same, so the patient experiences everything as being the same, although parts of his movements are already changing. By asking patients about these other aspects of the movement, they may learn about this and concentrate more on the aspects of the test movement as well. Summarizing the information gained out of the reassessment frequently reinforces this learning process.

During a treatment intervention

It is essential while performing a treatment technique such as passive mobilization to maintain communication. On the one hand, the physiotherapist wants to assess any changes in resistance to movement or motor responses – on the other hand, the therapist needs to know of any changes in symptom reaction to the movement. There may be no pain, or no pain to start with, but soreness may occur as the technique is continued; alternatively, while performing the technique there may be soreness or reproduction of the patient's symptoms, which behave in various ways:

1. The symptoms decrease and disappear (they may increase during the first 10–20 seconds and then decrease)

2. The symptoms may come and go in rhythm with the rhythm of the technique

3. An ache may build up which is not in rhythm with the technique.

The communication issues associated with determining the behaviour of symptoms during the performance of the technique are related to trying to help the patient understand what the differences might be, so that he can give a useful answer:

ET *Now that I have started performing the technique I must know straight away what is happening to the patient's symptoms.*

Q 'Do you feel any discomfort at all while I am doing this?'

A 'No, I can't feel any discomfort at all other than the stretching.'

ET *This state of affairs may change fairly quickly, so in about 10 seconds I will ask again.*

Q 'Still nothing?'

A 'No, I can feel a little in my left buttock now.'

Q 'And that wasn't there when I started?'

A 'Yes it was there, it's always there.'

Q 'Has it changed since I started?'

A 'Yes, it's slightly worse.'

ET *What I need to know now is whether this is a gradual build-up into an ache, or whether it is going to 'come and go' in rhythm with the technique. To make it easier for him, the question is better asked in such a way that he can choose between two statements.*

Q 'Does it come and go in rhythm with the movement, or is it a steady ache?'

A 'It's just a slight ache.'

ET *What I need to determine as quickly as possible is whether it is going to increase with further use of the technique, whether it will remain the same, or whether it will decrease and go.*

After a further 10 seconds, the question is asked:

Q 'Is it just the same or increasing?'

ET *The question in asked in this way because it is hoped that the symptoms will be decreasing and therefore it is better to influence the answer towards what is not wanted rather than to get a false answer suggested by me.*

A 'It's about the same.'

Ten seconds later:

Q 'How is it now?'

A 'It's less, I think.'

In another 10 seconds:

Q 'And now?'

A 'It's gone.'

ET *That's an ideal response. I also had the impression that I could move further into the range. I will record this response later.*

Treatment and education of bodily awareness

Communication is important not only during the application of passive movement techniques, but also during education of bodily awareness. The 34-year-old patient described in the communication examples of collaborative goal setting had a tendency to pull her shoulders in protraction and elevation.

Although it may seem time consuming, a different communication technique may have immediate effects on understanding and compliance.

Directive communication

Q 'You should not sit like this. That will certainly provoke pain. I think it is better that you take care in your daily life not to sit in so much tension. I will show you the exercise once again and I suggest you do this exercise three times a day and, of course, when it hurts as well.' (*shows the patient once again how to relax the shoulders more towards a neutral position*)

A 'Okay.'

Q 'I'll see you then next time.'

Next session:

Q 'How have you been since last time?'

A 'I still have pain.'

Q 'Have you been able to do that exercise I showed you last time?'

A 'Yes.'

Q 'Could you show me once again?'

A 'Em…, I don't know if I have done it right, could you show me again?'

In such cases the physiotherapist may be disappointed that the patient seems to have forgotten the exercise. However, this may be due to the timing within the session (in the last few minutes of the session) and the quality of communication.

Mirroring, guiding by asking questions, including reassessments

Q 'How are you now?'

A 'It hurts at my shoulder.'

Q 'Do you notice anything different about your posture?'

A 'No.'

Q 'I see that you have pulled your shoulder forwards and up.' (*mirrors the positions*)

A (*observes herself now*) 'Oh yes, that's right.' (*but does not change anything immediately*)

Q 'Would you be able to change something?'

A (*pulls shoulders very far down and in retraction*) 'Like this?'

Q 'Maybe a little bit less. (*Guides the movement.*) How does it feel now?'

A 'That feels fine.'

Q 'Anything that hurts you right now?'

A 'No.'

Q 'You mean nothing of the shoulder pain that you had right before?'

A 'No.'

Q 'Could you please pull your shoulder up and forwards, as you did before?'

A (*Performs the movement.*)

Q 'How does it feel right now?'

A 'That hurts at my shoulder.' (*But does not change automatically.*)

Q 'How about trying to relax your shoulder again.' (*Guides the movement, tactile.*)

A 'Now it's gone.'

Q 'Could you please do that again?'

A (*Pulls the shoulder up again.*) 'That hurts again.'

Q 'And if you change the position again?'

A (*Performs the movements without the aid of the physiotherapist.*) 'Now it is much better again.'

In this case the reassessment is not only the evaluation of the symptom responses, but also the patient automatically changing her movement behaviour as happened in the third repetition. To follow the sequence with cognitive reinforcement and explanation will often be useful.

Q 'I suggest you monitor yourself a bit during the daytime, this afternoon and tomorrow. Maybe you'll notice that you pull up your shoulder quite frequently. We all often move automatically, without thinking – I notice that with myself as well. Shall

I explain what happens to your body when you perform such movements?'

A   'Yes please.'

Q   (*Explains the principle of the bent finger; McKenzie 1981.*)

A   'Aha!'

Q   'Could you imagine that similar things happen in your shoulder?'

A   'Oh well, yes.'

Q   'I have explained a lot to you – however, I'm not sure if I've done a good job. Would you mind explaining to me in your own words what you've understood?'

A   'If I am sitting in such a tensed position the blood circulation is in trouble. If I move differently it is better.'

This has been a reassessment on a cognitive level. If the patient is invited to explain in her own words, the physiotherapist immediately understands if the explanation 'touched ground' and in the patient herself deeper understanding may be enhanced.

Q   'Then I would like to suggest that you focus on your shoulder a few times during the day, to check if you are pulling it up, particularly when you feel it is hurting again. Maybe you could try this simple exercise then. If this helps you, then we come closer to understanding your problem. However, if it does not help, then we have to look for alternatives. So please try it and feel free to tell me if you think it is successful or not.'

Next session:

Q   'How have you been since last time?'

A   'I have noticed that I have this silly habit of pulling my shoulder up. I've paid more attention to this and I feel it's getting better already.'

Q   'How did you notice that?'

A   'It does not hurt so much now and I am able to complete all the tasks that I have to do during the day.'

Retrospective assessments (after three to five treatments)

Frequently it is necessary to assess the progress in the patient's symptoms and signs compared with those at the first visit. The physiotherapist may also have employed various interventions, the effects of which need to be determined. Furthermore, it needs to be clarified collaboratively with the patient if the agreed treatment objectives are still relevant or if new goals need to be defined. The latter becomes especially important if the patient is supported towards resuming activities at work or in hobbies.

A valuable question is: 'How do you feel compared with before we began?' The answer enables the physiotherapist to see the progress in its proper perspective. It sometimes happens that a patient reports at each successive treatment to be feeling a bit better, yet at the fourth treatment session may say, 'Well…I'm not any worse.'

It is for reasons such as this that retrospective assessment must be made a routine part of the therapeutic process. Sometimes the patient may be asked to define the percentage of progress:

Q   'What do you think the percentage of improvement has been compared with when we began?'

For some patients it is difficult to think in these terms, in which case they may be asked:

Q   'Do think you are less than halfway to being completely better?'

A   'Oh no, I'm more than half better, thank you.'

The communication may then continue, for example, as follows:

Q   'That sounds good, tell me in what way are you better?'

A   'The aching doesn't bother me during the day now and when I get out of bed in the morning I don't feel stiff any more. Also I can put my socks on without any difficulty.'

Q   'That's good. Any symptoms left? How is your day?'

A   'I still feel it a bit after I've been sitting for a long time.'

Q   'Sitting for how long?'

A   '2–3 hours.'

Q   'Anything you can do about it then, once it comes on?'

A   'Well, as you suggested, I move my back or I put my arm or a pillow in my back while I'm sitting or I stand up and do this straightening exercise.'

Q   'Do you feel this allows you to sit for longer?'

A   'Yes, then I can get on with my work again.'

Q   'How's that in comparison with the first treatment?'

A   'Oh, then I could sit for only 10 minutes, so I think that's quite a step forward, isn't it?'

After the assessment of the symptoms, activity levels and the employment of self-management strategies, it is essential to assess the subjective effects of the treatment. The physiotherapist may ask, for example:

Q 'I have done various things in the first few sessions. Is there anything that you think has been especially helpful – is there anything that you feel I certainly should not do to again?'

Furthermore, it is often useful to reflect on the learning process:

Q 'From all the things we have discussed and done, which has been particularly useful for you? In other words, what have you learned from the therapy so far?'

A 'I understand now that my being in the same position for a long time may provoke pain. I've been working so hard over the last 2 years that I did not have time for my usual sports and when I was working I was concentrating so hard that I forgot about the stress on my body.'

Q 'Is there anything that is particularly useful to you to do now for this?'

A 'Well, I feel it is really useful to think of the movements of my back once I'm at work and I am already thinking of returning to my sports again.'

After having established this, a prospective assessment in which treatment objectives are redefined may be useful:

Q 'On which activities should we work together in the next period of treatment?'

A 'Well, I don't know, you're the therapist.'

Q 'You told me you wanted to go back to your sports – which sports?'

A: 'I would like to play golf and tennis again.'

Q 'Are there any particular movements that you think may be difficult?'

A 'I think at golf only the bending down to pick up a ball. At tennis I'm not so sure, the quick changes and the deep reaching at forehand – I don't know.'

Q 'Let's take these movements into the reassessment procedures and I think we should start to train them. Could you bring in a golf club with you the next time?'

Similar questions need to be asked with regard to working situations, before reassessing the physical examination tests.

Final analytical assessment

In this phase it is the objective not only to evaluate the overall therapeutic process so far, but also to anticipate possible future difficulties in order to enhance the patient's long-term compliance with the suggestions, instructions and self-management strategies (Sluys 2000).

Similar questions may be posed as described in retrospective assessment. The anticipation of future difficulties may take place as follows:

Q 'We have now looked back at the therapeutic process. I'm glad that I've been able to help you so far. In the future, where would you anticipate difficulties may arise again?'

A 'I don't know. I think if I stick to the exercises you taught me I should be in good shape, I guess.'

Q 'I think so. However, we are all only human, so it may be that you forget some of the exercises over time. Which exercise would you do first, just in case your back started to hurt again?'

A 'I guess I would start with the straightening exercises.'

Q 'When would you do them particularly?'

A 'I believe I would think of them after sitting or bending over.'

Q 'Anything else?'

A 'Well, if I bend over for a longer period, it is also helpful to tuck my belly in, so I think I should not forget about that one too.'

Q 'Are there any working activities which you think could cause you difficulties?'

A 'Well, I help out with a gardener at times – in spring we often put up fences and then I may lift a lot and may use a heavy sledgehammer.'

Q 'Oh, that may be important. Can you show me the way you would do this?'

Conclusion

Although this discussion about communication and its problems may seem lengthy, it merely touches the surface of the subject. Communication and the establishment of a therapeutic relationship nowadays have been declared an integral part of physiotherapy (WCPT 1999, Mead 2000). However, communication is both an art and a skill which needs careful attention and ongoing training in order to enhance the assessment and treatment process between the patient and the physiotherapist.

References

Alsop A, Ryan S: *Making the most of fieldwork education – a practical approach*, London, 1996, Chapman and Hall.

Bassett SF, Petrie KJ: The effect of treatment goals on patient compliance with physiotherapy exercise programmes, *Physiotherapy* 85:130–137, 1997.

Besley J, Kayes NM, McPherson KM: Assessing therapeutic relationships in physiotherapy: literature review, *New Zealand Journal of Physiotherapy* 39(2):81–91, 2011

Brioschi R: *Kurs: die therapeutische Beziehung*. Leitung: Brioschi R, Hengeveld E. Fortbildungszentrum Zurzach, 1998, Mai.

Burnard P: *Counselling Skills for Health Professionals*, London, 1994, Chapman and Hall.

Charmann RA: Pain theory and physiotherapy, *Physiotherapy* 75:247–254, 1989.

Chin A, Paw JMM, Meyer S, et al: Therapietrouw van cystic fibrosis patienten, *NTvF* 105:96–104, 1993.

de Haan EA, van Dijk JP, Hollenbeek Brouwer J, et al: Meningen van clienten over de kwaliteit van fysiotherapie: verwachting en werkelijkheid, *NTvF* 105:18–22, 1995.

French S: History taking in the physiotherapy assessment, *Physiotherapy* 74:158–160, 1988.

French S, Neville S, Laing J: *Teaching and learning – a guide for therapists*, Oxford, 1994, Butterworth-Heinemann.

Gartland GJ: Communication skills instruction in Canadian physiotherapy schools: a report, *Physiother Can* 36:29–31, 1984a.

Gartland GJ: Teaching the therapeutic relationship, *Physiother Can* 36:24–28, 1984b.

Grant RIE, editor: Manual therapy: science, art and placebo. In Grant RIE, editor: *Physical therapy of the cervical and thoracic spine*, New York, 1994, Churchill Livingstone.

Härkäpää K, Järvikoski A, Mellin G, et al: Health locus of control beliefs in low back pain patients, *Scand J Behav Ther* 18:107–118, 1989.

Hall AM, Ferreira PH, Maher CC, Latimer J, Ferreira M: The influence of the therapist-patient relationship on treatment outcome in physical rehabilitation: a systematic review, *Phys Ther* 90:1099–1110, 2010.

Hayes KW, Huber G, Rogers S, Sanders B: Behaviors that cause clinical instructors to question the clinical competence of physical therapist students, *Phys Ther* 79:653–667, discussion 668–671, 1999.

Hengeveld E: *Psychosocial issues in physiotherapy: manual therapists' perspectives and observations. MSc Thesis*. London, 2000, Department of Health Sciences, University of East London.

Hengeveld E: Compliance und Verhaltensänderung in Manueller Therapie, *Man Ther* 7:122–132, 2003.

Horton J, Bayne R, editors: *Counselling and communication in health care. Counselling and communication skills for medical and health care practitioners*, Leicester, 1998, BPS Books.

Jensen G, Shepard KF, Hack LM: The novice versus the experienced clinician: insights into the work of the physical therapist, *Phys Ther* 70:314–323, 1990.

Jensen GM, Shepard KF, Gwyer J, Hack LM: Attribute dimensions that distinguish master and novice physical therapy clinicians in orthopedic settings, *Phys Ther* 72:711–722, 1992.

Kendall NAS, Linton SJ, Main CJ, et al: *Guide to assessing psychosocial yellow flags in acute low back pain: risk factors for long-term disability and work loss*, Wellington, New Zealand, 1997, Accident Rehabilitation & Compensation Insurance Corporation of New Zealand and the National Health Committee.

Keogh E, Cochrane M: Anxiety sensitivity, cognitive biases, and the experience of pain, *J Pain* 3:320–329, 2002.

Kerssens JJ, Jacobs C, Sixma H, et al: Wat patienten belangrijk vinden als het gaat om de kwaliteit van fysiotherapeutische zorg. *NTvF* 105:168–173, 1995.

Klaber Moffet J, Richardson PH: The influence of the physiotherapist-patient relationship on pain and disability. *Physiother Theory Pract* 13:89–96, 1997.

Kleinmann A: *The illness narratives – suffering, healing and the human condition*, New York, 1988, Basic Books.

Klenermann L, Slade PD, Stanley IM, et al: The prediction of chronicity in patients with an acute attack of low back pain, *Spine* 20:478–484, 1995.

KNGF: *Beroepsprofiel Fysiotherapeut*, Amersfoort/ Houten, 1998, Koninklijk Nederlands Genootschap voor Fysiotherapie/Bohn Stafleu van Loghum.

Lawler H: The physiotherapist as a counsellor. In Gibson A, editor: *Physiotherapy in the community*, Cambridge, 1988, Woodhead-Faulkner.

Main CJ: *Communicating about pain to patients. Schmerzen, alles klar?* Zurzach, Switzerland, 2004.

Main CJ, Spanswick CC: *Pain management – an interdisciplinary approach*, Edinburgh, 2000, Churchill Livingstone.

Maitland GD: *Vertebral manipulation*, ed 5, Oxford, 1986, Butterworth-Heinemann.

Maitland GD: *Peripheral manipulation*, ed 3, Oxford, 1991, Butterworth-Heinemann.

Mattingly C, Gillette N: Anthropology, occupational therapy and action research, *Am J Occup Ther* 45:972–978, 1991.

May S: Patient satisfaction with management of back pain. Part 1: What is satisfaction? Review of satisfaction with medical management; Part 2: An explorative, qualitative study into patients' satisfaction with physiotherapy, *Physiotherapy* 87:4–20, 2001.

McKenzie R: *The lumbar spine: mechanical diagnosis and therapy*, Waikanae, New Zealand, 1981, Spinal Publications.

Mead J: Patient partnership, *Physiotherapy* 86:282–284, 2000.

Merry T, Lusty B: *What is patient-centred therapy? A personal and practical guide*, London, 1993, Gale Publications.

Philips HC: Avoidance behaviour and its role in sustaining chronic pain, *Behav Res Ther* 25:273–279, 1987.

Pratt JW: Towards a philosophy of physiotherapy, *Physiotherapy* 75:114–120, 1989.

Riolo L: Commentary to Sluys, Kok & van der Zee (1993), *Phys Ther* 73:784–786, 1993.

Roberts L, Chapman J, Sheldon F: Perceptions of control in people with acute low back pain, *Physiotherapy* 88:539–548, 2002.

Roberts L, Bucksey SJ: Communication with patients: what happens in practice? *Phys Ther* 87:586–594, 2007.

Rogers CR: *A way of being*, Boston, 1980, Houghton Mifflin.

Rotter J: Generalized expectancies for internal versus external control of reinforcement, *Psychol Monogr, General and Applied* 80:1–5, 1966.

Schachter CL, Stalker CA, Teram E: Towards sensitive practice: issues for physical therapists working with survivors of childhood sexual abuse, *Phys Ther* 79:248–261, 1999.

Schön DA: *The reflective practitioner. How professionals think in action.* Aldershot, 1983, Arena.

Schulz von Thun F: *Miteinander Reden – Störungen und Klärungen. Allgemeine Psychologie der Kommunikation*, Reinbek bei Hamburg, 1981, Rowohlt Taschenbuch Verlag.

Schwartzberg SL: *Self-disclosure and empathy in occupational therapy*, Invited Paper at Occupational Therapy Conference, Trinity College, 1992, Dublin.

Sim J: Focus groups in physiotherapy evaluation and research, *Physiotherapy* 82:189–198, 1996.

Sluys E: *Therapietrouw door Voorlichting – Handleiding voor Patiëntenvoorlichting in de Fysiotherapie*, Amsterdam, 2000, Uitgeverij SWP.

Sluys E, Hermans J: Problemen die patienten ervaren bij het doen van huiswerkoefeningen en bij het opvolgen van adviezen, *NTvF* 100:175–179, 1990.

Sluys EM, Kok GJ, van der Zee J: Correlates of exercise compliance in physical therapy, *Phys Ther* 73:771–786, 1993.

Stenmar L, Nordholm LA: Swedish physical therapists' beliefs on what makes therapy work, *Phys Ther* 77:414–421, 1997.

Stone S: Qualitative research methods for physiotherapists, *Physiotherapy* 77: 449–452, 1991.

The Age. 1982. 21 August.

Thomson D, Hassenkamp AM, Mainsbridge C: The measurement of empathy in a clinical and non-clinical setting. Does empathy increase with clinical experience? *Physiotherapy* 83:173–180, 1997.

Trede FV: Physiotherapists' approaches to low back pain education, *Physiotherapy* 86:427–433, 2000.

Van der Linden M: Therapeutische relatie: een specifieke of een non-specifieke factor, *NBMF-Nieuws* 1:12–15, 1998.

Vlaeyen J, Linton S: Fear avoidance and its consequences in chronic pain states: a state of the art, *Pain* 85:317–332, 2000.

Wall PD: The placebo and the placebo response. In Wall PD, Melzack R, editors: *Textbook of pain*, Edinburgh, 1994, Churchill Livingstone.

Watzlawick P, Beavin J, Jackson DJ: *Menschliche Kommunikation*, Bern, 1969, Huber Verlag.

WCPT: *Description of physical therapy*, London, 1999, World Confederation of Physical Therapy.

WHO: *ICF – International Classification of Functioning, Disability and Health*, Geneva, 2001, World Health Organization.

Wiegant E: Tussen intimiteit en sexueel misbruik, *FysioPraxis* 16:24–27, 1993.

Management of cervical spine disorders: A neuro-orthopaedic perspective

4

Robin Blake   Tim Beames

CHAPTER CONTENTS

Epidemiology of neck, head and arm pain . . . 116

Common syndromes in the cervical region
and their presentation 117

Clinical Reasoning and the
biopsychosocial model 118

Pain mechanisms 120

Subjective examination 131

Physical examination 132

Pre-cervical spine treatment screening 150

Treatment 155

Key words

Pain, sensitization, nerve, neuromatrix, output,
neurodynamics, nerve palpation

Introduction

This chapter aims to provide appropriate information to allow the clinician to assess and treat common
pain disorders affecting the cervical spine by using
a solid clinical reasoning approach. These disorders
include whiplash-associated disorder (WAD), headache and cervical nerve root lesion. The epidemiology will be discussed within a bio-psychosocial
paradigm demonstrating how features of each individual's pain experience can then be identified in
clinical interview and physical examination. Treatment will then be considered with reference to the
disorders above.

Epidemiology of neck, head and facial pain

The incidence of neck pain varies significantly from
fairly rare diagnoses of disc herniation with radiculopathy (0.055 per 1000 persons) to more common
self-reported neck pain (213 per 1000 persons).
From 30 to 50% of neck pain sufferers report
ongoing symptoms up to 12 months after onset with
an increased prevalence among women, peaking in
middle age (Hogg-Johnson et al. 2009). This indicates that we should be more effective with our
treatment and consider why such a large proportion
of people have ongoing pain.

Localized neck pain appears to be fairly rare
and neck pain is almost always reported as part of
either regional or widespread pain states (Natvig
et al. 2010). Those suffering with neck pain as
part of a more widespread pain state are also more
likely to have concurrent reduction of function.
This suggests that the clinician should maintain a
global or holistic perspective within their treatment
approach.

In WAD, up to 50% of people have ongoing neck
pain 1 year after the accident. In terms of the risk
factors following injury, greater initial pain, more
symptoms and greater initial disability predicted
slower recovery. There are very few prognostic
factors, however, that actually relate to the collision.
Psychological factors such as passive coping style,
depressed mood and fear of movement all relate to
slower or less complete recovery (Carroll et al.
2009a).

A large variation exists in the prevalence of neck pain in a working population with 27.1% reporting symptoms in Norway and 47.8% in Quebec. In Quebec between 11 and 14.1% of workers had to limit their activities as a result of their neck pain (Côté et al. 2009). Recovery is not influenced by physical demands from the job or other workplace characteristics. Those with a poorer prognosis were shown to: have little influence on their work situation; were blue collar workers as opposed to white collar workers; or had experienced prior neck pain or had taken previous sick leave, again pointing to the need for the practitioner to maintain a bio-psychosocial perspective and truly understand the individual (Carroll et al. 2009b).

Interestingly, no prevention strategies aimed at changing workstation set-up or ergonomics have been shown to reduce the incidence of neck pain in workers (Côté et al. 2009). There are, however, psychological protective factors. Having a job which allows for decision-making and where there is empowering leadership helps to reduce the incidence of neck pain (Christensen & Knardahl 2010). This health focused or salutogenic approach (Antonovsky 1996) considers the positive attributes in the person with neck pain and fits well with a collaborative approach that a clinician and their patient can utilize.

There is a prevalence of neck pain in people with metabolic syndrome (Mäntyselkä et al. 2010) and it is unsurprising that around 34% of people with head and neck cancer experience neuropathic pain, break-through pain and pain of non-malignant origin in the neck region (Williams et al. 2010). Clinicians should maintain strong clinical reasoning skills to incorporate this information and understand the multifactorial components of a pain state at all times (see Chapter 2).

Common syndromes of the cervical region and their presentations

Whiplash-associated disorders (WAD)

WAD are a common and sometimes disabling condition as a consequence, generally, of a motor vehicle accident. These conditions may be seen in the acute or chronic stages with many variations between. The full spectrum of physical and psychological impairments is given in the proposed adaptation of the Quebec Task force (QTF) classification (Sterling 2004). Jull and colleagues (2008) suggest that WAD is one of the most controversial musculoskeletal conditions, due to its physical and psychological complexity and that precise patho-anatomical diagnosis is commonly not available even with current imaging techniques.

Symptoms occur predominately in the posterior region of the neck, but may radiate to the head, shoulder, arm, interscapular and lumbar region (Barnsley et al. 1998). Headache, dizziness, loss of balance, visual disturbance, paraesthesia, anaesthesia and cognitive disturbance are common (Treleaven et al. 2003). Hypersensitivity is also a familiar symptom and can be present in a local form suggesting a relationship to nociceptive input, or over widespread body sites when the central nervous system (CNS) is implicated (Sterling et al. 2003a).

Headache

Headache is a common complaint. There are many proposed causes (The International Headache Society (IHS) 2004). It may be a primary disorder such as migraine, tension type or cluster type, or cervicogenic headache, referred to as a secondary kind of disturbance.

The main origins of cervicogenic headache are thought to be patho-anatomical and pathophysiological events occurring in the neuromusculoskeletal structures, but there may be considerable overlap with the primary types of headaches (Vincent 2011). Central nervous system sensitivity also plays an important role in all types of headache pain. In the differentiation procedure cervicogenic headache is usually unilateral and side-consistent while migraine can change sides within or between attacks (HIS 2004).

Cervical nerve root lesion

Cervical nerve root injuries are a common problem particularly in contact sports where they may be attributed to the 'stinger' or burner injury (Safran 2004). The mechanism of injury is considered to be tensile or compressive forces acting on either the nerve root or brachial plexus (Standaert & Herring 2009). As a result of this type of injury, there can be partial or total loss of motor, sensory and autonomic functions of the damaged nerves (Navarro et al. 2007). This means that this type of problem may present with varied symptomology.

It was commonly thought that in nerve root lesions causing radiculopathy, the underlying problem was due to compressive forces acting on the nerve root through disc herniation or foraminal stenosis (Levitz et al. 1997). Although this can happen it appears that the presence of new disruption is likely in only a small percentage of people suffering with radicular symptoms (Caragee et al. 2006). More recently it has been shown that a chemical influence may be more critical in the development of these symptoms (Winkelstein & DeLeo 2004), whereby the nerves become highly sensitized due to a local immune response (e.g. inflammation).

Clinical reasoning and the bio-psychosocial model

It is obvious from the epidemiological information on neck pain that the clinician needs to consider a broader reasoning approach than the traditional biomedical model will allow. Although the biomedical model is not wrong, as a paradigm it is insufficient to fully understand each person's neck pain experience (as shown in the differing epidemiology of neck pain). This is due to the differences that exist in genetic make-up, previous experiences, cultural backgrounds and socioeconomic situations, to name a few. The bio-psychosocial model takes on board all of this information, allowing the clinician to synthesize information from many different areas in a person's pain experience. The bio-psychosocial model requires that we consider the different interacting variables across biological, psychological and social domains (Engel 1978). This will allow some appreciation of the variety of responses to treatment of what may seem similar pathophysiology.

Using the bio-psychosocial paradigm to clinically reason requires the consideration of interactions of systems at many levels. For example, a person who experiences ongoing headache may notice a change in their mood. This could be as a result of the availability of one of the chemicals acting in their CNS, such as serotonin. The change in mood may affect how they function in society. They may avoid going out or it may affect the dynamics of their family. On another level the change in serotonin availability may have an effect on their overall sensitivity,

exhibited by increased sensitivity to different external stimuli like bright lights or loud noises. This demonstrates how relatively small changes at one system level can have repercussions at many other levels. A more holistic view of our patients and identification of the effect of their illness behaviours ties into the current appreciation of the WHO International classification of functioning, disability and health. This allows the integration of the knowledge that all biological systems and every system level are functionally interrelated in a hierarchical continuum, i.e. from microscopic to macroscopic and beyond.

To apply clinical reasoning to the patient on an individual basis requires a depth of knowledge and skills beyond anatomy, biomechanics and tissue healing. It should embrace knowledge from other models such as a current understanding of pain mechanisms and with that the mature organism model (Gifford 1998; Fig. 4.1) and the neuromatrix paradigm (Melzack 1989, 1990). In addition, understanding of psychology models would be beneficial. The fear-avoidance models have value in understanding relevant thoughts and beliefs in ongoing pain states (Vlaeyen & Linton 2000) and ties in with the idea of both education and the notion of graded exposure, which is often applied by movement therapists in rehabilitation. Information from models such as the evolutionary biology model may enhance the thought process for both the clinician and patient. An example of the clinical reasoning approach for WAD is given in Box 4.1.

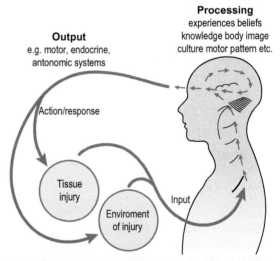

Figure 4.1 • The mature organism model (Gifford 1998), showing the input, processing and output domains and interactions in a circular model.

Box 4.1

Application of clinical reasoning to cervical conditions

A 26-year-old female with a 3-week history of WAD

Anatomy, biomechanics, tissue healing

What are the possible structures known to be damaged with WAD? What is the impact on alignment, joint function, muscle tone and nerve gliding? What are the time scales relating to aspects of tissue healing?

Pain mechanisms

What are the likely pain mechanisms present in this patient? Nociceptive contributions, e.g. inflammation; neuropathic elements, e.g. an ectopic impulse generating site; central sensitivity causing lowered threshold to normal stimuli; and output responses such as pain, movement changes and alteration of mood.

Mature organism model

What are this person's previous experiences of whiplash or injury especially involving pain? What are their current thoughts and beliefs regarding pain or the changes in their movement? How do the other responses such as the changes in immune system activity relate to their current problem and how will this affect their treatment?

Pain mechanisms can be integrated into the model for this individual.

Neuromatrix model

What are the ongoing inputs into the neuromatrix e.g. sensory, cognitive and affective on both conscious and unconscious levels? What are the subsequent responses and what makes up their individual neurotag? What effect would a change in brain representation for their neck have on the subsequent response and does this create an error or mismatch of information being processed in the neuromatrix regarding their WAD?

Psychology models

Are there clinical features where changes in thought may be apparent, e.g. rumination over the accident or a predilection for attributing the pain to a patho-anatomic cause?

Fear-avoidance of pain model

Is there fear of causing pain with movement and does this link with a belief that pain equates to tissue damage? How can these thoughts be challenged in order to grade the exposure of feared activities and regain activity levels and engagement in life areas?

Evolutionary biology model

Why has this individual chosen certain protective mechanisms e.g. holding the neck stiff to avoid movement and are these serving a useful purpose?

Working with an underlying conceptual model can guide treatment by allowing the synthesis of information and evidence into a unifying principle. This helps provide some understanding of the different enigmatic pain situations such as pain in the absence of nociception; the absence of pain in the presence of tissue damage; variability and unpredictability of individual responsiveness to identical treatments; and the lack of predictable relationships between pain, impairment and disability. Understanding more fully the relationship of interacting variables from biological, psychological and social domains should allow a more effective clinical diagnosis and appropriate treatment plan and intervention (Smart et al. 2008).

Despite several guidelines published for the management of different neck disorders it is necessary in the clinic for the clinician to apply these in the context of the individual and their current presentation by using high level reasoning, evaluation and therapeutic skills (Jull 2009). By recognizing the heterogeneity of our patients alternate pathways can be created to understand how best to individualize intervention. This may be achieved by grouping individuals into classification systems such as recognition of bio-psychosocial variables or through the development of clinical predication rules for certain conditions (Beneciuk et al. 2009a). Despite progress in the research of these scientific principles it is important that the therapist maintains a high level of independent reasoning regarding each individual presenting to them.

A definition for pain

Pain has been described as 'an unpleasant sensory and emotional experience associated with actual or potential tissue damage or described in terms as such' (Merskey & Bogduk 1994). However, with continuing understanding of pain, this definition could be considered insufficient to relate the full extent of what a neck pain experience encompasses. As a pain experience always involves the brain, it is necessary that clinicians and the general public become aware and are ready to accept that. A newer working definition that should allow this transition in understanding has been proposed, stating:

> Pain is a multiple system output activated by an individual pain neuromatrix. This pain neuromatrix is activated whenever the brain considers that the tissues are in danger and action is required…and that pain is allocated an anatomical reference in the virtual body.

(Moseley 2003)

Therefore, pain is a response produced by the neuromatrix as a consequence of potential or perceived threats to the individual's tissues. This means that the different brain areas (and other parts of the neuroimmune system) that communicate together to process this information subsequently create a response that includes the conscious perception of pain. Pain is not the only output from the neuromatrix; there will be changes in activity of other response systems. For example, there may be changes in the motor system seen through altered movements or in the sympathetic nervous system with abnormal sweating or increased heart rate. Many of these changes in the response systems or deviations from the expected norms can be picked up through a comprehensive assessment – both subjective and objective.

Moseley's pain definition also includes an understanding that brain changes have been measured in different pain states, such as in the primary somatosensory cortex (e.g. Flor et al. 1997a). These changes may be reflected in an alteration of the body's representation of the symptomatic body part in the brain (i.e. a change in the virtual body). Therefore, if we looked at the brain of someone with neck pain we are likely to find changes in many areas that represent the neck and neck movements. These changes in representation of the virtual body may also correlate with certain assessment techniques.

Pain mechanisms

Pain mechanisms have been categorized to allow a better understanding of the neurobiological changes responsible for generating or maintaining a pain experience (Gifford & Butler 1997). Through the

recognition of different signs and symptoms present during clinical interview and physical examination and the use of clinical reasoning skills the clinician should be able to pick up the dominant pain mechanisms (Smart et al. 2010). These include:

1. Input dominant mechanisms:
   ○ nociceptive pain
   ○ peripheral neuropathic pain
2. Centrally mediated mechanisms:
   ○ central sensitization
3. Output/response mechanisms.

It is important to understand some of the basic neurophysiology underpinning these categories in order to recognize them in your patient. As suggested in the known epidemiology and presentations of the common cervical problems, there may be varying elements of any/all pain mechanisms in each individual.

Placing pain mechanisms into a reasoning framework

The mature organism model (Gifford 1998), sometimes referred to as 'the circular model' (Butler 2000), allows integration of pain mechanisms into an understandable framework. It describes the continuous processing of information that allows us to be comfortable at any time and in any given environment. The model consists of multiple sensory inputs into the central nervous system. The CNS then processes this incoming information. Finally, there is an output or response created by the brain that may include changes in homeostatic regulation such as subtle changes in hormone levels or maybe the perception of pain. This correlates with the working definition of pain proposed by Moseley (2003), which incorporates the neuromatrix paradigm that will be discussed later.

Pain may be initiated and often maintained in any or all components of the model, i.e. input, processing or output (Box 4.2). Ongoing input from an unhealthy nerve, changes in thought processes regarding movement, or the response to circulating hormones can all contribute in maintaining a pain experience. This model is helpful for clinical reasoning and subsequent therapeutic education. It can be used as a tool to emphasize the different areas of a problem that need addressing and highlights where a particular treatment technique may specifically act.

Box 4.2

Using the mature organism model for a cervical nerve root lesion (see Fig. 4.1)

A 40-year-old man with a 2-month history of a right-sided cervical nerve root lesion

Input: ongoing firing of the nerve from an ectopic impulse generating site and changes in local sensitivity due to the lower activation threshold of the afferent system creating ongoing nociception; slowing of axoplasmic and blood flow in the brachial plexus possibly affecting tissue health of the neck and arm.
Processing: previous knowledge of a nerve root lesion; a belief that pain is a sign of further tissue damage; changes in the representation of the neck and arm in the brain; central sensitization.
Output: burning pain; altered movement – cradling of arm and limited movement of the neck; lack of sleep; change in mood – feeling low (Fig. 4.1).

Input dominant mechanisms

Nociception

Nociception is essentially the processing of noxious or dangerous stimuli, be it intense heat, strong mechanical pressure or chemicals in the local tissues. This is partly due to the transduction of those different types of stimuli by specific ion channels and receptors found on the end of peripheral nerves in our tissues (nociceptors). These nerves are generally known as nociceptive neurons due to their ability to pick up the noxious stimuli (Bear et al. 2001). By processing this potentially damaging stimuli and communicating this information (transmission) to the brain, nociceptive neurons allow some defense against threatening inputs to our systems (Woolf & Ma 2007). It is the brain that ultimately decides whether it is necessary to create a pain experience from this information – nociceptive pain. It is useful to remember that pain is often not an end product of nociception.

Types of nociceptive neurons

Sensory stimulation is communicated by a range of afferent neurons: Aβ, Aδ and C fibres. Noxious stimuli is generally transmitted on the slow conducting, relatively unmyelinated C fibres and thinly myelinated Aδ fibres (Woolf & Ma 2007), although some larger myelinated and faster conducting Aβ fibres may also act as nociceptive neurons. It may be beneficial to know the different classes and their relative responses to chemical mediators and growth factors and their central connectivity (Snider & McMahon 1998).

Location of nociceptive neurons

Nociceptive neurons are present in most body tissues, including skin, muscle, joints, internal organs, blood vessels and nerve connective tissue. They are most notably absent in the brain itself, except the meninges (the connective tissues of the central nervous system).

Activation of nociceptive neurons

Nociceptive neurons are activated by stimuli that have the potential to cause tissue damage. Tissue damage can result from strong mechanical stimulation, extremes of temperature, oxygen deprivation and exposure to certain chemicals. The membrane of nociceptive neurons contains ion channels and receptors (nociceptors) that are activated by these types of stimuli.

Nociceptors and nociception

Potentially damaging extremes of heat are picked up by different nociceptors located at the nerve endings (Dhaka et al. 2006). The most common being the TRPV1 channel, which under normal circumstances picks up noxious heat temperatures above 43°C and is responsible for the feelings brought about by touching chili peppers!

For conduction of an electrical impulse to occur there must be sufficient nociceptors opened through the stimulation, e.g. heat, to allow enough positively charged ions to flow into the nerve cell, thus causing depolarization and the creation of an electrochemical message, the action potential or, in the case of nociception, a danger message. Greater stimulation of a nociceptor causes greater intensity of its firing. Ultimately, nociception could be referred to as danger signalling or messaging.

Speed of messaging

The action potentials (nociception or danger messages) bring relative information towards the CNS

Table 4.1 Nerve fibre features

Type of nerve fibre	Myelination	Conduction velocity
Aβ	Thick	Fast
Aδ	Thin	Slow
C	Rudimentary/unmyelinated	Very slow

about the site and intensity of the stimulus. Aδ and C fibres conduct to the CNS at different speeds due to the differences in myelination. It is usually considered that there are two distinct sensory perceptions when creating nociception (e.g. when stubbing your toe very hard): a fast, sharp, first pain caused by activation of Aδ fibres followed by a duller, longer-lasting second pain due to activation of C fibres (Costigan et al. 2009). See Table 4.1 for a summary of the features of nerve fibres.

Transmission of messages via second order neurons

Primary afferent neurons (including the peripheral nociceptive neurons) transmit electrochemical impulses towards the dorsal horn of the spinal cord where they synapse with second order neurons. These second order neurons may be either nociceptive specific neurons or wide dynamic range neurons depending on the lamina that they synapse at and communicate nociceptive or non-nociceptive messages, respectively.

There are many ascending pathways that contribute to the messaging of nociceptive information that ultimately project to cortical and subcortical regions (Almeida et al. 2004). There is huge complexity of neuroanatomy that helps to form the sensory-discriminatory part of perception.

Mechanical nociception

With sufficient pressure or stretch, local mechanoreceptors will be activated causing nociception. It is not clear yet what the exact high threshold mechanotransducers are, although it is clear that noxious mechanical stimuli can activate nociceptors (Hu et al. 2006). Under normal circumstances when you stub your toe the nociceptors will be activated and send a message to the brain via second order nociceptive specific neurons. Many routine clinical tests

may create mechanical nociception, especially where overpressure is used to assess joint range or stability.

Ischaemic nociception

Following sustained postures there will be local changes in oxygenation of the tissues. This ultimately leads to a rise in hydrogen ions that are picked up by local acid sensing ion channels and TRPV1 receptors. These are found on the peripheral terminals of nociceptive neurons and if sufficiently stimulated will create nociception. This is often enough to motivate a change in behaviour without being aware of it, i.e. move. The motivation to move and promote blood flow and normalization of tissue oxygenation will reduce the ischaemic nociceptive process. For someone with neck pain that is exacerbated by maintaining prolonged postures, for example at their computer workstation, they can be easily helped by recommending regular movement, which will reduce the nociception caused by the ischaemia.

Inflammatory nociception

Following injury to tissues there will be an immune-mediated healing response. Local immune cells, macrophages, neutrophils and mast cells are excited and move into the damaged area. They release immune-signalling chemicals like tumour necrosis factor-α and interleukin-1β. Some of the immediate effects of the immune system will cause the blood vessels to become leakier and allow more immune cells to access the damaged area. They cause mast cells to break down releasing histamine, bradykinin, ATP and various proinflammatory cytokines (Costigan et al. 2009). This ultimately means that there are numerous chemicals circulating in the damaged area. This is commonly referred to as an inflammatory soup.

The various chemicals that make up the inflammatory soup activate their specific receptors on the nerve endings causing nociception. There are other cellular effects that include the alteration in the ion channel type, number and kinetics. This can create sensitivity in the nerves supplying the damaged tissue. This phenomenon is called primary hyperalgesia. Now less stimulation is required to activate the neuron (Juhl et al. 2008), i.e. the damaged area becomes more sensitive. This can be seen when jumping in a warm shower when you are sun-burned. It feels excessively hot on the damaged/burned area!

This is likely to be due to the lowering of the heat threshold necessary to activate the TRPV1 receptors on the ends of the sensitized nociceptive neurons.

Along with changes to sensitivity in the damaged tissues (primary hyperalgesia) there will also be an increase in sensitivity outside of the damaged area. This is known as secondary hyperalgesia. This indicates changes in CNS processing (Huang et al. 2006, Woolf & Salter 2000). If you examined sensibility to pin-prick examination in these areas it would be perceived as much more intense even though there is no underlying tissue damage.

Neurogenic contributions to inflammation

When the peripheral terminal of a particular C fibre, the peptidergic C fibre, is excited it creates an axon reflex. This is essentially a spread of activity (transmission of impulses) to neighbouring nerve endings. There is subsequent release of chemicals into the tissues, known as neurogenic inflammation. Neurogenic inflammation adds to the immune-mediated inflammatory process. It can sometimes be seen as redness and swelling away from the damaged area, in an innervation field for the excited nerve. There are obviously implications to ongoing tissue health if neurogenic inflammation persists. (See Butler (2000) for a more in-depth summary of these events.)

Summary of clinical patterns from inflammation

- Swelling and stiffness with diurnal variations
- Redness/local erythema
- Increased pressure in tissues
- Protective motor response
- Acute pain and background aching.

Box 4.3 summarizes the nociceptive patterns occurring in WAD.

Clinical detection of nociceptive mechanisms

Nociceptive pain has generally been considered to have a fairly close stimulus/response relationship such that aggravating/easing factors are reasonably well defined and testable on examination. It is considered that pain localized to the area of injury or dysfunction, localized pain on palpation and antalgic postures or abnormal movement patterns are more predictive of a dominant nociceptive pain process (Smart et al. 2010).

Box 4.3

Nociceptive patterns in WAD

25-year-old woman with an acute WAD

- Her symptoms include feelings of pain and stiffness particularly when waking and later in the evening
- There is limited movement of her neck in all directions with pain and increased motor response
- There is a feeling of weakness, particularly lifting the head off the pillow
- Some ongoing/residual aching throughout the day
- Responds well to anti-inflammatory medication

It is important to remember that nociception is not sufficient for a pain experience. This was suggested with ischaemic nociception due to sustained postures, where nociception often occurs without ever coming into our consciousness.

Pain associated with changes in the nervous system

The definition of neuropathic pain is controversial (Bennett 2003). For our purpose *peripheral neuropathic pain* is the term used to describe situations where pain originates with an identified lesion of the peripheral somatosensory system, including the nerve roots or peripheral nerve trunks (Merskey & Bogduk 1994).

Nee & Butler (2006) described the clinical manifestation of peripheral neuropathic pain in terms of positive and negative symptoms. Positive symptoms reflect an abnormal level of excitability in the nervous system including pain, paraesthesia, dysaesthesia and spasm. Negative symptoms indicate reduced impulse conduction in neural tissues and include hypoesthesia, anaesthesia and weakness.

Neuropathic pain is typically described as a deep, burning or aching and has been attributed to an increase in the sensitivity of the nervous system. Dysaesthesic symptoms are also often reported with more unfamiliar or abnormal sensations such as tingling or crawling (Asbury & Fields 1984).

Nerves aren't normally that sensitive

Nerves are designed to move, slide and glide. They are happy to be squeezed and stretched a bit. They can also cope with a lack of blood supply for short periods without complaint. This is mostly the same for the nerve root complex, which will be irritated (i.e. evoke nociception) by a lack of blood – ischaemia – but will generally not cause any lasting symptoms. This is certainly not the case in the presence of local inflammation. In this instance there will be increased responsiveness of the peripheral nerves and in particular the nerve root complex to movements and ischaemic changes (e.g. Dilley et al. 2005). This means that moving and placing pressure through the excited nerves will more easily cause nociception. The irritated nerve root complex will also create a greater intensity of firing or nociception. It is, therefore, unsurprising that this can cause pain out of all proportions to the lesion or injury.

Injuries to peripheral nerves

Injuries to the peripheral nerves cause changes in both the injured and the uninjured axons. These changes take place not only where the nerve has been injured but also along the axon of the nerve, at the central terminals, dorsal root ganglion and higher centers (Costigan et al. 2009).

There are many changes that underpin a pain state following injury to a nerve. These are mediated by the immune system (Thacker et al. 2007). Assuming that there is no loss of conduction there will ultimately be an increase in excitability and a reduction in the ability to control this (i.e. a loss of descending modulation) – essentially the brain wants to know what is happening and therefore arranges to receive more messages that are also much louder.

One important neurophysiological change present in nerve injury is the development of ectopic impulse generating sites. These are areas where ion channels insert into portions of the axon membrane devoid of myelin. Myelin is broken down during injury and results in different types and amount of channels and receptors being inserted into the membrane. This allows the generation of messages to many different kinds of stimuli in areas that do not normally have this ability, hence ectopic (Devor & Seltzer

1999). Therefore, these 'hot spots' may now signal nociception from areas along the nerve as opposed to just the peripheral terminals.

Ectopic impulse generating sites have been consistently shown to be present not only in nerve injury but following inflammation within the nerve. They are part of the neurophysiology that causes the nerve to become mechanosensitive (Dilley et al. 2005) and may be picked up during nerve palpation or movement testing such as with neurodynamics. Ectopic impulse generating sites can be present along the length of the axon following nerve injury and are in part dependent on the health of the nerve and the local axoplasmic flow (Dilley & Bove 2008).

Clinical note

Therefore, the more unhealthy or immobile the nervous system is, the greater the chance of developing ectopia – or where there is altered axoplasmic flow there is greater chance of the generation of ectopia which act as 'hot spots'. This is due to the increase in availability of ion channels and receptors. These are likely to be features in nerve root lesion but may also be present in WAD and headache.

Blood flow

Nerves are bloodthirsty. A pressure gradient exists around and in neural tissue to ensure the maintenance of adequate nutrition. The gradient must exist so that blood can flow into neural tissue and then out of the tunnel surrounding the nerve. This can obviously be perturbed (e.g. through inflammation, scar tissue or an overactive muscle) and as such the clinician may want to evaluate the state of the surrounding tissues in order to understand the impact to the local blood flow.

The dimensions of neural tunnels can diminish from encroachment of surrounding structures. In the example of the cervical intervertebral foramina, the extraneural narrowing of the foramina can result from swelling of the facet joints, protrusion or degeneration of the intervertebral disc, abnormal posture producing a 'closing' effect on the foramina, such as the 'poking chin' position where the upper cervical spine is kept in extension. Intraneural swelling will also reduce the space available for unhindered neural movement and blood flow.

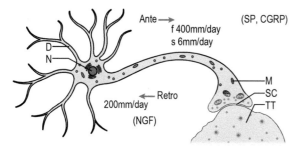

Figure 4.2 • Axoplasmic transport system: diagram. Axoplasmic transport system within a single neuron. D: dendrite; N: nucleus; M: mitochondria; SC: synaptic cleft; TT: target tissue; NGF: nerve growth factor; SP: substance; CGRP: calcitonin gene-related peptide (adapted from Butler 1991, p. 25 with permission).

Axoplasmic flow

Axoplasmic flow (Fig. 4.2) is the mechanism that allows cell components (e.g. ion channels, neurotransmitters held in pouches and mitochondria) to be transported to their functional sites and returned to the nerve cell for re-cycling. As with blood flow, unhindered axoplasmic flow is critical for nerve health (Delcomyn 1998). The thixotropic properties of axoplasm require regular bodily movements to maintain the flow. If there is insufficient movement then the axoplasm becomes thicker and the flow rate slows down, which will ultimately have an effect on the speed of recovery from nerve damage. This has obvious clinical implications i.e. the need to maintain some movement of the nervous system to maintain normal blood and axoplasmic flow.

Clinical tip

It is common in nerve root lesion, WAD and headache for someone to be relatively immobilized for a period of time. It may be beneficial therapeutically to maintain some movement in the nervous system to maintain normal health. This may come from pain-free neural mobilization exercises, such as sliders or from maintaining some activity, such as walking.

Clinical detection of peripheral neuropathic pain

Clinical tools such as the PainDETECT questionnaire and the Leeds Assessment of Neuropathic Symptoms and Signs (LANSS) have been found to be beneficial in helping to diagnose peripheral neuropathic pain (Bennett et al. 2007). These highlight the differences in the quality and behaviour of pain and dysesthesias as well as the signs and symptoms of allodynia, hyperalgesia and hyperpathia. However, other clinical signs have been suggested such as pain referred in a dermatomal/cutaneous distribution, pain/symptom provocation associated with subjective aggravating/easing factors and clinical tests associated with disturbance of neural tissue (e.g. neurodynamic testing) and pain/symptom provocation on palpation of relevant neural tissues (Smart et al. 2010).

Centrally mediated mechanisms, such as the development of central sensitization or representational changes in the brain, are also important in the generation and maintenance of neuropathic pain.

Centrally mediated mechanisms

Central sensitization

One consequence of both inflammation and nerve injury is the onset of the phenomenon central sensitization. This explains some of the common clinical signs that are present in cervical conditions such as the presence of allodynia (pain on normally non-painful stimulation) and secondary hyperalgesia (increased responsiveness to a normally painful stimulus outside of the original area of injury). If the clinician is able to pick up on this information then it will not only help to guide their treatment but minimize negative responses to treatment.

Central sensitization was proposed as a model to describe the different responses found to noxious stimulation in animals that had received prior noxious stimulation (Woolf 1994). It appeared they were more sensitive after repetitive testing and therefore the term sensitization was adopted to describe this phenomenon. The primary focus was originally of changes in the spinal cord but the same changes are known to occur in higher centers too.

The changes brought about by ongoing nociceptive stimulation include a lowering of the activation threshold at the pre- and post-synaptic membranes (i.e. primary afferent and second order neurons) at the dorsal horn, reduced descending inhibitory modulation and an increase in the descending facilitation. Ultimately this leads to an increase in the

Box 4.4

Central sensitization in headache

Man with 10-year history of headache
Current symptoms

Pain out of known anatomical fields that has spread since the onset. No obvious or reliable movements that exacerbate the pain. Symptoms may come on without warning and do not settle easily. Sensitivity to bright lights and loud noises. Possibly aggravated by stressful experiences or low mood. Suffers with irritable bowel syndrome.

Assessment demonstrates increased sensitivity to nerve palpation in facial nerves and bilaterally in the upper limbs.

Box 4.5

Brain areas commonly found to be part of a pain experience on brain imaging – example of nociceptive pain mechanisms

- Primary and secondary somatosensory cortices
- Primary motor cortex
- Insular cortex
- Anterior cingulate cortex
- Prefrontal cortex
- Thalamus
- Basal ganglia
- Cerebellum
- Amygdala
- Hippocampus

Unfortunately there is very little specific brain imaging research for cervical pain conditions. These areas are those generally found during experimental pain conditions i.e. during a controlled nociceptive stimulus. They may change considerably in people with ongoing pain problems.

response to normal stimuli or an amplification of the signaling in the nociceptive system (Latremoliere & Woolf 2009). Therefore, the brain is receiving louder/more intense messages to normal stimulation, as illustrated by the case in Box 4.4.

From a clinical point of view this means that normal movement can become painful even when there is no damage to the particular area. Also, neurosensory testing will likely reveal changes to light touch and pin-prick examination. Other proposed signs and symptoms are that the pain is diffuse, there is a distortion in the stimulus-response characteristics, spontaneous pain and pain associated with emotional and cognitive change. Also, previous failed interventions and tenderness on palpation are more signs of the presence of central sensitization (Smart et al. 2010).

Central sensitization has been found to be present in headache, WAD and neuropathic pain and musculoskeletal disorders with the presence of generalized pain hypersensitivity. It is also a phenomenon closely linked to irritable bowel disorder, depressive symptoms, chronic fatigue and joint pains (Woolf 2011). This suggests that picking up on these co-morbidities during the clinical interview will also act as guidance towards the diagnosis of the underlying pain mechanism.

The brain and pain

The CNS is the ultimate representational device. It has the ability to represent the whole body, embracing anatomy, physiology, movements, emotions and diseases. An understanding of pain and the role of the CNS in terms of the body-self neuromatrix have been proposed (Melzack 1990). The neuromatrix can be considered as a vast, interconnecting, highly flexible, plastic network of groups of neurons in the brain activated and sculpted by any and every lifetime activity and experience.

Essentially there is input into the body-self neuromatrix from sensory, cognitive and emotional influences. The consequent output from the brain is commonly called the neurosignature and involves firing in and between many different and individual brain areas. This subsequent neurosignature, also called a neurotag (Butler & Moseley 2003), includes changes in the regulation of many homeostatic, behavioural and perceptual systems. This fits with our current understanding of pain that considers pain to be a multiple output response (Moseley 2003) and the mature organism model that has been used to incorporate pain mechanisms (Gifford 1998).

Imaging studies demonstrates there is no single 'pain centre'. Many areas alight almost simultaneously during a pain experience (Tracey & Bushnell 2009) and wide variability exists within and between individuals (Ingvar 1999). See Box 4.5 for an example of the brain areas that make up the neuromatrix in an acute nociceptive experience.

Brain changes in pain

Recent studies have shown that there may be several distinct changes in the brain during a pain state. These include:

- Changes in the brain's representation of the body e.g. in the primary somatomotor (Tsao et al. 2008) and somatosensory cortices (Flor et al. 1997a)
- Decreased areas of gray-matter in different cortical areas e.g. dorsolateral prefrontal cortex (Apkarian et al. 2004)
- Altered resting brain dynamics e.g. changes in the default mode network (Baliki et al. 2006)
- Altered levels of neurotransmitters and/or receptors, e.g. in the brainstem in descending modulation (D'Mello & Dickenson 2008)
- Changes in immune activity, e.g. ongoing activation of microglia in the thalamus in neuropathic pain (Banati et al. 2001).

The changes expected as being present in neck pain, for instance in the somatosensory cortex, may be picked up through careful assessment. It may be that the patient describes an inability to imagine the symptomatic part clearly, which may reflect in a change in the representation of the neck. Other clinical tools such as two-point discrimination, left/right discrimination tasks or reasoning tasks such as the Iowa Gambling Task may become important in understanding what underlying brain changes are present and will give the clinician objective markers to use during treatment to document the progression of these changes (Box 4.6).

Other clinical changes such as an alteration in movement can be picked up through careful assessment or are often noticeable while just observing the patient. These may be related to both changes in the motor representations and alterations at spinal and tissue levels. More changes in the brain's output include altered mood, concentration, emotion, thoughts and activity of the stress systems. Each pain experience will be individual and as such the level of involvement of each of the response systems will vary widely both between individuals and as a pain state progresses.

Mirror neurons and context change

Mirror neurons are a huge revelation in terms of our understanding of the development of language,

---

Box 4.6

Example of clinical tests aimed at cortical functioning

Iowa gambling task – a psychological gambling task that uses four decks of cards to assess a person's emotional decision-making abilities (Bechara et al. 1994).

Two-point discrimination (TPD) – a psychophysical test of tactile acuity, whereby a pair of calipers are used to discriminate the minimal distance that a person can tell that they are being touched by two points. It is thought to give some understanding of the representational changes in the primary somatosensory cortex (S1) of the body part assessed (Lotze & Moseley 2007).

Left/right discrimination task – A motor imagery task that involves guessing right from left body parts in pictures that are rapidly presented. Thought to provide an indication of a person's ability to unconsciously plan movement for that part of the body (Moseley 2004b).

---

imitation and learning and are likely to be important in the assessment and treatment of our patient in the clinic. Essentially they are neurons that fire to both the observation of movement (i.e. mirror the movement) and to the execution of the same movement (Rizzolatti et al. 2001). Picking up changes in mood or movement may feel natural to some clinicians and this is likely to be a result of the activation of our mirror neuron system.

Different populations of neurons represent the same movement depending on the context that the movement is performed in or the desired goal of that movement (Iacoboni & Mazziotta 2007). This means that if a particular movement activates a pain neurotag then it could be possible that the same movement performed in a different context, and therefore activating a different population of neurons within the neuromatrix, will not activate a pain neurotag. In this case the brain is running the same movement but without creating a pain experience. Box 4.7 gives examples of how to change the context in which a movement is performed.

Output mechanisms

The brain is constantly making small adjustments to the regulatory/homeostatic systems in order to keep us in maximal comfort within our environment. This

> **Box 4.7**
>
> ## The use of context change in nerve root lesion/WAD
>
> There are numerous ways of changing the context of a movement and this should again be individual for the patient. The main objective would be to see whether a change in context for the same movement helped and subsequently changed the response. This could then be used as a basis for therapy and self-management strategies. In this case the brain would still be running the same movement representation and creating health for the tissues but without maintaining the pain experience and likely underlying sensitization.
>
> Neck rotation may be painful in sitting in a cervical nerve root lesion. There are many other ways of performing the same movement by changing the context within which it is performed:
>
> - Close eyes during rotation
> - Rotate in supine lying or 4-point kneeling
> - Passive rotation of the cervical spine
> - Imagine turning the neck
> - Watch the clinician perform the movement first
> - Try it with some distraction e.g. whilst talking/answering questions
> - Do the movement from below upwards i.e. keep the neck still and turn the trunk
> - Turn the neck in water
> - Turn the neck with some music on in the background
> - Turn the neck with the addition of SNAGs (sustained normal apophyseal glides).
>
> All this means that different populations of neurons – possibly different mirror neurons, will represent the same movement. This is one way of helping to discern the underlying pain mechanisms and guide the graded exposure strategy for rehabilitation.

is part of what we understand from the mature organism model and neuromatrix paradigm. It monitors the levels of different hormones and chemicals (interoception), thoughts, emotions, sensory inputs and perceptual inputs including pain experiences coming into the neuromatrix. The subsequent alterations in activity of the different regulatory systems (neurosignature) will be influenced by the perceived threat of the situation (Moseley 2007). If someone feels threatened, even at an unconscious level, then the brain will act by changing the activity in the different systems, affecting various physiological mechanisms and behavioural adaptive responses in order to deal with the stressor (Chrousos 2009).

This may be through a change in movement, mediated through the prefrontal and motor cortices or increase in heart rate due to altered activity in the sympathetic nervous system. As mentioned previously, in a pain state there will be measurable changes in many systems that are apparent as brain changes too. The common output systems that a clinician will be considering during assessment and related to a pain experience include:

- Sympathetic nervous system (SNS)
- Endocrine system
- Parasympathetic nervous system (PNS)
- Immune system
- Motor system
- Descending modulatory control
- Mood
- Language
- Respiratory system
- Pain
- Thoughts/beliefs.

Some of these will be apparent on observation of your patient, others may be more obvious during careful questioning, and others still may require specific examination.

Sympathetic nervous system

It is normal to be stressed during daily life and the SNS helps deal with these stresses. It is a fast acting system that works via two pathways: the sympatho-adrenal and sympathoneural axes.

The sympatho-adrenal axis works by activating the release of adrenaline/noradrenaline via the adrenal medulla. This results in systemic action and, as such, the effects will generally be widespread. The sympathoneural axis works as an efferent system via the peripheral nervous system to effect change locally by releasing adrenaline directly into the target tissues (including visceral organs) and so has a fast acting effect. Essentially, the SNS helps deliver blood to the necessary systems and it can be seen how mood is intimately linked with the body (see Gifford & Thacker 2002 for more in-depth analysis).

Adrenaline/noradrenaline does not cause pain in itself, but can magnify the sensitivity of alarm signals (Devor & Seltzer 1999). In chronic inflammation, nerve damage (ectopic impulse generating sites) and nerve root irritation there is an increase of ion channels picking up the local availability of circulating adrenaline (Navarro et al. 2007).

There are recent interesting developments which appear to show that it is not so much the centrally mediated changes which are controlled by the SNS but local changes in channel responses to circulating adrenaline. This means that the same amount of circulating adrenaline can have more potent effects on the tissues it supplies.

Endocrine response

Together with the SNS, the endocrine system is the other key stress response system. Sympathetic reactions are rapid and of short duration, the endocrine response can take slightly longer to respond due to the systemic, hormonal effect. Higher centres stimulate the hypothalamus (particularly during perceived threat), which releases corticotropin-releasing hormone. This in turn stimulates the pituitary gland to release the adrenocorticotropic hormone (ACTH) into the blood stream. ACTH activates the adrenal cortex to release glucocorticoids such as cortisol, a famous stress hormone, into the bloodstream.

A summary of the general actions caused by an increase in activation of the stress systems is generally summed up as a 'fight or flight' response (although this is a fairly simplistic view). This includes: increasing cardiovascular tone and respiration, increasing oxygenation, nutrition of the brain, heart and skeletal muscles, increased metabolism (including inhibition of reproduction and growth), facilitation of arousal, alertness, cognition and attention (Chrousos 2009). See also Box 4.8 for examples of the effects of stress response.

The general effects from the stress response systems are therefore to help liberate energy and deliver it to the areas and organs that most need them. With ongoing activation of these stress systems there is likely to be deleterious effects on the health of tissues and organs.

Parasympathetic nervous system (PNS)

The PNS is concerned with slowing and conserving energy. It helps digestion, storing of energy, cellular replenishment and reproduction (Butler & Moseley 2003). The PNS is involved in tissue healing, rest and repair.

Box 4.8

Example of changes in outputs within an ongoing stress response

If the stress response is ongoing e.g. in WAD there may be obvious alterations in:
- Slow healing of cuts and recovery from colds
- Difficulty in concentrating and memory recall
- Changes in sleep patterns and energy levels (e.g. fatigue)
- Digestive problems
- Altered libido.

These may all appear to be minor changes to the person with neck pain but will help to improve your overall understanding of the output/response mechanisms involved in their pain experience.

In persistent pain states there are changes to the representation of the PNS in the brain (Thayer & Sternberg 2010) – as has been found in sensory and motor areas. This will have knock-on effects on the function of the parasympathetic nervous system and could impact on general health and the balance between the stress systems.

 Clinical tip

Activation of the PNS is achieved by:
- Applying pain-free non-stressful treatment techniques
- Positive motivation
- Neuroscience education
- Relaxation techniques

Breathing exercises, e.g. the Buteyko technique, will promote a longer exhalation or pause before inspiration. This will preferentially activate the PNS and could be one way of trying to actively balance the activity in the sympathetic and parasympathetic nervous system. This will have direct effects on blood pressure, heart rate and respiratory rate (Kaushik et al. 2006).

The immune system

The immune system is a powerful protective system especially in disease and trauma. It also plays an important role in persistent pain. Glial cells in the brain (e.g. astrocytes and microglia) contribute to the onset and maintenance of pain states, particularly neuropathic pain (Thacker et al. 2007). In sickness there is a clear immune/pain link (Watkins & Maier 2000).

Communicating chemicals, such as the proinflammatory cytokines interleukin-1β, interleukin-6 and tumour necrosis factor-α, collectively mediate inflammatory responses. They are also important signalling proteins between the immune and central nervous system and may mediate effects through parasympathetic ganglia on vagal afferents. It is through this signalling that the brain can promote changes in behaviours and sensitivity (such as illness/sickness behaviour) in order to best manage the current experience.

Clinical tip

The major immune boosting behaviours are:
- Ability to develop coping skills
- Perception of stressors
- Perception of health: the healthier you think you are the better the immune profile
- Social interaction
- Family and medical support, with all people speaking the 'same'
- Language
- Beliefs
- Appropriate exercises
- Graded fitness training
- Humour

(Butler & Moseley 2003)

Motor system

Changes in the motor system can sometimes be seen even before your introduction to the patient. This may manifest as holding the neck in a forward position, protection of a limb, the facial expressions shown or the voice of the patient (Box 4.9).

In chronic pain states where central sensitivity is a dominant process, there will usually be unhealthy and unfit muscles, which may be a source of nociception. This may be maintained through an ongoing local immune response, altered axoplasmic flow of the nerve or a persistent axon reflex creating neurogenic inflammation creating ill-health of the tissues or from altered use and firing of the muscles.

Box 4.9

Example of motor impairment in WAD
- There may be decreased range of movement of the neck, shoulder and thoracic region, which can be extremely limited due to pain inhibition and protective muscular activity
- The principle factors causing limitation are the actual trauma to the anatomical and physiological components of movement, the severity and the resultant protective muscle spasm, initiated and maintained by the CNS
- Poor quality of active movement is another characteristic of whiplash injuries, and may remain well into the recovery phase
- There may also be a joint position sense error in WAD (Sterling et al. 2003b)

Descending modulatory control

During a pain experience there are changes to the descending modulatory pathways. This was referred to as one of the processes responsible for central sensitization. There is tonic and phasic facilitatory and inhibitory modulation of the afferent and efferent pathways. There may be an increase in the facilitation of afferent processing and a reduction in the inhibition (disinhibition). This will cause a general amplification of the incoming signals to the brain, which will then respond accordingly (Mason 2005). A similar effect occurs in the efferent pathways, exciting the motor cells and maintaining muscle activity. This may, for example, be seen in a brisk response to reflex testing.

Some of the therapeutic methods employed by manual therapists include techniques that aim to effect a change in descending modulation (Box 4.10). This may be through traditional manual therapy techniques or appropriate education to effect a change in the facilitatory tone. These act via a top-down process, possibly through changes in thoughts or beliefs as a result of experiencing some pain relief or hearing reassuring information. By considering these components of the pain experience and the concept of affecting change directly on the outputs generated by the brain it can be helpful in guiding the therapist towards an appropriate treatment plan.

There are many other changes in the response systems including mood changes, altered cognitions

Box 4.10

Strategies to effect change in descending modulation

Encouraging descending inhibition in cervical nerve root lesion and subsequent release of e.g. endorphins and enkephalins:

- Give specific education regarding their problem
- Give a timescale for recovery
- Empowering techniques to settle the pain
- Laughter
- TENS
- Acupuncture or electroacupuncture
- Social support.

There are obvious links to boosting the positive function of the healing systems – the immune and parasympathetic nervous system.

Box 4.11

Examples of questioning relating to a suspected nerve root lesion

Ask for signs of dizziness, diplopia, drop attacks, dysphasia and dysphagia. These may implicate CNS involvement or cervical arterial dysfunction and require consideration in terms of clinical testing i.e. appropriateness/necessity to assess cranial nerve function or need for further medical investigations prior to physical intervention.

Do they experience any dysaesthesias such as crawling, worm-like or tingling sensations? These symptoms are more likely to implicate neuropathic pain mechanisms. There may be other pain quality and spatial characteristics that allow identification of neuropathic from non-neuropathic pain and therefore, of possible underlying mechanisms (Dworkin et al. 2007). These may also be identified in questionnaires.

What is the pattern of night symptoms e.g. pain that is of a variable nature, alleviated with some movement may be indicative of neuropathic pain. However, sleep that is grossly disturbed due to pain being worse at night is one warning sign of metastatic spinal cord compression (red flag).

What about other considerations such as the person's ability to:
- Concentrate
- Short-term memory recall
- Work out difficult problems.

These are all abilities that have been implicated to change in people with neuropathic pain conditions. They are measurable both through assessment and correlate with changes found on brain imaging (Moriarty et al. 2011). They highlight examples of what can make up the possible individual pain experience and possible directions for therapies in the future.

and changes language to name a few but are beyond the scope of this chapter.

Examination of the cervical region

Subjective examination

The most important element of the subjective examination is the communication between the patient and therapist. Maitland had many attributes but communication was, considered by many, to be the greatest of all. This topic is described in great detail elsewhere (e.g. Jones & Rivett 2004). The subjective examination is a great opportunity for the patient to tell their own story, in any way they choose. It is the therapist's job to listen attentively to the patient and make them feel comfortable telling their story.

Where necessary you may have to ask essential questions yet unanswered or direct the conversation (see Box 4.11 for examples). Ultimately you should remain empathetic and open. It is unwise to lead the patient along your own questioning path, as this is likely to run towards a favourite clinical hypothesis or miss valuable information.

By the end of the subjective examination the clinician should have a working hypothesis with which to guide their physical examination. It is likely that the patients will also have formulated their own hypothesis related to the questioning and it is beneficial to ask for their thoughts on this.

Planning the physical examination

Before commencing the physical examination the key points highlighted during the subjective interview must be considered:

- What will be the extent of the examination related to severity and irritability of the problem?
- Where irritability is the main factor, minimal (if any) tests will be performed with the principle desire to find easing or relieving postures, movements or other self-administered

management such as medication or the application of heat. It is likely that some education will be required or a consideration of that person's current beliefs regarding their problem

- It would be counterproductive to perform a physical examination that aggravates the problem. Therefore, the physical assessment could be considered in terms of titrating the appropriate dose of assessment for your patient. It is important to understand this concept in light of the potential latency of symptoms found in neuropathic pain problems or that creating sensory input will amplify the present state of central sensitization. The patient may be fine following your assessment but their symptoms may flare up days, or even a few weeks, later, purely as a result of an excessive dose of physical assessment. Hopefully the therapist will no longer ask what the patient did to aggravate themselves under the assumption that because they were fine immediately after the assessment, it wasn't due to the assessment itself!

- The severity of the problem helps identify those people who are more likely to proceed into chronicity. This has been shown to be the case in WAD where ongoing moderate/severe symptoms correlate with changes in physical parameters and psychological distress (Sterling et al. 2006)

- Consider the minimum amount of physical examination required to provide relevant data to prove or disprove a current hypothesis of an underlying pain state, for example, neurosensory testing to confirm the presence of central sensitization. Box 4.12 outlines some considerations for physical examination of underlying pain mechanisms.

Physical examination

The aims of the physical examination are to:

1. Support or reject hypotheses identified in the subjective examination in terms of the likely underpinning pain mechanisms, e.g.:
   a. recognizing the presence of a mechanical nociceptive contribution originating in the cervical spine or a local inflammatory problem

> ### Box 4.12
>
> ### Considerations for physical examination of underlying pain mechanisms
>
> - Nerve root disorders can have a latency effect of between 2/3 days and a few weeks due to changes in the processing and sensitization. It is important to consider the relationship of this with the likely response to the physical examination.
> - What should you avoid/or need to examine if someone is in danger of ramping up the nociceptive system.
> - Someone with widespread pain and altered beliefs may be harmed more than benefitted with manual therapy that could trigger or sustain central sensitization (Nijs & Van Houdenhove 2009).

   b. adaptive/maladaptive movement or behaviour due to a change in the motor output
   c. a change in mechanosensitivity in the nervous system indicative of a peripheral neurogenic pain mechanism
   d. the contribution of CNS sensitivity
   e. consideration of other output mechanisms and their effect on the pain problem e.g. activation of the sympathetic nervous system during testing
2. Find the least provoking postures and movements
3. Look at current function and functional limitation
4. Confirm or rule out the need for caution and decide when physical intervention is inappropriate.

Starting out the physical examination

Find out whether the patient is happy to undergo a physical examination and briefly what this is likely to entail. Make sure your patient understands the importance of their feedback from the testing and that they should keep you informed regarding their responses. It is often wise to begin with symptom-free movements when possible. Try not to give them too much information as this may bias their responses. When movement is unnecessary/unwise then some form of neurological assessment will give information to reason the underlying pain mechanisms, such as an increase in sensitivity.

Observation

Observation of your patient begins during your introductions or possibly before. If they have adopted a particular posture is this to alleviate their symptoms or just normal for them (remember the role of your mirror neurons in understanding both the movement of the patient and their current emotional state)? In which case would you want to alter it? This should guide your assessment and ultimately your treatment by showing the most comfortable position.

It is sad to think how many patients have been forced to alter an antalgic posture e.g. retracting the chin in order to regain what is thought by the therapist to be an optimal posture, when they are appropriately resting in their safe/comfortable and relieving position due to an irritable nerve root lesion i.e. adopting a poking chin with some ipsilateral side flexion of the neck and elevation of the shoulder. An antalgic posture provides a huge amount of relevant information for the judicial therapist.

Functional assessment

This is an ideal time for the patient to demonstrate their main functional problems while respecting the symptoms. Ultimately this is what brought them to see you, e.g. the difficulty in turning their head whilst reversing the car. It is unnecessary to evaluate every possible movement and in some instances is likely to make your patient worse. It will also show your patient that you are interested in their problem and have listened thoroughly. It is possible to incorporate context change strategies within this part of the assessment.

Testing positions

The testing positions will relate to the need to respect the severity and irritability of the disorder but also the functional considerations. Contextual change of a movement is thought to cause different neuronal populations within the neuromatrix to fire with the consequent result being a different neurotag that no longer involves pain as one of the outputs.

Ongoing analysis of your patient and reassessment

During your patient assessment you are constantly monitoring their response. This may be a verbal response but often takes the form of non-verbal reactions such as withdrawing a limb, grimacing, an increase in sweating and colouration of the skin. All of these are important signs guiding your evaluation to assessment and firming your clinical reasoning. These clinical signs or outputs are likely to be what you monitor during reassessment/re-evaluation.

It is not necessary to reassess function immediately after treatment. Assuming you have chosen the appropriate technique there should be a positive change. The change you are most interested in is one that has been maintained beyond the first seconds following treatment. This may mean reassessing 15–20 minutes after treatment or waiting until your follow-up appointment. There are occasions when a judicial and professional examination with appropriate feedback will reduce the fear or worry of the complaint and therefore shows as a reduction of sensitivity, possibly mediated as a reduction in the descending facilitation.

Physical examination of the nervous system

Data retrieved through physical examination of the nervous system will help in refining your current hypothesis regarding your patient's current diagnosis, including an understanding of the underlying pain mechanisms (Dworkin et al. 2007). Clinicians with good manual skills and strong clinical reasoning should be able to identify pathophysiological changes (Greening & Lynn 1998). Mechanosensitivity of nervous system may be assessed through palpation of the peripheral nerves and passive and active neurodynamic testing. These can be combined with the assessment and comparison of the sensitivity and health of adjacent tissues. This will guide the clinician's understanding of possible nociceptive elements driven by neighbouring tissues, local sensitivity of the nervous system or the presence of central sensitization.

Conduction abilities of the nervous system are traditionally assessed through manual muscle, reflex and sensibility testing. It is also possible to examine cranial nerve function or the representation of the body in the brain through assessment of two-point

Box 4.13

Brief summary of neurological examination techniques that can be performed at the bedside

Neurological examination may include:

Manual muscle testing (MMT) – aims to assess the strength of individual muscles and groups of muscles isometrically or isotonically and therefore give an indication of the conduction properties of the motor system and possible changes present. Changes may indicate alterations in the contractile material and/or the processes leading to activation, including those at cortical level, e.g. premotor and supplementary motor regions and the primary somatomotor cortex. The presence of pain will affect the accurate measurement of muscle strength.

Reflex testing – is used to assess the health of the nervous system through sensory and motor connections and also the general sensitivity of the CNS. Reinforcement techniques can be used to maximize the response when it is difficult to elicit or diminished. A brisk deep tendon reflex is thought to show overactivity of spinal reflex mechanisms. Absent of diminished responses are likely to show an inability of the afferent stimulus in accessing the spinal cord or the efferent volley in accessing the muscle (Dick 2003).

Sensory testing – can be performed in order to give gross information regarding the afferent properties of the nervous system through light touch performed with a tissue or piece of cotton wool. More detailed sensory testing can be performed using validated measuring tools such as Semmes-Weinstein monofilaments that are used in quantitative sensory testing (e.g. Siao & Cros 2003). Sensibility to hot/cold/vibration may also be used as part of the assessment and guides the clinician in terms of the underlying changes in sensibility and sensitivity of the sensory system including cortical processing. Common findings in nerve root lesion

manifesting with negative symptoms are reduced sensibility to light touch and pin-prick examination and may correlate with changes in MMT or reflexes.

Two-point discrimination (TPD) – TPD tests both the quantity of innervated sensory receptors (Novak & MacKinnon 2005) but also the patients' cognitive function (Lundborg & Rosen 2004).

There is an excellent reliability of two-point discrimination between examiners (Dellon et al. 1987); however, to our understanding there has been little research looking at TPD in cervical pain problems. It has been used for many years to document the progress in recovery following maxillofacial surgery, as well as hand surgery. Recently there has been good evidence to show significant disturbance in TPD in LBP (Moseley 2008) and CRPS and that this disturbance is related to cortical changes in the representation of the symptomatic body part (Pleger et al. 2006). Therefore, this technique may be used as a part of the examination of psychophysical functioning of the patient with headache, nerve root lesion and whiplash.

Clonus – is a test that places rapid and repeated movements through a limb e.g. the ankle. The examiner is watching for a clonic response where the limb begins to fight/extend against the test movement (hyperreflexia). This is thought to be indicative of a lesion of the corticospinal tract or spinal cord.

Babinski – tests the primitive reflex of the foot and toe response to a firm stroke up the outside of the foot. If there is fanning of the toes with upward movement of the hallux this is suggestive of a pyramidal tract lesion.

---

discrimination and testing of left/right discrimination. See Box 4.13 for a brief summary of common neurological examination techniques.

Due to a lack of a gold standard test for most disorders, a battery of tests including motor and sensory elements should be the most valid way of identifying these changes (Novak & MacKinnon 2005). The next section will concentrate on palpation of the peripheral nerves and neurodynamic testing.

Palpation of peripheral nerves

Nerves are hard, rounded and, due to their outer covering of mesoneurium, feel slippery to the touch.

Some nerves are visible, especially when the adjacent joint component is positioned to load the nerve. Many nerves are sufficiently prominent to allow direct palpation. The three trunks of the brachial plexus are an example of easily identifiable and superficial peripheral nerves that the clinician may decide to palpate. Abnormal or increased sensitivity is a frequent finding in this area following WAD and nerve root lesions and may require sensitive handling.

Nerves can also be palpated indirectly where muscle and fascial tissues cover them. This is possible when palpating the median nerve through the wrist flexor muscles in the forearm.

Palpation can be performed transversely over the nerve or with static pressure directly onto the nerve.

This depends on the size and location of the nerve and a reasoned approach. Placing the nerve on some slight load, as with a neurodynamic test position, may allow it to become more prominent and places a greater mechanical load and pressure change through the nerve trunk. This method can also be used to differentiate a local nociceptive process from nerve trunk mechanosensitivity whereby a perceived change in response to nerve palpation with altered neurodynamic positioning is more indicative of mechanosensitivity of the nervous system than local nociceptive processes.

Response to nerve palpation

The response should be compared to the asymptomatic/less symptomatic side. Palpation in the lower limbs can be used when central sensitization is suspected or the pain problem is highly irritable or severe. This should give a wider perspective of the mechanosensitivity of the nervous system.

Normal responses to palpation of a nerve will naturally vary amongst and within individuals through the day but will also vary due to internal and external factors. The same nerve trunk may also vary slightly in its response at different sites due to the change in relative connective tissue or conductive tissue present (Butler 2000).

A relevant increased response may present as feeling more marked or may even provoke a change in behaviour, such as withdrawal of the limb, a grimace or exclamation. When the response reflects negative symptoms then the feeling is less marked or absent in comparison to the asymptomatic side.

Palpation related to peripheral neuropathic pain

There is some experimental support for nerve palpation as a diagnostic aid towards finding the primary source of a neurological lesion (Durkan 1991). Injured nerves often hurt when subjected to mechanical forces; this must be due a combination of local – for example the presence of an ectopic impulse generating site – and central changes, such as central sensitization. This mechanosensitivity can be present even without an identified nerve lesion when there is local inflammation surrounding the nerve (Dilley et al. 2005). Sensitivity to palpation must be seen as a reflection of processes throughout the nervous system, including thoughts and beliefs

such as the expectation of the consequences of touching a nerve.

Palpation of the upper limb nerve trunks and brachial plexus has reasonable reliability (Jepsen et al. 2006; Schmid et al. 2009). Someone with a painful cervical radiculopathy is highly likely to have an increased response to nerve trunk palpation (Hall & Quintner 1996). Increased response to palpation of the median nerve along its tact has been documented in people with WAD (Greening et al. 2005). Unilateral migraine and tension-type headache also display mechanosensitivity to nerve palpation of the supraorbital nerve on the symptomatic side along with increased sensitivity to palpation of nerve trunks bilaterally in the upper limbs, indicating a predominance of central changes indicative of central sensitization (Fernández-de-las-Peñas et al. 2008, 2009).

Palpation of the nerves of the head, neck and upper limb

The clinician is likely to be guided by the distribution of the symptoms in terms of which nerves/nerve trunks they palpate. Headache symptoms may require palpation of the facial and occipital nerves, whereas a nerve root lesion may require assessment of the peripheral nerve trunks of the upper limb.

To understand widespread sensitivity and central sensitization is appropriate to assess palpation away from the symptomatic site such as in the lower limbs prior to assessment over the symptomatic area. This helps to give some understanding of what to expect for the patient. See Box 4.14 for an outline of clinical symptoms found in headache.

The trigeminal nerve (V)

The trigeminal nerve is the sensory supply to the face, the greater part of the scalp, the oral and nasal cavities and motor supply to the masticatory muscles. Fibres in the sensory root are mainly axons of the trigeminal (semilunar) ganglion. From the ganglion three nerves arise: the ophthalmic, maxillary and mandibular nerves.

Palpation of the trigeminal nerve is most effective where it becomes superficial as shown in Figure 4.3. It is useful to consider palpating these nerves with headache and facial pain problems.

The ophthalmic nerve becomes superficial through the supraorbital fissure.

Box 4.14

Example of clinical signs found in headache

Palpation of the occipital nerves on the symptomatic side provokes a marked response. There is also some tenderness to palpation into the ipsilateral upper limb found at the brachial plexus and upper arm. There is side-to-side difference in the response to palpation.

Sensory testing of the head and face showed hyperalgesia to pin-prick examination, particularly laterally and superiorly to the greater occipital protruberance on the symptomatic side.

The greater occipital nerve becomes superficial at the superior nuchal line lateral to the greater occipital protruberance and the *lesser occipital nerve* can be located more laterally. Palpation of these nerves can be considered for both headache and WAD. See Figures 4.4 and. 4.5 and Box 4.15.

Palpation of the cervical nerve roots and the brachial plexus

Palpation of the intervertebral foraminal area is achieved by the identification of the pointed

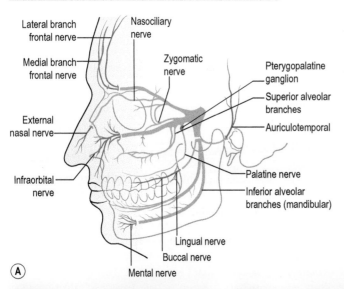

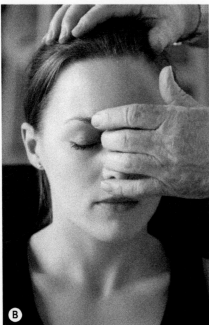

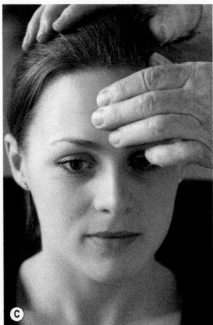

Figure 4.3 • A Schematic diagram of the trigeminal nerve (reproduced from Clemente 1975 with permission). **B** Palpation of lacrimal nerve (a branch of the ophthalmic nerve) at the supraorbital fissure. **C** Palpation of the frontal (supraorbital) nerve.

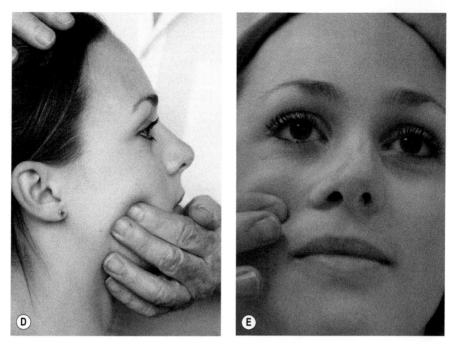

Figure 4.3 • cont'd D Palpation of the maxillary nerve at the infraorbital fossa. **E** Palpation of the mandibular nerve at the mental foramen.

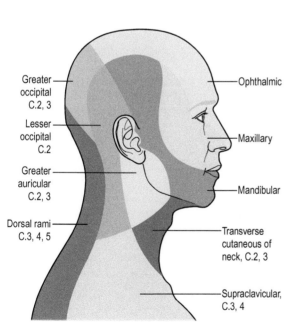

Greater occipital C.2, 3

Lesser occipital C.2

Greater auricular C.2, 3

Dorsal rami C.3, 4, 5

Ophthalmic

Maxillary

Mandibular

Transverse cutaneous of neck, C.2, 3

Supraclavicular, C.3, 4

Figure 4.4 • Cutaneous nerve supply of the face, scalp and neck (reproduced from Williams et al. (1989) Gray's Anatomy, 37e, with permission from Elsevier). This can provide useful guidance when performing neurosensory testing.

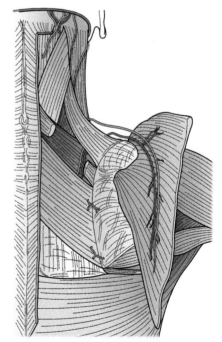

Figure 4.5 • Occipital and auricular nerves. Dissection of the upper back. The trapezius has been reflected and segment of rhomboideus has been removed.

Box 4.15

Neurodynamic response in headache

Testing the occipital nerve reproduced headache symptoms. These are altered through structural differentiation by using the test same but in a slump position.

The positive test response correlates with the raised mechanosensitivity found with nerve palpation over the occipital nerves.

tubercles on the end of the transverse processes of the cervical vertebrae. The application of the classical anteroposterior unilateral vertebral pressure technique is ideal for this purpose (Fig. 4.6). The sternocleidomastoid muscle should be displaced during the procedure. The actual nerve root is difficult to identify in this location, as it lies between scalenus anterior and medius, so the principle of indirect nerve palpation may be applied.

The three trunks of the brachial plexus are clearly detected between scalenus anterior and

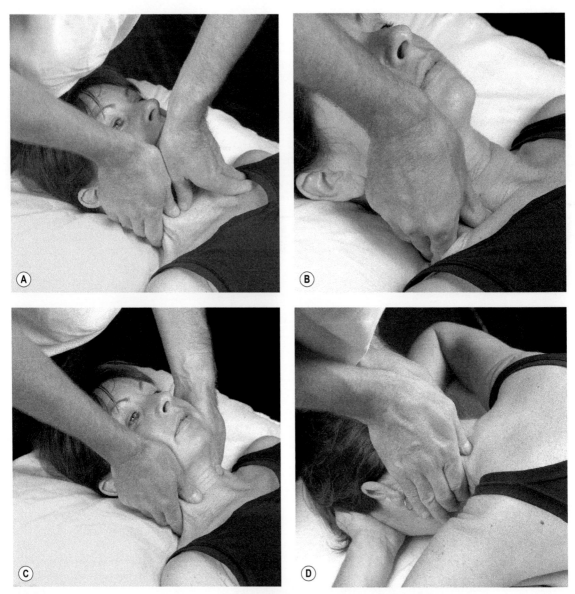

Figure 4.6 • A unilateral anteroposterior vertebral pressure. **B** Bilateral anteroposterior vertebral pressure.
C Anteroposterior unilateral vertebral pressure in upper thoracic area. **D** Anteroposterior unilateral vertebral pressure.

medius to where the trunks pass under the medial one-third of the clavicle. By applying contralateral lateral flexion to the neck or shoulder girdle depression the nerve trunks become more prominent (Fig. 4.7).

The cords of the brachial plexus can be discovered and palpated in the axilla as they encapsulate the axillary artery. It is therefore useful to be able to palpate pulsatile structures to help use as a guide for locating the nerves (Fig. 4.8).

Palpation of the median and ulnar nerves in the upper arm next to the brachial artery is illustrated in Figure 4.9. The median nerve lies anterior to the ulnar nerve in this situation.

Palpations of the major nerves of the upper extremity are illustrated in Figures 4.10–4.13 and are described in detail in The sensitive nervous system (Butler 2000).

Neurodynamic testing

Another technique used to assess the mechanosensitivity of the nervous system is neurodynamic testing (Dilley et al. 2005). In contrast to the assessment of the nervous system's ability to accept pressure exerted on nerves through palpation, neurodynamic testing examines mechanosensitivity to specific movements. More recently it has also been suggested that neurodynamic tests assess the representation for specific movements of body parts, i.e. cortical representation or the movement neurotag. Therefore the mechanosensitivity found during testing may be mediated peripherally or centrally or, likely, both.

There are many base tests that have been designed in order to bias an emphasis towards specific nerve tracts and movements. However, it is necessary to be able to adapt these to make the assessment individual for the patient with neck pain. This may include changes in the start position, order of movements of the test and the use of structural differentiation.

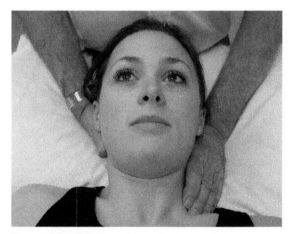

Figure 4.7 • Palpation of nerve trunks.

Palpations of the major nerves of the upper extremity

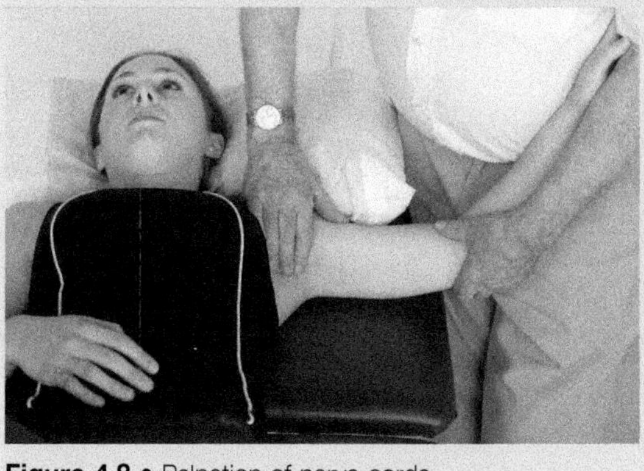

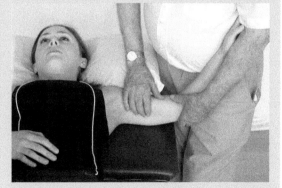

Figure 4.8 • Palpation of nerve cords.

Figure 4.9 • Palpation of median and ulnar nerve in the upper arm.

Continued

Palpations of the major nerves of the upper extremity—cont'd

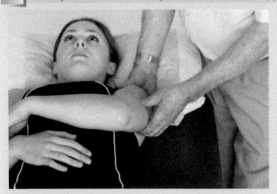

Figure 4.10 • Palpation of the radial nerve in the radial groove.

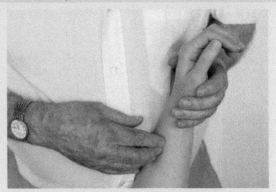

Figure 4.11 • Palpation of the radial sensory nerve at the distal anterolateral part of the radius.

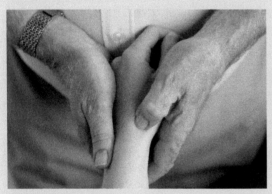

Figure 4.12 • Palpation of the radial sensory nerve over the scaphoid.

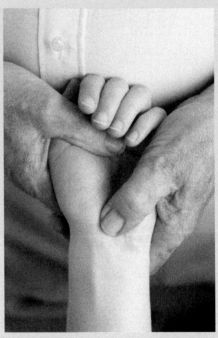

Figure 4.13 • Palpation of the median nerve at the carpal tunnel – an example of indirect palpation.

Responses to neurodynamic testing

During testing it is important to compare the range and quality of movement and compare, where possible, the symptomatic with the asymptomatic/less symptomatic side. A change in the available movement is often due not to specific restriction in the nerve but to a protective motor response, possibly brought on by the increase in mechanosensitivity to stretch and pressure (van der Heide et al. 2001).

It is important to watch for antalgic postures and subtle changes in the muscles as these may be the first overt signs which help you to understand the patient's willingness to be moved. This may include a slight withdrawal of the limb but is mostly a noticeable increase in resistance to the movement.

Other signs that may be apparent are the reproduction of symptoms, which needs to be monitored carefully and should be noted after the test. Be open with your questioning and allow your patient to inform you of the response and the area of symptoms. This will allow some comparison with what you know to be normal. The aim is not always to reproduce pain, especially for someone with more severe or irritable symptoms. In this case, neurodynamic testing may be used to explore relieving positions and allow the patient to have some control over their problem. This works especially well during a functional assessment.

Using structural differentiation in neurodynamics

A change in response to structural differentiation, i.e. an addition or subtraction of a joint component away from the symptomatic area, can help support or refute a clinical diagnosis. It is thought that a change in response, whether increased or decreased, reflects a change in the load through the nerve and subsequent mechanosensitivity (Coppieters et al. 2005). This should be used as a guide and not by itself to confirm the presence of peripheral neuropathic pain or more correctly, mechanosensitivity of the nervous system.

Neurodynamics relating to cervical conditions

Neurodynamic testing is a great assessment technique for ruling out cervical radiculopathy due to its high sensitivity and low specificity (Rubinstein et al. 2007). Positive responses to upper limb neurodynamic testing of the median nerve have also been shown in people with WAD (Greening et al. 2005, Sterling et al. 2003b, Sterling & Pedler 2009). The responses to testing slump in a long sitting position are significant for migraine and headache (von Piekartz et al. 2007).

Furthermore, it has been shown that pain catastrophizing predicts the pain intensity perceived by the individual during neurodynamic testing (Beneciuk et al. 2010) and provides another link to the need

to consider a bio-psychosocial approach with your patient.

Neurodynamic testing for people with unilateral arm and/or neck pain is moderately reliable (Schmid et al. 2009). There is also a high reliability between trials in terms of symptom reproduction and onset of symptoms during testing (van der Heide et al. 2001). We believe that if neurodynamic examination is performed well as a part of a clinical reasoning approach it can be an extremely useful tool in ascertaining the underlying mechanosensitivity of the nervous system. It can be used as a good clinical guide to document changes in mechanosensitivity over a period of time. Neurodynamic tests for the craniocervical nerves are shown in Figure 4.14 and for the occipital and auricular nerves in Figure 4.15.

The nerve roots, trunks and cords of the brachial plexus

The classical upper limb neurodynamic tests (ULNT) with structural differentiation are shown in Figures 4.16–4.19.

The classical upper limb neurodynamic tests (ULNT) with structural differentiation

Box 4.16

Neurodynamic testing of a suspected cervical nerve root lesion

ULNT1 demonstrates limited elbow extension due to a protective muscle response and reproduction of symptoms. These are alleviated with cervical side flexion towards the symptomatic side.

Nerve palpation of the median nerve in the upper arm caused an increased response that was subsequently reduced with the release of a loading component of the neurodynamic test.

Altering the test and/or start position

It may be appropriate, especially with more severe pain problems such as a nerve root lesion, to adapt the base test and find ways to help reduce the symptoms. A cradle position allows support for the arm and is useful when the patient is unhappy with it flat on the bed (Fig. 4.20).

Text continued on p. 150

The neurodynamic tests for the craniocervical nerves: trigeminal nerve

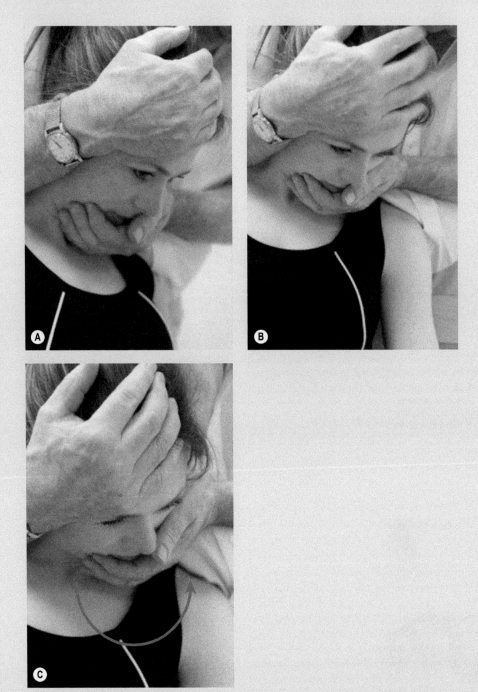

Figure 4.14 • A Start position involves cupping around the mandible in cervical flexion. **B** This is followed by contralateral cervical side flexion. **C** The addition of lateral glide of the mandible or alternatively opening and closing of the mouth can be included.

A neurodynamic test: occipital and auricular nerves

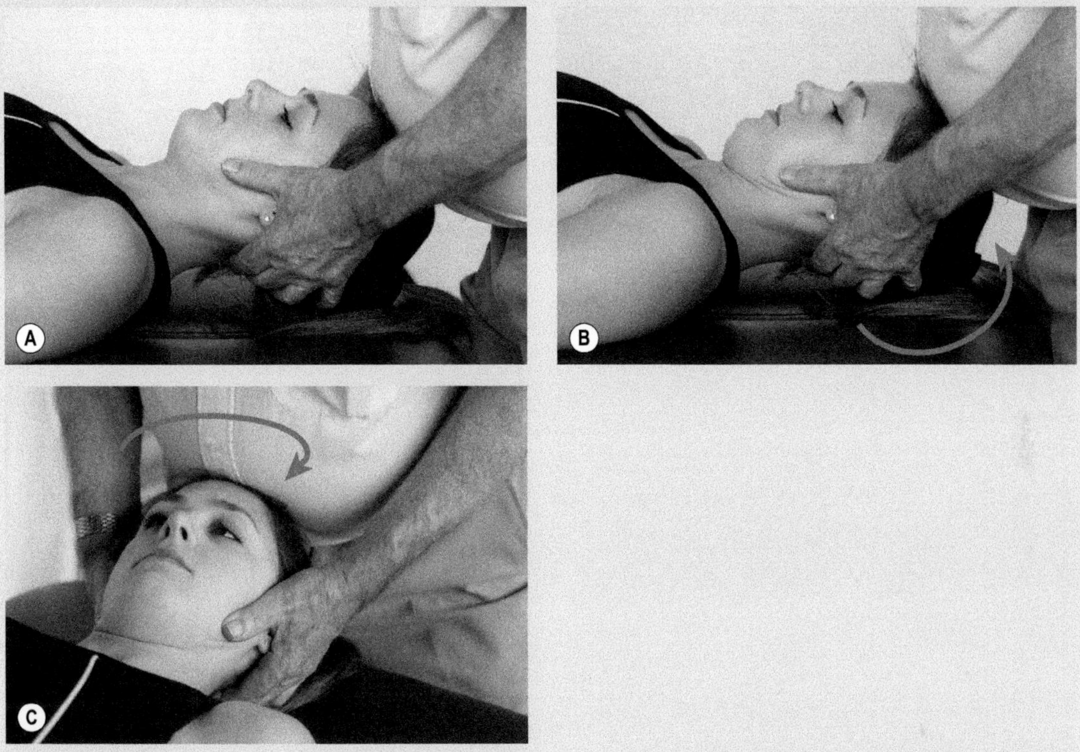

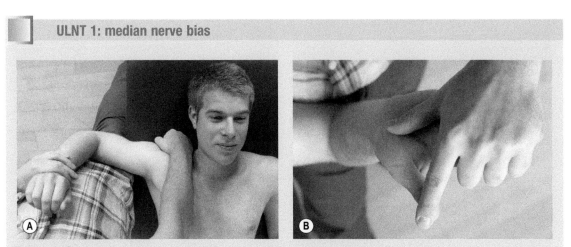

Figure 4.15 • **A** Start position cupping the occiput bilaterally with thumbs gently resting on the maxilla. **B** Upper cervical flexion is achieved through supination of the forearms. **C** Contralateral cervical lateral flexion can be performed. A common structural differentiation manoeuvre is to ask the patient to flex their knees either at the beginning or end of the test. If there is a change in symptoms then there is a greater indication of underlying mechanosensitivity.

ULNT 1: median nerve bias

Figure 4.16 • **A** Start position for the ULNT1 (median nerve bias) with the shoulder in abduction to the point where you begin to feel elevation in the shoulder girdle. **B** The hand position (using a gun grip) enables control of thumb, finger and wrist extension and then forearm supination, during the test.

Continued

ULNT 1: median nerve bias—cont'd

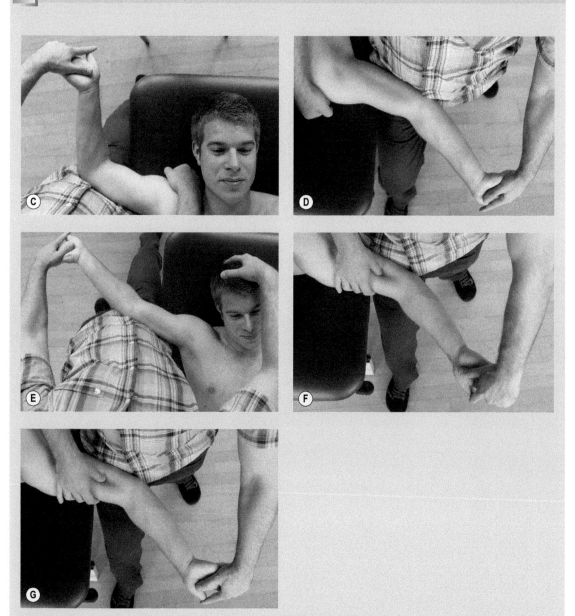

Figure 4.16 • cont'd C Lateral shoulder rotation. The anterior thigh of the examiner maintains the shoulder in abduction and gives some added comfort and support for the upper arm (as though there is an extension of the surface of the examining couch). **D** The last movement in the base test is elbow extension. The point at which the clinician begins to feel resistance should be the stopping point. With practice this should correlate closely with the point at which the patient feels the need to stop. One possible method of structural differentiation is to change a joint component away from the symptomatic area such as with ipsilateral cervical side flexion for symptoms felt in the arm. This presumes to affect the underlying nervous tissue and not other structures adjacent to the symptoms. **F** Palpation of the median nerve in the upper arm in a neurodynamic position can be used as another form of differentiation. **G** Adding flexion of the hand and wrist can further differentiate this palpation technique. If the response differs, this should rule out the presence of local nociceptive processes and confirm mechanosensitivity of the nervous system.

ULNT2a: median nerve bias

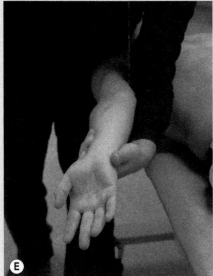

Figure 4.17 • A Start position with the patient lying diagonally on the bed with the test shoulder over the side of the bed. **B** Support the upper arm and position your anterior thigh on the superior aspect of the shoulder. It is common for a patient to side flex the cervical spine away from the examiner's thigh and this should be corrected where necessary. **C** Then add gentle depression to the shoulder girdle to the point of slight resistance. **D** Extend the elbow. **E** Using the 'inside' arm reach under the medial aspect of the arm and whilst holding the wrist apply whole arm lateral rotation.

Continued

ULNT2a: median nerve bias—cont'd

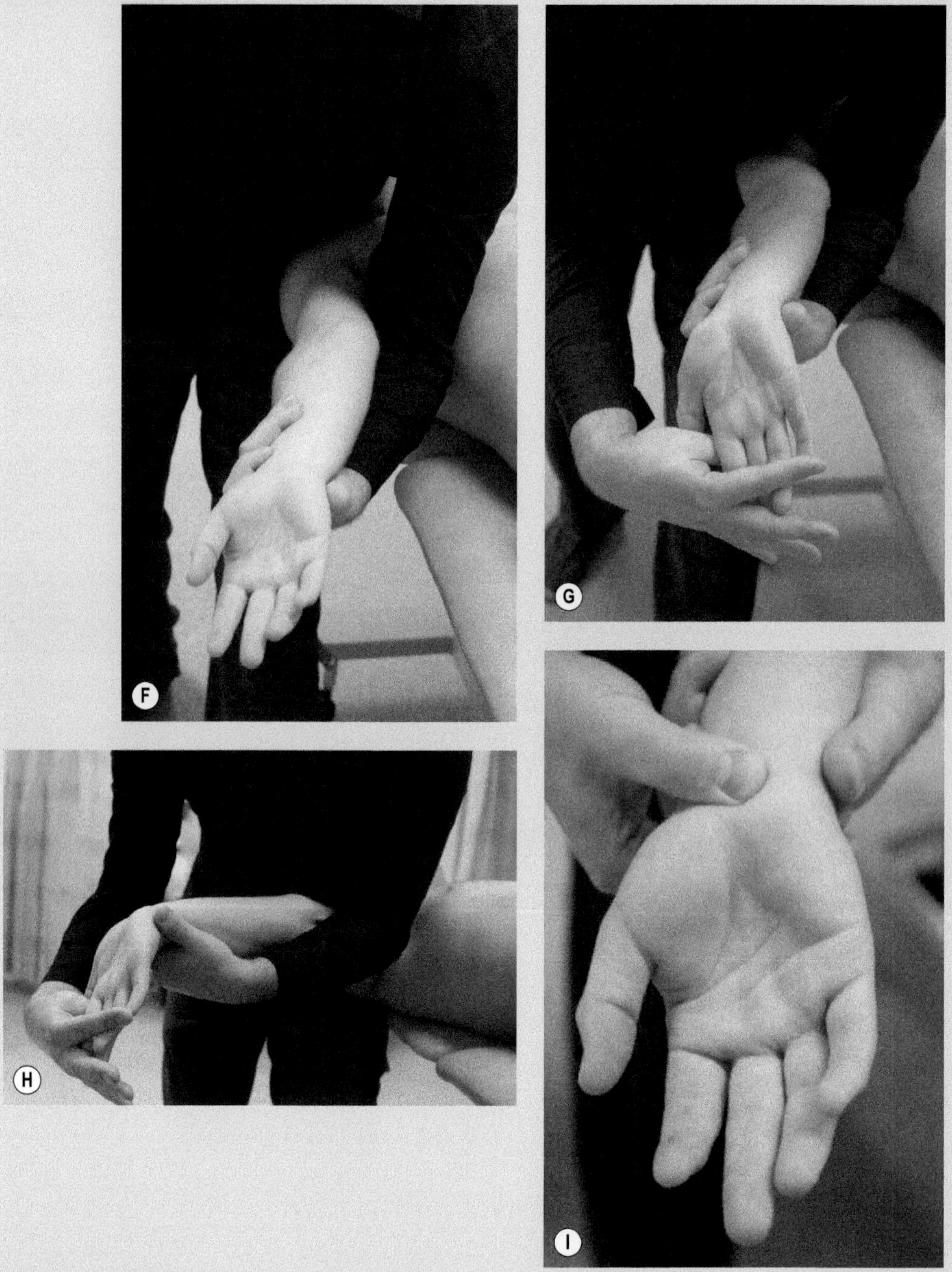

Figure 4.17 • cont'd F The examiner's arm should be in a position whereby it simultaneously helps maintain elbow extension and whole arm lateral rotation. **G** Place your thumb into the web space and gently apply wrist and thumb extension. With greater ranges of wrist extension bring your outside elbow towards the inside one. **H** If required you may add shoulder abduction. Common structural differentiation techniques are to release a small amount of shoulder depression or wrist extension, depending on the site of symptoms. **I** You may add nerve palpation in this test position as required. This shows indirect palpation of the median nerve at the carpal tunnel.

ULNT2b: radial nerve bias

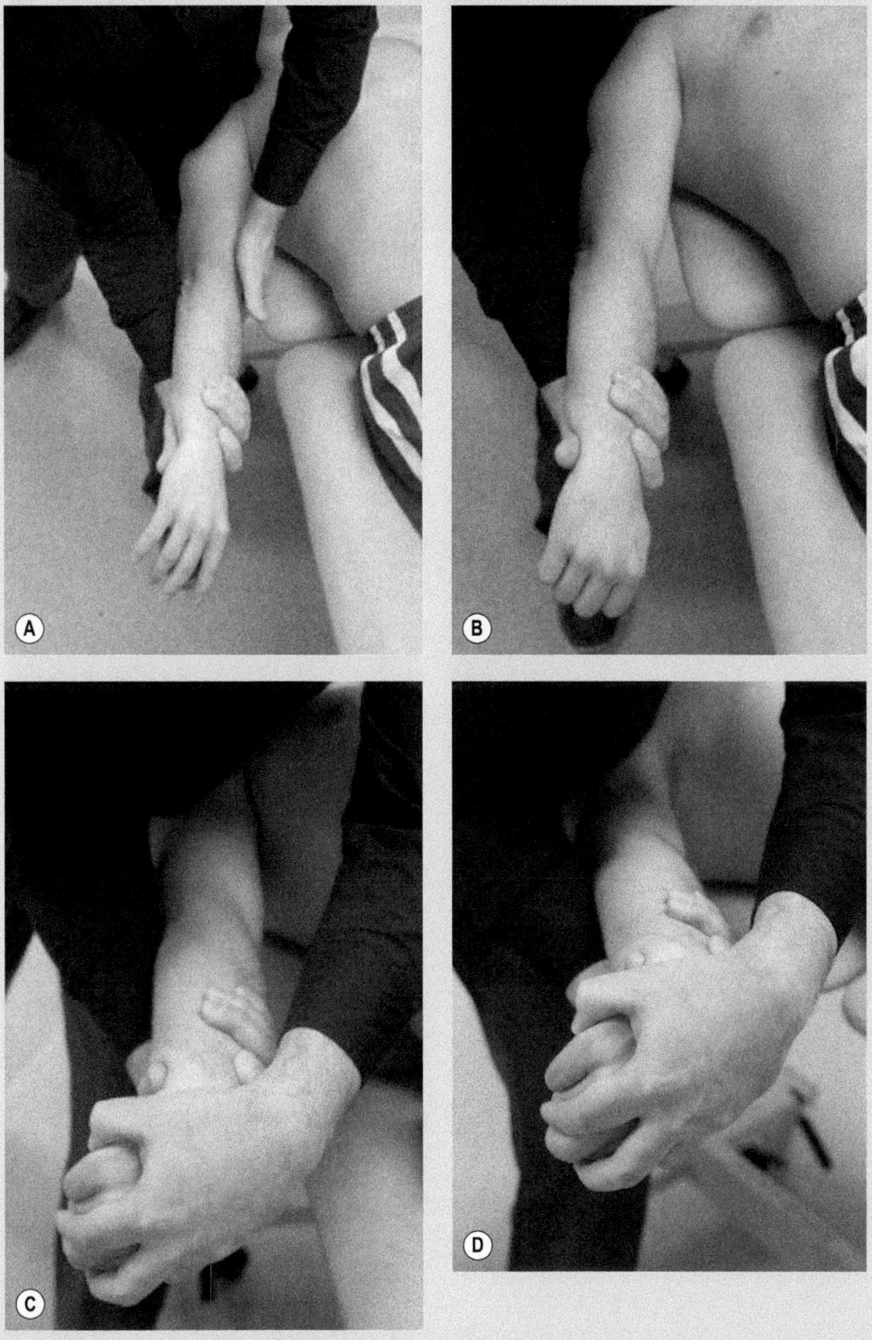

Figure 4.18 • A This test begins in the same start position as for the ULNT2a and includes shoulder girdle depression followed by elbow extension. **B** Then using the 'outside' arm and coming under the lateral aspect of the patients arm, hold the wrist and internally rotate the whole upper limb. Your arm should help to maintain both the elbow extension and the internal arm rotation in this position. **C** Ask your patient to hold their thumb and form a fist, then by reinforcing this position gently add wrist flexion. **D** If required you may then add shoulder abduction. The radial nerve can be palpated at the upper arm, elbow and distal forearm. Common structural differentiation techniques are to release the shoulder girdle depression or wrist flexion, depending on the location of the symptoms.

ULNT3 – ulnar nerve

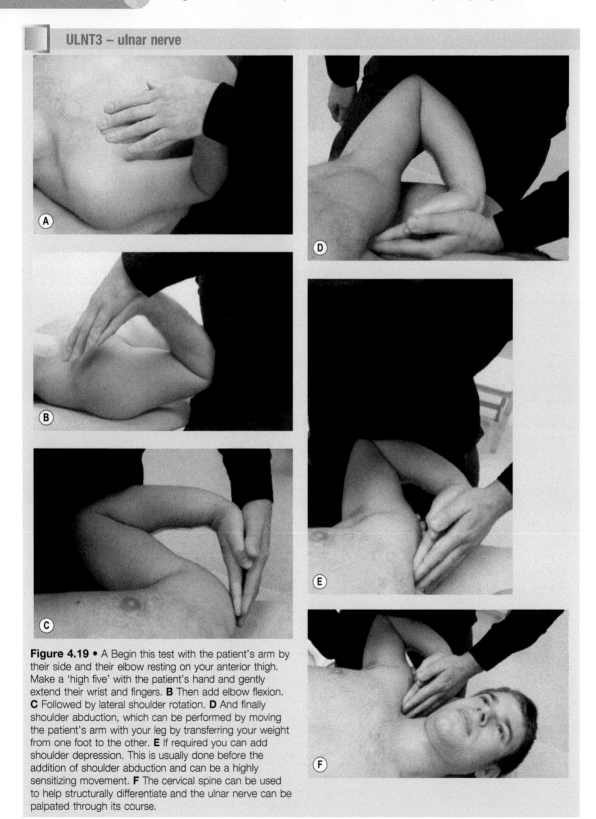

Figure 4.19 • **A** Begin this test with the patient's arm by their side and their elbow resting on your anterior thigh. Make a 'high five' with the patient's hand and gently extend their wrist and fingers. **B** Then add elbow flexion. **C** Followed by lateral shoulder rotation. **D** And finally shoulder abduction, which can be performed by moving the patient's arm with your leg by transferring your weight from one foot to the other. **E** If required you can add shoulder depression. This is usually done before the addition of shoulder abduction and can be a highly sensitizing movement. **F** The cervical spine can be used to help structurally differentiate and the ulnar nerve can be palpated through its course.

Altering the test and/or start position

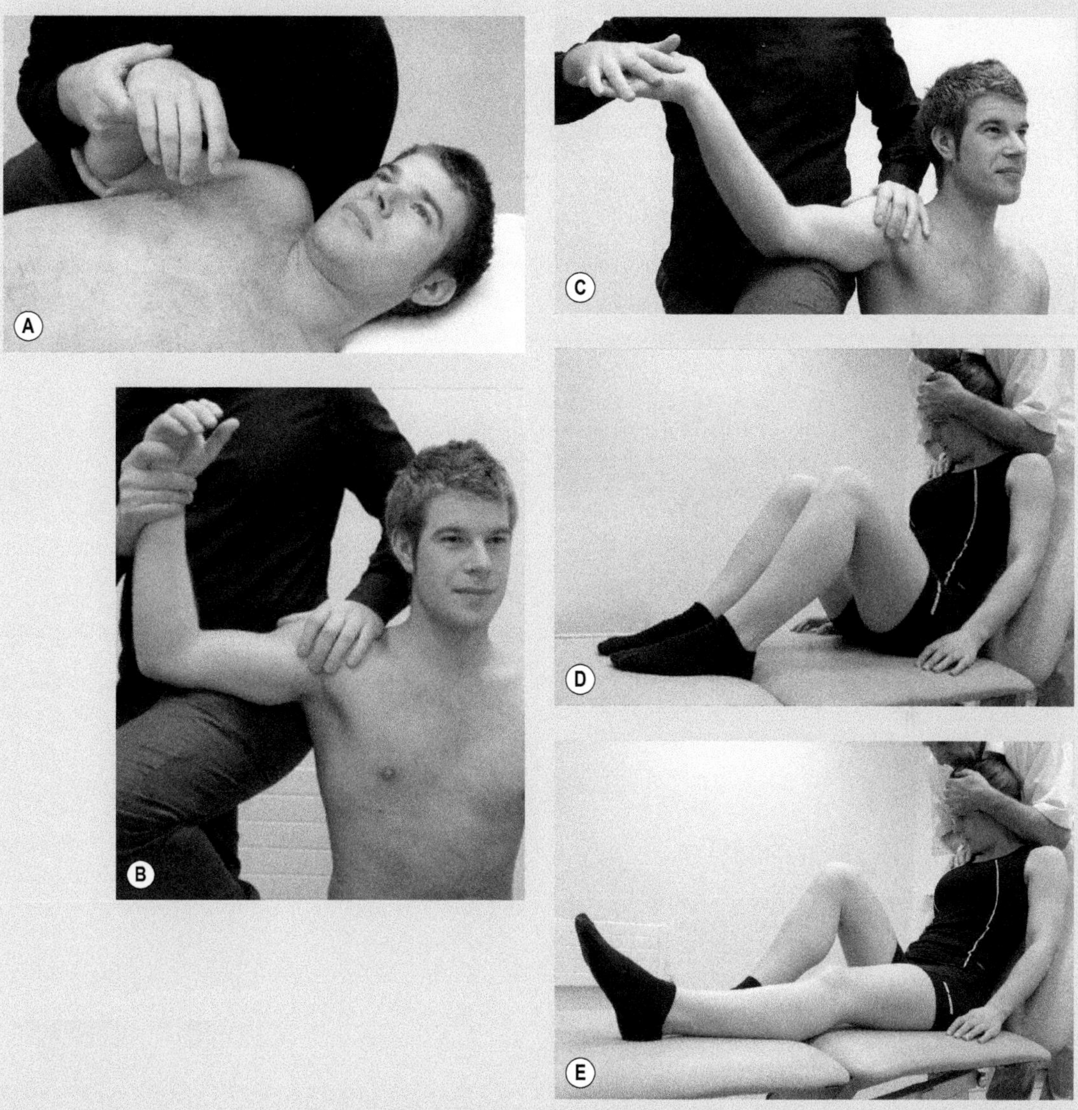

Figure 4.20 • A Cradle position. In this you can elevate the shoulder, alter the position of the neck or manoeuvre their elbow and wrist. It is sometimes appropriate to perform this in a supported sitting position in order to keep the patient as comfortable as possible. B It may also make more sense to adapt the base tests and start in a different position e.g. sitting, especially if this fits into functional description. C An example of the ULNT1 test being performed passively in sitting. It is very easy to ask the patient to perform a test actively and help guide them when a structural differentiation manoeuvre is desired. D Another example of a change in the starting position is to perform a neurodynamic test for the trigeminal nerve in a long sitting slump position. E The leg is being used as a way of exploring structural differentiation for this test. This applies the principle of the nervous system as a continuum.

Pre-cervical spine treatment screening – implications for examination

Cervical arterial dysfunction (CAD)

As part of the clinical interview, therapists are asked to identify any precautions or contraindications for treatment. Screening for vertebrobasilar artery insufficiency is commonly suggested in the presence of specific subjective symptoms (Box 4.17). The presence of CAD, which may be attributed to upper cervical instability, is considered to be one risk of manual therapy techniques to the cervical spine.

Guidelines for screening patients for risk of neurovascular complications of manual therapy have been available for many years (Taylor & Kerry 2010). In spite of the large number of papers devoted to CAD, there is no consensus of opinion as to the validity and reliability of the guidelines. Due to the medicolegal implications and the need to follow clinical guidelines, despite the lack of evidence, functional testing may be necessary – the minimum comprising a judicious sustained rotation of the cervical spine. If in doubt the patient must be referred for further medical tests before commencing the treatment (Kerry et al. 2008). However, extreme caution should be shown when presented with a

Box 4.17

Subjective symptoms possibly indicating the presence of CAD

- Headache and neck pain – which obviously present a problem when clinically reasoning
- History of migraine
- Visual disturbances
- Hearing disturbances
- Tingling or numbness in the face or around or in the mouth
- Dizziness or feeling of spinning around
- 'Gravitational' dizziness
- Double vision
- Speech or swallowing difficulties
- Sudden black-outs and falls to the floor
- Nausea or vomiting
- Hoarseness
- Clumsiness or limb weakness
- Loss of memory

(Kerry et al. 2007)

case where there is subjective data that is likely to prove CAD. It is the authors' opinion to err on the side of the caution with CAD testing.

Clinically, the type of tests selected will closely relate to the patients description of the aggravating factors (e.g. end of range cervical rotation or extension). The intensity of the tests should be taken only to, or just before, the onset of symptoms, in the first instances. These tests constitute important physical 'markers'.

Craniovertebral instability

Craniovertebral instability has been attributed as one possible cause of CAD and as such the discerning clinician should be aware of it. If you encounter patients displaying the symptoms noted below then craniovertebral instability is suggested as a necessary measure. A good depth of knowledge and use of clinical reasoning should guide the clinician when confronted with these symptoms, for example, craniovertebral instability testing could be a consideration for headache and WAD.

Symptoms and signs of cervical instability

Symptoms and signs of instability include (Gibbon & Tehan 2006):

1. Facial paraesthesia secondary to dysfunction of the connections of the hypoglossal nerve. Dysfunction ventral ramus as a cause of neck–tongue syndrome (Lance & Anthony 1980) and the dorsal ramus producing facial numbness
2. C1–C2 instability causing abnormal pressure on cervical nerves
3. Vertebrobasilar artery compromise (Savitz & Caplin 2005, Thanvi et al. 2005)
4. Cord compression (Rao 2002).

Clinical testing of craniovertebral instability

In the past certain classical tests have been proposed to test for cervical instability. These include the Sharp-Purser for the transverse ligament, the lateral flexion rotatory tests for the alar ligaments and the longitudinal cranial assessment for the tentorial membrane (Fig. 4.21). It is the authors' opinion that if there is a suspicion of cervical instability then it would be unwise to use these clinical tests due to the inherent danger to the patient.

Clinical testing of craniovertebral instability

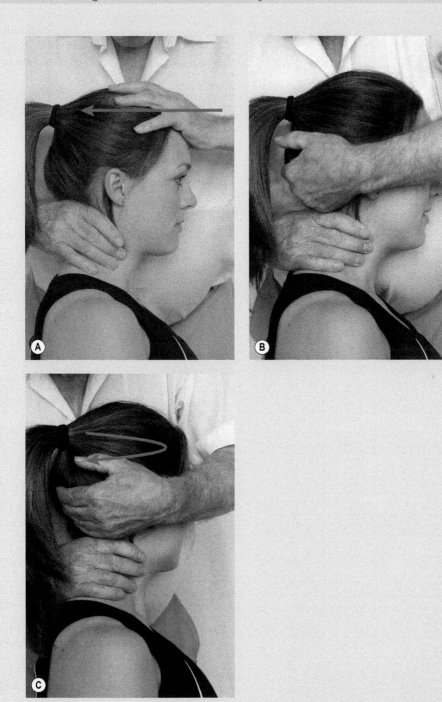

Figure 4.21 • A Sharp-Purser test. Fixing at C1/2 and anteroposterior tanslation of the occiput above by placing gentle pressure through the forehead. **B** Alar ligament test. Fix upper cervical spine and rest the head in the crook of the elbow. **C** Rotation towards testing shows rotation of the head to the right to test the left alar ligament.

Examination of the cervical spine through mobilization techniques

Passive mobilization

Manual examination techniques have a place in the physical examination of cervical pain disorders. Traditional passive joint palpation techniques, such as passive accessory intervertebral movements (PAIVMS), can assist in the clinical reasoning process. For instance, a unilateral posteroanterior palpation of a C5 that elicits a pain response should be viewed with consideration of the relative stimulus-response predictability i.e. what is the relationship between the extent of the response and how this varies with each repetition of the palpation? If there is fairly close stimulus/response predictability then it is more indicative of underlying nociceptive mechanisms. It should also encompass prior reasoning of the possible underlying pain mechanisms i.e. whether central sensitization is likely to be present.

 Posteroanterior unilateral vertebral pressure ⌐

Starting position

The patient lies prone with his forehead resting comfortably on his hands. The physiotherapist stands towards the side of the patient's head. She places the tips of her thumb pads, held back to back and in opposition, on the posterior surface of the articular process to be mobilized. Her arms should be directed 30° medially to prevent the thumbs from slipping off the articular process. The fingers of the uppermost hand rest across the back of the patient's neck and those of the other hand rest around the patient's neck towards his throat. Most of the contact is felt with the underneath thumb (Figure 4.22).

Method

Oscillatory pressure directed posteroanteriorly against an articular process if done very gently will produce a feeling of movement, but to prevent any lateral sliding at the point of contact, a gentle constant pressure directed medially must be maintained. If the movement is produced correctly there will be small nodding movements of the head but no rotary or lateral flexion movement.

As with other techniques involving pressure through the thumbs, this movement must not be produced by intrinsic muscle action.

Local variations

When mobilizing the first cervical vertebra, the physiotherapist needs to lean over the patient's head so as to direct the line of her thumbs towards the patient's eye. In the lower cervical area, the line is directed more caudally.

The second, third and fourth articular processes are far easier to feel accurately than are the remainder. The first cervical vertebra can be felt laterally, and the lower articular processes can be felt if the thumbs are brought in under the lateral border of the trapezius.

The symbol ⌐ indicates that the unilateral pressure on the vertebra is directly posteroanterior. There are two common variations to this direction that are used in treatment. Under circumstances where pain is quite severe, the direction is angled slightly away from posteroanterior as indicated by the symbol ⌐. The second variation, used when the joint is still and pain is minimal, is to angle the pressure more medially, endeavouring to increase the range. The angle is indicated by the symbol ←→; it is a very important examination procedure, especially for the upper cervical spine.

These directions can be varied still further by inclining them cephalad and caudad as indicated by the requirements of pain or stiffness.

Precautions

The only precaution is to perform the techniques very gently, especially in the upper cervical region. It is

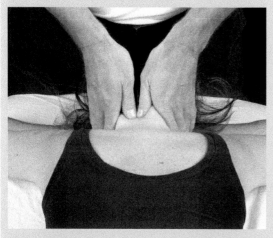

Figure 4.22 • Posteroanterior unilateral vertebral pressure ⌐.

Posteroanterior unilateral vertebral pressure ⌐—cont'd

seldom realized how effective these techniques can be while still being performed very gently.

Uses

Application of this technique is the same as for the previous technique, except that it is used for unilateral symptoms on the side of the pain. The medially directed technique is especially important for upper cervical disorders, particularly when aimed at restoring a full range of pain-free movements to prevent or lessen recurrences.

The testing position for cervical palpation can be changed according to patient comfort or the need to mimic functional movement. It would be far more predictive of a local nociceptive process if the same posteroanterior palpation evoked the same response in both a supine and a sitting position. If there is some variance then the therapist should be considering how this could be incorporated into their treatment, in terms of context change and altered firing of the pain neurotag.

Mobilization linked to context change

One further way of analyzing movement of the cervical spine is through passive physiological techniques, such as passive physiological intervertebral motion (PPIVMS). Again these can help to cement a reasoning process. It may be that these physiological techniques alter the current pain neurotag and can be used as one method within a graded exposure approach in the treatment of a functional impairment.

Rotation ↺

Starting position

The position described is for a 'rotation' to the left. This particular starting position is chosen because it is the most suitable position for learning feel, and because it is the starting position for the manipulative technique described later.

The patient lies on his back so that his head and neck extend beyond the end of the couch. The physiotherapist stands at the head of the couch and places her right hand under the patient's head and upper neck, with the fingers spread out over the left side of the occiput and adjacent neck. The thumb extends along the right side of the neck, with the thenar eminence over the right side of the occiput. She grasps the chin with the fingers of her left hand, while the palm of the hand and the forearm lie along

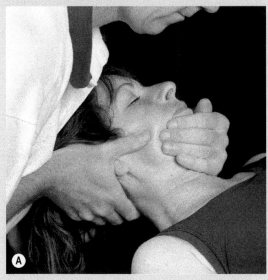
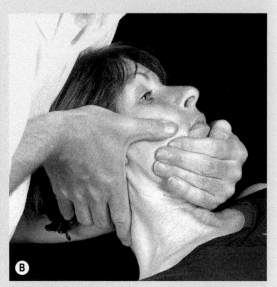

Figure 4.23 • A, B Rotation Grades I and II C Rotation Grade III.

Continued

Rotation ↻—cont'd

the left side of the patient's face and head just anterior to the ear. The patient's head should be held comfortably yet firmly between the left forearm and the heel of the right hand, and also between her left hand and the front of her left shoulder.

When oscillatory movements are being performed near the beginning of the rotation range, the physiotherapist stands head-on to the patient and the occiput is centred in the palm of her right hand. When the movements are performed at the limit of the range, she moves her body to the right until she is facing across the patient, and moves her hand further

around the occiput towards the ear. The head should at all times be comfortably supported from underneath. The physiotherapist should crouch over the patient so that she hugs the patient's head. The position of the patient's head and neck may be raised or lowered to position the joint being treated approximately midway between its flexion and extension limits. A position of flexion is shown in the diagrams.

The starting position finally adopted should be the one where the grasp with either arm should be able to perform the movement on its own (*Fig. 4.23*).

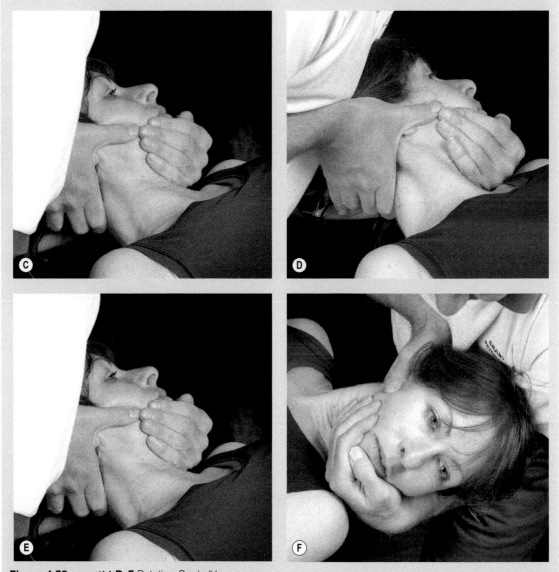

Figure 4.23 • cont'd D–F Rotation Grade IV.

Rotation ↺—cont'd

Method

The position is taken up by turning the head to the left with a synchronous action of both hands. It is most important that the fingers of the right hand should produce as much movement of the occiput as the left hand produces with the chin. This turning movement of the patient's head can be likened to the movement of a barbecue chicken as it revolves on a spit. In most other techniques the oscillatory movement is produced by body movement, but with rotation the physiotherapist's trunk remains steady and the rotation is produced purely by the physiotherapist's arm movement. The movement of the left arm is glenohumeral adduction with the elbow passing in front of the trunk.

Particular care needs to be exercised to be sure that a normal rotation is being produced and not a rotation distorted by deformity or muscle spasm. The range at which the oscillation is done should be kept at the limit of the normal movement obtainable.

Local variations

The upper cervical vertebrae are more readily mobilized with the head and neck in the same plane as the body. To mobilize the lower cervical vertebrae, the neck needs to be held in a degree of neck flexion. The lower the cervical level being mobilized, the greater the angle of neck flexion required for successful movement of that vertebral joint. The level being mobilized can be isolated somewhat by using the index finger of the occipital hand to hold around the vertebra above the joint.

Precautions

If a patient feels neck discomfort on the side of the neck to which the head is turned during or following this technique, it will readily disappear in a few minutes with active neck movements.

Although it may seem reasonable at times (when the technique is very gentle and symptoms are localized to the neck) to do rotation towards the side of pain, it should rarely be done in this direction as a strong manipulation when pain is referred from the neck.

Rotation should never be used in treatment if it produces any sign of dizziness, and to this end it is wise to do an exploratory rotation before carrying out rotary treatment.

Uses

Rotation is one of the most valuable mobilizing procedures for the cervical spine. It is frequently the first technique chosen when treating symptoms of cervical origin, and is of greatest value in any unilateral distribution of pain of cervical origin. In such cases, the procedure is carried out with the patient's face being turned away from the painful side.

Changing the context of a movement, as previously suggested, may give weight to a hypothesis and guide treatment. Painful and restricted cervical rotation assessed in a traditional supine position may be eased with a SNAG performed in sitting (see Fig. 4.24). This could be due to altered descending modulation, firing of a neurotag, or possibly relief through segmental inhibition.

Mobilization techniques have a role to play in the diagnosis and treatment of cervical pain disorders but should be viewed in relation to how the fit into the bio-psychosocial perspective of the individual.

The treatment of the cervical region

Ultimately treatment is not about sticking to set algorithms. Due to the individual nature of pain, no single treatment will be sufficient for each common complaint. It is therefore necessary to remain flexible. If pushing on a certain point on the neck relieves the patient's pain or by them holding a particular area then you should have the flexibility to accept that and incorporate it into your treatment. This is used to great effect with Brian Mulligan's SNAGs (sustained natural apophyseal glides; 2010). These techniques ultimately empower the patient to have some self-control over their pain problem. These techniques also lead well from the assessment into an individually tailored treatment approach.

Understanding the local pathophysiology and interacting components within each person's pain experience and maintaining a bio-psychosocial perspective will help to determine the specific intervention that will be most appropriate and beneficial. This next section documents some of these treatment approaches that will help the common cervical conditions and their underlying pain neurobiology.

Information and communication

Part of the rehabilitation process is to promote the patients' health literacy skills. Health literacy is the degree to which individuals have the capacity to

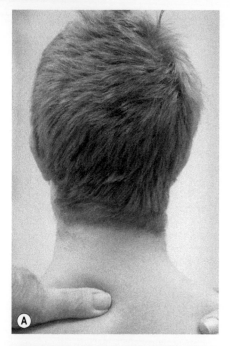

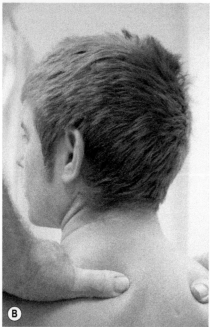

Figure 4.24 • A, B Example of active cervical left rotation with the addition of a transverse mobilization of T1 to the right as an assessment or treatment technique for someone struggling to turn his head.

obtain, process and understand basic health information and services needed to make appropriate health decisions. In general those with lower health literacy have a lower health status, which ultimately impacts on the health economics and both the prevalence and prognosis of neck pain. Improving health literacy could enhance the ability and motivation of the patient to solve their pain problems by applying their knowledge of health and accessing healthcare in a self-efficacious and appropriate manner (Ishikawa & Kiuchi 2010).

The information you impart and how you go about communicating it is vitally important. Communication is not only your verbal instructions but also the non-verbal aspects. These include your handling skills, touch of the patient and the careful way you perform techniques. This should allow continued positive feedback to your patient that will be apparent in their presentation and will enable them to understand their pain problem more fully.

Clinical note

Use of the word pain is common in a clinical setting with therapists often referring to it on numerous occasions. There is, however, substantial evidence that this will evoke unwanted arousal, particularly in someone experiencing pain. It may be that just hearing the word 'pain' or seeing it written will be sufficient to activate a pain experience or at least increase a patient's level of sensitivity (e.g. Asmundson et al. 2005, Dehghani et al. 2003, Flor et al. 1997b). This supports the need for clinicians to maintain a careful and measured approach when communicating with their patients, particularly if this includes imparting information regarding pain.

Shaping beliefs through pain education

Part of a clinical reasoning approach incorporates the use of psychology models or the concept of cognitive and affective domains within the neuromatrix paradigm. This includes a need to understand a person's attitudes and beliefs regarding their pain experience. Some of the factors that commonly relate to the disability and chronicity of a disorder are catastrophization regarding their pain and attributing it to a patho-anatomical cause, which in the light of known pain neurobiology is insufficient and sometimes incorrect.

Interest in the provision of education regarding pain neurobiology, helped by the book *Explain pain* (Butler & Moseley 2003), has grown recently. With suitable pain education it is possible for someone to change their belief that pain is a good indicator of tissue damage and can lessen their pain catastrophization (Meeus et al. 2010). Along with these changes in pain attitudes and beliefs there are likely to be improvements in physical markers that relate to both the underlying mechanosensitivity and the subsequent motor response, even without any physical interventions (Moseley 2004a, 2004b). This ultimately shows a beneficial change in the outputs from the brain; possibly reflecting altered descending modulation and a change in the activation of motor processing areas.

Education of pain neurobiology commonly includes an understanding of pain mechanisms such as nociception, the processes relating to central sensitization and brain changes in pain (Moseley 2004b). As expected with an individually tailored approach, the amount and type of information should be reasoned to best suit each patient.

Brief education has a positive effect on the health literacy in people suffering acute WAD (Oliveira et al. 2006). This includes a change in the use of medication, seeking ongoing interventions and a person's self-efficacy. Benefit is also seen when education is provided to people with chronic WAD (Van Oosterwijck et al. 2011).

However, with the advent of promising results following pain education, there appears to have been a worrying trend for some therapists to consider education sufficient in the treatment of people with pain problems. They have essentially become 'hands off' therapists. This is not only sad for manual therapy but shows a distinct lack of understanding of the benefit that certain therapeutic techniques have in aiding the diagnosis of underlying pain mechanisms (e.g. as seen in the use of neurodynamic techniques) or that can be directed towards affecting changes of specific elements of a pain experience (e.g. passive mobilization techniques creating hypoalgesic effects).

Passive mobilization techniques

Passive cervical mobilization techniques have been found to create hypoalgesic effects. They also activate the sympathetic nervous system (Vicenzino et al. 1998, Sterling et al. 2001, Skyba et al. 2003, Schmid et al. 2008). Both can effect modulation of nociceptive processing. The modulatory effects created are extrasegmental and can last up to 24 hours following the intervention. This suggests that passive mobilization can be directed to segments above and below the most painful area and help to reduce the impact of ongoing nociception (Box 4.18).

These responses to passive mobilization techniques are likely to be mediated by higher centres creating descending inhibition (Wright 2002, Souvlis et al. 2004). There appears to be less of a direct effect on the motor system and it is thought that changes shown in it are more of a reflection on the modulation of pain.

Given the extrasegmental effects it would be beneficial to begin mobilization above or below the most painful area, in the knowledge that there should still be a modulatory effect on their neck pain. The dismissal of more peripheralistic viewpoints regarding the effects of passive joint mobilization allow for the therapist to have flexibility in treating their patient effectively, i.e. it is more than moving a stiff segment.

Specific mobilization treatments

The cervical lateral glide technique (Fig. 4.26) has been used as a treatment technique due to its capacity to elicit hypoalgesia in painful musculoskeletal conditions (Sterling et al. 2010, Vicenzino et al. 1996, 1998, Coppieters et al. 2003). The technique should not be provocative (Elvey 1986).

This technique may be performed either as a basic localized translation or as a pulling technique whereby the therapist hooks their fingers onto the opposite side of the neck and draw the neck towards the position of their hand.

Selecting the correct technique

Ultimately the selection of the most appropriate specific passive mobilization technique will be dictated by the patient's requirements and the clinical skills of the therapist. It may be necessary for the patient to focus on the area that is being treated;

Box 4.18

Passive mobilization of the cervical spine in acute WAD

Acute WAD, presenting with left-sided neck pain that is exacerbated with all movements towards the left and cervical extension. There is some residual aching particularly first thing in the morning and later in the day. An initial hypothesis is that there is some resolving local inflammation and mechanical contribution to nociception.

Left unilateral C4 posteroanterior palpation evokes a pain response but there is a less marked response both above and below. There is a close stimulus/response predictability to palpation i.e. each time the area is palpated it evokes much the same response. This stimulus/response pattern is also seen through cervical movements that only slightly vary during the day.

Treatment of a gentle, slow and rhythmical passive mobilization technique (e.g. grade II) using the same posteroanterior inclination may be used but directed at the levels either side of the most symptomatic area. This will create an inhibitory/gating effect and help to reduce the ongoing nociception (Fig. 4.25).

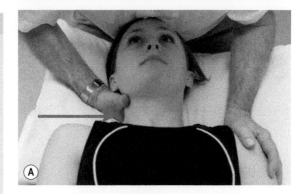

(A)

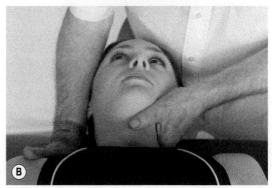

(B)

Figure 4.26 • A Lateral glide. This technique may be performed either as a basic localized translation or as a pulling technique whereby the therapist hooks their fingers onto the opposite side of the neck and draws the neck towards the position of their hand. **B** Lateral glide alternate grip. The fingers hook around the neck to draw towards the side of the mobilizing arm.

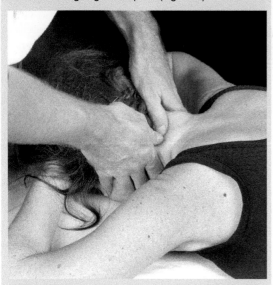

Figure 4.25 • Unilateral pressure posteroanterior with medial inclination on C2, III.

however, there is always a possibility that this may reinforce any hypervigilance.

When using these techniques to help a pain experience the treatment should be comfortable. This may allow the subconscious to reduce the vigilance maintained by the perception of an ongoing threat

(e.g. pain that is always associated with this area and the belief that the pain is a good indicator of tissue damage). If the perceived threat reduces then there will likely be changes in descending modulatory control and the subsequent neurotag relating to the neck. However, there are still a lot of unknowns regarding the possible processes that affect mobilization techniques and that may become apparent in the future.

The correct testing position

Finding the correct testing position depends very much on patient comfort and functional considerations. It may be impossible to assess or treat them in prone, as is commonly suggested, particularly when they have severe pain or breathing difficulties in this position. Conversely, this might be a position of comfort and as such would be a sensible starting position.

For example, it may be appropriate to begin a mobilization technique for someone with a nerve root lesion in an upright/supported sitting position, avoiding neck extension. In essence this incorporates the principle of context change and is likely to cause a change in the output from the neuromatrix – i.e. a different neurotag!

Incorporating context change into treatment

Brian Mulligan (2010) defined SNAGS as sustained natural apophyseal gliding movements (see Fig. 4.27). They are accessory mobilizations performed through movement in order to provide a pain-free movement. They provide an ideal opportunity to assess someone with neck pain in a functional position, e.g. cervical rotation in sitting that correlates with that person's current functional impairment of turning the neck when reversing a car.

SNAGS and other similar techniques are ideal to offer as a self-treatment strategy, therefore boosting the individual's control of their pain problem.

Manual therapy and central sensitization

It is important to understand whether central sensitization is a dominant mechanism underpinning a pain experience prior to the use of manual therapy. By applying more afferent stimulation through already sensitized nociceptive pathways it is likely that the therapist will only serve to amplify the current sensitization and underlying changes (Nijs & van Houdenhove 2009). It would be more appropriate in these circumstances to consider other treatment approaches aimed at reducing the central sensitization prior to the application of local manual therapy. This may include education and drug therapy aimed at reducing the amplification of the nociceptive system or techniques that aim to create lateral cortical inhibition such as sensory-discrimination and left/right discrimination training.

Manipulation

There is a high incidence of adverse events experienced by patients following cervical manipulation, with up to one in five patients experiencing mild or transient effects following treatment (Kerry et al. 2008). Cerebral vascular accidents are five times more likely to occur in someone who has received cervical manipulation up to one week prior to the event. Also, people suffering from vertebral artery stroke are five times more likely to have received cervical manipulation up to 1 week prior to the stroke. This information suggests the judicial evaluation of the use of manipulation prior to the use of cervical manipulation and as such is an approach that the authors would not choose.

However, the grade V manipulative techniques advocated by Maitland, which consider all aspects of safety, may be practised by physiotherapists.

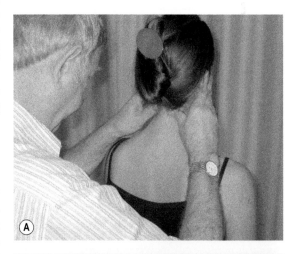

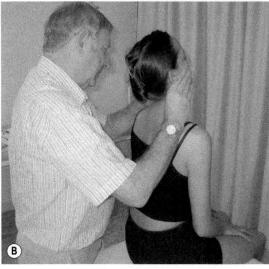

Figure 4.27 • A, B The examiner performs a SNAGS technique in the upper cervical region in order to facilitate a pain-free cervical extension.

They are appropriate to use when activation of a local neuroimmune response or neural silencing are desired; the proviso being that when the nerve begins to fire following the silent period, there may be an increase in the symptoms due to nociceptive firing.

Treatment with reference to neurodynamics

Treating the containers

One of the objectives of treatment of abnormal neurodynamics is to improve and maintain the health and mobility of the tissues comprising the containers, in combination with direct mobilization of the nervous system. The neural containers are considered to be the interfacing tissues of the nervous system, commonly known as the nerve bed (i.e. the tissues in which the nerve lies). This consists of any structures adjacent to the nervous system, such as muscles, tendons, bones, ligaments, fascia and blood vessels (Shacklock 2005).

From the neurodynamic aspect, nerves slide through the tunnels, while tunnels move over nerves. Movements of the nerve bed such as stretching, shortening, bending, twisting and turning produce similar effects on the nervous system. The nerve can also move independently from the nerve bed and requires appropriate movement to maintain health, e.g. axoplasmic and blood flow.

It may be necessary to treat the container tissues prior to commencing any neurodynamic techniques such as sliders or tensioners. This is particularly the case when the interfacing tissues directly affect the movement, pressure changes or health of the nerves (e.g. through local inflammation, muscle spasm or scarring).

Neural mobilization techniques

In recent times, neurodynamic mobilizing techniques have been divided into 'sliders' and 'tensioners' (Coppieters & Butler 2008). Sliders consist of simultaneously increasing the load of the nervous system at one joint whilst decreasing the load at another joint (Butler 2000, Coppieters et al. 2004, Shacklock 2005). During these manoeuvres there is large amplitude of movement of the nerve

(Coppieters et al. 2009) and, most likely, little change in intraneural pressure. These techniques are generally chosen for more sensitive conditions where the objective is to get some movement and health without increasing symptoms in the nervous system. This may create hypoalgesia or local sympathetic activation and should be less threatening for the patient. They can also be seen as another form of context change that will alter the neurotag.

Tensioners are the more traditional and aggressive techniques where movements place progressive load through the nervous system. These would be equivalent to using movements of the base test as a treatment and are more likely to be used in the later stages of rehabilitation where the patient needs to become accustomed to more load through the system. Tensioners have been shown to cause a change in thermal sensitivity and possible hypoalgesic effects and should be used with these effects in mind (Beneciuk et al. 2009b).

Slider technique for the median nerve (ULNT1) is illustrated in Figure 4.28. As elbow extension is added there is simultaneous subtraction of wrist extension. This is then repeated in the reverse

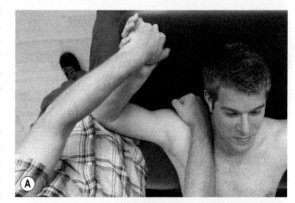

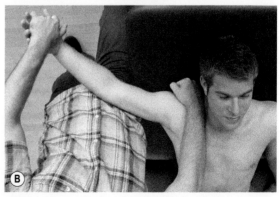

Figure 4.28 • A, B Slider technique for the median nerve.

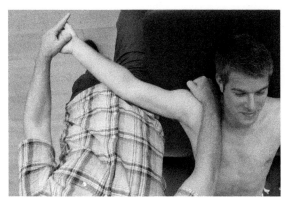

Figure 4.29 • Tensioner.

Slider technique using elbow flexion

A and B show a slider technique using elbow flexion with shoulder girdle depression in the cradle position that can be used for a possible nerve root lesion. This is to create a sense of support and allow some relaxation.

In C, it would be easy to make it functional (e.g. feeding) or bring in some distraction to allow some modulatory effects. It can be great for your patient to laugh during your treatment session – don't forget the role of the endogenous drug cabinet (opioids, endorphins, enkephalins)! It is another form of context change within a treatment that will affect the neurotag.

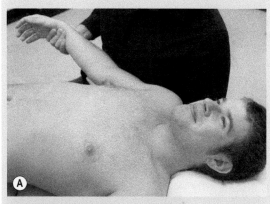

Ⓐ

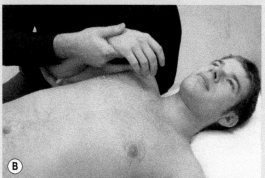

Ⓑ

direction in a slow, oscillatory manner. This may be useful for nerve root disorders in which there is sensitivity of the upper limb nerve trunks.

Figure 4.29 shows how the base ULNT1 test can be incorporated into a neural mobilization treatment as a tensioner. The movement will still be oscillatory, depending on the desired needs of the patient. It will enable progressive loading through the nerve trunks and a graduated exposure to these positions.

When the patient is recovering from adverse neurodynamic problems, a combination of slider and tensioner techniques can be performed since the normal nervous system continually functions through these means, i.e. both sliding through the nerve bed and loading the nerve when placed in a stressed position. It is important for the clinician to clinically reason when this may be appropriate. A slider technique is illustrated in Figure 4.30.

Clinical tip

Neural mobilization techniques in combination with passive mobilization of the cervical spine have been shown to have immediate clinical benefits in people with nerve-related neck and arm pain (Nee et al. 2012). This approach also demonstrates that there is a low incident of adverse events due to the treatment. It is reasonable to suggest that this approach should be considered in order to help reduce mechanosensitivity and improve the health and function of someone with neuropathic pain.

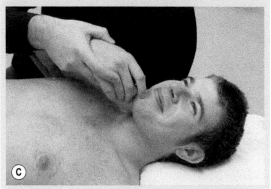

Ⓒ

Figure 4.30 • A Slider technique using elbow flexion. **B** Slider technique: cradle position. **C** Slider technique: relaxation.

Massage

Massage should be considered an important part of your treatment modalities. This may include massage directly over nerve trunks in order to create a gating/inhibitory effect of the pain problem. The same caution should be shown in the presence of allodynia as with other manual techniques. However, massage or desensitization techniques on the border of a sensitized or allodynic area may provide beneficial inhibitory effects.

More vigorous/stronger techniques may be more appropriate after any sensitivity has reduced sufficiently to be able to cope with them or as a progression when the patient is getting used to accepting greater force or load being placed on their tissues.

Self-treatment and management

Self-treatment and management will be included in most of the treatment options. This will promote self-efficacy and hopefully enhance the beneficial effects proposed through the various treatment approaches. Ideally the patient should clearly understand what they are doing and why. This means spending sufficient time educating them and ensuring that the self-treatment is performed appropriately. It is imperative that the patient feels they can ask any further questions and is a good idea to ask what their understanding of the problem is following the delivery of treatment.

Figure 4.31 shows a self-mobilizing slider technique for the radial nerve using the neck ipsilateral rotation with elbow extension and can be used to maintain health of the nervous system.

Figures 4.32 and 4.33 illustrate self-management of cervical rotation using a towel or the hand to change the context of the movement and hence the motor output from the neuromatrix.

Treatment dose and ongoing intervention

In the same way that a doctor would prescribe medication and consider the appropriate dose, they would also think about the possible side-effects or adverse events caused by taking the medication. This should be no different for the manual therapist delivering a particular intervention. These calculations should be based on the current hypothesis and understanding of the mechanisms underpinning the pain problem. With a highly sensitive condition you

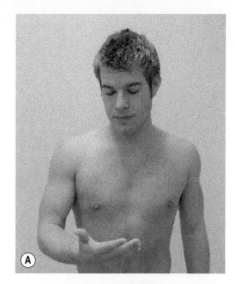

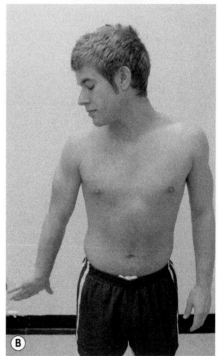

Figure 4.31 • A, B Self-mobilizing slider technique for the radial nerve using the neck ipsilateral rotation with elbow extension.

need to deliver far less treatment (lower dose). This means less time and fewer repetitions of a treatment and most likely a less forceful technique.

For a more stable condition it may be prudent to deliver far more. To gain lasting effects, it will be beneficial to give the patient some self-management

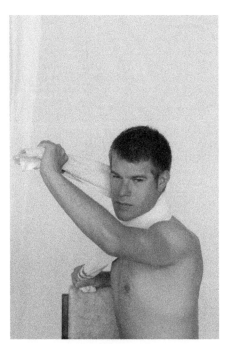

Figure 4.32 • Self-management of cervical rotation using a towel.

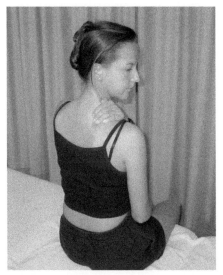

Figure 4.33 • Self-management of cervical rotation using the hand.

techniques or to see them for ongoing appointments at reasonably regular time intervals. Although one risk factor for someone proceeding onto a chronic condition is the over-reliance of a passive intervention, i.e. they don't take ownership of their own care.

For the more severe and sensitized states, there is no benefit in seeing the patient numerous times

> **Box 4.19**
>
> **Graded exposure for WAD that includes restricted and painful cervical rotation**
> - Perform left/right discrimination tasks for the neck
> - Imagine performing cervical rotation
> - Passive rotation of the neck in supine
> - Cervical rotation SNAGS in sitting
> - Active cervical rotation with the eyes closed
> - Rotation of the trunk, keeping the neck still
> - Active rotation in the car, imaging the car moving
> - Short drives in the car
> - Longer drives in the car, including driving past the crash site
>
> These are some ideas of how to grade the exposure of cervical rotation and include contextual challenges and return to functional activities.

for the delivery of manual therapy. In this case it is far more important to gain some stability in the condition first. This may come through education, drug therapy and appropriate self-management.

Graded exposure in order to progress treatment

Progressing treatment can be achieved through a graded exposure approach. This essentially includes some form of pacing within contextual changes and challenges. It should encompass the functional limitations and goals of the individual. The ultimate aim is to change the current pain response (neurotag) and gradually expose the individual (and hence the brain) to more challenging activities. These activities include changes in how a movement is performed and recognizing that changing the emotional context or thoughts and beliefs regarding the movement may be a part of achieving this. This obviously ties into the concept of the neuromatrix paradigm and the different input domains. The end goal for the patient would be for them to have the freedom and flexibility to run any movement without creating a pain experience. An example of graded exposure treatment for WAD can be found in Box 4.19.

There are many other treatment options and techniques that are at the disposal of manual therapists and we encourage clinicians to maintain a healthy interest in these but hope that treatment will include strong clinical reasoning skills and an understanding of the underlying pain mechanisms.

Case study 4.1

Management of cervical nerve root lesion

Subjective examination

Social history

Pat is a 50 year-old publican who has run her own public house in the Yorkshire Dales for the past 10 years. The establishment also has six self-contained holiday letting apartments. She is extremely busy and is able to carry out most of the widely varying tasks needed to maintain the profitable running of the business.

Present history

Five weeks ago the sharp neck pain ① came on with a jolt as a low flying Tornado jet flew overhead. Initially the pain subsided within 2 days or so but returned 2 weeks later. This time the neck pain got worse, spreading into the left scapular region, as a dull ache ② and a heavy achy feeling in the left upper limb ③ with pins and needles in the hand ④. Pat reported the neck becoming stiffer and increasingly painful to move. Refer to the body chart in Figure 4.34, which illustrates the categories of pain described above.

Symptom behaviour

Pat described the very worse time being at night. She finds it difficult, if not impossible, to find any position which eases the symptoms for any length of time. The GP has prescribed diclofenac, which has helped to reduce symptoms at night to some extent.

Pat finds many general and household activities difficult to achieve without causing pain, for example putting on a coat, making beds, reaching high shelves and any lifting is out of the question. When she performs these activities they aggravate her pains for several minutes and these can last considerably longer if she 'pushes' it.

When asked, have you found any way of reducing the pain and heaviness? She replied 'Yes, I get some relief by resting in a comfortable high-back arm chair with my head and arms fully supported. I also get some ease by supporting the arm across the front of my body, rather like a sling. In these positions, relief is only short-lived'.

Past history

She suffered a similar episode 10 years ago but the symptoms were much less severe. The cause was described as a minor whiplash. She had left-sided neck pain with some referral of pain into the upper arm. Physiotherapy treatment consisted of cervical manual traction with active exercises. Full symptomatic recovery took 6 weeks. Pat has had a stiff neck on about three other occasions since, which lasted for a few days each time.

Medical history

Pat is a healthy, fit person with no history of any serious illnesses. There was no subjective indication of possible 'red flags' or CAD.

Working hypothesis

This currently looks like a peripheral neuropathic pain problem due to the presenting patterns e.g. symptom description, distribution, night pain and her relieving positions. It is possible that there is a learned response maintained from her previous experience and therefore regulated by a neuroimmune interaction.

Planning the physical examination with clinical reasoning models

Due to the moderate to high severity and irritability of the disorder it is more appropriate to undertake a minimum of testing that aims towards finding non-provoking postures and movements. It is important to assess the integrity of the nervous system and aim to support or reject the current hypotheses concerning the underlying pain mechanisms:

1. **Relieving positions**

   The subjective examination suggests the head, neck and arms must be fully supported before attempting any active or passive movements. Supporting the arm to create relief has been described as a way of attaining relief from the neuropathic pain disorders (Gifford 2001). A common position adopted is the 'arm overhead' position as a way of attaining short-term relief. This has been called the 'shoulder abduction relief sign' (Fast et al. 1989), and has been shown to significantly reduce intraforaminal pressure on the C5, C6 and C7 nerve roots (Farmer & Wisneski 1994). This suggests underlying mechanosensitivity to pressure and load through the nervous system.

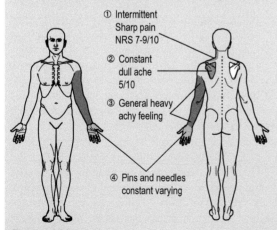

① Intermittent Sharp pain NRS 7-9/10

② Constant dull ache 5/10

③ General heavy achy feeling

④ Pins and needles constant varying

Figure 4.34 • Body chart.

Case study 4.1—cont'd

A change in Pat's posture seems wholly appropriate in her current circumstance.

2. **Nerve palpation**

Palpation of the peripheral nerves throughout their length and of the surrounding tissues will help to ascertain any heightened sensitivity and discriminate nociceptive process with neuropathic ones. In the sensitized nerve, palpation in one part may cause neurological symptoms to spread in both directions along the nerve tract (Butler 2000). With widespread sensitivity of the nervous system e.g. through either the whole of one side of the body or the whole of the upper limb, this is suggestive of central sensitization and should be approached with respect for the effect this could have on assessment and treatment, particularly when using manual techniques.

It is important to palpate the trunks of the upper limb but remain respectful of any sensitivity that may be apparent in the brachial plexus. Although there is likely to be a small component of central sensitization, this does not seem to be the overriding issue therefore quickly palpating outside of the known peripheral nerve trunks or distal to the current problem will help to establish this.

3. **Movement testing, including neurodynamic tests with structural differentiation tests**

It is important to consider the testing position for Pat. For her the most appropriate position to begin testing would be sitting, preferably in a high back chair, in her most comfortable and supported position.

Movements such as light depression of the shoulder girdle, possibly causing a small increase in symptoms, will give some reference of her sensitivity to movements. Changes in the position of either hand or wrist during this test bring in an element of structural differentiation and a greater understanding of the underlying neuropathic component. If the symptoms alter it is more suggestive of a neurogenic origin. It is unnecessary and unwise to try to increase all symptoms, as a reduction in the symptoms will help to establish whether there is a neurogenic involvement.

4. **Neurological examination**

A neurological examination is required in order to confirm or rule out the need for caution. In conditions where it is suspected that neurological dysfunction is likely to be present, as is the case of a cervical nerve root lesion, 'bed-side' manual examination of the nervous system is essential in order to ascertain the health and sensitivity of the nervous system. This will also aid in guiding provision of appropriate treatment by building a picture of the change in nervous system function, including the processing of sensory information, motor output and cortical or representational changes.

For Pat it is appropriate to perform a sensory assessment and test reflexes, clonus and Babinski. At the present time a motor assessment is unlikely to provide further information without aggravating her condition.

5. **Thoughts and beliefs**

It is worth asking Pat her opinion regarding the problem. This will guide the provision of education, including the feedback from the specific tests that are performed during the assessment.

Physical examination

Present pain: the symptoms expressed on the body chart (Fig. 4.34) were all present.

Pat sat in a slouched position with her head and neck in a few degrees of flexion and contralateral right lateral flexion. The left shoulder girdle was elevated and protracted. This antalgic posture suggests that she is unconsciously trying to offload her nervous system. It is likely that passive techniques away from the affected side or unloading the nervous system are most appropriate.

Even the slightest amount of passive movement of the neck towards the midline increased the symptoms, so was immediate abandoned. Asking Pat to come out the 'slouched' position only increased the symptoms marginally.

Relieving positions in sitting

Cervical: The combined movement of flexion and contralateral flexion very slightly reduced the symptoms.

Thoracic: Rotation of the thorax to the right was approaching full range without increase of symptoms. Thoracolumbar slump relieved symptoms moderately.

Shoulder girdle: With the left forearm supported in 90° flexion, shoulder girdle elevation was the most relieving movement and position.

Left shoulder: With the forearm still in the supported position, symptoms were somewhat eased with assisted active flexion/abduction to about 100° of movement. Right shoulder movements were virtually full.

Palpation in sitting

There was marked tissue tenderness on the left anterolateral aspect of the cervical area between C5 and T1; even with light touch of the tissues in this area there was some nerve-like symptoms referring into the left upper arm. When palpated the nerve trunks of the brachial plexus above the clavicle were also tender to touch and referred symptoms into the

Continued

Case study 4.1—cont'd

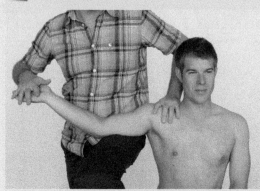

Figure 4.35 • ULNT 1 on the right upper limb.

arm and hand. This was markedly different from the right side, which was unremarkable and comfortable to palpate.

Neurodynamic testing

ULNT 1 test in sitting increased the symptoms at minus 40° of elbow extension. These are relieved with a small amount of active shoulder elevation. In Figure 4.35, ULNT 1 on the right upper limb was tested with sensitizing movements. Six repetitions of elbow flexion to extension were performed with no definite change of symptoms.

Tests in supine

The most comfortable position for Pat was with the head-end of the couch raised 10°, her head resting on two pillows and her upper limbs also supported on pillows. In this position light palpation of the cervical region was repeated with less referral of systems into the left arm.

The left hand was placed behind the head. There was an increase in symptoms on lifting the left arm, but once in position the symptoms gradually reduced by 10%. This 'hand-behind-head' position was tolerated for about 10 seconds. To bring the arm back down required the assistance of the other arm.

Neurological testing

Light touch: There was slight hyperaesthesia through the whole of the left arm but only allodynia over the tissues in the left anterior triangle of the neck. The lateral side of the left hand was more sensitive (hyperaesthetic) than the medial side. The right side was unremarkable.

Pin-prick: There was mild hyperalgesia throughout the left arm but this was pronounced over the left anterior triangle region. The right side was unremarkable.

Reflexes: Deep tendon reflexes for biceps and triceps were performed and were slightly brisker on the left side for both.

Clonus and Babinski: Nothing remarkable was found for both tests.

Thoughts and beliefs

Pat was fairly confident that the problem was due to her nerves and was happy to have found partial relief through some of the small movements attempted. She was slightly concerned about how sensitive her left arm was but happy that this correlated with the current picture of her sensitive nervous system.

Clinical reasoning

When considering the evidence from the examination it points towards irritation and sensitization in and around the nerve root complex. Cervical postures and movements where Pat was unable to extend and laterally flex to the ipsilateral side indicate an intervertebral foraminal compression problem on the left side of the neck. The causes of the symptoms may be due to soft tissue trauma to the structures surrounding the intervertebral foraminae, and the concomitant inflammation producing extra or intraneural swelling and chemical irritation to neural tissue. The consequence of this compression is likely to result in the formation of ectopic impulse generation sites, impaired axoplasmic and blood flow through the damaged nerve fibres and general mechanosensitivity, including an element of central sensitization.

Prognosis

Butler (2000) suggests that prognosis is one of the most difficult hypothesis categories. Many clinical factors are involved: the individual's rate of healing from previous injuries, whether they have had similar injuries in the past, how the current episode compares with those of the past, if there is evidence of family problems and how severe and irritable the disorder is. The affective and cognitive factors play an important role in the prognostic process. Pat looks as though she has some positive prognostic factors and so is likely to respond well.

As regard to a cervical nerve root disorder, typically the worst period is the first 1–2, or at worst, 4 weeks. Thereafter, the condition usually subsides gradually with occasional temporary setbacks (Gifford 2001) – to quote:

> ...for patients, the 'good news' is that the symptoms do settle, the 'bad news' is that it can take up to 3 months or more to recover full function.
>
> Gifford (2001)

Our clinical experience for a severe nerve root lesion is that it can take more than a year to recover full function.

Case study 4.1—cont'd

Treatment aims and plan

1. Treatment of the neural interfacing structures; mobilization of 'tunnel' sites to increase tunnel dimension; passive mobilization techniques to encourage segmental inhibition.

2. Direct mobilization of the nervous system through slider and tensioner techniques, including sensitizing and differentiating procedures, to maintain health of the nervous system.

3. Using contextual change to effect a change in the representation of movement in the neck and the subsequent output of the pain neurotag. Fit this into a graded exposure paradigm that ties into providing the brain and tissues with suitable challenges to give them back the freedom and flexibility to maintain good function.

4. Neurobiological education that is specific to the changes relevant to Pat's neuropathic pain problem, including a provision of a prognosis.

5. Self-treatment techniques including sliders and tensioners, SNAGS and self-management techniques that correlate with Pat's relieving positions.

6. Improve general health and fitness to encourage health support for the healing process.

7. Discussion with GP the use of neuropathic pain medication, as appropriate.

Treatment 1 (day 1)

After the examination Pat reported a slight increase of symptoms. The treatment consisted solely on finding and practicing relieving positions and movements.

'Cradling' the left arm across the front of the body with the right arm supporting the weight of the affected limb was practised. In this position two exercises were attempted: 1) gentle assisted active shoulder raising movements in the most comfortable plane of motion; and 2) shoulder girdle elevation. This was to relieve pressure on the nerve roots and to allow the probable immune response to settle a little. Also, it gives Pat something active and empowering to do, creating some confidence that she has the ability to settle her pain.

Pat was advised to sleep with two or more pillows and experiment with various positions of the affected arm in an attempt to ease the symptoms. She was given some brief education regarding the nerves and the increase in their sensitivity, including why she was experiencing night pain. She was advised to move a little at night where possible, if she had woken, in order to promote an increase in blood flow to the nerves.

Treatment 2 (day 3)

Pat returned for re-evaluation and treatment. The main subjective problems were heightened symptoms at night with loss of sleep and general arm activities,

especially reaching up and putting a coat on. The left arm felt heavy, weak and achy. The neck was still held in an antalgic posture of flexion and contralateral lateral flexion.

Pat thought the pain relieving position helped to ease the pain a little and she had slept for longer periods before waking. Otherwise her condition was unchanged.

Re-assessment of the physical parameters

Cervical: Pat was automatically sitting up 'straight' with her head and neck in some degree of flexion and contralateral lateral flexion. She was able to move her head into the midline without an immediate increase in pain and into 5° of ipsilateral cervical left rotation before areas ① and ② increase.

Shoulder girdle: with the left arm supported, shoulder girdle elevation reached about half range before pain increased in area ①. This was relieved slightly with further elbow flexion.

Left shoulder: with the arm still supported, the left arm was lifted through the plane of flexion/abduction to 100° before areas ③ and ④ increased in intensity.

ULNT1 in sitting: in the supported position the left elbow was able to extend to minus 30° before symptoms in areas ③ and ④ were heightened. These were reduced through a small amount of shoulder elevation.

Neurological testing: light touch and pin-prick examination remained the same.

Technique 1

• Position: supported supine.
• Method: cervical lateral glide from right to left for C5, C6 and C7, Grade II 3 × 6 on each segment.

There was no tenderness elicited during the techniques. The reassessment: symptoms in areas ① and ② were slightly reduced.

A cervical lateral glide technique from right to left is shown in Figure 4.36. The patient found this technique quite relieving therefore the procedure was repeated.

Technique 2

• Position: supported ('cradle') supine position with 2 pillows for the neck.
• Method: slider to the left shoulder girdle and elbow. Involving passive shoulder girdle depression towards neutral with simultaneous elbow flexion, followed by shoulder elevation to half range and extension of the elbow to 90° flexion – six repetitions of slow and rhythmical passive movements within a pain-free range were performed (see Fig. 4.37). Again, Pat found this

Continued

Case study 4.1—cont'd

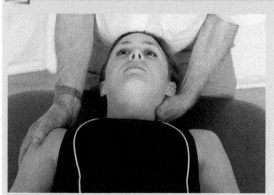

Figure 4.36 • A cervical lateral glide to the left.

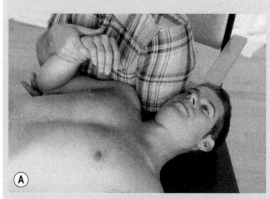

Ⓐ

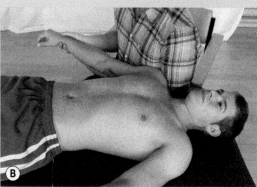

Ⓑ

Figure 4.37 • **A, B** The cradle position and slider using shoulder depression/elevation with elbow flexion/extension.

relieving and particularly found that the pins and needles sensation in the left hand reduced during the treatment. This treatment technique was repeated.

Reassessment in sitting following treatment

Pat reported that the left arm felt lighter and she could hold her head up without increasing pain in the neck.

There was evidence that the antalgic posture of her head had improvement and that she was holding her left arm straighter i.e. didn't need to keep it in a flexed position. She could turn her head 10° to the left before bringing on ① and ②.

A home exercise programme was discussed. Pat would continue to regularly support the left arm and begin gentle slider exercises that incorporate the shoulder girdle and elbow. These were to be performed in a supported position. Gentle neck rotation movements from midline to the right were included with emphasis placed upon the importance of pain-free movements. Pat was warned against working too much until the problem had stabilized.

Treatment 3 (day 6)

Pat reported the she had slept better and that the relieving movements and positions had reduced symptoms quicker than before. The symptoms were still present in all areas but the intensity had diminished. Although the arm did not feel so heavy she still had pins and needles in the left hand and the neck pain remained, especially when turning to the left and looking up.

Re-assessment of the physical parameters

Pat's sitting posture was no longer slouched and her neck and head were held in a neutral position without an increase in symptoms.

Cervical: her cervical movements had improved. Left rotation had reached 10/15° before areas ① and ② were exacerbated. Extension was now approximately 10° and then symptoms in the left arm increased.

Shoulder girdle: elevation was full while a small amount of depression from neutral position was achieved before an increase in pain.

Left shoulder: flexion/abduction equalled 110° and was comfortable.

ULNT 1 in sitting: this was tested on the right upper limb first: resistance elicited at −20° elbow extension. In this position there was a 'dragging' feeling in areas ① and ②, which was relieved with a release of wrist extension.

Then left ULNT 1 was carried out with each component taken through a virtually pain/symptom-free range of movement: shoulder abduction 70°, hand and wrist extension −20°, forearm supination full range, lateral shoulder rotation 50° and elbow extension reached −60° before an increase in symptoms, which reduced with the release of wrist extension. Immediately afterwards the heavy feeling and pins and needles returned for about 10 minutes before subsiding.

Neurological testing: there was a reduction in the allodynia, with some hyperaesthesia around the left anterior triangle.

Case study 4.1—cont'd

Nerve palpation: there was a marked response to nerve palpation on the left side at the brachial plexus and into the nerve trunks in the upper arm but no difference between the sides in the lower arm.

Treatment plan

As the symptoms are subsiding and movements of neck and shoulder complex have improved it's time to gradually increase the scope and intensity of treatments whilst avoiding any increase in pain and other symptoms. To start to regain further cervical extension while avoiding any increase in arm symptoms, the Mulligan SNAGS technique may be successful. This is likely to be achieved through the recruitment of gating and descending inhibition along with an increased sense of self-efficacy.

Technique 1

Position: sitting

Method: SNAGS unilateral to C6, C7 and T1 on the left side with active cervical extension before any local or referred symptoms occurred. Each segment was treated three times. The C6 mobilization produced the most comfortable active extension, reaching 20° of symptom-free movement. The C6 SNAG technique was repeated with three repetitions of six movements. A further small increase in cervical extension was achieved. This SNAGS technique also helped the left upper limb flexion/abduction movement to reach 120° before areas ③ and ④ started to appear.

Now that the movements of the left shoulder had improved, Pat was able to use self-SNAGS techniques for the neck and shoulder region at home, at regular intervals – not forgetting the 'no pain rule.'

Technique 2

Position: supported supine

Method: slider for the shoulder girdle and elbow through their full range of movement but the shoulder still resting in 15° of abduction.

Reassessment following treatment

Areas ① and ② were only present toward the end of range of cervical rotation to the left and shoulder girdle depression. Areas ③ and ④ are still present more as a low grade 'hum'.

Self-exercise programme

1. Regular shoulder girdle movements in all symptom free directions.
2. Self-SNAGS for cervical extension and rotation as a way of grading the exposure to the limited and painful movements (care must be taken not to progress into extension too quickly when there is a suspicion of an inflamed nerve root where you are

closing the intervertebral foramen and possibly irritating the nerve).

3. Active sliders incorporating shoulder girdle and elbow movements.
4. Encourage Pat to take her dog out for walks, but advise her to take care not to be dragged by the lead. This is to help her general fitness and boost her immune system.
5. Now that the symptoms, including pain, are subsiding, she must not overdo her work in her business as the healing of the nerves are in an early stage. This fits into the concept of graded exposure with regards to her work.

Treatments 4–8 (days 10–30)

Subjective

Over the next 20 days the symptoms gradually subsided with a few minor setbacks. The pins and needles were still present but more intermittently.

Pat's life was returning to normal. She was sleeping soundly, managing to carry out most of the tasks required to run the inn, but was still avoiding the heavy work of lifting and tending to fires.

Physical assessment

Pat's posture was very good and her cervical movements were mostly normal with the exception of extension, which tended to reproduce the dull scapular pain when taken to the limit of the movement.

The left upper limb movements were good and she could achieve all functional activities, such as putting a coat on, without difficulty. There remained some mild sensitivity to nerve palpation of the nerve trunks in the brachial plexus. However, neurodynamic test responses were similar between sides with a greater response to testing on the left at the same end point of testing.

Progression of treatment

1. Passive mobilization techniques were progressed, utilizing unilateral posteroanterior mobilization of the mid and lower cervical spine and lateral gliding movements, in both directions, progressing in duration and intensity to allow a graded exposure of load through Pat's tissues.
2. SNAGS were used mainly as self-treatment techniques to maintain the gains she achieved and the freedom and flexibility of movement for her neck.
3. ULNT 1 sliders were progressed by changing the position of the head and neck and

Continued

Case study 4.1—cont'd

incorporating this into the shoulder or elbow movements that were more functional. Tensioner techniques were applied during later treatment sessions.

4. Active exercises: the principles of graded exposure and changing the context of movements for the neck and shoulder were employed to assist in recovery. One example was exercising the upper

limbs and cervicothoracic region in a 4-point kneeling position.

5. General fitness activities: advise a gradual and sensible increase in household work within Pat's pain-free tolerance; recommend outside activities such brisk walking and hill climbing (there are plenty of hills in the Yorkshire Dales where Pat lives!)

References

Almeida TF, Roizenblatt S, Tufik S: Afferent pain pathways: a neuroanatomical review, *Brain Res* 1000:40–56, 2004.

Antonovsky A: The salutogenic model as a theory to guide health promotion, *Health Promot Int* 11(1):11–18, 1996.

Apkarian AV, Sosa Y, Krauss BR, et al: Chronic pain patients are impaired on an emotional decision-making task, *J Neurosci* 24(46):10410–10415, 2004.

Asbury A, Fields H: Pain due to peripheral nerve damage: an hypothesis, *Neurol* 34:1587–1590, 1984.

Asmundson G, Wright K, Hadjistavropoulos D: Hypervigilence and attentional fixedness in chronic musculoskeletal pain: consistency of findings across modified stroop and dot-probe tasks, *J Pain* 6(8):497–506, 2005.

Baliki M, Chialvo DR, Geha PY, et al: Chronic pain and the emotional brain: specific brain activity associated with spontaneous fluctuations of intensity of chronic back pain, *J Neurosci* 26(47):12165–12173, 2006.

Banati R, Cagnin A, Brooks DJ, et al: Long-term trans-synaptic glial responses in the human thalamus after peripheral nerve injury, *NeuroReport* 12(16):3439–3442, 2001.

Barnsley L, Lord S, Bogduk N: The pathophysiology of whiplash, *Spine* 12:209–242, 1998.

Bear MF, Connors BW, Paradiso MA: *Neuroscience: exploring plain*, ed 2, 2001.

Bechara A, Damasio AR, Damasio H, et al: Insensitivity to future consequences following damage to

human prefrontal cortex, *Cogn* 50:7–15, 1994.

Beneciuk JM, Bishop MD, George SZ: Clinical prediction rules for physical therapy interventions: a systematic review, *Phys Ther* 89:114–124, 2009a.

Beneciuk J, Bishop MD, George SZ: Effects of upper extremity neural mobilization on thermal pain sensitivity: a sham-controlled study in asymptomatic participants, *J Orthop and Sport Phys Ther* 39(6):428–438, 2009b.

Beneciuk J, Bishop MD, George SZ: Pain catastrophizing predicts pain intensity during a neurodynamic test for median nerve in healthy participants, *Man Ther* epub, 2010.

Bennett G: Neuropathic pain: a crisis of definition, *Anaesth Analg* 97:619, 2003.

Bennett MI, Attal N, Miroslav MB, et al: Using screening tools to identify neuropathic pain, *Pain* 127:199–203, 2007.

Butler DS: *Mobilisation of the nervous system*, Melbourne, 1991, Churchill Livingstone.

Butler DS: *The sensitive nervous system*, Adelaide, Australia, 2000, NOI Publications.

Butler DS, Moseley GL: *Explain pain*, Adelaide, Australia, 2003, NOI Publications.

Caragee E, Alamin T, Cheng I, et al: Are first-time episodes of serious low back pain associated with new MRI findings? *Spine J* 6:624–635, 2006.

Carroll LJ, Holm LW, Hogg-Johnson S, et al: Course and prognostic factors for neck pain in whiplash-associated disorders (WAD), *J Manipulative Physiol Ther* 32(2S):S97–S107, 2009a.

Carroll LJ, Hogg-Johnson S, Côté P, et al: Course and prognostic factors for neck pain in workers, *J Manipulative Physiol Ther* 32(2S):S109–S116, 2009b.

Christensen JO, Knardahl S: Work and neck pain: a prospective study of psychological, social, and mechanical risk factors, *Pain* 151:162–173, 2010.

Chrousos G: Stress and disorders of the stress system, *Nature Rev Endocrinol* 5:374–381, 2009.

Clemente C: *Anatomy*, Urban and Schwarzenbuerg, 1975, Munich.

Coppieters M, Strappaerts K, Wouters L, et al: The immediate effects of a cervical lateral glide treatment technique in patients with neurogenic cervicogenic pain, *J Orthop Sports Phys Ther* 33:369–378, 2003.

Coppieters MW, Barthomeeusen KE, Strappaerts KH: Incorporating nerve-gliding techniques in the conservative treatment of cubital tunnel syndrome, *J Manipulative Physiol Ther* 27(9):560–568, 2004.

Coppieters MW, Kurz K, Mortensen TE, et al: The impact of neurodynamic testing on the perception of experimentally induced muscle pain, *Man Ther* 10:52–60, 2005.

Coppieters MW, Butler DS: Do 'sliders' slide and 'tensioners' tension? An analysis of neurodynamic techniques and consideration regarding application, *Man Ther* 13(3):213–221, 2008.

Coppieters M, Hough A, Dilley A: Different nerve-gliding exercises induce different magnitudes of median nerve longitudinal excursion: an in-vivo study using dynamic ultrasound imaging, *J Orthop Sports Phys Ther* 39:3, 2009.

Costigan M, Scholz J, Woolf C: Neuropathic pain: a maladaptive response of the nervous system, *Annu Rev Neurosci* 32:1–32, 2009.

Côté P, van der Velde G, Cassidy JD, et al: The burden and determinants of neck pain in workers, *J Manipulative Physiol Ther* 32:S70–S86, 2009.

Dehghani M, Sharpe L, Nicholas M: Selective attention to pain-related information in chronic musculoskeletal pain patients, *Pain* 105:37–46, 2003.

Delcomyn F: *Foundations of neurobiology WH Freeman*, New York, 1998.

Dellon A, MacKinnon S, Crosby P: Reliability of two-point discrimination measurements, *J Hand Surg (Am)* 12(5 Pt.1): 693–696, 1987.

Devor M, Seltzer Z: Pathophysiology of damaged nerves in relation to chronic pain. In Wall PD, Melzack R, editors: *Textbook of pain*, Edinburgh, 1999, Churchill Livingstone.

Dhaka A, Viswanath V, Patapoutian A: TRP ion channels and temperature sensation, *Annu Rev Neurosci* 29:135–161, 2006.

Dick J: The deep tendon and abdominal reflexes, *J Neurol Neurosurg and Psychiatry* 74:150–153, 2003.

Dilley A, Bove G: Disruption of axoplasmic transport induces mechanical sensitivity in intact rat C fibre nociceptors axons, *J Neurophysiol* 586:593–604, 2008.

Dilley A, Lynn B, Pang SJ: Pressure and stretch mechanosensitivity of peripheral nerve fibres following local inflammation of the nerve trunk, *Pain* 117:462–472, 2005.

D'Mello R, Dickenson AH: Spinal cord mechanisms of pain, *Br J Anaesth* 101(1):8–16, 2008.

Durkan J: A new diagnostic test for carpal tunnel syndrome, *J Jt and Bone Surg* 73A:536–538, 1991.

Dworkin R, Jensen M, Gammaitoni A, et al: Symptom profiles differ in patients with neuropathic versus non-neuropathic pain, *J Pain* 8(2):118–126, 2007.

Elvey RL: Treatment of arm pain associated with abnormal brachial plexus tension, *Aust J Physiother* 32:224–230, 1986.

Engel G: *The biopsychosocial model and the education of health professionals*, 1978, Annals NY Academy of Sciences, pp 169–181.

Farmer J, Wisneski R: Cervical nerve root compression. An analysis of neuroforaminal pressure with varying head and arm positions, *Spine* 19(16):1850–1855, 1994.

Fast A, Pirakh S, Marin E: The shoulder abduction relief sign in cervical radiculopathy, *Arch Phys Med Rehabil* 70(5):402–403, 1989.

Fernández-de-las-Peñas C, Coppieters MW, Cuadrado M, et al: Patients with chronic tension-type headache demonstrated increased mechano-sensitivity of the supra-orbital nerve, *Headache* 48:570–577, 2008.

Fernández-de-las-Peñas C, Arendt-Nielsen L, Cuadrado M, et al: Generalized mechanical pain sensitivity over nerve tissues in patients with strictly unilateral migraine, *Clin J Pain* 25:401–440, 2009.

Flor H, Braun C, Elbert T, et al: Extensive reorganization of primary somatosensory cortex in chronic back pain patients, *Neurosci Lett* 224:5–8, 1997a.

Flor H, Knost B, Birbaumer N: Processing of pain- and body-related verbal material in chronic pain patients: central and peripheral correlates, *Pain* 73:413–421, 1997b.

Gibbon P, Tehan P: HVLA thrust techniques: what are the risks? *Int J Osteopath Med* 9(1):4–12, 2006.

Gifford L: Pain, the tissues and the nervous system: a conceptual model, *Physiotherapy* 84:27–33, 1998.

Gifford L: Acute low cervical nerve root conditions: symptom presentation and pathological reasoning, *Man Ther* 6(2):106–115, 2001.

Gifford L, Butler D: The integration of pain science into clinical practice, *Hand* 10(2):86–95, 1997.

Gifford L, Thacker M: A clinical overview of the autonomic nervous system, the supply to the gut and mind-body pathways. In Gifford L, editor: *Topical Issues in Pain 3*, Falmouth, 2002, CNS Press.

Greening J, Lynn B: Minor peripheral nerve injuries: an underestimated source of pain? *Man Ther* 3(4):187–194, 1998.

Greening J, Dilley A, Lynn B: In vivo study of nerve movement and mechanosensitivity of the median nerve in whiplash and non-specific

arm pain patients, *Pain* 115:248–253, 2005.

Hall T, Quintner J: Responses to mechanical stimulation of the upper limb in painful cervical radiculopathy, *Aust J Physiother* 42:277–285, 1996.

HIS (The International Headache Society): Headache Classification Subcommittee. The International Classification of Headache Disorders, ed 2, *Cephalalgia* 24(suppl. 1):1–151, 2004.

Hogg-Johnson S, van der Velde G, Carroll LJ, et al: The burden and determinants of neck pain in the general population, *J Manipulative Physiol Ther* 32:S46–S60, 2009.

Hu J, Milenkovic N, Lewin GR: The high threshold mechanotransducer: a status report, *Pain* 120:3–7, 2006.

Huang J, Zhang X, McNaughton PA: Inflammatory pain: the cellular basis of heat hyperalgesia, *Curr Neuropharmacol* 4:197–206, 2006.

Iacoboni M, Mazziotta JC: Mirror neuron system: basic findings and clinical applications, *Ann Neurol* 62:213–218, 2007.

Ingvar M: Pain and functional imaging. *Philos Trans Roy Soc Lond B: Biol Sci* 354(1387):1347–1358, 1999.

Ishikawa H, Kiuchi T: Health literacy and health communication, *Biopsychosocial Med* 4:18, 2010.

Jepsen J, Laursen L, Hagert C-G, et al: Diagnostic accuracy of the neurological upper limb examination 1: Inter-rater reproducibility of selected findings and patterns, *BMC Neurol* 6:8, 2006.

Jones M, Rivett D: *Clinical reasoning for manual therapists*, Edinburgh, 2004, Butterworth Heinemann.

Juhl GI, Jensen TS, Northholt SE, et al: Central sensitisation phenomena after third molar surgery: a quantitative sensory testing study, *Eur J Pain* 12:116–127, 2008.

Jull G: the primacy of clinical reasoning and clinical practical skills, *Man Ther* 14:353–354, 2009.

Jull G, Sterling M, Falla D, et al: *Whiplash, headache and neck pain*, Edinburgh, 2008, Churchill Livingstone Elsevier.

Kaushik RM, Kaushik R, Mahajan SK, et al: Effects of mental relaxation and slow breathing in essential hypertension, *Complement Ther Med* 14:120–126, 2006.

Kerry R, Taylor A, Mitchell J, et al: *Manipulation Association of*

Chartered Physiotherapists. *CAD information document*, Nottingham, 2007, University of Nottingham.

Kerry R, Taylor A, Mitchell J, et al: Cervical arterial dysfunction and manual therapy: A critical literature review to inform professional practice, *Man Ther* 13:278–288, 2008.

Lance J, Anthony M: Neck-tongue syndrome on sudden turning of the head, *J Neurol, Neurosurg Psychiatry* 43(2):97–101, 1980.

Latremoliere A, Woolf C: Central sensitization: a generator of pain hypersensitivity by central neural plasticity, *J Pain* 10(9):895–926, 2009.

Levitz C, Reilly P, Torg J: The pathomechanics of chronic, recurrent cervical nerve root neurapraxia: the chronic burner syndrome, *Am J Sports Med* 25(1):73–76, 1997.

Lotze M, Moseley GL: Role of distorted body image in pain, *Curr Rheumatol Rep* 9:488–496, 2007.

Lundborg G, Rosen B: The two-point discrimination test – time for a reappraisal? *J Hand Surg (Br)* 29B(5):418–422, 2004.

Mäntyselkä P, Kautiainen H, Vanhala M: Prevalence of neck pain in subjects with metabolic syndrome – a cross-sectional population-based study, *BMC Musculoskelet Disord* 11:171, 2010.

Mason P: Deconstructing endogenous pain modulation, *J Neurophysiol* 94:1659–1663, 2005.

Meeus M, Nijs J, Van Oosterwijck J, et al: Pain physiology education improves pain beliefs in patients with chronic fatigue syndrome compared with pacing and self-management education: a double-blind randomized controlled trial, *Arch Phys Med Rehabil* 91:1153–1159, 2010.

Melzack R: Phantom limbs, the self and the brain, *Can Psychol* 1–16, 1989.

Melzack R: Phantom limbs and the concept of a neuromatrix, *Trends Neurosci* 13:88–92, 1990.

Merskey H, Bogduk N: *Classification of chronic pain, ed 2, IASP Task Force on Taxonomy*, Seattle, 1994, IASP Press.

Moriarty O, McGuire B, Finn D: The effect of pain on cognitive function: a review of clinical and preclinical research, *Prog Neurobiol* 93:385–404, 2011.

Moseley GL: A pain neuromatrix approach to patients with chronic pain, *Man Ther* 8(3):130–140, 2003.

Moseley GL: Why do people with complex regional pain syndrome take longer to recognise their affected hand? *Neurol* 62:2182–2186, 2004a.

Moseley GL: Evidence for a direct relationship between cognitive and physical change during an education intervention in people with chronic neck pain, *Eur J Pain* 8:39–45, 2004b.

Moseley, GL: Reconceptualising pain according to modern pain science, *Phys Ther Rev* 12:169–178, 2007.

Moseley GL: I can't find it! Distorted body image and tactile dysfunction in patients with chronic back pain, *Pain* 140:239–243, 2008.

Mulligan B: *Manual therapy, NAGS, SNAGS, MWMS etc.*, ed 6, Minneapolis, 2010, Orthopedic Physical Therapy Products.

Natvig B, Ihlebæk C, Grotle M, et al: Neck pain is often part of widespread pain and is associated with reduced functioning, *Spine* 35(23):E1285–E1289, 2010.

Navarro X, Vivó M, Valero-Cabré A: Neural plasticity after peripheral nerve injury and regeneration, *Prog Neurobiol* 82:163–201, 2007.

Nee RJ, Butler, D. 2006. Management of peripheral neuropathic pain: integrating neurobiology, neurodynamics and clinical evidence, *Phys Ther Sport* 7:36–49.

Nee R, Vicenzino B, Jull G, et al: Neural tissue management provides immediate clinically relevant benefits without harmful effects for patients with nerve-related neck and arm pain: a randomised trial, *J Physiother* 58(1):23–31, 2012.

Nijs J, Van Houdenhove B: From acute musculoskeletal pain to chronic widespread pain and fibromyalgia: Application of pain neurophysiology in manual therapy practice, *Man Ther* 14:3–12, 2009.

Novak C, MacKinnon S: Evaluation of nerve injury and nerve compression in the upper quadrant, *J Hand Ther* 18:230–240, 2005.

Oliveira A, Gevirtz R, Hubbard D: A psycho-educational video used in the emergency department provides effective treatment for whiplash injuries, *Spine* 31:1652–1657, 2006.

Pleger B, Ragert P, Schwenkreis P, et al: Patterns of cortical reorganization parallel impaired tactile discrimination and pain intensity in complex regional pain syndrome, *NeuroImage* 32:503–510, 2006.

Rao R: Neck pain, cervical radiculopathy and cervical myelopathy, *J Bone Joint Surg* 840(10):1872–1881, 2002.

Rizzolatti G, Leonardo Fogassi L, Gallese V: Neurophysiological mechanisms underlying the understanding imitation of action, *Nat Rev Neurosci* 2:661–670, 2001.

Rubinstein SM, Pool JJM, van Tulder MW, et al: A systematic review of the diagnostic accuracy of provocative tests of the neck for diagnosing cervical radiculopathy, *Eur Spine J* 16:307–319, 2007.

Safran M: Nerve injury about the shoulder in athletes, part 2: long thoracic nerve, spinal accessory nerve, burners/stingers, thoracic outlet syndrome, *Am J Sports Med* 32:1063–1076, 2004.

Savitz S, Caplan L: Vertebrobasilar disease, *N J Med* 352:2618–2626, 2005.

Schmid A, Brunner F, Wright A, et al: Paradigm shift in manual therapy? Evidence for a central nervous system component in the response to passive cervical joint mobilisation, *Man Ther* 13:387–396, 2008.

Schmid A, Brunner F, Luomajoki H, et al: Reliability of clinical tests to evaluate nerve function and mechanosensitivity of the upper limb peripheral nervous system, *BMC Musculoskelet Disord* 10:11, 2009.

Shacklock M: *Clinical neurodynamics: a new system of musculoskeletal treatment*, Edinburgh, 2005, Butterworth Heinemann Elsevier.

Siao P, Cros D: Quantitative sensory testing, *Phys Med Rehabil Clin N Am* 14:261–285, 2003.

Skyba D, Radhakrishnan R, Rohlwing L, et al: Joint manipulation reduces hyperalgesia by activation of monoamine receptors but not opioid or GABG receptors in the spinal cord, *Pain* 106:159–168, 2003.

Smart KM, O'Connell NE, Doody C: Towards a mechanisms-based classification of pain in musculoskeletal physiotherapy? *Phys Ther Rev* 13(1):1–10, 2008.

Smart KM, Blake C, Staines A, et al: Clinical indicators of 'nociceptive', 'peripheral neuropathic' and 'central' mechanisms of musculoskeletal pain. A Delphi survey of expert clinicians, *Man Ther* 15:80–87, 2010.

Snider WD, McMahon SB: Tackling pain at the source: new ideas about nociceptors, *Neuron* 20:629–632, 1998.

Souvlis T, Vicenzino B, Wright A: Neurophysiological effects of spinal manual therapy. In Boyling JD, et al, editors: *Grieve's modern therapy*, Edinburgh, 2004, Churchill Livingstone, pp 367–379.

Standaert C, Herring S: Expert opinion and controversies in musculoskeletal and sports medicine: stingers, *Arch Phys Med Rehabil* 90:402–406, 2009.

Sterling M: A proposed new classification system for whiplash associated disorders – implications for assessment and treatment, *Man Ther* 9:60–70, 2004.

Sterling M, Jull G, Wright A: Cervical mobilisation: concurrent effects on pain, sympathetic nervous system activity and motor activity, *Man Ther* 6:72–81, 2001.

Sterling M, Jull G, Vicenzino B, et al: Sensory hypersensitivity occurs soon after whiplash and is associated with poor recovery, *Pain* 104:509–517, 2003a.

Sterling M, Jull G, Vicenzino B, et al: Development of motor system dysfunction following whiplash injury, *Pain* 103:65–73, 2003b.

Sterling M, Jull G, Kenardy J: Physical and psychological factors maintain long-term predictive capacity post-whiplash injury, *Pain* 122:102–108, 2006.

Sterling M, Pedler A: A neuropathic pain component is common in acute whiplash and associated with a more complex clinical presentation, *Man Ther* 14:173–179, 2009.

Sterling M, Pedler A, Chan C, et al: Cervical lateral glide increases nociceptive threshold but not pressure and thermal pain in chronic whiplash associated disorders: A pilot randomised controlled trial, *Man Ther* 15(2):149–153, 2010.

Taylor AJ, Kerry R: A 'system based' approach to risk assessment of the cervical spine prior to manual therapy, *Int J Osteopath Med* 13:85–93, 2010.

Thacker MA, Clark AK, Marchand F, et al: Pathophysiology of peripheral neuropathic pain: immune cells and molecules, *Anesth Analg* 105:838–847, 2007.

Thanvi B, Munshi SK, Dawson SL, et al: Carotid and vertebral artery dissection syndrome, *Postgrad Med J* 81(956):383–388, 2005.

Thayer JF, Sternberg EM: Neural aspects of immunomodulation: focus on the vagus nerve, *Brain Behav Immun* 24:1223–1228, 2010.

Tracey I, Bushnell MC: How neuroimaging studies have challenged us to rethink: is chronic pain a disease? *J Pain* 10(11):1113–1120, 2009.

Treleaven J, Jull G, Sterling M: Dizziness and unsteadiness following whiplash injury –characteristic features and relationships with cervical joint position error, *J Rehabil* 34:1–8, 2003.

Tsao H, Galea MP, Hodges PW: Reorganization of the motor cortex is associated with postural control deficits in recurrent low back pain, *Brain* 131:2161–2171, 2008.

van der Heide B, Allison G, Zusman M: Pain and muscular responses to a neural tissue provocation test in the upper limb, *Man Ther* 6(3):154–162, 2001.

Van Oosterwijck J, Nijs J, Meeus M, et al: Pain neurophysiology education improves cognitions, pain thresholds, and movement performance in people with chronic whiplash: a pilot study, *J Rehabil Res Dev* 48(1):43–58, 2011.

Vlaeyen JWS, Linton SJ: Fear-avoidance and its consequences in chronic musculoskeletal pain: a state of the art, *Pain* 85:317–332, 2000.

Vincent MB: Headache and neck, *Curr Pain Headache Rep* 15:324–331, 2011.

Vicenzino B, Collins D, Wright A: The initial effects of cervical spine physiotherapy treatment on the pain and dysfunction of lateral epicondylalgia, *Pain* 68:69–74, 1996.

Vicenzino B, Collins D, Benison H, et al: An investigation of the interrelationship between manipulative therapy induced hypoalgesia sympathoexcitation, *J Manipulative Physiol Ther* 21:448–453, 1998.

von Piekartz HJM, Schouten S, Aufdemkampe G: Neurodynamic responses in children with migraine or cervicogenic headache versus a control group. A comparative study, *Man Ther* 12:153–160, 2007.

Watkins LR, Maier SF: The pain of being sick: implications of immune-to-brain communication for understanding pain, *Annu Rev Psychol* 51:29–57, 2000.

Williams JE, Yen JT, Parker G, et al: Prevalence of pain in head and neck cancer out-patients, *J Laryngol Otol* 124(7):767–773, 2010.

Williams PL, Warwick R, Dyson M, et al, editors: *Gray's anatomy*, 37e, Edinburgh, 1989, Churchill Livingstone.

Winkelstein B, DeLeo J: Mechanical thresholds for initiation and persistence of pain following nerve root injury: mechanical and chemical contributions at injury, *J Biomech Eng* 126(2):258–263, 2004.

Woolf C: Central sensitization: implications for the diagnosis and treatment of pain, *Pain* 152:S2–S15, 2011.

Woolf, CJ: *The dorsal horn: state dependent sensory processing and the generation of pain. Textbook of Pain. P. D. Wall and R. Melzack*, Edinburgh, 1994, Churchill Livingstone.

Woolf C, Ma Q: Nociceptors: noxious stimulus detectors, *Neuron* 55:353–364, 2007.

Woolf C, Salter MW: Neural plasticity: increasing the gain in pain, *Science* 288:1765–1769, 2000.

Wright A: Pain-relieving effect of cervical manual therapy. In Grant R, editor: *Physical therapy of the cervical and thoracic spine*, New York, 2002, Churchill-Livingstone, pp 217–238.

Management of thoracic spine disorders

5

Peter Wells   Kevin Banks

CHAPTER CONTENTS

Clues in subjective examination to thoracic
spine involvement 176

Chronic conditions 178

Improvement of remote symptoms and
signs after mid thoracic spine treatment 185

Patient examples 186

Examination to determine the use of
passive mobilization techniques and
associated interventions 189

Examination and treatment techniques 202

Key words

Sympathetic nervous system, recurrent meningeal
(sinu-vertebral) nerves, neurodynamics, costovertebral,
costotransverse, hypogastric nerve, ilio-inguinal nerve,
genitofemoral nerve, SLR, neck pain, shoulder pain

Introduction: thoracic spine and the Maitland Concept

The 'open', non-dogmatic principles of the Maitland
Concept and the emphasis on believing the patient

have been invaluable in helping manipulative
physiotherapists to treat patients with complex,
multi-area, multi-symptomatic presentations.

An example is the case of Mrs B, presenting with
thoracic and chest pain; neck and scapula pain; headache and facial pain; and low back pain and sciatica
(Fig. 5.1). The physiotherapist who regards these as
separate problems presenting concurrently would,
in the opinion of this author, do better to regard
each of them as a part of one problem, with separate
and discrete structural and neurological inputs.

To reach this conclusion, it is firstly necessary, as
Maitland et al. (2005) stated, to believe the patient.
As obvious as this seems, this view is frequently
bypassed in favour of the belief that anyone with as
many areas of pain but no medically diagnosable
disease must, at the least, be exaggerating or worse,
are neurotic or making it up.

The following scenario is all too common:

> Therapist: Right, Mrs B, I understand you are
> complaining of a number of problems but I see you
> have been referred to me with your neck problem.
> I can't also start looking into your back and leg
> pain and the other areas. I'm going to have to
> concentrate on one problem area, that is the worst,
> and see if we can sort this out first.
> *Is there, perhaps, a note of frustration and even
> disbelief in the therapists voice?*
> Therapist's thinking: How could anyone have so
> many areas of pain, discomfort, paraesthesia and
> stiffness?! Is this a psychological problem?

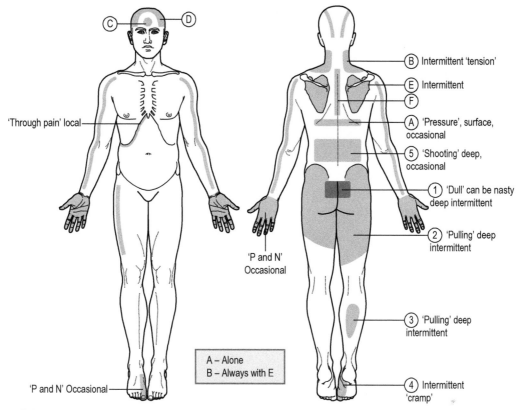

Figure 5.1 • Thoracic and chest pain, neck and scapula pain, headache and facial pain and low back pain and sciatica.

The likelihood is that, yes, it has become increasingly a psychological problem, because the individual has carried it for so long and no one has really helped and now the patient has the creeping suspicion that no one believes them. Whilst the biopsychosocial model is an essential concept in understanding and managing complex, ongoing pain problems, the **bio** aspect is often underplayed in attributing these sorts of problems to mainly psychological factors. The therapist who believes the patient and shows they believe them, sympathizes and then discusses the possible underlying mechanisms driving their problem (including wayward sympathetic nervous system activity) in words the patient can understand, initiates a therapeutic approach, which is likely to succeed.

Finally, this enjoinder to 'believe the patient' places a heavy yet appropriate demand on the therapist. It is, firstly, that they will develop the knowledge, skills and experience to make a diagnosis which fits all the known aspects of the patient's often complex problems, as Maitland et al. (2005) stated, 'Make the features fit'. Secondly, it is vital

to offer the patient a broad range of passive techniques to both assess and treat the appropriate areas of the spine, with constant ongoing re-assessment. In these cases it is important to include the thoracic spine, recognizing the fundamental role the thoracic region has in so many benign musculoskeletal problems.

It goes without saying, of course, that teaching the patient coping strategies, as well as an appropriate exercise programme for strength, stability and flexibility, is an intrinsic part of any physiotherapeutic and pain management programme.

The literature also supports this notion that the thoracic region can be a source of many complex and non-specific, debilitating pain conditions, as in the case of Mrs B (Fig. 5.1).

Briggs et al. (2009a, 2009b) have carried out systematic reviews of reports of thoracic spine pain prevalence, incidence and associated factors for thoracic spine pain in adult working populations and in general populations (including children and adolescents). In a systematic review (Briggs et al. 2009a) of 52 reports on adult populations meeting appropriate inclusion criteria, most show an average of 30% prevalence of thoracic spine pain reported in most occupational groups ranging from manual labourers to drivers to performing artists.

In another systematic review of 33 reports meeting inclusion criteria (Briggs et al. 2009b), the 1-year incidence of thoracic spine pain in the general population was reported as being between 15 and 27.5% and was associated with concurrent musculo-skeletal pain, growth, lifestyle, backpack use and posture, as well as with psychological and environmental factors.

In a case study design, Cleland & McRae (2002) reported on a 50-year-old patient with chronic regional pain syndrome (CRPS 1); effective management was achieved with 10 treatment sessions over a 3-month period directed towards thoracolumbar segmental and neurodynamic impairment. The key inclusions in management, as well as activity and exercise, included thoracolumbar mobilization techniques (see Figs 5.28, 5.30 and 5.31) and neural mobilization using slump long sitting with a sympathetic emphasis (see Fig. 5.60).

Cleland et al. (2002) in a randomized controlled trial using 12 healthy subjects, further explored the effects of the slump long sitting technique with sympathetic emphasis (SLSSE) and costovertebral joint mobilization (see Fig. 5.61) on sympathetic activity to try to explain how such a therapeutic technique may be effective in the management of sympathetically maintained pain. Cleland et al. (2002) were encouraged by the greater changes in foot skin temperature and conductance in the experimental group compared with the control group. The results suggest a link between the SLSSE technique and sympathetic activity in the lower extremity, despite the changes attributable to the technique alone not being statistically significant.

Clues in the subjective examination to thoracic spine involvement

Symptoms at and around thoracic spine levels, and in areas neurally related to T1–12

These areas include those which, because of the location and even perhaps the type and behaviour of

the symptoms, are sometimes thought to be visceral, as opposed to a somatic musculoskeletal, in origin. Examples include:

- Left-sided chest pain of approximately 4th–8th thoracic spine level referral, suggesting cardiac origin (Fig. 5.2)
- Right-sided infracostal pain from approximately 9th thoracic level, suggesting gall bladder disease (Fig. 5.3)
- Right-sided hypogastric and groin pain originating from the T12 /L1 levels, the hypogastric nerve and the ilio-inguinal nerve suggesting appendicitis
- Similarly, patients presenting, either by self-referral or who have been referred by a medical practitioner or, for example, a sports coach, with diagnosis such as 'groin strain' (of T12/L1 origin?) or 'pulled muscle' (costovertebral joint sprain) (Figs 5.4–5.6)
- Left-sided chest upper chest pain with some radiation down into the inner aspect of the left upper arm and axilla, from T1, T2 levels suggesting cardiac involvement, such as angina pectoris (Fig. 5.7)
- Acute radiating chest pain at any thoracic level, related to chest movement as in breathing and especially severe when coughing and sneezing, suggesting a pleural origin (Fig. 5.8).

Just as the somatic may simulate the visceral, so the visceral may simulate the somatic, or the two may co-exist. An example of the latter was a woman who, for a few years, had suffered occasional bouts of severe anterior upper abdominal pain (Fig. 5.9). Thorough medical screening had detected no visceral pathology and she was referred for physiotherapy.

Her condition was totally relieved on two separate occasions by thoracic mobilization (see Figs 5.28–5.31). A year later, she was re-referred by a medical practitioner with similar pain. Two treatments, the second being on a Friday, did not follow the previous pattern of response – that of marked relief of symptoms – and she was told that if after the weekend she was no better, then she should return to the referring physician for further investigation. That weekend she became very ill, collapsed and on admittance to her local hospital underwent emergency surgery for acute peritonitis. She made a full recovery.

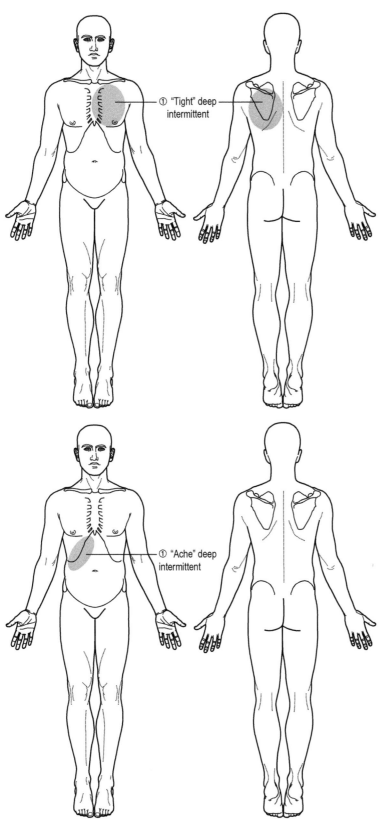

Figure 5.2 • Left-sided chest pain of approximately 4th to 8th thoracic spine level referral, suggesting cardiac origin.

① "Tight" deep intermittent

Figure 5.3 • Right-sided infra-costal pain from approximately 9th thoracic level, suggesting gall bladder disease.

① "Ache" deep intermittent

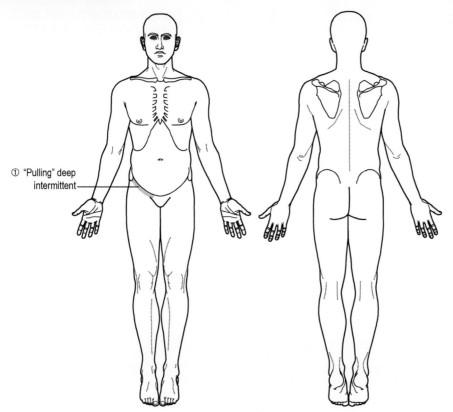

① "Pulling" deep intermittent

Figure 5.4 • 'Groin strain' (of T12/L1 origin?) or 'pulled muscle' (costovertebral joint sprain).

Chronic conditions, which are not resolving with treatment

Pain in areas of the body and benign pain conditions that do not suggest direct thoracic neural referral, which have become chronic and have not responded to reasonable treatment, frequently have an association with the thoracic spine. Wherever the site of the problem is, there will usually be a report of stiffness, aching, discomfort or frank pain in the vertebral areas of thoracic 4–7. A re-assessment of progress can be made after appropriate mobilization of the area of the thoracic spine has been added to the treatment plan.

Patient example

A 40-year-old lady who had undergone repeated gynaecological procedures for groin and pubic pain (Fig. 5.10) with no lasting relief of her symptoms became symptom-free following a short course of mobilization and manipulation at the thoracolumbar junctions (T12/L1), mid-thoracic manipulation and neurodynamic mobilization techniques in side-lying

targeting the ilio-inguinal and genitofemoral nerves (see Figs 5.28-5.31, 5.45, 5.62).

Evidence from the literature also supports the narrative that conditions which are amenable to thoracic spine mobilization can be identified from their symptom presentation, symptom history and behaviour.

Conroy & Schneider (2005) presented a case report of a 28-year-old patient with pain across both shoulders and bilaterally down both arms. These main symptoms were associated with bilateral hand tingling, headache and stiffness in the thoracic spine, along with long-standing back and left leg pain and anxiety. Symptoms were associated with prolonged sitting in lectures, with little relief on movement or position change. Symptom onset was associated with an intense study period. Visceral and serious pathology were excluded. Needless to say, comparable movement impairments were found in and around the thoracic and cervical spine on physical examination (see Figs 5.16–5.21, 5.26 & 5.27; Chapter 4) and mobilization techniques (see Figs 5.28–5.31) of the mid-thoracic spine along with postural alignment and muscle balance activities

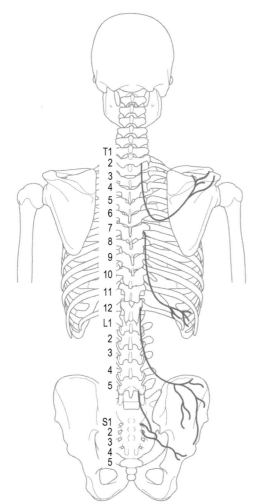

Figure 5.5 • Posterior primary rami of T2, T7 and T12 and the areas they supply.

ensured symptom relief and restoration of cervical and thoracic spine movement.

Jowsey & Perry (2009), in an original article, reviewed the suggested mechanisms of 'T4 syndrome' as described by Conroy and Schneiders (2005). They also carried out a double blind controlled trial to establish the effects of a grade III posteroanterior rotatory joint mobilization technique (see Fig. 5.29), applied to T4, on sympathetic activity in the hand of a sample of healthy subjects.

T4 syndrome is characterized by upper extremity paraesthesia and pain with or without symptoms into the neck and/or head (Conroy & Schneiders 2005). The typical presentation is glove distribution of paraesthesia in one or both hands (Fig. 5.11). The suggestion has always been that the sympathetic nervous system provides the mechanism which links the thoracic spine to the referred symptom pattern associated with T4 syndrome, and that the sympathetic nervous system mediates the hypoalgesic effects of spinal manipulative therapy through the dorsal periaqueductal grey in the mid-brain.

The study by Jowsey & Perry (2009) demonstrated a significant difference in skin conductance in the right hand of the sample subjects (and less so in the left) after T4 mobilization compared with a sample of individuals in a placebo group. This indirect measure of a sympathoexcitatory effect may explain the mechanisms by which passive mobilization techniques localized to the T4 spinal segment result in a relief of typical glove distribution symptoms and associated movement restrictions in some patients.

Cleland & McRae (2002), in their case report, describe the management of a 50-year-old woman who presented 8 weeks after an internal fixation of a tibia/fibula fracture with lower extremity complex region pain syndrome 1 (CRPS 1), as mentioned earlier. Her symptoms comprised an intense burning pain throughout the right lower extremity with an inability to weight bear because of severe allodynia. Other features of CRPS were also evident, such as swelling, sweating and redness. The body chart also showed evidence of a band of pain across her lower thoracic spine at the level of T12/L1. Intervention during 10 sessions over 4 months included desensitization and graded exposure to weight bearing along with thoracolumbar mobilization and a neural mobilization technique of SLSSE (see Figs 5.60 & 5.61). A follow-up after treatment was discontinued and later, after a year, revealed a sustained improvement in pain and function.

Fruth (2006) reported on the case of a patient with posterior upper thoracic pain and limited cervical and trunk and shoulder active range of movement. Symptom relief, cervical, thoracic and shoulder mobility restoration and a return to pre-injury activities were effected by seven sessions of mobilization techniques of the costovertebral and costotransverse joints of ribs 3–6 and periscapular trigger point release (see Figs 5.32, 5.40 and 5.64) along with postural correction and a stabilization home exercise programme.

Knowledge of presentation of visceral pathology (Fig. 5.9) can also help the therapist in determining the visceral or somatic origins of symptoms associated with the chest, rib cage, thoracic region, abdomen, loin, groin and both upper and lower extremities (Table 5.1; Fig. 5.12).

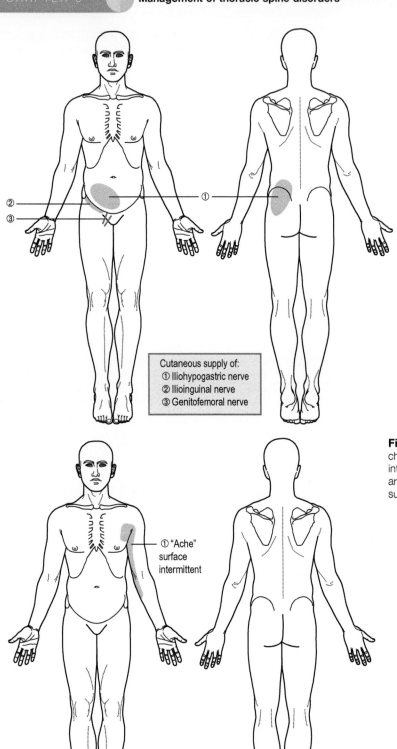

Figure 5.6 • Further example showing 'groin strain' (of T12/L1 origin?) or 'pulled muscle' (costovertebral joint sprain).

Cutaneous supply of:
① Iliohypogastric nerve
② Ilioinguinal nerve
③ Genitofemoral nerve

Figure 5.7 • Left-sided chest upper chest pain with some radiation down into the inner aspect of the left upper arm and axilla from T1, T2 levels, suggesting cardiac involvement.

① "Ache" surface intermittent

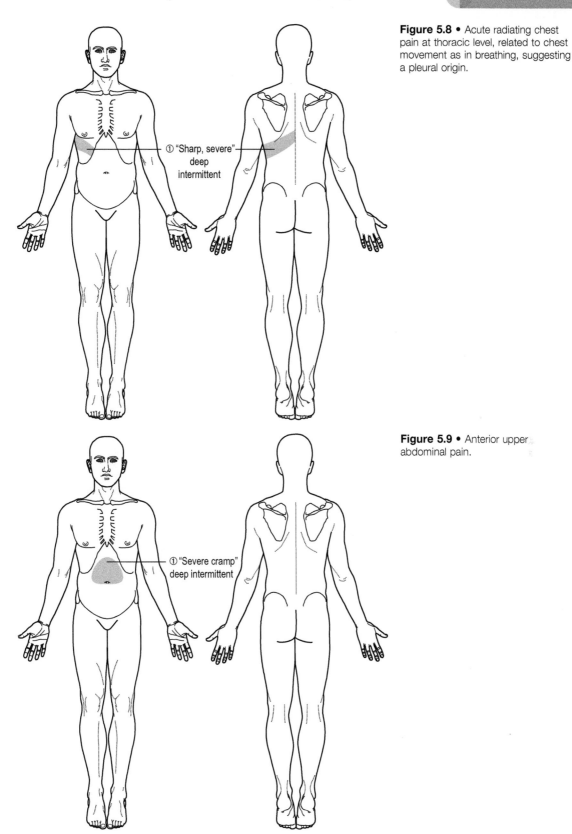

Figure 5.8 • Acute radiating chest pain at thoracic level, related to chest movement as in breathing, suggesting a pleural origin.

① "Sharp, severe" deep intermittent

Figure 5.9 • Anterior upper abdominal pain.

① "Severe cramp" deep intermittent

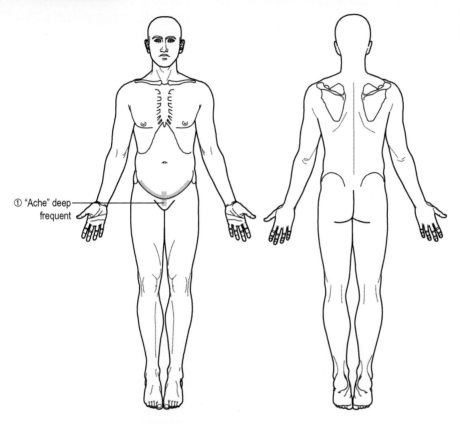

Figure 5.10 • Groin and pubic pain.

① "Ache" deep frequent

Table 5.1 Comparison of systemic/visceral and neuromusculoskeletal (NMSK)/somatic pain (Goodman & Snyder 1995, Evans 1997)

Systemic/visceral	NMSK/somatic
Awakened at night	Unloading of joint
Deep ache, throbbing, colic, nausea	reduces pain
Reduced by pressure	Pulling, stretching,
Constant or waves/spasms of pain	stiff, sharp
Slow to change (secretory, vasoregulated)	Trigger points accompanied by
Less related to physical activity	nausea and
Associated signs/symptoms include:	sweating
Wind	Quicker to change/
Feeling of malaise	impulse
Jaundice	generated
Migratory arthralgias	Movement/
Skin rash	position/
Fatigue	mechanical
Weight loss	stress related
Low grade fever	Onset related to
General muscular fatigue	physical stress
History of infections	
Changes in eating and bowel habits	

Michael et al. (2009), in an orthopaedic overview of thoracic pain, emphasize the need to explore thoracic spine pain as a 'red flag' and to ensure thorough screening for other red flags indicating serious pathology (Box 5.1).

The importance of differential diagnosis of thoracic pain is also stressed by Michael et al. (2009) so as not to miss:

- Deformity due to Scheuermann's disease or idiopathic scoliosis, especially in children and young adults
- Infections such as vertebral osteomyelitis presenting with pain, pyrexia and local tenderness
- Tumours (primary – benign or malignant and secondary metastatic). Patients with known tumours should be treated as suspicious for metastases, especially if the pain is predominantly constant, unremitting and felt at night
- High velocity injury or osteoporotic fractures
- Degenerative conditions associated with neurogenic claudication and stenotic impairments.

Box 5.2 shows the format for the subjective examination of the thoracic spine.

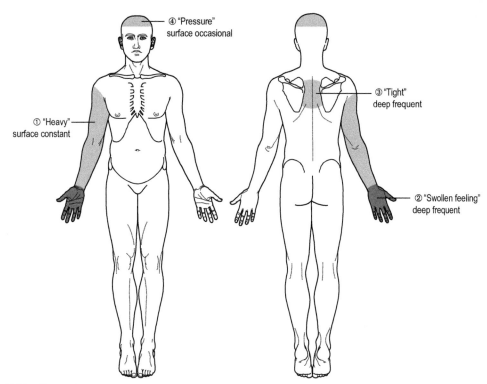

Figure 5.11 • T4 syndrome.

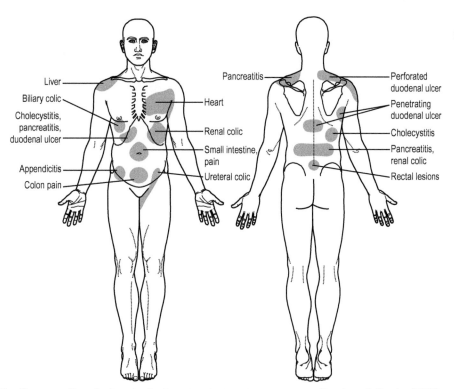

Figure 5.12 • Common sites of referred pain. Reproduced with kind permission from Goodman & Snyder (1995).

Box 5.1

Red flag signs

- Age of onset < 20 years or > 55 years
- Constant progressive, non-mechanical pain [no relief or worsening with bed rest]
- Thoracic pain
- Past medical history of malignant tumour
- Prolonged use of corticosteroids
- Drug abuse, immunosuppression, HIV
- Systematically unwell
- Unexplained weight loss
- Widespread neurological symptoms [including cauda equina syndrome]

(Michael et al. 2009)

- Structural deformity
- Fever

Signs and symptoms of serious spinal pathology requiring emergency referral (Greene 2001)

- Difficulty with micturition
- Loss of anal sphincter tone/faecal incontinence
- Saddle anaesthesia about anus, perineum or genitals
- Gait disturbance

Box 5.2

Thoracic spine: subjective examination

'Kind' of disorder

Establish why patient has been referred for or sought treatment:

1. Pain, stiffness, weakness, instability, etc.
2. Acute onset
3. Post-surgical, trauma, MUA, support, traction, etc.

History

Recent and previous (see 'History' below)
Sequence of questioning about history can be varied

Area

Is the disorder one of pain, stiffness, recurrence, weakness, etc.?
Record on the 'body chart':

1. Area and depth of symptoms indicating main areas and stating types of symptoms
2. Paraesthesia and anaesthesia
3. Check for symptoms all other associated areas, i.e.:
   (i) other vertebral areas
   (ii) joints above and below the disorder
   (iii) other relevant joints.

Behaviour of symptoms

General

1. When are they present or when do they fluctuate and why (associate/dissociate with day's activities, bed/pillow, inflammation)?
2. Effect of rest on the local and referred symptoms (associate/dissociate with day's activities, bed/pillow, size/content, inflammation). (Compare symptoms on rising in the morning with end of day.)

3. Pain and stiffness on rising: duration of.
4. Effect of activities. (Beginning of day compared with end of day.)

Particular

1. What provokes symptoms – what relieves (severity – irritability)?
2. Any sustained positions provoke symptoms?
3. Are quick movements painless?
4. Where is pain felt on full inspiration, expiration, coughing or sneezing?

Special questions

1. Does the patient have bilateral tingling in the feet, or any disturbance of gait (cord signs).
2. General health and relevant weight loss. (Medical history.)
3. Have recent X-rays been taken?
4. What tablets are being taken for this and other conditions (osteoporosis from extensive steroid therapy)?

History

1. Of this attack
2. Of previous attacks, or of associated symptoms
3. Are the symptoms worsening or improving?
4. Prior treatment and its effect
5. Socioeconomic history as applicable.
   HIGHLIGHT MAIN FINDINGS WITH ASTERISKS

Improvement of signs and symptoms in areas remote from the thoracic spine after passive mobilization of the mid-thoracic spine region

It is a common, clinically observed experience that where a benign painful musculoskeletal condition, such as headache, chronic sciatica or persistent paraesthesia in the upper limb, has not responded to treatment as expected, or where progress has stalled, the introduction of passive mobilization applied to the thoracic region between T4 and T8 (and especially T5/6) has an immediate and marked effect in improving symptoms and comparable signs.

For example, in some cases of cervicogenic headache where movement testing and palpation at the O–C1,C1–2 and C2–3 levels have revealed marked movement restriction, both physiological and accessory, the palpation findings including resistance to movement change markedly immediately following passive mid-thoracic mobilization. In turn, the pain related to these movements and the headache is reduced. This would seem to show that the factor seeming to limit movement, initially assessed as inert tissue resistance, was in fact intense, localized muscle spasm and that the locking effect of this spasm had been reduced by passive thoracic mobilization. These findings are supported by the results of the randomized controlled trial where thoracic manipulation (see Fig. 5.45) was shown to be effective in reducing neck pain, improving dysfunction and neck posture and neck range of motion of patients with chronic mechanical neck pain up to 6 months' post treatment (Lau et al. 2011).

Lau et al. (2011) support Cleland et al. (2005), who established that thoracic manipulation reduces perceived neck pain. In a randomized clinical trial, results suggested that thoracic manipulation (see Fig. 5.45) has an immediate analgesic effect on patients with mechanical neck pain.

Similar effects have been observed and reported in relation to other common musculoskeletal dysfunctions and features.

Boyles et al. (2009) found a statistically significant decrease in self-reported pain measures and disability in a sample of patients with sub-acromial impingement syndrome after being treated with thoracic spine thrust manipulation (see Figs 5.45 and 5.46). This effect was noted at 48 hours follow-up. The explanation given for this effect is the possibility that biomechanical changes in thoracic posture brought about by the manipulation may affect range of shoulder motion.

Strunce et al. (2009) also reports the use of thoracic spine or upper ribs high velocity thrust manipulation techniques (see Fig. 5.44) in a sample of patients whose main complaint was shoulder pain. The results of this study suggest that such an intervention has an immediate effect on shoulder pain and range of movement of the shoulder, therefore suggesting that physiotherapists should be aware of the regional interdependence of the thoracic spine, ribs and shoulder.

Berglund et al. (2008), in a survey of examination findings in samples of patients with and without elbow pain, found that there was a significant presence of cervical and thoracic spine pain, on examination, in the group with lateral elbow pain compared with the group without (70% and 16% respectively). The results indicate that there is a significant prevalence of pain and dysfunction in the cervical and thoracic spine in patients with lateral elbow pain. As a consequence, it is essential that physiotherapists include the cervical and thoracic spine in the assessment of patients with lateral elbow pain.

The author of this chapter has experience of many instances whereby chronic groin pain has been attributed to musculotendinous injury whereas, in fact, symptoms have been relieved by passive mobilization of the thoracolumbar spine (see Fig. 5.31) and neurodynamic mobilization of the ilio-inguinal and genitofemoral nerves (Fig. 5.6). Gilmore (1995) presented a paper on 'Gilmore's groin' a musculotendinous lesion that is successfully treated surgically. The author recalls a colleague, however, who differentially diagnosed a patient problem as 'Gilmore's groin' rather than thoracolumbar referral through careful assessment and recognition that features did not fit a pain referral situation. The need for referral for a surgical opinion was concluded because the patient had:

* Previous incidents of 'groin strain'
* No comparable signs in the thoracolumbar region
* Local deep 'soreness' on moderate resistance to hip abduction
* Pain on gentle lower abdominal hollowing (transverse abdominal activation producing strain at the fascial attachments)

- No comparable signs on sacroiliac joint (SIJ) pain provocation testing
- No comparable neurodynamic signs.

Therefore it is as important for physiotherapists to be able to identify where there is no evidence of comparable signs in regions of possible referred pain as well as to be able to recognize when comparable signs are, in fact, present.

Patient examples: manipulative procedures applied to the thoracic spine

Mrs W

A middle-aged woman had undergone a sympathectomy with the aim of reducing her excessive (axillary) perspiration. Following the operation she had developed upper and mid-thoracic girdle pain, varying in intensity but frequently severe. This was accompanied by neck pain, headache, shoulder and arm pain and paraesthesia (Fig. 5.13).

Previous treatment of her cervical spine and shoulder by a therapist had not improved her symptoms. The problem had been with her for more than a year. By chance, she had read a chapter in a book on neurodynamics (Butler 2000) and she said, 'some of the descriptions in the book of patients' problems sounded like mine'.

On examination, she appeared to have a complex pain problem driven by disordered sympathetic activity. Amongst other things, she was extremely hypersensitive to touch and pressure, exhibiting hyperaesthesia, hyperalgesia and allodynia, especially in the upper thoracic spinal area, the associated chest and ribs and anteriorly at the cervical spine.

Cervical and thoracic movements were painfully limited (see Fig. 5.6 and Chapter 4) and neurodynamic tests as well as the sitting slump test and sympathetic slump test were comparable in their partial symptom reproduction and limitation in range of movement (see Figs 5.49–5.61).

Following a detailed examination (Box 5.2; see also Box 5.4) and a discussion of the possible mechanisms underlying her pain and other symptoms, a

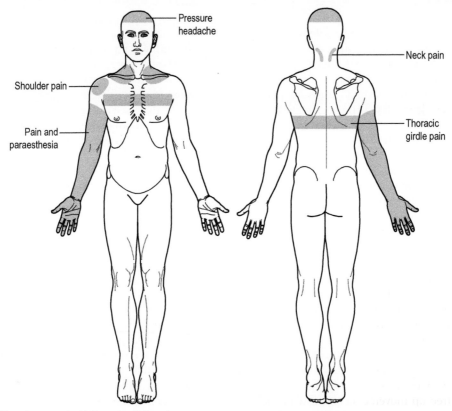

Figure 5.13 ● Upper and mid thoracic girdle pain.

Box 5.3

Examples of self-mobilization exercises

1. Thoracic rotation
   A Cervicothoracic: upright sitting, rotation left with opposite hand on right side of face giving gentle overpressure at end of range. Repeat for right rotation
   B Mid and low thoracic: sitting, rotation left, holding chair-back with right hand to pull further left for end of range stretch. Repeat for right rotation.
2. Thoracic extension
   Crook lying, with small firm polystyrene roll under thoracic spine-varying levels, extending over the roll (chin tucked in to protect cervical spine).
3. Thoracic side flexion
   Sitting on chair, stretching down to one side, fingers toward floor, stretching opposite side at mid and low thoracic. Repeat to opposite side.

---

treatment plan was devised and explained to the patient. As well as advice and a home programme of self-mobilization exercises (see examples in Box 5.3), which were gradually introduced, treatment centred mainly on graduated passive mobilization and eventually some manipulation of the thoracic spine and the ribs, posteriorly, laterally and anteriorly (see Figs 5.28–5.32 & 5.45–5.47).

Additionally, mobilization of her cervical spine particularly with the patient lying supine with initially gentle mobilization of the cervical spine and neural tissues from the anterior aspect (see Fig. 5.48, and Chapter 4, lateral glide) proved not only very potent but also effective in reducing her symptoms and freeing up active movement. Furthermore, neural mobilization techniques including those for the upper limb (see Chapter 4) and intermittent or 'slider' slump mobilization in sitting and long sitting (see Figs 5.49–5.60) were added with ongoing re-assessment to determine the most comparable movement directions and combinations (see Figs 5.17–5.21).

There was a steady improvement in all her symptoms, with occasional fallbacks. When her symptoms appeared 'stirred up', recovery was restored with a 'settling down' treatment, in which the same technique with perhaps one or two exceptions were used with a lower grade to calm and ease the situation. Following this we would press on with variations of a group of techniques, all the time aiming to free up movements and combinations of comparable movements to achieve symptom-free

mobility in all functional directions (for example: side flexion with rotation towards and then away; flexion with rotation).

Treatment had been spread over many months, never more frequently than once each week because the patient lived some distance away. Contact was maintained by telephone for advice and support. She dealt with minor exacerbations using self-mobilizing stretches (for example: using the back of a chair in sitting to lever over for flexion and extension and then rotation; lying supine, stretching over a roll at and below mid-thoracic region; cervical side flexion in median nerve bias upper limb neurodynamic position with the palm of the hand against a wall). A final retrospective re-assessment after 2 months without treatment saw her leading a normal life, virtually symptom free.

Miss A

A young woman was being treated for neck and circumferential arm pain and tingling in one hand, of glove distribution (Fig. 5.14). Passive mobilization and a self-help programme, including active movement of the cervical spine, designed to restore joint and neural tissue mobility and to activate stabilizing control of muscles in the region, had led to some improvement in the condition but that had 'plateaued'. The author of this chapter was asked to review her condition and treatment. Three things struck a chord, especially when going over her examination. Firstly, she reported feeling frequent itching over her back to one side at a level of approximately the 4th, 5th and 6th ribs. Secondly, her hand on that side, compared to the other hand, was a faint dusky blue colour. Thirdly, comparing her hands side by side, the affected hand had lost its skin creases with an overall mild puffy swelling. On palpation her thoracic spine between thoracic 4 and 6 was extremely tender on light and moderate palpation and the three ribs at the same side at those levels were prominent posteriorly and extremely sensitive to pressure (p. 207). The treatment emphasis was shifted to passive mobilization of the mid-thoracic region including the ribs (see Figs 5.28–32), at approximately the thoracic 4th–6th level. Immediately following the first treatment to this area, the itching feeling across her back disappeared, her hand resumed its normal colour and the puffy swelling reduced. A few further treatments resolved the problem.

Interestingly, a few weeks following her discharge she telephoned to say she had experienced a mild

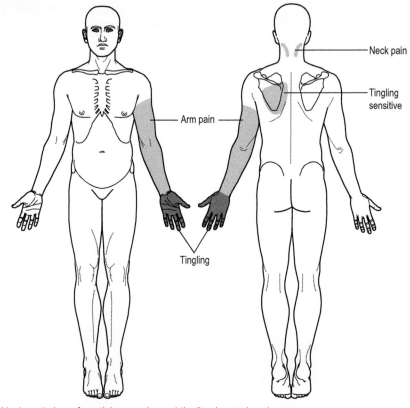

Figure 5.14 • Neck and circumferential arm pain, and tingling in one hand.

recurrence of her pain and her hand swelling and discolouration. She had been at a party and a friend had approached her and slapped her on the back. She said she *immediately* felt arm and upper back discomfort, and the discolouration of her hand recurred. One further treatment directed at her thoracic spine and ribs resolved the problem, and she remained symptom free.

The features of this patient's disorder and her management are not uncommon. The correct approach when using passive mobilization techniques is firstly to build up a group of techniques (anything up to a dozen; see Figs 5.28–5.40 & 5.48) which enable the patient to gradually tolerate more and varied movement inputs to the thoracic spine, almost like a conscious graded exposure to movement. Secondly, to ensure that detailed examination and analysis of movements, including palpation and segmental mobility testing where required (see Figs 5.16–5.32), identify all relevant impairments which the therapist should then aim to clear. Thirdly, that the movement capacity of the thoracic spine is sufficient to ensure full functional activity as required by the individual. So, comparable signs should be

cleared using techniques which incorporate combinations of movement in the thoracic spine, passive segmental mobilization in functional or combined positions, inclinations and angulations of accessory movement, neural mobility in stressed positions such as long sitting slump, and active postural alignment correction and muscle activated stability in order that the positional health of the thoracic spine tissues is sustained.

Thoracic mobilization/ manipulation: when to incorporate techniques to directly address neurodynamic signs/symptoms in the healing process of a lumbar disc lesion

In other words, in the timescale of treatment of, for example, sciatic pain, when should techniques such as passive straight leg raise (SLR) and slump test (see Figs 5.63, 5.49–5.59) components be carefully introduced?

Initially, with moderate to severe lumbar disc lesions, the behaviour of symptoms and signs is often erratic. For example, pain distribution and severity vary markedly from hour to hour, depending on the individual's posture and activities. Frequently sciatic pain (or that of, for example, the femoral nerve) persists, often with disabling severity, beyond the time when the disc healing is advancing well. At such a point, decided by the therapist aware of a typical time-scale of progress, passive mobilization of the mid-thoracic region (T5–7) will afford further insight into the clinical picture and some indication of when neurodynamic treatment techniques might, with careful ongoing re-assessment, be added.

To take an example, it is 4 weeks after the onset of a typical low lumbar disc trauma, resulting in sciatica and paraesthesia down the leg. The passive SLR manoeuvre has been used only to assess/reassess the result of the passive and active lumbar manoeuvres being employed (see Chapter 6). The slump test has not yet been attempted. The therapist feels that symptoms and their behaviour and signs have plateaued.

At this point if passive mobilization is carried out, with the patient in prone lying, typically posteroanterior central mobilization techniques and transverse movements around thoracic 5,6,7 levels (see Figs 5.28 and 5.30), the resultant change (or lack of it) in passive SLR will provide useful information. Firstly, if the SLR in terms of range of pain-free movement or reduced pain with movement remains unaltered, this will indicate that mechanically and neurologically the pain sensitive structures of the spinal canal, intervertebral foraminae and beyond are not yet amenable to direct neural mobilization. In other words, given that the treatment itself is not the cause of the stalemate, then it would be wise to stick to the present regime, assuming this already involves both active and passive movement manoeuvres and detailed advice/explanation. Should, however – and this is the most likely outcome at this stage – the range of passive movement of the SLR be increased with less pain immediately following the thoracic procedures, then some judicious exploratory variations of the passive SLR with the following may be added or substituted in the treatment: knee flexion/extension, foot plantarflexion/dorsiflexion and with less or more hip flexion/adduction.

Keer (1993), in an abstract of a research paper, provided evidence of significant changes in SLR in patients with low back pain after the administration of passive joint mobilization to the mid-thoracic spine. The message here is that if a patient with low back pain and reduced SLR is not responding to treatment as expected, an exploratory treatment of thoracic mobilization my effect a change in SLR.

In addition, if the sitting slump test (see Fig. 5.60) has not been carried out, it may be the time to explore this, both for the added assessment information it provides but also as an eventual additional treatment modality to help restore pain-free functional movement.

Analysis of role of detailed examination in determining when to use thoracic passive mobilization techniques and associated interventions

Edmondston & Singer (1997) reviewed the anatomical and biomechanical features of the thoracic spine as a knowledge support for manual therapists during patient physical examination. The evidence from the biological and clinical sciences and other evidence (Cleland et al. 2002, Butler 2000) are presented in the form of the symbolic permeable brick wall to highlight how decisions can be made by linking theoretical knowledge to clinical practice and vice versa (Table 5.2).

Physical examination

Box 5.4 lists the physical examination tests that are used, although not every listed movement is required for every patient.

Observation

Observation of the thoracic spine is often unremarkable. Postural adaptations such as rounded shoulders, pseudowinging of the scapulae, poking chin, flat thorax, kyphosis and scoliosis of the thoracic spine may be evident. However, these observations need to be related to the patient's signs and symptoms to be of significance.

Table 5.2 The 'brick wall model' of clinical reasoning applied – knowledge of the thoracic spine supporting clinical practice

Theoretical knowledge	
Research evidence	**Clinical evidence**
The thoracic spine exhibits regional variations in mobility	For active movements and PPIVMs [Passive Physiological Intervertebral Movements] examine the upper thoracic spine [T1–4] with the cervical spine, examine the mid thoracic spine separately [T4–10], examine the lower thoracic spine with the lumbar spine [T10–12]
Thoracic curvature determines overall spinal posture, influencing mobility and function of other regions of the spine, pelvis and shoulder girdle The stability of the thoracic spine is enhanced greatly by the rib cage and its articulations The resting length of antagonistic muscle groups will influence cervicothoracic posture The thoracic curvature increases with postural adaptation and age. This will add greater stiffness to segmental mobility of the thoracic spine and create compensatory changes in the lumbar and cervical spines Degenerative changes in the intervertebral discs, facet joints and costovertebral joints occur regionally within the thoracic spine. In particular in the upper and lower thoracic spine Physiological movements in the thoracic spine require simultaneous coupling between intervertebral joints and rib articulations Rotation in the thoracic spine is coupled with ipsilateral lateral flexion and lateral translation	Patients with lumbar/pelvic, neck/shoulder dysfunction may have contributing impairments in the thoracic spine Mobility of the costovertebral and costotransverse joints will have a significant effect on thoracic spine and shoulder girdle mobility Poking chin posture is a common feature of muscle imbalances in the cervicothoracic region On observation, stiffness in the thoracic spine presents as flattening of a region of the mid thoracic spine associated with prominence of segments above and below where increased flexion occurs Thoracic extension, side flexion and rotation will be restricted because of this adaptation The flattened section of the thoracic spine will be stiff during active, passive accessory and passive physiological movement testing The thoracic spine is a common source of local and referred pain which will manifest as tenderness, pain and stiffness with palpation examination and segmental mobility testing examination and treatment techniques should include evaluation of combined physiological movements and exploration of accessory movements in physiological positions to ensure comparable signs are 'cleared'
The sympathetic chains and ganglion lie in close proximity to the costovertebral joints in the thoracic spine. This interface is a potential site of neural irritation and sensitivity The mid thoracic spine is an area where relative mobility of the pain sensitive structures in the spinal canal is less. These tension points are where there is convergence of movement of the spinal canal towards mobile segments. T6 being one such case	Examination of long sitting slump with a sympathetic emphasis and at the same time testing mobility of the costovertebral joints will be a means of reproducing symptoms of a sympathetic nature, such as heaviness in the arm, glove distribution of paraesthesia and sweating Evaluating the slump test will identify whether segmental restrictions around the mid thoracic tension point is contributing to neurodynamic impairment within the thoracic spine

Present pain

Before starting examination of active functional movements of the thoracic spine the patient should always be asked whether he has any symptoms at present, and if so what and where they are. It is important that the assessment of the pain (symptoms) responsive to movement starts here.

Functional demonstration (and differentiation where appropriate)

Although the patient may not be able to perform a specific functional demonstration reproducing his symptoms, there may be a few cases when a functional demonstration or an 'injuring movement' will be useful to the manipulative physiotherapist.

Box 5.4

Thoracic spine: physical examination

Observation

Posture, willingness to move.

Brief appraisal

Movements

Movements to pain or move to limit

F, E; LF L and R in F and E, Rot^n L and R in F and E, pain and behaviour, range, countering protective deformity, localizing, over-pressure, intervertebral movement (repeated movement and increased speed).

When applicable, sitting

Neck movements should be tested for upper thoracic pain. Cervical rotation may need to be superimposed onto thoracic rotation for testing upper thoracic joints.

Sustained E, LF towards pain, Rot^n towards pain (when necessary to reproduce referred pain)

Tap test (when F, E, LF and Rot^n & tap are negative)

Compression and distraction (when F, E, LF & Rot^n & tap are negative)

Combined movement tests

Active peripheral joint tests

First rib.

Intercostal, costovertebral

PPIVM T_4–T_{12} F, E, LF, Rot^n

Canal (slump sitting) tests.

Supine

Passive neck F; range, pain (back and/or referred)

SIJ (ankylosing spondylitis)

First rib

Neurological examination (sensation)

Passive peripheral joint tests.

Side lying

PPIVM C_7–T_4 F, F, LF, Rot^n. T_4–T_{12} Rot^n

Prone

'Palpation'

Temperature and sweating

Soft-tissue palpation (muscle & interspinous space)

Position of vertebrae and ribs especially 1st rib

Passive accessory intervertebral movement, costovertebral and intercostal movement (↕, ⟶, ⟵, ↴ spine and ribs)

Combined PAIVM tests with physiological movement positions

Isometric tests for muscle pain.

Examination of other relevant factors

Other tests

Check 'case notes' for reports of relevant tests (X-rays, blood tests).

HIGHLIGHT IMPORTANT FINDINGS WITH ASTERISKS

Instructions to patient

(i) Warning of possible exacerbation

(ii) Request to report details

(iii) Instructions in 'back care' if required.

One example is the patient who is able to reproduce his chest pain by taking a deep breath, as mentioned earlier. In other cases it may be possible to differentiate the vertebral level responsible for the patient's symptoms using the functional demonstration. For example, when a patient has symptoms in the upper thorax area posteriorly, it is often difficult to determine whether the symptoms are arising from the cervicothoracic junction (or even C5/6 or C6/7) or the upper thoracic intervertebral joints. The procedure to differentiate between them if pain is reproduced by rotation is detailed below.

1. With the patient seated and facing straight ahead towards the physiotherapist, he is asked if he has any symptoms (Fig. 5.15A).

2. Assuming that his symptoms can only be provoked at the end of the range of rotation, he is asked to turn his head fully to the right with his trunk still facing straight ahead. If he feels no change in symptoms, the physiotherapist applies over-pressure to the cervical rotation by pressing her right forearm behind his right shoulder and her right hand behind the back of his head on the right side, while also placing her left hand against his left zygomatic arch. In this position she is able to apply over-pressure to the cervical area without movement of his shoulders. This is not testing cervical rotation to the exclusion of any thoracic rotation, as the upper thoracic spine does also rotate somewhat. Nevertheless, it is a useful attempt at differentiating (Fig. 5.15B).

3. Once the pain response with over-pressure to cervical rotation is assessed, the patient is asked to rotate his thorax to the right without there being any rotation of the head to the right. The

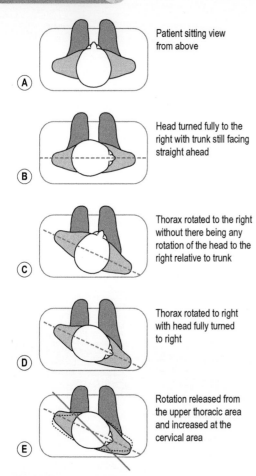

Patient sitting view from above

Head turned fully to the right with trunk still facing straight ahead

Thorax rotated to the right without there being any rotation of the head to the right relative to trunk

Thorax rotated to right with head fully turned to right

Rotation released from the upper thoracic area and increased at the cervical area

Figure 5.15 • A Patient sitting, view from above. **B–E** Various rotation positions.

physiotherapist applies over-pressure to the thoracic rotation by applying further rotary pressure through his shoulders (Fig. 5.15C).

4. With the pain response noted when over-pressure is applied to the thoracic rotation, the patient is then asked to turn his head fully to the right and any further change in symptoms is noted. If there is a change of symptoms when the cervical spine is rotated to the right, then movement of the cervical spine must be involved in the patient's symptoms (Fig. 5.15D).

5. While in the position described above, the physiotherapist changes her application of over-pressure from the upper thoracic area to cervical rotation to the right while at the same time allowing the patient to release the upper thoracic rotation slightly, and the change in symptoms is assessed. With this change of

over-pressure, the emphasis of the rotation is released from the upper thoracic area and increased at the cervical area (see Fig. 5.15E).

Brief appraisal

When the functional demonstration provides valuable information about the sources of the patient's symptoms, the manipulative physiotherapist should briefly appraise the areas involved to give clues to further examination. From the example above, if the thoracic spine appears to be involved more, detailed examination of this area can commence. The cervical spine should also be tested quickly so that it can be excluded or cleared of involvement.

Thoracic rotation

Thoracic rotation can be assessed in many different positions, but the first position chosen should be that indicated by the patient in response to the question, 'Is there any turning or twisting movement which *you* find provokes your symptoms?'. It may be that he responds by demonstrating his golf swing. Under these circumstances it is necessary to determine at what point in the movement is the pain provoked, so that the passive movement can be assessed more specifically.

Rotation can also be assessed in the standing position, with or without the help of outstretched arms or folded arms. Such rotation is more likely to detect movement of the lower thoracic spine.

With the patient in the sitting position and with his arms folded, ask him to 'hug' himself; rotation can be tested in the erect or extended position of the thoracic spine, and this can be compared with the same rotation but performed in the flexed position. Over-pressure to the movement can be performed by continuing the rotation via pressure against the scapula and pectoral areas (Fig. 5.16A).

Upper thoracic rotation can be performed in the sitting position, with the patient clasping his hands behind his occiput and the physiotherapist stabilizing his lower thoracic area. In this position, if the patient turns his head and shoulders to the left with his head kept in a static position in relation to his shoulders, the main movement will occur in the upper and middle thoracic spine.

Thoracic flexion, extension

Upper thoracic flexion and extension are included in the examination of neck movements, and lower

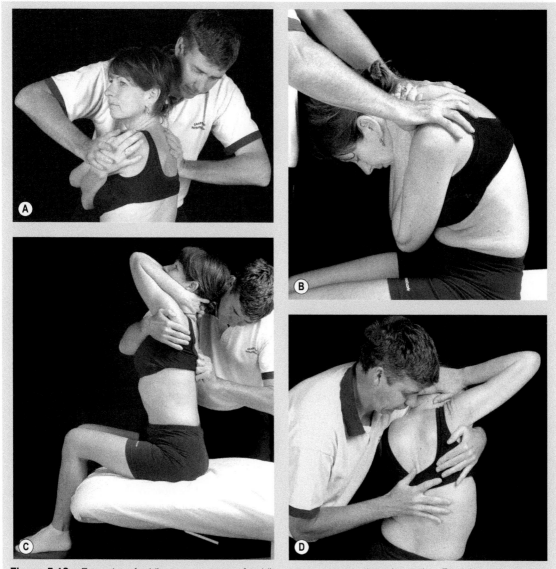

Figure 5.16 • Examples of adding over-pressure: **A** adding over-pressure to thoracic rotation; **B** adding over-pressure to thoracic flexion; **C** adding localized over-pressure to thoracic extension; **D** adding localized over-pressure to thoracic lateral flexion.

thoracic flexion and extension are included in the examination of lumbar spine movements. Mid-thoracic flexion and extension are examined by asking the patient to clasp his hands behind his head whilst in the sitting position, and point his elbows forwards so that they come together.

Flexion

Having adopted the above position, the patient is then instructed to curl his elbows into his groin to produce thoracic flexion. The therapist notes the range of movement, symptom response and quality of movement. If necessary, over-pressure can be added via the supraclavicular and suprascapular areas. The therapist stands in front of the patient and places her hands over the top of his shoulders with her fingers posteriorly and her thumbs anteriorly. Over-pressure is applied in the direction of the continuing arc of flexion. Over-pressure directed cranially, horizontally or caudally can put emphasis on the upper, middle and lower parts of the thoracic spine respectively (Fig. 5.16B).

Extension

The same starting position as for flexion is adopted, with one exception: the patient places one or both feet on a chair in order to flex the lumbar spine. The patient is instructed to direct his elbows upwards. The therapist notes the range, symptom response and quality of movement. If necessary, over-pressure can be added by the therapist, who stands by the side of the patient and places an arm under both his axillae and across his sternum. She places the other hand on his thoracic spine to localize the over-pressure, at the same time side-flexing her trunk in the direction of the thoracic extension (Fig. 5.16C).

Thoracic lateral flexion

Lateral flexion of the upper and lower thoracic spine is included in the examination of the cervical and lumbar spines, respectively. To localize lateral flexion to the mid-thoracic spine in sitting, the patient is asked to place his hands behind his head and direct his elbows away from his body. He is then instructed to curl his elbows into his side. The range, symptom response and quality of movement are noted. Over-pressure can be applied locally at each intervertebral level by the manipulative physiotherapist standing by the right side of the patient. Taking right lateral flexion as an example, she places her right axilla on his right shoulder and holds under his left axilla with her right hand. Her left thumb is then placed against the side of each spinous process of the thoracic spine in turn, and she bends her knees to increase the thoracic lateral flexion (Fig. 5.16D).

When applicable tests

Combined movement tests

If, at this stage of examination, the patient's symptoms have not been reproduced or comparable signs have not been found, then applicable tests such as combined movements can be used. The sequence of

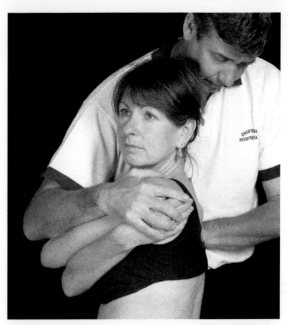

Figure 5.17 • Over-pressure added to thoracic rotation to the left.

combined movements should reflect the patient's functional limitations.

The following example is but one of many sequences of combined movements that can be used in the examination of the thoracic spine. In the example, thoracic rotation to the left is the starting position, to which is added in turn lateral flexion to the left, lateral flexion to the right, extension and flexion.

1. With the patient sitting he is asked to turn fully to the left, and when the physiotherapist has added over-pressure to this movement his symptoms are assessed (Fig. 5.17).

2. While over-pressure is maintained for rotation to the left, the physiotherapist laterally flexes the patient's trunk to the left while at the same time assessing changes in symptoms. It is important, during the movement of lateral flexion to the left, that the same strength of pressure to the rotation is maintained. This is not as easy as it may seem; with her right axilla stabilizing his right shoulder she must follow his lateral flexion (Fig. 5.18).

3. The physiotherapist then laterally flexes his trunk to the right, again using her right axilla to stabilize and control the lateral flexion, while noting changes in symptoms. Once more, it is

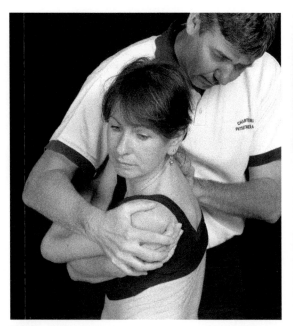

Figure 5.18 • Adding lateral flexion to the left to the rotation to the left.

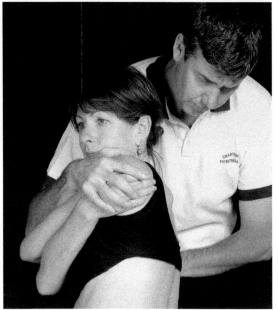

Figure 5.19 • Adding lateral flexion to the right to the rotation to the left.

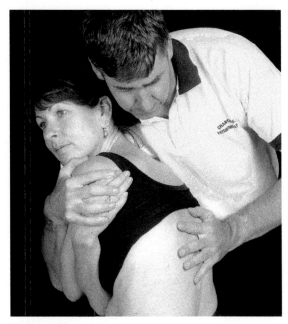

Figure 5.20 • Adding flexion to rotation to the left.

thoracic spine and assesses the changes in symptoms (Fig. 5.20).

5. To the sustained over-pressure to the thoracic rotation to the left, the physiotherapist then adds thoracic extension at the appropriate level while noting changes in symptoms. To produce the extension, the physiotherapist uses her right forearm as a fulcrum while using her two hands to extend the patient's thoracic spine (Fig. 5.21).

Compression movement tests

All of the physiological movements can be performed both with and without compression. The patient sits with his arms folded, and the physiotherapist stands behind him and stabilizes his thorax with her body, applying the compression by putting her forearms around in front of his shoulders and grasping over his supraspinous fossa area with her hands. She then uses her hands in conjunction with her upper sternum (at approximately his T3 level) to increase her body weight gradually, thus pushing through his thoracic spine towards the floor.

Localized oscillatory movements of flexion, extension, lateral flexion and rotation can then be performed while the compression is maintained. It is uncommon in the thoracic spine that the addition

necessary to retain the same strength to the rotary over-pressure (Fig. 5.19).

4. To the sustained over-pressure of the thoracic rotation to the left, the physiotherapist then adds flexing at the appropriate level of the

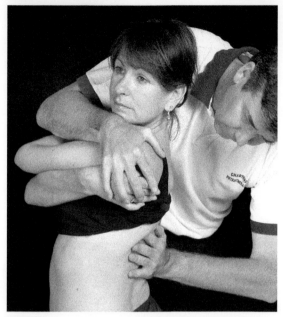

Figure 5.21 • Adding extension to the rotation to the left.

of compression makes any difference to the pain response found when the same movement or movements were performed without compression.

Tap test

If active movements are full and symptom free, the patient sits on the plinth with the spine flexed and each spinous process of the thoracic spine and the rib angle are tapped with a reflex hammer. One spinous process or rib angle may exhibit exquisite tenderness over and above any of the others. In some cases, this resonance effect may be a way of detecting bone demineralization, stress fracture or bone tumour.

Slump test

This test should form part of the examination of the thoracic spine. However, it is essential to remember that this test causes pain at approximately the T8/T9 area in at least 90% of all subjects. If the patient does experience pain at T8 or T9 and it is for this pain that he seeks treatment, and if the pain is increased during the slump test, then the only way in which a decision implicating the canal structures as a component of the cause of his disorder can be made is to balance it against the physiotherapist's

knowledge and experience of what is within the considered norms for this test.

The long sitting slump can be used as an adaptation of the slump test to emphasize the testing of the mobility of the canal structures of the thoracic spine. In this position and with the addition of trunk side flexion to the left, for example, the ribs can be examined and treated on the right. This is a means of influencing the sympathetic chains via the slump position and movement of the costovertebral joints.

Other neurodynamic tests such as the upper limb neural tests (ULNTs), SLR, prone knee bend (PKB) and passive neck flexion (PNF) may also be considered as part of the thoracic spine examination.

Palpation

The patient lies prone with his arms by his side or over the edge of the couch to widen the interscapular space.

Areas of sweating and temperature changes

It is not uncommon to find areas of increased temperature situated centrally in the thoracic spine. These areas do not indicate information of either mechanical or pathological origin.

The presence of any localized areas of sweating is determined first. Temperature changes are assessed by wiping the backs of the fingers or hands over the thoracic area, particularly in the area between the angles of the ribs or the left and right sides. It is not uncommon to find 9 cm areas situated centrally which do not indicate inflammation of either mechanical or pathological disorders.

Soft-tissue changes

Thickening of the interspinous tissue and the tissues in the interlaminar trough area is extremely informative. The thickening can be totally lateral, and can be expected to be found on the same side and at the appropriate intervertebral level as unilateral pain. The thickening can extend over more than one level on the same side, or it can be on the left side of, say, T5/6 and the right side of T4/5 and T6/7. The texture of the thickenings can clearly sort them into new and old changes. This sorting is far more difficult in the low lumbar area.

Quite often thoracic physiological combined movements and movements under compression are pain free. However, palpation anomalies can always be found. At a first consultation, if a patient has upper abdominal pain of skeletal origin it is common for all physiological movements to be pain free even when combined movements and movements under compression are tested. However, palpation anomalies can always be found, provided the examination is perceptively performed and related to the history of progression of the disorder. This reliability makes palpation a skill that should be learned by all general surgeons.

Bony changes and position tests

The two most common findings when examining the position of the spinous processes in relation to each other in the thoracic spine are:

1. A spinous process that feels more deeply set than its abnormally prominent adjacent spinous process above. This is the most informative finding, indicating either that it is the source of a patient's symptoms or that it is a disadvantaged intervertebral area which has the potential to cause symptoms if placed under excessive stress.

2. One spinous process displaced to one side in relation to the spinous process above and below.

This only indicates rotation of the vertebra when it is confirmed by establishing that one transverse process is more posteriorly positioned in comparison with the vertebra's transverse process on the opposite side. That is to say, if the spinous process of T6 is displaced to the right, this displacement only indicates rotation of the vertebra if the transverse process of T6 on the left is more prominent (or posteriorly positioned) than the transverse process of T6 on the right. This is rarely the case, and it is surprising to find how often a patient's symptoms, when related to this malalignment, are found to be on the same side as that to which the spinous process is deviated.

When one spinous process is deeply set and the adjacent spinous process above is prominent, pressure over the prominent spinous process usually provokes a superficial sharp pain while pressure over the sore deeply set spinous process, if firm and sustained, produces a very deeply felt pain. These findings indicate that the joint between them is abnormal and is the possible site of origin of symptoms.

Passive accessory intervertebral movements (PAIVMs)

The two main movements to be tested in the thoracic spine are posteroanterior central vertebral pressure and transverse vertebral pressure, and these are described on pages 201–202 and 204. As has been stated before, these movements can be varied both in the point of contact that produces them and in the inclination of movement. The other movement that is important for examination purposes by palpation is posteroanterior unilateral vertebral pressure, which is described on pages 206–207. It is also essential that costovertebral and intercostal movements are assessed for their range and pain response. These are described, respectively, on pages 207–208.

In earlier editions of this book, in the chapter regarding selection of techniques, the suggestion was made that the direction of transverse pressures should be performed initially towards the side of pain. This statement is based on the fact that the technique opens the intervertebral space on the side of pain, thus avoiding provoking pain. This is not to say that the technique should never be performed in the opposite direction, and nor should provoking the pain be the aim, as will now be explained.

It is sometimes very useful to assess responses one day after the examination and treatment and use of the 'D-plus-1' response should be made in chronic disorders when other test movements are uninformative. Therefore, when a patient with a chronic skeletal disorder causing unilateral referred pain is examined at the first consultation, part of the palpation examination that should be emphasized is the use of transverse pressure from the side of the referred pain against the spinous process of three or four adjacent vertebrae at the appropriate level. The aim is to endeavour to provoke the referred pain. If this is not achieved at the first consultation, its repetition may sensitize the joint at fault and thus make the same transverse pressure provoke the referred pain at the second consultation – i.e. on 'D-plus-1' (D+1).

Differentiation test by palpation

When transverse pressure on, say, T7 to the right provokes the patient's pain, it may be necessary to determine whether the symptoms are arising from the T7/8 intervertebral joint or the T7/6 intervertebral joint. The technique for doing this has been described fully on page 205.

Passive range of physiological movements of single vertebral joints (PPIVMs)

As has been stated before, the oscillatory testing movement is performed more slowly (as a general rule) than it is when used as a treatment technique. This is only because sometimes the through-range quality of movement is less easily appreciated with quicker movements. The end-of-range feel can sometimes be determined by applying an over-pressure component to the testing oscillatory movement.

The movements are described below for the selected intervertebral levels.

C7–T4 (flexion)

Starting position

With the patient sitting, the physiotherapist stands in front of him and slightly to the patient's right. She rests her left hand over his right shoulder with the middle finger positioned between two spinous processes, while the index finger palpates the upper margin of the spinous process of the upper vertebra and the ring finger palpates the lower margin of the lower spinous process. To produce a firm yet comfortable grasp with the left hand, the pad of the thumb is placed in the supraclavicular fossa. The right hand and forearm are placed over the top of the patient's head so that they lie in the sagittal plane. The fingers and thumb grasp the occiput near the nuchal lines, and the wrist is flexed to permit firm pressure on the front of the head by the forearm (Fig. 5.22).

Method

Movement of the patient's head is controlled by the physiotherapist's right hand and forearm. All scalp looseness must be taken up by the grasp between the fingers and forearm to permit complete control of the patient's head and make him feel that support of his head can be left to the physiotherapist.

As the amount of movement that can be felt at this level is much less than elsewhere in the vertebral column, two complementary actions are necessary to produce the maximum intervertebral movement. First, the oscillation of the head and

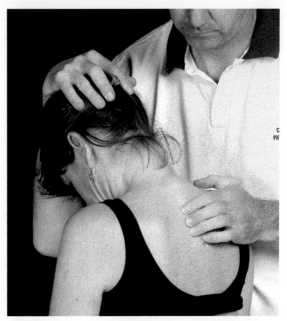

Figure 5.22 • Intervertebral movement. C7–T4 (flexion).

neck needs to be through a range at least of 30° performed near the limit of forward flexion. Secondly, because the lever producing movement is long, pressure by the three palpating fingers over the spine will help to localize movement as the head is moved back through a range of 30°.

The intervertebral movement is felt by the ring, middle and index fingers as the spinous processes move away from and towards each other during the back and forth movements of the head and neck.

C7–T4 (flexion/extension)

An alternative method for testing flexion, which is more convenient if rotation and lateral flexion are also to be tested, is performed with the patient lying on his side.

Starting position

The patient lies comfortably on his right side, near the forward edge of the couch, with his head resting on pillows. The physiotherapist stands in front of the patient, cradling his head in her left arm with her fingers covering the posterior surface of his neck, her little finger reaching down to the vertebral level being examined. She stabilizes his head between her left forearm and the front of her left shoulder. Next she leans across the patient, placing her right forearm along his back to stabilize his thorax, and palpates the under-surface of the interspinous space with the pad of her index or middle finger facing upwards (Fig. 5.23).

Method

With her left arm, the physiotherapist flexes and extends the patient's lower neck as much as possible. The spine above C6 and the head are not flexed or extended, because movement in this area makes movement in the test area less controlled and less isolated. The patient's head and neck are moved only until the particular joint tested has come to the limit of its range.

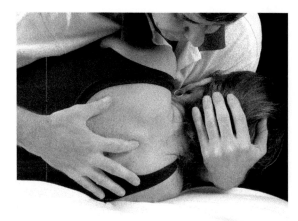

Figure 5.23 • Intervertebral movement. C7–T4 (flexion/extension).

C7–T4 (lateral flexion)

Method

The starting position is identical with that described for flexion/extension. The purpose of this method is to achieve lateral flexion at the particular joint being tested, and therefore the head does not laterally flex but rather is displaced upwards. Lateral flexion is produced by the physiotherapist lifting the patient's head with a hugging grip of his head, the majority of the lift being achieved by the ulnar border of her left hand against the underside of his cervicothoracic junction (Fig. 5.24). To test lateral flexion in the opposite direction, the patient must lie on his other side. The palpating finger feels for movement between the two adjacent spinous processes. The upper process moves first, and when the lower process starts to move this will signal the extent of the lateral flexion at this particular intervertebral level.

C7–T4 (rotation)

Method

The starting position is again the same as for flexion/extension. To produce the rotation properly, it is necessary to concentrate on moving the joint being examined without causing any tilting or flexing of the head and neck. Movement of the upper spinous process in relation to its distal neighbour is palpated through the pad of the physiotherapist's index or

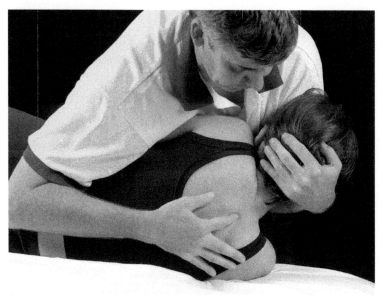

Figure 5.24 • Intervertebral movement. C7–T4 (lateral flexion).

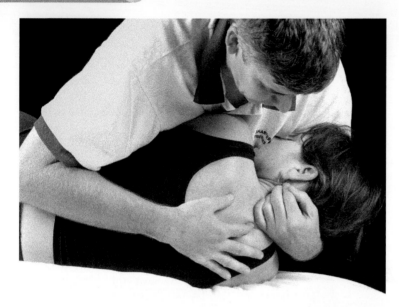

Figure 5.25 • Intervertebral movement. C7–T4 (rotation).

middle finger, which is facing upwards against the underside of the interspinous space.

With the patient's head cradled between the physiotherapist's left forearm and shoulder, and his lower neck firmly gripped in the ulnar border of her hand between the little finger and the hypothenar eminence, she rotates his lower cervical spine towards her. This is achieved by elevating her scapula to its highest point while maintaining a stable thorax (Fig. 5.25). As the movement is difficult to achieve accurately, more care is needed than with the other movements tested in this area.

T4–11 (flexion/extension)

Starting position

The patient sits with his hands clasped behind his neck while the physiotherapist, standing by his left side, places her left arm under his left upper arm and grasps his right upper arm in her supinated hand. She places her right hand across his spine just below the level being tested, and the pad of the tip of the middle finger in the far side of the inter-spinous space to feel adjacent spinous processes.

Method

While the patient relaxes to allow his thorax to be flexed and extended, the physiotherapist takes the weight of his upper trunk on her left arm.

To test flexion, she lowers his trunk from the neutral position until movement can be felt to have

taken place at her right middle finger; the patient is then returned to the neutral position by lifting under his arms. The oscillatory movement through an arc of approximately 20° of trunk movement is facilitated if the patient is held firmly and if the physiotherapist laterally flexes her trunk to the left as she lowers the trunk into flexion. This makes the return movement one of laterally flexing her trunk to the right rather than lifting with her left arm.

The extension part of the test is carried out in much the same way, except that the physiotherapist assists the trunk extension with the heel and ulnar border of her right hand. In doing this she must be careful to keep the pad of her middle finger in a constant position between the adjacent spinous processes. Movement of the patient's trunk is from the neutral position into extension. It is important to remember that it is movement at only one joint that is being examined, and therefore large trunk movements are not necessary; in fact they detract from the examination.

T4–11 (lateral flexion)

Starting position

The patient sits and holds his hands behind his neck or crosses his arms across his chest while the physiotherapist stands side-on behind his right side reaching with her right arm to hold high around and behind his left shoulder. She grips his trunk firmly between her right arm and her right side in her left

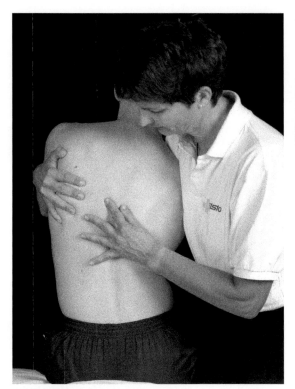

Figure 5.26 • Intervertebral movement. T4–11 (lateral extension).

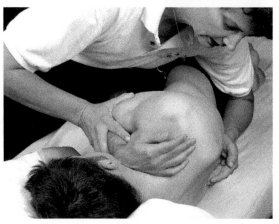

Figure 5.27 • Intervertebral movement. T4–11 (rotation).

axilla. This high grasp with the right hand is necessary for examination of the higher levels; as the examination extends below T8, so the grasp needs to be taken down to the lower scapular area. She places the heel of her left hand on the right side of his back at the level being examined, spreads her fingers for stability, and places the tip of the pad of her flexed middle finger in the far side of the interspinous space of the joint to be tested (Fig. 5.26).

Method

The physiotherapist laterally flexes the patient's trunk towards her by displacing his trunk away from her with the heel of her left hand and her costal margin, and laterally flexing his upper trunk by lifting her right arm and pressing downwards with her right axilla. She palpates for the interspinous movement through the pad of her middle finger, ensuring that during the lateral flexion her finger moves with the spine, maintaining even contact against the spinous processes. The palpating finger feels the space between the spinous processes open and close as the patient's trunk is laterally flexed and returned to the neutral position.

Lateral flexion in the opposite direction can be palpated without a change of position simply by laterally flexing the patient's trunk the other way. However, it is more accurate to change sides and reproduce the technique on the opposite side.

T4–11 (rotation)

Starting position

Although rotation can be tested in the sitting position, it is more easily and more successfully tested when the patient is lying down. The patient lies on his left side with his hips and knees comfortably flexed while the physiotherapist, standing in front of the patient, leans over his trunk to cradle his pelvis between her left side and her left upper arm. This position stabilizes the patient's pelvis. The physiotherapist's forearm is then in line with the patient's spine, and her hand reaches the level where movement is to be examined. She then places her left hand on his spine with the pad of her middle finger facing upwards against the under-surface of the interspinous space to feel the bony margins of the adjacent spinous processes. With her right hand, she grasps as far medially as possible over the patient's suprascapular area and places her forearm over his sternum or grasps the patients elbow over his sternum (Fig. 5.27).

Method

The patient's trunk is repeatedly rotated back and forth by the physiotherapist's right forearm and hand through an arc of approximately 25°. Care must be taken to ensure that the movement does not include scapulothoracic movement. To examine movement in the upper thoracic intervertebral joints, the arc of movement should be performed just behind the frontal plane. As lower intervertebral joints are examined, the arc of rotation used to assess movement moves backwards until an arc of rotation between 40 and 60° from the frontal plane is used to examine the movement between T10 and T11. The palpating finger must follow the patient's trunk movement, and when movement occurs at the joint being examined, the upper spinous process will be felt to press into the pad of the middle finger, which is facing upwards. When the lower spinous process starts to move, this is the extent of rotation at the intervertebral level.

Examination and treatment techniques

Passive mobilization techniques can be used for the treatment of disorders associated with thoracic and related pain and also in examination to establish the direction and dosage of treatment technique.

Mobilization

Posteroanterior central vertebral pressure (↕)

Starting position

The patient lies prone, either with his forehead resting on the backs of his hands or with his head comfortably turned to one side and his arms lying by his sides on the couch. The position depends on the amount of chest tightness created by the 'arms up' position, which is usually reserved for upper thoracic mobilization.

If the patient is on a low couch, the physiotherapist's position for mobilizing the upper thoracic spine (approximately T1–5) needs to be at the head of the patient with her shoulders over the area to be mobilized to enable the direction of the pressure to be at right angles to the surface of the body. The pads of the thumbs are placed on the spinous process, pointing transversely across the vertebral column, and the fingers of each hand are spread out over the posterior chest wall to give stability to the thumbs. As the spinous processes are large, the thumbs may be positioned tip to tip or with the tips side by side in contact with the upper and lower margins of the same spinous process. To gain the best control and feel of movement with the least

discomfort to the patient, the pressure should be transmitted through the thumbs so that the interphalangeal joints are hyperextended. This enables the softest part of the pad to be flat over the spinous processes, with a slight degree of flexion in the metacarpophalangeal joints. Not only is this more comfortable for the patient, but it hinders the physiotherapist's intrinsic muscles from producing the pressure.

To mobilize the mid-thoracic spine (T5–9), the physiotherapist should stand at the patient's side with her thumbs placed longitudinally along the vertebral column so that they point towards each other. The fingers can then spread out over the posterior chest wall, to each side of the vertebral column above and below the thumbs.

It may be more comfortable (and this is far easier to do if the patient is lying on a low couch) for the physiotherapist to stand to one side of the patient, approximately at waist level and facing his head, and place the pads of the thumbs on the spinous process pointing across the vertebral column. The fingers of each hand can then spread over opposite sides of the posterior chest wall for stability.

For the lower thoracic spine (T10–12), the physiotherapist's position depends upon the shape of the patient's chest. Either of the latter two positions described above may be used, but the essential factor is that the direction of the pressure must be at right angles to the body surface at the level. This means that the shoulders may need to be anywhere between vertically above the lower thoracic spine and vertically above the sacrum (Fig. 5.28). If the patient has difficulty lying prone because extension is painful, a small pillow under the chest will assist. The physiotherapist's position must also allow pressure to be applied to the spinous process using the anteromedial aspect of the fifth metacarpal, similar to that described in Chapter 6, for the lumbar spine. However, it may be essential to avoid direct contact between the pisiform and the spinous process for the sake of comfort (Fig. 5.28).

Method

The mobilizing is carried out by an oscillating pressure on the spinous processes, produced by the body and transmitted through the arms to the thumbs. It is important that this pressure is applied by the body weight over the hands and not by a squeezing action with the thumbs themselves. The fingers, which are spread out over the patient's back, should not exert any pressure but act only as stabilizers for the

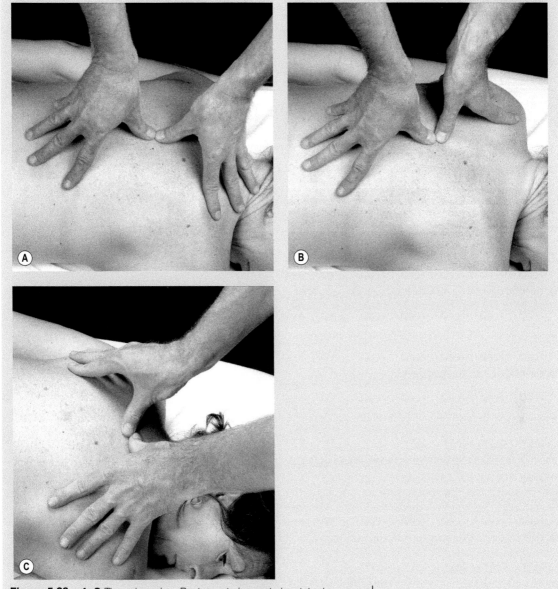

Figure 5.28 • A–C Thoracic region. Posteroanterior central vertebral pressure ↕.

thumbs. It is easy to dissipate the pressure and lose the effectiveness of the thumbs by faulty use of the fingers.

If the physiotherapist's elbows are kept slightly flexed and the thumbs maintained in the position of hyperextension of interphalangeal joints and slight flexion of metacarpophalangeal joints, the pressure can be transmitted to the pads of the thumbs through this series of strong springs. This springing action at the joints can readily be seen as the body weight is applied during the mobilizing.

Local variations

The degree of pressure required in the upper thoracic spine to produce movement is far greater than that required in the cervical spine, and slightly stronger than that required for the remainder of the thoracic spine.

The degree of movement possible in the middle and lower thoracic spine is considerable, and it is here that it is easiest to learn a feeling of movement. The degree of movement possible in the upper thoracic spine is considerably limited, and this is particularly so between T1 and T2.

Uses

Posteroanterior central vertebral pressure is as useful for the thoracic spine as rotation is for the cervical spine. In all symptoms arising from the thoracic vertebrae, it is worth trying this procedure first.

'Central pressure' is more likely to be successful with symptoms that are situated in the midline or evenly distributed to each side of the body, but it should also be tried for unilateral symptoms, particularly if they are ill-defined or widespread in their distribution.

Examples of treatment include: glove distribution symptoms, page 186 and Figure 5.14; thoracic backache, page 174 and Figure 5.1; and traumatic girdle pain, pages 185–186.

Rotary posteroanterior intervertebral pressures

Starting position

The patient lies prone with his arms by his side while the manipulative physiotherapist stands alongside the patient (in this case by his right side). She places her right hand between the spine and his right scapula, and her left hand between the spine and his left scapula, and transmits pressure through the lateral surface of the hypothenar eminence near the pisiform bone. To reach the final position, the first step is to place the ulnar border of each hand in a line across the patient's back in parallel lines, the right hand being slightly caudad to the joint to be mobilized and the left hand slightly distal to the joint to be mobilized. At this preliminary stage the physiotherapist's forearms are also directed across the patient's back at right angles to the vertebral column, and her pisiform bone is tucked into the space between the paravertebral muscles and the spinous processes. The next step entails taking up the slack in the soft tissues. This is achieved by applying both posteroanterior and rotary pressures; the rotary pressure is achieved by changing the direction of the forearms, in a swinging or twisting fashion, from across the body to somewhat caudad (the right arm) and cephalad (the left arm) as well as laterally. The final stage is that of being certain

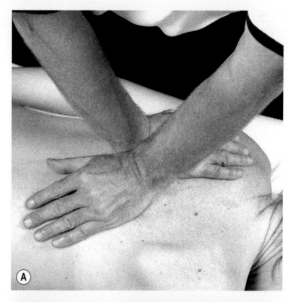

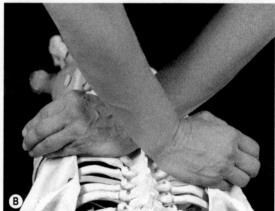

Figure 5.29 • A Intervertebral movement, rotary posteroanterior movements T1– clockwise. **B** Movement shown on a skeleton T10/anticlockwise.

that all of the slack has been taken up and that the pisiform bones are now opposite each other at the same intervertebral level (T6/7; Fig. 5.29A).

Method

When used as a mobilization, the technique consists of an oscillatory movement with three directions; posteroanterior, cephalad and caudad, and lateral. It can be performed as a very localized movement by using the pisiform as the main contact point through which the pressure is transmitted, or it can be performed much more comfortably over a wider area by utilizing the base of the palm of the hand together with the thenar and hypothenar eminences.

The technique can be performed rhythmically with increasing and decreasing posteroanterior pressure in time with the patient's breathing rhythm.

It can also be used as a manipulative thrust, usually at the end of the patient's expiration. There are times when the technique can be usefully employed in the lumbar spine.

Uses

The technique can be selected when movement is desired in a posteroanterior direction but the spinous processes are too tender for direct contact.

The ranges of movement of single costovertebral, costotransverse and intervertebral joints are quite small, and yet if this technique is performed through the palm of the hand as described above, quite considerable movement between three or four contiguous levels can be achieved. This can produce immediate comfort and improvement in movement (Fig. 5.29B).

Transverse vertebral pressure (←→)

Starting position

When the middle and lower thoracic vertebrae are to be mobilized with transverse pressures, the patient lies prone with his arms hanging over the sides of the couch or by his side to aid relaxation of the vertebral column. The head should be allowed to rest comfortably by being turned to one side, preferably towards the side where the physiotherapist stands. However, as this head position tends to produce some degree of rotation in the upper thoracic vertebrae, it is better for the patient to adopt the 'forehead rest' position when these vertebrae are to be mobilized in order to eliminate any rotation. Alternatively, some couches have a hole to allow the head to remain centrally placed. In some cases it may be useful to rotate or derotate the spine using the head position to produce the movement. If the mobilization technique needs to be performed strongly as a Grade IV1, it may help to ask the patient to face towards the manipulative physiotherapist.

The physiotherapist stands at the patient's right side at the level of the vertebrae to be mobilized, and places her hands on the patient's back so that the pads of the thumbs are adjacent to the right side of the spinous processes while the fingers are spread over the patient's left ribs. The left thumb acts as the point of contact and is fitted down into the groove between the spinous process and the paravertebral muscles, so that part of the pad of the thumb is pressed against the lateral aspect of the spinous process on its right-hand side. It is essential to have as much of the pad in contact with the spinous process as is possible. To prevent the thumb sliding off the spinous process, the palmar surface of the metacarpophalangeal joint of the index finger must be firmly brought down on top of the interphalangeal joint of the thumb. This is a valuable position to learn to adopt, as its stability is of value in other techniques. The right thumb, acting as reinforcement, is placed so that its pad lies over the nail of the left thumb. This thumb relationship is chosen because considerable effort is required to keep a single thumb comfortably against the spinous process.

The fingers of both hands should be well spread out over the chest wall to stabilize the thumbs, and the wrists need to be slightly extended to permit the pressure to be transmitted through the thumbs in the horizontal plane. Because of the slightly different functions required of the left and right thumbs, the left forearm is not as horizontal as the right forearm (Fig. 5.30).

Method

The pressure is applied to the spinous process through the thumbs by the movement of the trunk; alternate pressure and relaxation is repeated continuously to produce an oscillating type of movement of the intervertebral joint. For the gentler grades of mobilizing, very little pressure is needed. When stronger mobilizing is used, movement of the patient's trunk is involved and timing of pressures should coincide either with the patient's rolling or, in order to make the technique stronger, to go against the rolling.

Local variations

The upper thoracic spinous processes (T1–3/4) are readily accessible but have a limited amount of movement, T1 being almost immovable. The lower thoracic vertebrae (T8/9–12) are more easily moved and do not require great pressure. Local tenderness in these two areas is comparatively negligible. Mobilization of the mid-thoracic spine is made difficult by the relative inaccessibility of the spinous processes and natural tenderness, and when a painful condition is superimposed on this natural tenderness, adequate mobilization may be very difficult. Where stronger techniques are required to be performed for longer periods, better effect may be

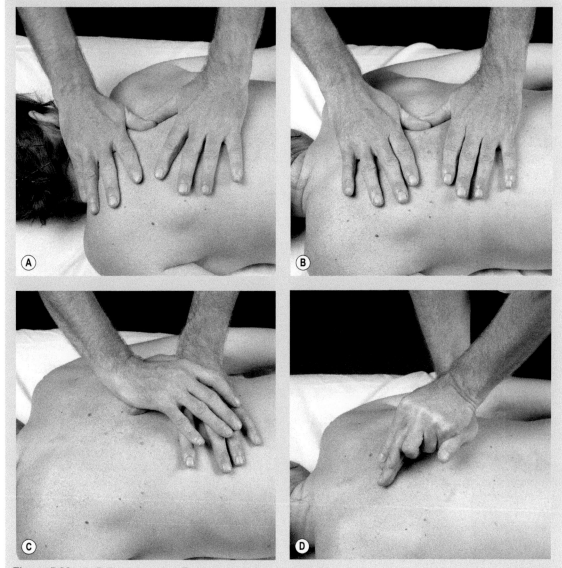

Figure 5.30 • A–D Thoracic region. Transverse vertebral pressure ←•→.

gained by reinforcing the contact thumb with the pisiform of the opposite hand rather than with the opposite thumb pad. In this way, the fingers can be spread over the chest wall and the movement can be produced through the thumb and hand via the therapist's trunk.

Uses

This technique is particularly useful for pain of unilateral distribution in the thoracic area. In such cases the pressure is best applied against the side of the spinous process that is away from the pain, applying the pressure towards the patient's painful side. When using this technique it is frequently necessary to mobilize the ribcage by a posteroanterior pressure directed through the angle of the rib. If progression is needed, the manipulative physiotherapist may need to clear the joint signs by using pressure on the spinous process on the painful side and towards the pain-free side.

Examples of treatment include pain simulating cardiac disease, page 175; scapula pain, page 176;

thoracic backache; traumatic girdle pain, page 185; and abdominal pain and vague pains, page 175.

Posteroanterior unilateral vertebral pressure (↓↱)

Starting position

The patient lies prone with his head turned to the left and his arms hanging loosely over the sides of the couch or by his side.

To mobilize the left side of the middle or lower thoracic spine (approximately T5–12), the physiotherapist stands on the left side of the patient and places her hands on the patient's back so that the pads of the thumbs, pointing towards each other, lie over the transverse processes. The fingers of the left hand spread over the chest wall pointing towards the patient's head, while the fingers of the right hand point towards his feet and the thumbs are held in opposition. By applying a little pressure through the pads of the thumbs, they will sink into the muscle tissue adjacent to the spinous processes until the transverse process is reached. The metacarpophalangeal joint of the thumb needs to be slightly flexed and the interphalangeal joint must be hyperextended to enable the pad of the thumb to transmit the pressure comfortably. When a much finer degree of localization of the pressure is required, the thumbnails should be brought together so that the tips of the thumbs make a very small but comfortable point of contact. In this position, the metacarpophalangeal joints of the thumbs are brought much closer together to lie directly above the thumb tips. The physiotherapist's shoulders and arms, with slightly flexed elbows, should be in the direct line through which the pressure is to be applied, and this is at right angles to the plane of the body surface.

Because of the curve of the thoracic spine, it is necessary when mobilizing the upper levels (T1–4) to stand either at the patient's head or towards the shoulder of the side being mobilized to accommodate the necessarily altered angle of the physiotherapist's arms. It is advisable to use the largest amount of the pad of the thumb that can be brought into contact with the transverse process, to enable the pressure to be administered as comfortably as possible (Fig. 5.31).

Method

A very steady application of pressure is necessary to be able to move some of the muscle belly out of the way and make bone-to-bone contact. As this

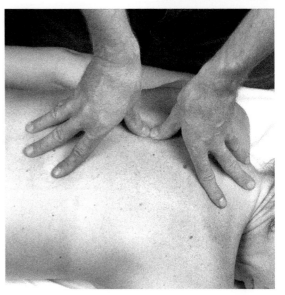

Figure 5.31 • Thoracic region. Posteroanterior unilateral vertebral pressure ↓↱.

procedure can be quite uncomfortable for the patient, care must be given to the position of the arms and hands to enable a spring-like action to take place at the elbows and the thumbs. This reduces the feeling of hardness and soreness between the physiotherapist's thumbs and the patient's transverse process that is present if the pressure is applied by intrinsic muscle action.

Once the required depth has been reached, the oscillating movement at the intervertebral joint is produced by increasing and then decreasing the pressure produced by trunk movement.

Local variations

Because of the structure and attachments of the ribcage, it is not possible to produce very much movement with this mobilization.

Some people may find it easier to carry out the mobilization using the hands (as described for the lumbar spine) instead of the thumbs, but this should be discouraged as the thumbs have a greater degree of 'feel' and can localize the mobilization more accurately. They also cause much less discomfort to the patient – a factor of considerable importance. When the hands are used, the technique is frequently more vigorous than is required.

Uses

Posteroanterior unilateral vertebral pressure is used, almost entirely, for unilateral distributed pain arising

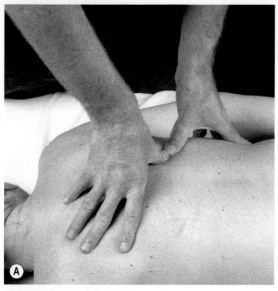 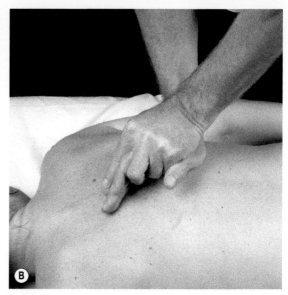

Figure 5.32 • A Posteroanterior unilateral costovertebral pressure using thumb. **B** Posteroanterior unilateral costovertebral pressure using hands ⤵.

from the thoracic spine, and the technique is done on the painful side. Unless the patient's pain is severe, it is less likely to produce a favourable change in the patient's signs and symptoms if it is done on the side away from the pain. When this technique is used in the presence of spasm the pressure must be steadily applied and not hurried, in order to allow time for the spasm to relax.

Posteroanterior unilateral costovertebral pressure (⤵)

Starting position

The patient lies prone with his arms by his side or hanging over the sides of the couch, and the physiotherapist stands at the side of the patient where the mobilization is to be effected. The physiotherapist's thumbs are placed along the line of the rib at its angle so that the maximum area of contact can be made between the thumbs and the rib (Fig. 5.32A). Alternatively, the whole ulnar border of the hand and little finger may be used to produce the movement (Fig. 5.32B).

Method

An oscillatory movement is transmitted to the rib by the thumbs or hands, and the range of movement produced at one rib angle is compared with that produced at the rib angles above and below. The

pain produced by the movement of the faulty rib is also compared with the pain (if any) produced at the rib above and the rib below. Similarly, both the range of the movement and the pain should also be compared with the ribs on the opposite side of the body.

Local variations

First rib. Examination of the first rib is somewhat different from that of the other ribs as the technique can be applied in three ways due to a greater area of the rib being palpable.

1. The pressure can be applied against the rib posteriorly through the trapezius muscle, and the direction of the pressure is not only posteroanteriorly but is also inclined towards the feet (Fig. 5.33).

2. Alternatively, the physiotherapist can place her thumbs underneath (anterior to) the muscle belly of the trapezius and the direction of the pressure can be inclined a little more towards the feet as well as being posteroanteriorly directed (Fig. 5.34).

3. For the next technique that mobilizes the first rib, the patient lies supine while the physiotherapist, standing at the patient's shoulder level of the side to be treated, applies the pressure to produce the oscillatory anteroposterior and caudad movement on all

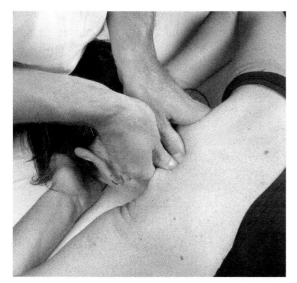

Figure 5.33 • Pressure applied against the first rib posteriorly through the trapezius.

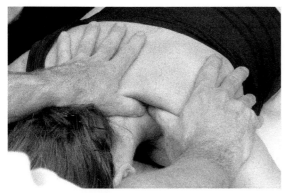

Figure 5.34 • Pressure applied against the first rib posteriorly under the trapezius.

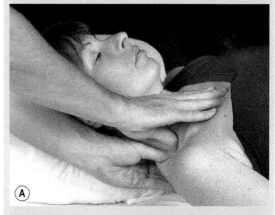

(A)

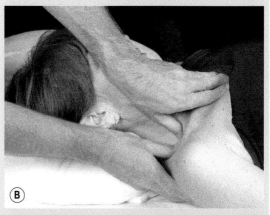

(B)

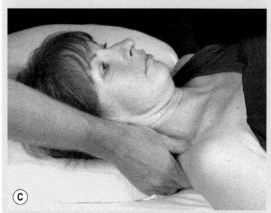

(C)

Figure 5.35 • **A–C** Pressure applied to the first rib anteriorly.

parts of the first rib that are palpable (Fig. 5.35). The symbol for this technique is ⤴ R1.

Other ribs. All of the ribs can be examined throughout their entire length by thumb palpation, including the costochondral junctions and the junction with the sternum. The freedom of movement between adjacent ribs can also be tested, but as these are not part of the vertebral column they are not described in this book. They are, however, described in *Peripheral manipulation* (Maitland 1970).

A technique performed with the patient supine is described below.

Uses

Whenever treatment is applied to the thoracic intervertebral joints, the inclusion of mobilization of the ribs should be considered for two reasons:

1. It is frequently difficult to assess whether a patient's pain arises from the intervertebral joint, the costovertebral joint or the costotransverse joint. Therefore, if mobilization of the thoracic intervertebral joint is not producing adequate improvement when used on a patient, mobilization of the rib at its angle should be added to the intervertebral mobilization.

2. If the rib is moved as a treatment technique, it must also create some movement at the intervertebral joint. This combination may hasten the rate of progress.

If pain is in a referred area of the ribcage, the symptoms may be arising from some abnormality between adjacent ribs. Palpation will reveal abnormalities of position and of movement between adjacent ribs. This aspect of treating costal pain is described in *Peripheral manipulation* (Maitland 1970).

Thoracic spine: rotation to the right (T2–12)

Starting position

The patient lies supine with his arms folded across his chest, resting his hands on the opposite shoulders (Fig. 5.36). The physiotherapist stands on the right-hand side of the patient, taking hold of the left shoulder with the left hand and the left iliac crest with the right hand (Fig. 5.37). The trunk is then rolled towards the therapist so that the left shoulder comes off the couch, exposing the thoracic spine.

The right hand is then placed so that the flexed interphalangeal joint of the thumb is placed over the transverse process of the thoracic vertebrae to be rotated, allowing the fingers to lie across the thoracic spinous process.

The contact hand is positioned in such a way as to allow the thumb to be flexed at the interphalangeal joint and adducted and slightly opposed at the metacarpo-interphalangeal joint so that it lies in contact with the palm of the hand, the proximal phalanx being in line with the index finger.

The index finger of the right hand is placed over the spinous process of the vertebrae being rotated (Fig. 5.38). The patient's trunk is then rolled backwards over the right hand, and the therapist leans over the patient so that the patient's flexed forearms are tucked into the physiotherapist's chest (Fig. 5.39).

Method

The mobilization is then carried out by the physiotherapist rolling the patient's trunk over the right hand. This is done in an oscillating manner.

Mobilization of the ribs (R2–12)

The same position is adopted as above, with the exception that the right hand is placed so that the right flexed thumb is over the angle of the rib, allowing the fingers to be directed towards the thoracic spinous processes. The index finger is in contact with the spinous process of the vertebrae, to whose transverse process the rib is attached (Fig. 5.40).

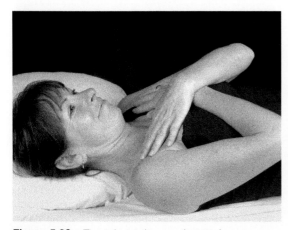

Figure 5.36 • Thoracic rotation – patient supine.

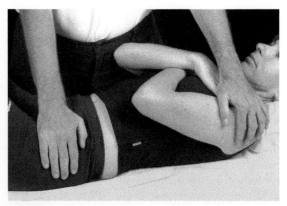

Figure 5.37 • Thoracic rotation – reaching across to hold the patient.

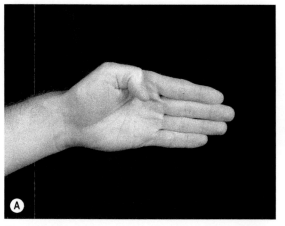
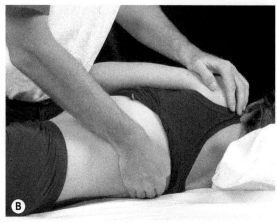

Figure 5.38 • Thoracic rotation. **A** Hand position. **B** Hand position on spine.

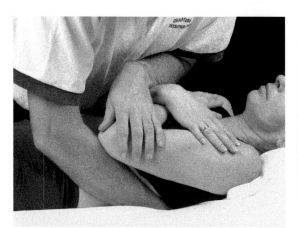

Figure 5.39 • Thoracic rotation. Final starting position.

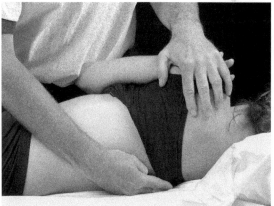

Figure 5.40 • Costovertebral mobilization.

Thoracic traction

An example of treatment is thoracic backache, page 176.

Traction can be administered to the thoracic spine just as readily as it can to the cervical and lumbar areas, and the guiding principles are exactly the same. However, it is true to say that it is less frequently successful than it is in either of the other two areas, and this may be due, at least in part, to the presence of the thoracic cage.

The principle is to position the vertebral column so that the particular joint to be treated is in a relaxed position midway between all ranges. The amount of pressure to be used is guided first by movement of the joint, with further changes in tension made in response to changes in the patient's symptoms as outlined for cervical traction. Further

treatments are guided by changes in symptoms and signs.

Upper thoracic spine (TT ↗)

Starting position

The patient lies on his back with one or two pillows under his head to flex the neck until the intervertebral level to the treated is positioned midway between flexion and extension. A cervical halter is then applied in the same way as has been described for cervical traction in flexion. If a lower level is to be treated and if the strength of the traction needs to be very firm, it may become necessary to apply some form of counter-traction. A belt is fitted around the pelvis and is attached to the foot end of the couch to stabilize the distal end of the vertebral column. The halter is then

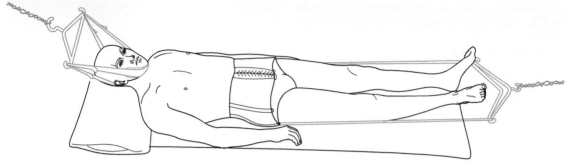

Figure 5.41 • T1–10 traction with counter-resistance (TT ↗).

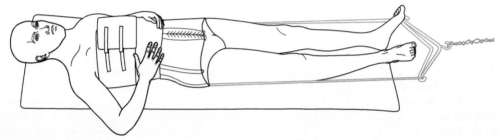

Figure 5.42 • T10–12 traction (TT ⟶).

attached to its fixed point so that the angle of the pull on the neck will be approximately 45° to the horizontal. The actual angle used varies with the amount of kyphosis present in the upper thoracic spine, and it should be an angle that will allow the thoracic intervertebral joint to be moved longitudinally while in a position midway between its limits of flexion and extension. To relieve strain on the patient's lower back during the period when the traction is being applied, his hips and knees may be flexed (Fig. 5.41).

Method

The traction can be adjusted from either end or from both ends, but whichever method is used, care must be taken to ensure that friction between the patient's trunk and the couch is reduced to a minimum. This can be done while the traction is being applied by gently lifting the weight of the patient's thorax or pelvis off the couch and allowing it to relax back into a new position. Friction is almost completely eliminated by a couch whose surface is in two halves that are free to roll longitudinally. Releasing the traction does not present any problem, but it is advisable to release slowly.

Lower thoracic spine (TT ↗)

Starting position

For the lower thoracic spine, a thoracic belt similar to that used for lumbar traction is used in place of the cervical halter. Traction is usually more effective if it is carried out with the patient supine, but it can be done with him prone.

The thoracic belt is applied to hold the chest above the level of the spine to be treated, and it is then attached to its fixed point. After this the pelvic belt is applied and attached to its fixed point. The direction of the pull is then longitudinal in the line of the patient's trunk, but pillows may be needed to adjust the position of the spine so that the joint being moved is relaxed midway between flexion and extension (Fig. 5.42).

Method

Traction is applied from either end or from both ends, but again care is required to reduce friction to a minimum both at thoracic and at pelvic levels. As mentioned previously, a roll-top couch eliminates friction. A simple, cheap and extremely effective roll-top couch is described below.

Releasing the traction should be done steadily, and the patient should rest for a short time before standing.

Intermittent variable traction can also be used in this area of the spine, and the details of times for 'rest' and 'hold' periods are the same as have been discussed for the cervical spine.

Local variations

The thoracic kyphosis varies considerably from person to person, and the positioning of the patient is controlled by this curve. Theoretically, the direction of the pull may be thought of as being at right angles to the upper and lower surfaces of the intervertebral disc at the level that is being moved. The kyphosis usually influences the position for upper thoracic traction more than for the lower thoracic spine.

Precautions

A check must be kept on the patient to ensure that the traction does not cause any low-back pain.

As with the cervical traction in flexion, it is possible for the head halter in upper thoracic traction to cause occipital headache, but this can be eliminated by the means already described.

Uses

Traction is of greatest value in patients who have widely distributed areas of thoracic pain, particularly if they are associated with radiological degenerative changes in the thoracic spine. It is also of value for patients whose thoracic symptoms do not appear to be aggravated by active movements of the spine or when neurological changes are present. Similarly, it is the treatment of choice for patients with severe nerve-root pain. Whenever mobilizing techniques have been used in treatment without achieving the desired result, traction should be tried.

Sometimes a patient is able to guide the therapist as to what to do because his body tells him what it wants (and what it doesn't want). Figure 5.43 is a perfect example of such a case. The patient's disorder had been very difficult to help in that progress gained at a treatment session was not retained well enough. The disorder was at the level of T6/7, and had been responding to extremely gentle traction. One day the patient said that he needed the traction, but he also needed to have the vertebra pushed backwards and towards the left while having the levels above twisted to the right. Figure 5.44 shows how the position was obtained while the mobilizing

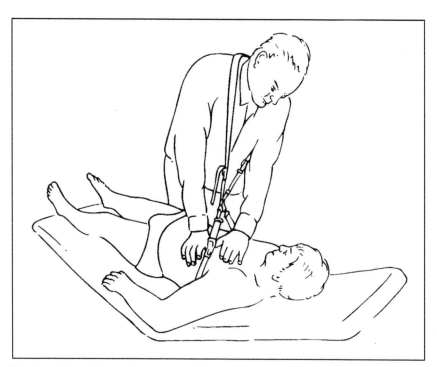

Figure 5.43 • Traction of the mid-thoracic spine combined with localized T6/7 mobilization via the sternum.

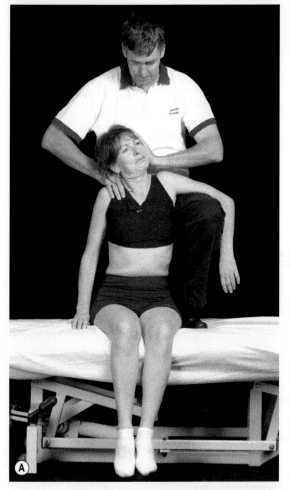

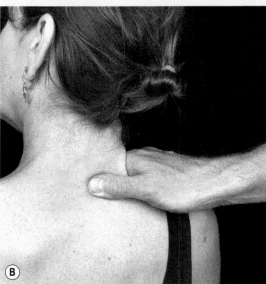

Figure 5.44 ● **A** and **B** Intervertebral joints C7–T3.

was produced through the patient's sternum. He claimed that he was 60% better after the first of these treatments, and 80% better after the second. At his suggestion, treatment was discontinued, and on review 12 months later he showed no signs of recurrence.

Grade V manipulation overview

Evans & Lucas (2010) reviewed the definitions of manipulation in its specific sense as:

> High velocity, low amplitude passive movements that are applied directly to the joint or through leverage.
>
> (CSP 2006)

> A manual procedure that involves a direct thrust to move a joint past the physiological range of motion, without exceeding the anatomical limit.
>
> (Gatterman & Hansen 1994)

The key features of a grade V manipulation technique are:

Action (by the therapist to the patient)

- A force is applied to the patient at a specific joint or spinal segment.
- The direction of force is perpendicular to the surface of the joint.
- The magnitude of this force increases to a peak over a finite period of time (100–200 ms; Herzog 2000).

Mechanical response (occurring within the patient)

- The force applied (100–150N in the cervical spine; Herzog 2000) produces motion at the joint.
- The joint motion always included articular surface separation.
- The velocity of joint motion is variable.
- The sum displacement of the articulating bones is usually zero.
- Cavitations occur within the affected joint (the formation and activity of bubbles or cavities within synovial fluid, formed when tension is applied to the fluid as a result of local reduction in pressure; Evans & Breen 2006).

The clinical prediction rules to identify patients with neck pain likely to respond to thoracic manipulation (Cleland et al. 2007) include:

- Duration of symptoms less than 30 days
- No symptoms distal to the shoulder
- Looking up does not aggravate symptoms
- Fear-avoidance beliefs questionnaire (FABQPA) score less than 12
- Diminished upper thoracic kyphosis
- Cervical extension range less than 30°.

Proposed mechanisms of effect of spinal manipulation (Evans & Breen 2006):

- Mechanical release of entrapped and painful intraarticular material
- Relaxation of hypertonic muscle
- Mechanoreceptor pain gating
- Descending pain suppression
- Stimulus re-interpretation
- Disruption of restrictive articular and periarticular adhesions
- 'Unbuckling' of motion segments.

Clinical reasoning considerations for thoracic spinal manipulation:

Indications

- Is there segmental stiffness, which has not responded to strong mobilization?
- Is there evidence of locked segmental motion with active movement and with passive physiological and accessory movement testing?

Precautions (Maitland 1986)

- Careful and thorough assessment (C/O and P/E).
- Mobilize before manipulation.
- Never manipulate through protective spasm.
- Always inform the patient of your intentions and give them the choice to stop whenever they wish to.
- Avoid repeated manipulations over long periods of time.

Contraindications (Gibbons & Tehan 2001)

Absolute contraindications

- Bone:
  - any pathology that has led to significant bone weakening
  - tumour, e.g. metastatic deposits
  - infection, e.g. tuberculosis
  - metabolic, e.g. osteomalacia

  - congenital, e.g. dysplasia
  - iatrogenic, e.g. long-term steroids
  - inflammatory, e.g. severe rheumatoid arthritis
  - traumatic, e.g. fracture.
- Neurological:
  - cord compression
  - cauda equina compression
  - nerve root compression with increasing neurological deficit.
- Vascular:
  - aortic aneurysm
  - bleeding into joints e.g. severe haemophilia.
- Lack of diagnosis.
- Lack of patient consent.
- Patient positioning cannot be achieved because of pain, resistance, or protective spasm.

Relative contraindications (at risk for adverse reactions)

- Adverse reactions to previous manual therapy
- Disc herniation or prolapse
- Inflammatory arthritides
- Pregnancy
- Spondylosis with osteophytes potentially causing nerve root or vascular compromise
- Spondylolisthesis/instability in the direction of the manipulation
- Osteoporosis
- Anticoagulant or long-term corticosteroid use
- Advanced degenerative joint disease
- Psychological dependency upon high velocity low amplitude (HVLA) thrust techniques
- Ligamentous laxity
- Arterial calcification.

Best practice involves the receiving of informed consent to carry out the intervention and should include information to the patient that clearly explains:

- What the procedure entails
- The known benefits
- The known risks
- Known adverse responses
- Alternative interventions
- Supporting evidence in the literature.

The manipulation procedure should include:

- An attention to detail in per-manipulation screening to establish relevant impairments and limitations.

- Support the decision to manipulate with evidence from the literature on clinical prediction rules, conditions known to respond to manipulation, and features of the clinical presentation which indicate that manipulation will achieve the desired outcome.
- Carry out a risk benefit analysis to ensure there are no structural, pathological or patient consent issues, which may put the patient in danger of adverse response or damage.
- Obtain consent.
- Choose the most appropriate manipulation for the patient and therapist with attention to patient and therapist positioning and localization of forces.
- Carry out any pre-manipulation checks in the pre-manipulation, 'set up' position (that is any evidence of vascular, neurological or other structural compromise and/or patient distress/choice to go no further.
- Perform the action of the thrust to effect localized cavitations wherever possible.
- Re-assess immediately the effects of the manipulation on subjective and objective asterisks.
- Inform the patient of possible treatment soreness.

Principles and guidelines for manipulative thrust of the thoracic spine

As in other areas of the spine, the mobilization techniques described can be performed as very rapid small-amplitude thrusts. These may be general in distribution, covering more than one intervertebral level (as in rotary PAs described on p. 204), or they can be performed in a much more localized manner so that the emphasis of the movement is focused, as much as is possible, on a single intervertebral level. These more localized manipulative techniques are now described for the thoracic spine.

Intervertebral joints C7–T3 (lateral flexion ⌒)

Starting position

The patient sits well back on a medium-height couch while the physiotherapist stands behind. To provide the patient with comfortable support, the physiotherapist places her left foot on the couch

next to the patient's left buttock, rests the patient's left arm over her left thigh, and asks the patient to relax back against her. Localization of the manipulation is achieved by firmly placing the tip of the right thumb against the right side of the spinous process of the lower vertebra of the intervertebral joint. Pressure is applied horizontally in the frontal plane by this thumb, while the fingers spread forward over the patient's right clavicular area. These fingers also stabilize the vertebra. The next step is to flex laterally the patient's head to the right until the tension can be felt at the thumb. While maintaining the lateral flexion tension, the middle position between flexion and extension is found by rocking the neck back and forth on the trunk. After determining this position, rotation (face upwards) is added in small oscillatory movements until the limit of the rotary range is found. The therapist then positions both forearms to work opposite each other (Fig. 5.44).

Method

The manipulation consists of a sudden short-range thrust through the right thumb transversely across the body, while a counter-thrust is given by the operator's left hand against the left side of the patient's head.

Intervertebral joints T3–10 (PAs ↕)

Starting position

The patient lies supine without a pillow and links his hands behind his neck while the physiotherapist stands by his right side. By grasping the patient's left shoulder in her right hand and both elbows in her left hand, the physiotherapist holds the patient in this position; she releases her hold on the shoulder and leans over the patient to palpate for the spinous process of the lower vertebra forming the intervertebral joint being manipulated. Still holding the patient in this position, the physiotherapist makes a fist with the right hand by flexing the middle, ring and little fingers into the palm but leaving the thumb and index finger extended. A small pad of material grasped in the fingers will give added support. This fist is then applied to the patient's spine (the thumb points towards the head) so that the lower spinous process is grasped between the terminal phalanx of the middle finger and the palmar surface of the head of the opposed first metacarpal. The patient is then lowered back until the physiotherapist's right hand is wedged between the patient and the couch. The weight of the patient's trunk is taken on the flat of the dorsum of the hand (not on the knuckles), and the forearm should project laterally to avoid interference with movement of the patient's trunk. If the surface of the couch is too hard, it will be difficult for the physiotherapist to maintain her grip on the spinous process. To achieve firm control of the patient's trunk, his elbows should be held firmly and pressed against the physiotherapist's sternum. However, when a patient has excessively mobile joints it may be necessary for him to grasp his shoulders with opposite hands while keeping the elbows in close apposition rather than clasping the hands behind the neck. The patient's upper trunk is then gently moved back and forth from flexion to extension in decreasing ranges until the stage is reached where the only movement taking place is felt by the underneath hand to be at the intervertebral joint to be manipulated (Fig. 5.45).

Method

Pressure is increased through the patient's elbows, causing stretch at the intervertebral joint, and the manipulation is then carried out by a downward thrust through his elbows in the direction of his upper arms. This thrust is transmitted to the patient's trunk above the underneath hand. The thrust may be given as the patient fully exhales.

Intervertebral joints T3–10 (longitudinal movement ←→)

Starting position

The patient sits well back on the couch and grasps his hands behind his neck, allowing his elbows to drop forwards. The physiotherapist stands behind the patient and threads her arms in front of his axillae to grasp over the dorsum of his wrists. When grasping his wrists, she encourages his elbows to drop forwards while at the same time holding his ribs firmly from each side with her forearms. She then turns her trunk slightly to one side to place her lower ribs against his spine at the level requiring manipulation. While feeling for movement with her ribcage, she flexes and extends his thoracic spine above the level to be manipulated until the neutral position between flexion and extension is found for the joint to be treated (Fig. 5.46).

Method

The physiotherapist lifts the patient's trunk in the direction of the long axis of the joint being treated, and makes a final adjustment of the flexion/extension

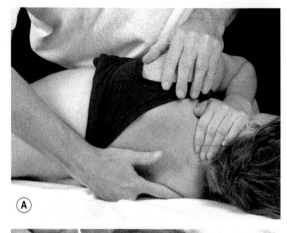

(A)

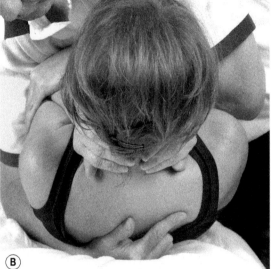

(B)

Figure 5.45 • A and **B** Intervertebral joints T3–10 (Pas ↕).

position to ensure that the mid-position has been retained. The manipulation then consists of a short-amplitude sharp lift.

Some degree of extension may be added into this technique. This extra movement is achieved by a very small movement with the therapist's ribs against the patient's spine, performed at the same time as the lift is executed through the arms.

Intervertebral joints T3–10 (rotation ↺)

Starting position

If rotation to the left is to be performed, the patient sits on the edge of the couch near the right-hand end while the physiotherapist stands behind his right side. The patient hugs his chest with his arms and turns his trunk to the left. For the mid-thoracic area, the physiotherapist reaches with her left arm around his arms to grasp his right shoulder while placing the heel of her right hand along the line of the right rib above the joint to be manipulated. She cradles his left shoulder in her left axilla (Fig. 5.47A). For the lower thoracic levels, she grasps around his chest under his arms to reach his scapula.

This time she places the ulnar border of her right hand along the line of the ribs (Fig. 5.47B). With both techniques she then takes the movement to the limit of the range, taking up all slack.

Method

The manipulation consists of a synchronous movement of the physiotherapist's trunk and an extra pressure through her right hand. With her trunk she carries out an oscillatory rotation back and forth at the limit of the rotary range. At the same time she maintains constant pressure with either the heel of her right hand or its ulnar border exerting an extra rotary push at the limit of the rotation. The manipulation consists of an over-pressure at the limit of the range, being done in a very small amplitude and very sharply.

Additional examination and treatment techniques for thoracic disorders

Cervical anteroposterior unilateral vertebral pressure (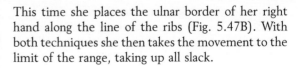)

Starting position

The patient lies supine. A pillow is not used unless the patient has a 'poking-chin' postural abnormality. The physiotherapist stands by his head and makes

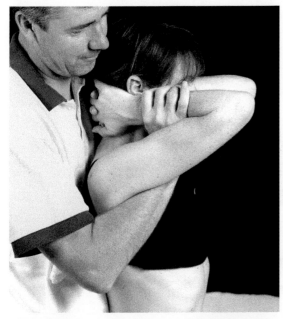

Figure 5.46 • Intervertebral joints. T3–T10 (longitudinal movement).

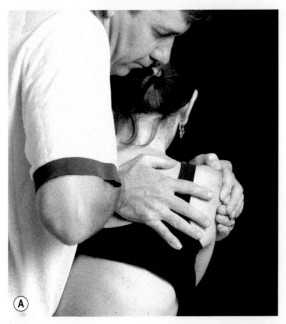

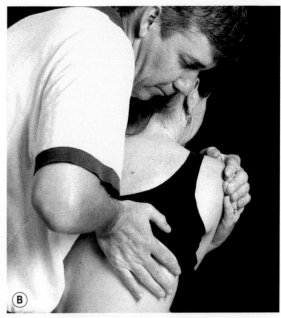

(A)   (B)

Figure 5.47 • Intervertebral joints. T3–10 (rotation). **A** Mid-thoracic area. **B** Lower thoracic area.

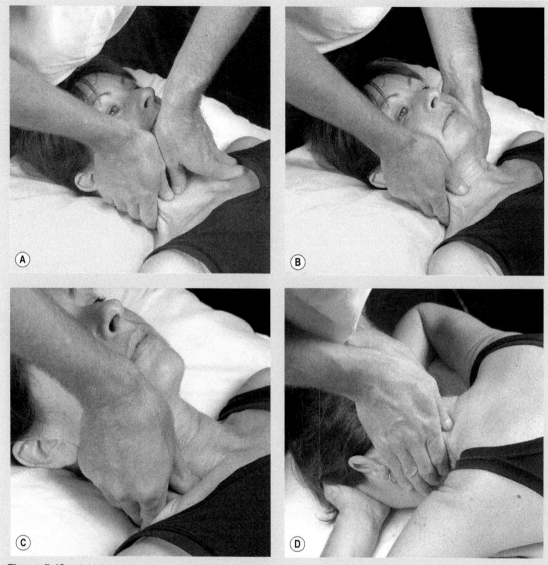

Figure 5.48 • **A** Unilateral anteroposterior vertebral pressure. **B** Bilateral anteroposterior vertebral pressure.
C Anteroposterior unilateral vertebral pressure in upper thoracic area. **D** Anteroposterior unilateral vertebral pressure.

a broad contact medial to the transverse process of the vertebra to be mobilized with both thumbs. The thumbs should be used with care, as direct bone-to-bone contact can be uncomfortable. She spreads her fingers around the adjacent neck area for stability while positioning her shoulders above the joint being treated (Fig. 5.48A).

Method

The oscillatory anteroposterior pressures are performed very gently, and the movement must be produced by the physiotherapist's arms and trunk. Any effort to produce the movement with intrinsic thenar muscle action will produce discomfort immediately.

This technique is not a comfortable one to use unless great care is taken. Also, the muscles lying over the area make direct contact rather difficult, and care should be taken to see that the thumbs are positioned medial to the transverse process. This means that at some levels the muscle belly needs to be moved to one side.

Local variations

This technique can be performed either unilaterally or bilaterally, as is shown in the diagrams (Fig. 5.48A and 5.48B). The intervertebral level to which one can reach varies enormously from patient to patient. In the stocky, heavily built patient with a short, thick neck, extending down into the thoracic area is almost impossible. Conversely, in the long-necked, slim person enough space is allowed to reach down to approximately T3 (Fig. 5.48C). With all patients, the technique can be used as high as C1.

Anteroposterior movement can be produced with the patient lying prone. The patient rests his forehead in his palms, and the physiotherapist grasps around the sides of the neck to hook the palmar surface of the pads of her fingers medial to the transverse process area. It is easy to localize the joint to be mobilized by the accurate placement of the fingers (Fig. 5.48D).

Precautions

The only precaution necessary is to avoid discomfort from undue pressure.

Uses

Application of this technique is reserved for patients whose symptoms, felt anterolaterally, can be reproduced by anteroposterior pressure on the side of the pain. Pain referred to the ear or throat can often be reproduced by this technique. Anterior shoulder pain, scapula pain (Cloward 1959) and headache associated with irritation of the stellate ganglia of the sympathetic chain may also be reproduced by this technique. Under all these circumstances, the described technique could be the treatment of choice.

Slump test

The test is called the slump test for two reasons. The first is that when the patient is sitting and the examiner wants him to adopt the position described below (point 2), most patients respond accurately and quickly to the instruction to slump. The second reason is that the action of adopting the test position parallels a test used by architects and engineers for assessing the consistency of wet concrete, which is also called the slump test.

With the patient sitting on the examination couch, the therapist proceeds as follows:

1. The patient is asked to sit well back until the posterior knee area is wedged against the edge

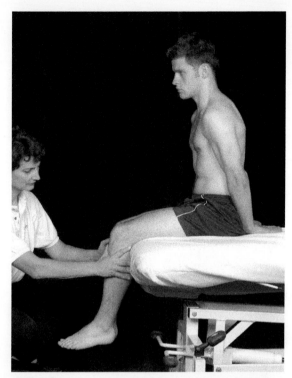

Figure 5.49 ● The slump test: pain response while sitting well back.

of the examination couch so that uniformity of the test position is maintained. In this erect sitting position, he is asked to report any pain or discomfort (Fig. 5.49).

2. He is then asked to let his back slump through its full range of thoracic and lumbar flexion, while at the same time preventing his head and neck from flexing. Once he is in this position, gentle over-pressure is applied to the shoulder area to stretch the thoracic and lumbar spines into full flexion. The direction of pressure is a straight line from T1 to the ischial tuberosities, as though increasing the convexity of a bow by shortening its string (Fig. 5.50). Any hip extension that might take place, as would be the case if the convexity increased markedly, must be prevented by bringing the patient's shoulders closer to his knees. Any pain response in this position is noted (Fig. 5.51).

3. Having established a 90° hip flexion angle he is asked to flex his head and neck fully, approximating his chin to his sternum. Sufficient over-pressure is applied to the neck flexion position to ensure that the whole spine

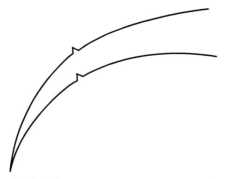

Figure 5.50 • Effect of over-pressure on spine during slump test.

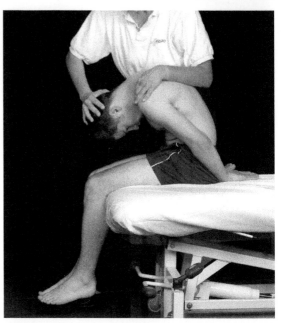

Figure 5.52 • Fully flexed spine, from head to sacrum.

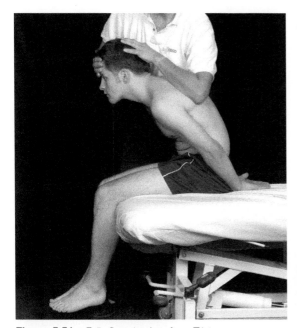

Figure 5.51 • Fully flexed spine, from T1 to sacrum.

from head to ischial tuberosities is on equal stretch. The range with pain response is recorded (Fig. 5.52). Next, the over-pressure maintaining the head and neck flexion is maintained by the physiotherapist's chin (Fig. 5.53) and then her left hand is free to palpate his spine (Fig. 5.54).

4. With the whole spine maintained in flexion with over-pressure, he is asked to extend his left knee as far as possible, and while he is holding it in this position the range and pain response is noted (Fig. 5.55).

5. The next step is to add active dorsiflexion of the ankle to the knee extension and note the pain response (Fig. 5.56).

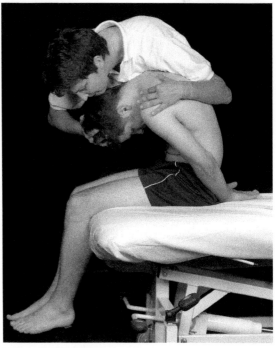

Figure 5.53 • Maintenance of over-pressure with physiotherapist's chin.

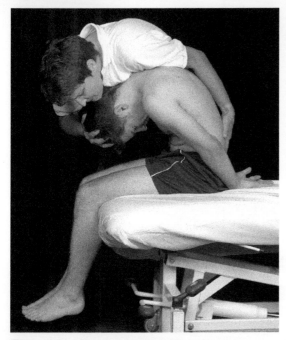

Figure 5.54 • Palpation of spine while maintaining over-pressure at the cervical spine.

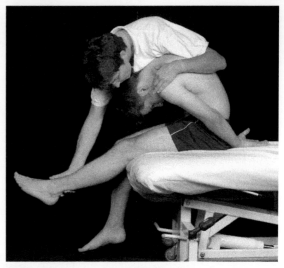

Figure 5.55 • Knee extension with entire spine under over-pressure during slump test.

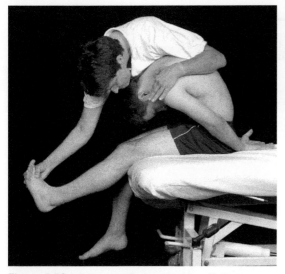

Figure 5.56 • Active dorsiflexion of ankle, with knee extension and spine over-pressure.

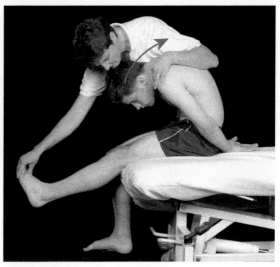

Figure 5.57 • Raising of neck to neutral position in slump test.

6. While the neck flexion to knee extension position is maintained, and being sure that the symptoms are stable and consistent, the physiotherapist retains the same over-pressure to thoracic and lumbar flexion while at the same time releasing some of the neck flexion, allowing the patient's head to be raised to the neutral position (Fig. 5.57) or extended (Fig. 5.58). He is asked to state clearly what happens to the symptoms. In the fully slumped position he may not have a full range of knee extension. If he is unable to extend his knee fully he i s then asked, when neck flexion has been released, if he can extend his knee further. In this new position the range is noted and any pain response recorded (Fig. 5.59).

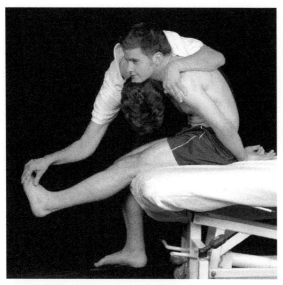

Figure 5.58 • Head and neck extended in slump test.

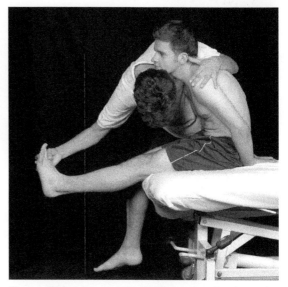

Figure 5.59 • Assessment of further knee extension and ankle dorsiflexion with head and neck extended.

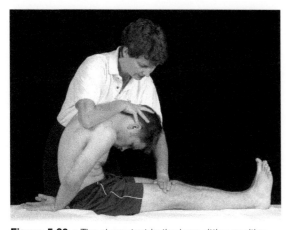

Figure 5.60 • The slump test in the long-sitting position.

This test is effective for all levels of the spine, and should form part of the examination for cervical disorders just as much as for lumbar disorders. When firmer over-pressure is required for the assessment, the procedure can be carried out in the long-sitting position – that is, with the patient sitting on the couch with his legs stretched straight in front of him (Fig. 5.60).

In making a judgement as to the findings of the test, *the pain responses, particularly in relation to releasing the neck flexion component, are the most important.* A pain-free lack of 30° of knee extension can be normal, as can pain felt centrally at the T9, T10 level (Maitland 1980).

An immediate relief of the symptoms on releasing neck flexion indicates involvement of the canal's pain-sensitive structures and, although there may be some restriction of knee extension due to hamstring tightness, this range would be unaffected by releasing the neck flexion. Having extended the cervical spine, which slackens the canal structures, the patient may then be able to gain further extension of the knees. Again, this clarifies the extent to which hamstring tightness is restricting knee extension. There may be some hamstring restriction as well as a canal component to a patient's symptoms. With a patient who is generally very mobile, it is necessary to reach full flexion by getting his head down between his knees. If he is very stiff, this will not be possible and one can expect the canal structures also to be tight. This is seen in people who can, on flexion in standing, hardly reach their knees (they may even comment that at junior school they had difficulty touching their toes), and this stiffness will remain regardless of their exercising. If the source of this restriction is neural, cervical flexion and extension will change the symptomatic response, while in the flexed position. Although some people cannot fully straighten their knees in the slumped position, it does not mean that the range is abnormal; it may be normal *for them*. It is the pain response and the change in knee extension with the release of neck flexion that is important.

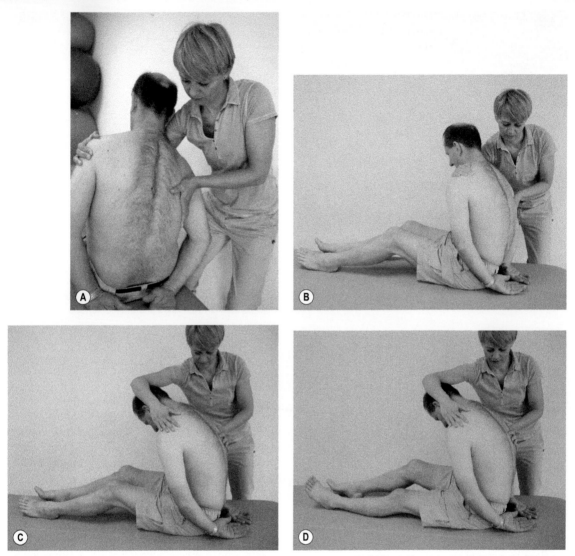

Figure 5.61 • The slump long sitting technique with sympathetic emphasis (SLSSE). **A** Thoracic sideflexion right. **B** Add rotation right. **C** Add neck flexion. **D** Patient actively extends one knee then the other knee.

The long sitting slump technique can be adapted further to include a sympathetic emphasis. Sympathetic chain emphasis is produced by the addition of contralateral trunk lateral flexion with the patient in the long sitting slump position. The therapist can help the patient to maintain this position as they actively bend and straighten their knee or flex and extend their cervical spine to effect reproduction of symptoms or neural mobilization. Additionally, with the patient in the SLSSE, as described above, the therapists hand can be placed against offending rib(s). The rib(s) can then be mobilized using direct

pressure against them and to reproduce symptoms (see Figs 5.60 & 5.61).

PKB/Slump

Starting position

The patient is positioned in side lying, trunk parallel to the edge of the bed, the leg to be tested in hip extension and knee flexion, the other leg being held by the patient in 90° of hip and knee flexion.

The therapist stands behind the patient level with the pelvis. With one hand the therapist stabilizes the

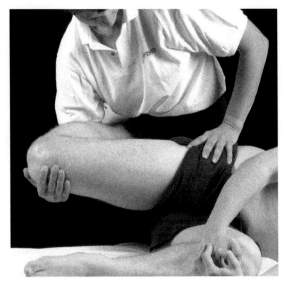

Figure 5.62 • Slump in side lying. Reproduced from Banks & Hengeveld (2010) with permission from Elsevier.

patient's pelvis to prevent lumbar extension. The therapists other hand supports the patient's knee and lower leg (Fig. 5.62).

Method

Whilst stabilizing the patient's pelvis, the therapist extends the patient's hip to pain or limit and then adds medial rotation of the hip to pain or limit to tension the ilio-inguinal (and genitofemoral) nerve(s).

A change in the patient's symptoms and range of hip medial rotation with the addition and subtraction of cervical flexion will indicate involvement of the ilio-inguinal (genitofemoral) nerve (s) in the symptom response.

Straight leg raising (SLR)

Starting position

The patient lies supine towards the side of the bed to be tested.

The therapist stands by the side of the patient at the level of the patient's knee, facing the patient's head. One of the therapist's hands keeps the knee in full extension whilst the other supports under the patient's heel.

Method

The therapist then lifts the patient's straight leg with the hip in neutral adduction/abduction and

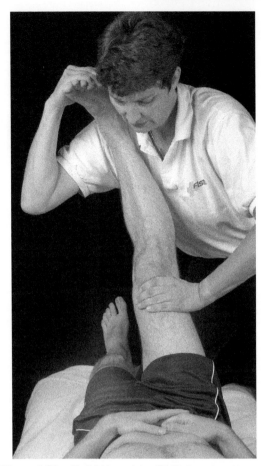

Figure 5.63 • Straight leg raising (SLR). Reproduced from Banks & Hengeveld (2010) with permission from Elsevier.

neutral rotation with the foot relaxed. On reaching the point of onset of back or thoracic pain or the limit of SLR, the patient's leg is then rested on the therapist's shoulder. The therapist then dorsiflexes the patient's ankle. A change in back or thoracic pain with this manoeuvre of the foot will support the hypothesis that neural tissue is involved in the symptom response (Fig. 5.63).

Anteroposterior sternochondral/costochondral joint mobilization

Starting position

The patient lies supine near the edge of the bed on the side to be treated. The therapist stands by the side of the bed at the level of the sternochondral/costochondral joint to be mobilized. The therapist's

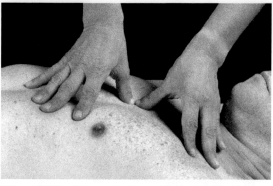

thumbs are placed adjacent to each other across the line of the sternochondral/costochondral joint. The therapist's fingers spread out over the chest for added stability.

Method

The therapist leans over the patient. The therapist's elbows are slightly bent and tucked in. The therapist's body produces the movement through the therapist's thumbs to the joint (Fig. 5.64).

Figure 5.64 • Anteroposterior costal movement.
Reproduced from Banks & Hengeveld (2010) with permission from Elsevier.

References

Banks K, Hengeveld E: *Maitland's Clinical companion: an essential guide for students*, Edinburgh, 2010, Churchill Livingstone.

Berglund KM, Persson B, Denison E: Prevalence of pain and dysfunction in the cervical and thoracic spine in persons with and without lateral elbow pain, *Man Ther* 13:285–299, 2008.

Boyles R, Ritland B, Miracle B, et al: The short term effects of thoracic spine thrust manipulation on patients with shoulder impingement syndrome, *Man Ther* 14:375–380, 2009.

Briggs A, Smith A, Straker L, et al: Thoracic spine pain in the general population: prevalence, incidence and associated factors in children, adolescents and adults. A systematic review, *BMC Musculoskelet Disord* 10(77):1–12, 2009a.

Briggs A, Bragge P, Smith A, et al: Prevalence and associated factors for thoracic spine pain in the working population: a literature review, *J Occup Health* 51:177–192, 2009b.

Butler D: *The sensitive nervous system*, Adelaide, 2000, NOI Group.

Cleland J, Childs J, McRae M, et al: Immediate effects of thoracic manipulation in patients with neck pain: a randomized clinical trial, *Man Ther* 10:127–135, 2005.

Cleland J, Childs J, Fritz J, et al: Development of a clinical prediction rule for guiding treatment of a subgroup of patients with neck pain: use of thoracic manipulation, exercise and patient education, *Phys Ther* 87(1):9–23, 2007.

Cleland J, Durall C, Scott S: Effects of slump long sitting on peripheral sudomotor and vasomotor function: a pilot study, *J Man Manip Ther* 10(2):67–75, 2002.

Cleland J, McRae M: Complex regional pain syndrome 1: management through the use of vertebral and sympathetic trunk mobilisation, *J Man Manip Ther* 10(4):188–199, 2002.

Cloward R: 'Cervical discography: a contribution to the etiology and mechanism of neck, shoulder and arm pain', *Ann Surg* 150:1052, 1959.

Conroy J, Schneider A: Case report: the T4 syndrome, *Man Ther* 10(4):292–296, 2005.

CSP: Definition of manipulation, *Chartered Society of Physiotherapy* 2006.

Edmondston S, Singer K: Thoracic spine: anatomical and biomechanical considerations for manual therapy, *Man Ther* 2(3):132–143, 1997.

Evans P: The T4 Syndrome. Some basic science aspects, *Physiotherapy* 83(4):186–189, 1997.

Evans D, Breen A: A biomechanical model for mechanically efficient cavitation produced during spinal manipulation: pre-thrust position and neutral zone, *J Manipulative Physiol Ther* 29(1):72–82, 2006.

Evans D, Lucas N: What is 'manipulation'? A reappraisal, *Man Ther* 15:286–291, 2010.

Fruth S: Differential diagnosis and treatment in a patient with posterior upper thoracic pain, *Phys Ther* 86(2):254–268, 2006.

Gatterman M, Hansen D: The development of chiropractic nomenclature through consensus, *J Manipulative Physiol Ther* 17(5):302–309, 1994.

Gibbons T, Tehan P: Patient positioning and spinal locking for lumbar spine rotation manipulation, *Man Ther* 6(3):130–138, 2001.

Gilmore O: Gilmore's groin, *Physiotherapy in Sport* XVIII(1): 14–15, 1995.

Goodman C, Snyder T: *Differential diagnosis in physical therapy*, ed 2, Philadelphia, 1995, WB Saunders.

Greene G: Red flags: essential factors in recognizing serious spinal pathology, *Man Ther* 6(4):253–255, 2001.

Herzog W: *Clinical biomechanics of spinal manipulation*, New York, 2000, Churchill Livingstone.

Jowsey P, Perry J: Sympathetic nervous system effects in the hand following a grade III posteroanterior rotatory mobilisation technique applied to T4: a randomised, placebo-controlled trial, *Man Ther* 15: 248–253, 2009.

Keer R: Abstract: Effects of passive joint mobilisation in the mid-thoracic spine on straight leg raising in patients with low back pain, *Physiotherapy* 79(2):86, 1993.

Lau H, Chui T, Lam T: The effectiveness of thoracic

manipulation on patients with chronic mechanical neck pain – A randomised controlled trial, *Man Ther* 16:141–147, 2011.

Maitland G: *Peripheral manipulation*, Upper Saddle River, NJ, 1970, Prentice Hall.

Maitland G: Movements of the pain-sensitive structures in the vertebral canal in a group of physiotherapy students, *S Afr J Physiother* 36:4–12, 1980.

Maitland G: *Vertebral manipulation*, ed 5, Oxford, 1986, Butterworth Heinemann.

Maitland G, Hengeveld E, Banks K, et al: *Maitland's Vertebral manipulation*, ed 7. Edinburgh, 2005, Butterworth Heinemann Elsevier.

Michael A, Newman J, Rao A: The assessment of thoracic pain, *Orthopaedics and Trauma* 24(1): 63–73, 2009.

Strunce J, Walker M, Boyles R, et al: The immediate effects of thoracic spine and rib manipulation on subjects with primary complaints of shoulder pain, *J Man Manip Ther* 17(4):230–236, 2009.

Management of lumbar spine disorders

6

Elly Hengeveld   Kevin Banks

CHAPTER CONTENTS

Introduction 228

Demedicalization and the conceptualization
of non-specific low back pain (NSLBP) 229

Scope of practice of physiotherapists with
regard to NSLBP 234

Clinical reasoning. 244

Examination of the lumbar spine:
subjective examination 255

Physical examination. 269

Treatment 308

Case studies. 320

Key words

Demedicalization, non-specific low back pain,
lumbago, competencies, hypothesis, prognosis, best
practice

Introduction

Low back pain is characterized by pain and discomfort localized below the costal margin and above the inferior gluteal fold, with or without leg pain (Burton et al. 2009). Low back pain is a part of everyday life in Western industrialized countries and will affect 80% of all adults in their lifetime (Nachemson &

Jonsonn 2000). Acute low back pain normally settles within 4–6 weeks, but the majority of people often will experience recurrence at some time or other (Burton et al. 2009). In a small percentage of cases pain becomes persistent and impacts significantly on healthy living and health care costs (Burton et al. 2009).

Although the latter may seem a relatively small percentage, the prevalence of chronic disability due to (non-specific) low back pain (NSLBP) increased significantly in Western industrialized countries in the last two decades of the 20th century. This has led to a discussion on the basic assumptions and paradigms regarding causes of the pain and disability, treatment and research involved (Borkan et al.1998, Waddell 2004) and to the development of programmes to the secondary prevention of chronic disability due to low back pain.

If serious pathologies, such as cancer, fractures, visceral pathologies, systemic inflammation, infection or severe neurological deficits can be ruled out as a source of the pain, it has been suggested NSLBP should be de-medicalized and patients' complaints should be grouped according to symptoms into four categories (see Table 6.1; International Paris Task Force on Back Pain: Abenhaim et al. 2000).

Several guidelines have been developed over the years (Airaksinen et al. 2004, Van Tulder et al. 2006, Vleeming et al. 2008), in which it has been recommended to stay as active as possible and to reduce rest or bed rest to a minimum (Abenhaim et al. 2000). The role of physiotherapeutic care has been discussed in relatively broad terms, but without detailed description and recommendation of the

Table 6.1 Abenhaim et al. (2000) defined four categories of non-specific low back pain based on patients' complaints. Recommendations have been given for the treatment of the different categories

1. Low back pain, with no radiation
2. Low back pain radiating no further than the knee
3. Low back back radiating further than the knee, with no neurological signs
4. Low back pain radiating to entire leg dermatome with or without neurological signs

kind of passive movements and exercises in acute, subacute and chronic phases of NLSBP. Nevertheless, the Paris Task Force on Low Back Pain suggests in subacute intermittent and recurrent low back pain to encourage patients to follow an active exercise programme, as well as in chronic low back pain to perform physical, therapeutic or recreational exercises (Abenhaim et al. 2000). Furthermore, the Paris Task Force concludes that scientific evidence exists in favour of strength training, stretching and fitness, which must be based on a medical assessment by a competent professional and on the patient's compliance to the prescribed course of action (Abenhaim et al. 2000, p.3S).

Demedicalization and conceptualization of NSLBP

Demedicalization

Sheehan (2010), among others, recognized the need to de-medicalize low back pain and emphasized the need for such a condition to be managed in the community rather than hospitals. Waddell (2004) recognized the inadequacies of a back pain revolution driven by the biomedical model of diagnosis and treatment. Waddell also made the medical communities aware of the consequences of medicalization of low back pain and its psycho-socioeconomic impact on Western industrialized populations. He suggested following a bio-psychosocial paradigm in the management of low back pain disorders (Waddell 1987). Chronic NSLBP is associated with a combination of physical, cognitive, social, behavioural, life style and neurophysiological factors. The latter with changes in processes of the peripheral and

central nervous system. Taken these factors together, they have the potential to maladaptive cognitive behaviours (as fear avoidance, catastrophizing, unfavourable beliefs), pain behaviours (as communication and avoidance), and movement behaviours, leading to a vicious circle of ongoing pain sensitization and disability (O'Sullivan 2011).

Burton et al. (2009) recommended that the focus of prevention and management of NSLBP is directed towards physical activity and education. National strategies on prevention and management of low back pain have also placed conservative measures at the forefront of policy (Briggs & Buchbinder 2009, NICE 2009). Briggs & Buchbinder (2009) also recognized that the most important aspect of low back pain lays in its consequences rather than in the mere the fact that it exists. NICE (2009) highlights the need for individualized, patient-centred, needs-based management of NSLBP.

Policy makers therefore need to re-think what de-medicalization means to health care professions, to individual people, to populations, particularly in Western industrialized countries and to societies as a whole. Furthermore, it seems necessary to analyze those factors contributing to NSLBP and disability and conceptualize them in subgroups for treatment and better-aimed research efforts (Kent et al. 2009a).

One may learn from history how to approach such a dilemma in relation to health care, healthy living, promotion of healthy life expectancy as well as the financial and governmental consequences of low back pain in society. Low back pain was formally known as 'lumbago' or 'muscular rheumatism' (Gowers 1904). In the modern era lumbago is being used as a partner term for low back pain on many health care web pages. The term lumbago is a term which may suit de-medicalization well. It is non-threatening and places the condition in its true context of non-specificity. Compare this with terms like 'slipped disc', 'degenerating vertebrae', 'trapped nerve' etc., which are all terms used specifically for a non-specific condition. The consequences of the term lumbago are also less impacting on the individual. Moseley (2004) demonstrates a strong association between a sense of threat (e.g. knowledge that you have been told you have a crumbling disc) and pain perceptions. The road to de-medicalization is, therefore, in the terminology used. Lumbago seems to be fashionable again as a means of explaining pain experienced between the costal margins and the inferior gluteal folds.

The best way to treat low back pain, as reported by the HEN (Health Evidence Network) associated with WHO/Europe (2000), is:

> ... by staying active, returning to work, and exercising at an appropriate and increasing intensity. Anti-inflammatory and muscle relaxant drugs offer effective pain relief.
>
> (WHO/Europe 2000, p. 1)

And the recognition that:

> Back pain and its consequences are not isolated physical problems, but are associated with social, psychological, and workplace-related factors such as stress, worry, and anxiety; effective prevention and treatment must take these into account. Dealing with this situation can play a decisive role in preventing the development of chronic back pain.
>
> (WHO/Europe 2000, p. 1)

A shift in culture about low back pain therefore needs to continue to evolve. This shift should move away from a reductionist, biomedical model, in which numerous interventionist pathways as medications, radiological examinations, injections and surgical interventions, may heighten patients' expectations and demands, ultimately leading to a dependency upon all different interventions. The alternative model should be based upon the viewpoint that low back pain is a problem of painful movements and movement-sensitivity, even though structural changes and some pathology may be present. In this model it is essential to consider the following aspects:

* Support recovery from injury or strain
* Gradually expose or reintroduce the structures and the patient to loading
* Condition the lumbar spine and associated structures
* Gradually condition to recover capacity and performance
* Use movement as a painkiller-evidence
* Use passive movement to support tissue and cellular function, as well as to introduce sensomotor learning processes towards active movement
* Creating independency and self-advocacy rather that creating dependency.

Policy makers also need to recognize which health care professions are best placed to lead on design of individual exercises and activity programmes and the delivery of non-threatening, de-medicalized information about lumbago and its potential consequences. As stated in an Australia based study, it seems that professions linked to manual therapy more likely connect subgroups of NSLBP to different treatment needs than primary care medical practitioners (Kent et al. 2009b). Health care professions such as physiotherapy are now mature enough to lead on policy supported by medical needs such as prescription medication and diagnostic imaging (rather than the other way round). Physiotherapists are best placed to ensure that individuals who experience lumbago move quickly from health care support back into healthy living. In effect, lumbago has become a public health issue rather than a medical issue.

The route to de-medicalization of NSLBP, therefore, is:

* Health care led supported by medical practitioners, who are skilled in guiding patients towards an active life style
* Early transition from health care needs to healthy living
* An emphasis on management to restore physical capacity and performance with less emphasis on biomedical diagnosis, medication and diagnostic imaging
* Embed the management of low back pain within the public health domain rather than the domain of health services
* Non-specific classification as, for example, using the term lumbago as well as the development of research classifications related to movement capacity and performance to guide research endeavours.

Conceptualization

As discussed in the previous paragraph, it seems necessary to define de-medicalization of NSLBP in greater depth. As a consequence, the conceptualization of the factors contributing to the development and maintenance of NSLBP, including its clinical assessment and treatment, should be investigated. This should be discussed in systematic studies and clinical practice. Also it appears that decisions on a political level are necessary whereby health care professions should play a pivotal role in the prevention and treatment of NSLBP and associated disability.

Some studies have been designed around the question of how clinicians perceive the nature of NSLBP.

Kent et al. (2009a) concluded, based on questionnaire information from 544 attendees at major conferences on low back pain in Europe and Australia, that consensus between different groups of clinicians existed on the following points:

- NSLBP is more likely to be an expression of numerous conditions rather than one single condition. This has implications for systematic studies. Currently many studies include heterogeneous cohorts of persons with NSLBP. Therefore, external validity of the studies suffer and will lead to only limited generalizability to clinical practice.
- Most respondents preferred to sub group NSLBP on the basis of a cluster of symptoms and signs rather than based on patho-anatomic changes.
- Pain, physical impairment (range of movement [ROM], muscle strength), activity (ability to perform activities of daily living e.g. sitting, walking standing, lifting), participation (abilities to perform social roles such as in work, family, hobbies, social contacts) and psychosocial function (e.g. depression, anxiety, coping, fear avoidance beliefs) were considered essential aspects of clinical assessment of the patients concerned and needing different, individualized approaches to treatment.

Furthermore in another Australia based study, it appears that primary clinicians such as manual therapists, chiropractors and osteopaths often link the subgroups to different treatment needs more than to medical practitioners (Kent et al. 2004).

Clinical tip

The authors of this chapter propose that an alternative model of NSLBP should be based upon the viewpoint that low back pain is a problem of painful movements and movement sensitivity, even if at times some structural changes and pathology may be present.

Clinical assessment

The clinical assessment of persons with low back and/or leg pain should encompass various aspects of clinical analysis regarding pathobiological processes, movement analysis and contributing psychosocial factors. Furthermore, the clinician needs to incorporate different paradigms or perspectives in their clinical reasoning processes in order to be able to develop a comprehensive, meaningful, individualized treatment programme for the patient.

If a person presents with low back and/or leg pain, the clinician should consider *all* of the following points:

- The presenting dysfunction, referring to nociceptive pain mechanisms, which are in direct relationship to patho-anatomical and pathophysiological dysfunctions in bodily tissues ('endorgan-dysfunction', Apkarian & Robinson 2010).
- Within this perspective, the clinician is evaluating whether serious pathologies such as cancer, fractures, visceral pathologies, systemic inflammation, infection or severe neurological deficits may be present, which require specialized medical care. If serious pathologies can be ruled out, possible tissue processes may need to be considered as a precaution to (physiotherapeutic) treatment. Additionally, in the absence of contra-indications and precautions to physiotherapeutic treatment, the physiotherapist may have certain structures in mind, which may be contributing to the clinical pattern of the movement disorder of the patient, while considering treatment options (e.g. it may be possible in the treatment of a movement disorder of a person, that physiotherapists select, next to other techniques, rotation of the lumbar spine as a first treatment technique, because of the recognition of a movement disorder based on a discogenic dysfunction).
- If serious pathologies can be ruled out, the central core of clinical assessment should be the analysis of the movement disorder, the movement capacity and the movement potential of the patient (Cott et al. 1995; see also Chapters 1 and 2 of volume 2).
- The movement diagnosis may be expressed in the terms of levels of functioning as described in the International Classification of Functioning, Disabilities and Health (ICF; WHO 2001). Information on the movement capacity and restrictions may be found mainly during the subjective examination and observation of these, while the more specific physical examination procedures will inform the NMS-physiotherapist about the level of local movement (dys)functions (impairments).

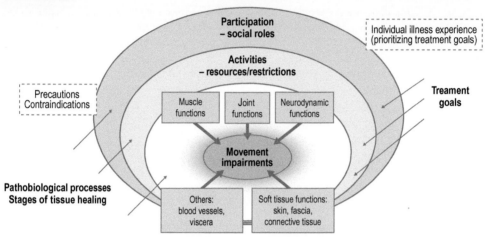

Figure 6.1 • The analysis of movement dysfunctions should incorporate the current movement capacities of a person on function, activity and participation levels as described in the International Classification of Functioning, Disabilities and Health (ICF, WHO 2001). Adapted from Hengeveld (1999) with permission.

- Information regarding movement capacities on the levels of function, activity and participation serves as a basis for the collaborative definition of treatment goals with the patient. Pathobiological processes may define precautions to the therapeutic objectives, while psychosocial aspects of the individual illness experience may be decisive in the treatment priorities and the integration of other therapeutic measures as for example patient education and the development of coping strategies as a means of patient-empowerment (Fig. 6.1).

- Although numerous practice guidelines recommend the assessment of functional activity levels and psychosocial contributing factors, it appears that between various primary care professions considerable difference is present in the utilization of assessment tools and in the focus on activity levels. In a study between physiotherapists, manipulative physiotherapists, osteopaths, chiropractors, general medicine and musculoskeletal medicine it was shown that the assessment of pain and physical impairment, as for example ROM, was a more common denominator between professional disciplines, while activity limitations and psychosocial function were less commonly assessed, with marked differences between groups. It has been recommended to standardize procedures, including the assessment of activity levels and psychosocial factors, as this information may be prognostically important and useful for outcome assessment. Furthermore the information from activity levels and psychosocial factors should aid in the identification of subgroups, requiring different treatment (Kent et al. 2009b)

- In order to enhance standardization in assessment, the International Paris Task Force on Back Pain summarized criteria to assess and decide upon meaningful therapeutic goals regarding optimal mobility and optimal performance of activities of daily living. They are based on selected functional and quality of life indexes, such as The Nottingham Health profile, Health Assessment Questionnaire, Sickness Impact Profile, SF-36, Roland Morris Questionnaire, Oswestry, Quebec Back Pain Disability scale (Quebec Task Force on Spinal Disorders, 1987), Dallas Pain Questionnaire (Abenhaim et al. 2000).

- Criteria for optimal mobility:
  - able to walk for several hours or several kilometres
  - capable of remaining seated for several hours; however, within a lifestyle where sitting is interrupted regularly and preferably where sitting does not occur for the majority of the day
  - able to remain standing for more than 1 hour
  - not having to go to bed or lie down to rest; not having to get out of, or turn over in, bed because of pain
  - capable of climbing several flights of stairs

- able to go down stairs frequently
- able to travel for over 2 hours; able to open a car door; get in and out of cars.
- The criteria of optimal performance of activities of daily living are listed as follows (Abenhaim et al. 2000):
  - lean forward without difficulty; lean over a sink for 10 minutes
  - bend over, kneel and crouch without difficulty; pick up objects from the ground without support
  - get dressed and undressed, putting on socks/ stockings and shoes without difficulty
  - use the toilet
  - wash oneself completely without difficulty, wash one's hair, brush one's teeth, get in and out of the bath tub
  - eat a meal without difficulty
  - run errands without difficulty; pick up bags weighing at least 2 kg without difficulty
  - do housework without difficulty or resting, do the laundry, vacuum, move tables, make the bed, bend over to clean the bathtub, not avoiding heavy housework
  - stretch out one's arm to lift heavy or light objects located on the ground or above one's head; reaching a high shelf; carrying a large valise.

Individualized assessment of persons with low back pain may encompass more activities than the ones listed above; however, it seems appropriate to include questions and observations about these activities in clinical examination procedures.

- Contributing psychosocial factors. Numerous psychosocial factors ('yellow flags') that hinder or enhance complete recovery to full function have been described over the past few decades (Kendall et al. 1997, Watson & Kendall 2000, Waddell 2004). Those hindering recovery have been described in an acronym 'ABCDEFW', which does *not* indicate a ranking in relative importance (Kendall et al. 1997). This list of yellow flags is quite extensive, but in relation to the physiotherapeutic treatment of movement disorders and pain the following psychosocial factors may be conclusive:
  - 'perceived disability'
  - 'beliefs and expectations' with regard to the causes of the problem, as well as the possible treatment options

- confidence in own capabilities to control pain and/or well-being
- sense-of-control over own well-being
- movement behaviour during daily life activities, when the pain occurs
- opinions of other clinicians
- level of activities and participation
- reactions of social environment (boss, spouse, colleagues, friends).

A detailed description of these contributing psychosocial factors can be found in Chapter 8.

The assessment of psychosocial risk factors and resources should be an integral part of the assessment of persons with low back pain as they are mostly expressions of normal human illness experiences and may have a considerable effect on short-term and long-term treatment outcomes. Contrary to some guidelines, they should be taken into consideration within the first encounter with the patient. Particularly a sense of helplessness needs to be addressed early in treatment. An individualized programme of self-management strategies, in which the patient experiences a sense of control over the pain and/or well-being, needs to be incorporated in the initial therapeutic sessions.

Treatment/advice to the patient

The Paris Task Force on Low Back Pain suggested that patients' complaints of NSLBP are categorized into four groups (Table 6.1) and should be differentiated into acute, sub-acute or chronic pain (Abenhaim et al. 2000). They recommend the following approach with regards to bed rest, activity and exercises:

- Acute phase of pain (lasting less than 7 days). Bed rest is contraindicated for the groups 1–3. For group 4, bed rest should only be authorized if the pain indicates it. If bed rest is authorized, it should be intermittent rather than continuous. After 3 days of bed rest the patient should be strongly encouraged to resume their activities.
- In sub-acute phases (lasting between 4 and 12 weeks) and in chronic phases, bed rest is not only contraindicated, but should be stopped in patients still resting in bed at this stage.

The task force did not recommend any exercises or functional restoration for the acute phases of

NSLBP in the first 7 days, but for sub-acute and chronic phases they found sufficient scientific evidence to recommend patients to follow an active exercise programme.

However, the recommendations to the kind of exercises and movement approaches have been kept in general terms, such as strength training, stretching and fitness, in which no movement concept was found to be more superior to another.

Furthermore no distinction seems to be made if the acute pain is of a recurrent nature or occurring for the first time. Recurrences of acute NSLBP and disability need to be prevented (Burton et al. 2009) and the clinician should evaluate in which circumstances recurrences develop, in order to be able to define an adequate individualized (behavioural-) movement therapy programme aimed at the prevention of such episodes.

It is suggested that low back pain should be treated in the primary care setting, with a focus on a concept of reduced activity, rather than resting, recommending patients to stay as active as possible and to take NSAIDs if necessary for a period of 7–10 days, provided that no special 'red flags' indicative of more serious pathology are present (CSAG 1994). In addition, Waddell (2004) suggested examining a patient within 48 hours, treating patients with medication or manipulative therapy and, further, to follow the guidelines of the Clinical Standards Advisory Group (CSAG 1994). However, in a study with audiotaped interviews and questionnaires with 1-month follow-up, Turner et al. (1998) conclude that providers typically addressed medical issues, but did not (or only inconsistently) assess functional limitations related to pain and did not discuss how to resume normal activities, although this was a highly rated goal for most patients. Physicians often did not adequately reassure patients that serious conditions were ruled out, nor did they consistently address worries by the patient. In fact, at times patients felt more insecure about the (self-) management of their problem than before the consultation.

It appears that deliberate measures should be taken by the primary care clinician to provide the patient with a sense of control over the pain. This probably is best obtained within a single session with a specialist of movement rehabilitation and pain management, as for example a physiotherapist specialized in musculoskeletal (MSK) rehabilitation (manipulative physiotherapist).

Referral of patients with acute low back pain

If the pain and disability do not settle as quickly as desired, a second opinion in the primary care setting should be considered. This opinion could be provided by a family doctor with special interest and expertise in back pain or by a physiotherapist, chiropractor or osteopath (Waddell 2004).

If patients, in whom specific pathologies have been ruled out, do not improve and remain off work after 3–6 weeks, they should be referred to rehabilitation services, in which physiotherapy has a key role to play. However, rehabilitation is often only considered after medical treatment is complete or has failed (Waddell 2004). The restoration of movement functions appears to be considered an automatic process, in which patients are expected to resume their normal level of activities and assume their participatory roles in society on their own. Although quite a number of persons with back pain may do so, it is essential to recognize those individuals, who do not resume their normal levels of activity within the expected time of recuperation and to refer them to a physiotherapist.

Only if patients should be investigated and treated for specific pathology should they be referred to specialist services (CSAG 1994). However, Waddell (2004) argues that they should be referred with a clear and explicit goal in mind, being the exclusion of more serious problems, pain control or rehabilitation. The choice of specialist, the facilities they provide and the outcome measures should reflect these goals. As Waddell states: 'there is no point referring a patient to a surgeon and judging success in surgical terms if what the patient really needs is rehabilitation' (p. 444).

The Clinical Guidelines for the Management of Acute Low Back Pain (RCGP 1999) summarize the process of diagnostic triage and referral recommendations, as described in Box 6.1.

Scope of practice of physiotherapists regarding NSLBP

With the conceptualization of NSLBP, physiotherapists may need to (re-)consider their scope of practice, both in the emphasis of clinical work and in the development of subgroups of patient classifications needing different approaches of movement therapy.

Box 6.1

Clinical guidelines for the management of acute low back pain (RCGP 1999)

Diagnostic triage:

- Simple backache (no specialist referral required)
  - Presentation between 20 and 55 years
  - Symptoms in lumbosacral, buttocks, thighs areas
  - 'Mechanical' pain
  - No other problems with general health
- Nerve root pain (usually no specialist referral necessary first 4 weeks, provided the problems resolves)
  - Unilateral leg pain worse than low back pain
  - Radiates to foot or toes
  - Numbness and paraesthesia in same distribution
  - SLR reproduces leg pain
  - Localized neurological signs
- Red flags for possible serious spinal pathology (consider prompt investigation or referral in less than 4 weeks)
  - Presentation under age 20 or onset over 55
  - Non-mechanical pain
  - Thoracic pain
  - Past history of carcinoma, steroids, HIV
  - General health: unwell, weight loss
  - Widespread neurological symptoms or signs
  - Structural deformity

- Cauda equine syndrome (emergency referral)
  - Sphincter disturbance
  - Gait disturbance
  - Saddle anaesthesia
- Assessment
  - Carry out diagnostic triage
  - X-rays are not routinely indicated in simple backache
  - Consider psychosocial yellow flags
- Simple backache – treatment
  - Drug therapy: NSAIDs, avoid strong opoids if possible
  - Do not recommend or use bed rest as a treatment
  - Some patients may be confined to bed for a few days as a consequence of their pain, but this should not be considered as a treatment
  - Advice on staying active as possible, continue normal daily life activities, advice to increase physical activities progressively over a few days or weeks. This includes work: returning to work as soon as possible
  - Consider manipulative treatment for patients who need additional help with pain relief or failing to return to normal activities
  - Referral for reactivation/rehabilitation should be considered for patients who have not returned to ordinary activities and work by 6 weeks

Pillars of physiotherapy practice

It is essential that physiotherapists remain aware of the overall scope of their profession and the possibilities it offers in treating patients suffering from pain, and to not reduce their work to active exercises aimed at muscle strengthening, stretching or general fitness, just because many reviews have qualified studies of these aspects of human movement therapies as acceptable evidence.

In the UK the scope of practice of physiotherapists is defined by four pillars of practice and the fostering and development of such being massage, exercise and movement, electrotherapy and kindred methods of treatment (Chartered Society of Physiotherapy 2008). As stated in numerous places in this book, there is ample evidence for passive movement, therapeutic touch and physical applications being equivalent to active therapies, and in certain cases it even may be better to start with these treatment forms before embarking on an active movement programme. In relation to low back pain, evidence suggests that the following should be included in the current best practice for the management of NSLBP:

- Staying active and work productive
- Engaging in physical activity and exercise
- Being informed and educated about low back pain in a non-threatening way
- Simple analgesic and NSAID support
- Timely manipulation and acupuncture (NICE 2009).

All these recommendations (apart from prescribing, which is an extended scope practice) fall within the four pillars of practice.

Paradigms

Furthermore, it is important to note that every intervention aimed at anatomical structures or to enhance movement will also influence emotional or other aspects of a person.

In a discussion on paradigms, Coaz (1993) argues that physiotherapists may implicitly be working within a bio-psychosocial paradigm, although their explicit viewpoint may be a biomedical one. He states that the perspective of the average physiotherapist and especially of manual therapists is focused on bones, muscles, connective tissue and sometimes on circulatory problems in which emotional dimensions hardly reach the awareness of the physiotherapist. However, Coaz (1993) argues that physiotherapists:

> ... have an access to and influence emotional aspects, even when this does not reach the consciousness of the physiotherapist – and neither the consciousness of the patient. (p. 4)

It seems that since this statement numerous studies have dealt with the bio-psychosocial viewpoints on the physiotherapeutic work. However, it is possible, in spite of the increasing number of studies, that physiotherapists still work more implicitly than explicitly within a bio-psychosocial paradigm (Hengeveld 2001). When the bio-psychosocial effects are being reflected and conceptualized, they can be deliberately integrated in treatment rather than being an implicit, intuitive aspect. In fact, it is recommended that physiotherapists develop a phenomenological viewpoint to their work, in which they guide patients from individual illness experience and illness-behaviour towards an individual sense-of-health and health promoting behaviours with regards to movement functions and general well-being (Hengeveld 2001).

International Federation of Orthopaedic Manipulative Physiotherapists' competencies and scope of practice

Physiotherapists also need to be clear therefore about where their role in the management of low back pain begins and ends. Best practice management of low back pain demands that physiotherapists acquire, foster and develop a broad and deep knowledge and skills clinical framework supported by professional, analytical and reflective attributes (IFOMPT 2008).

The physiotherapists' scope of practice for low back pain should encompass the dimensions and competencies detailed by the International Federation of Orthopaedic Physical Therapists (IFOMPT 2008; see Box 6.2). This should be viewed within the specific context of manipulative and movement therapies related to neuromusculoskeletal low back pain.

Treatment objectives

In the development of treatment, the physiotherapist, in collaboration with the patient, should define short-term and long-term treatment goals, which ideally should lead to optimum movement functions, overall well-being and purposeful actions in daily life, in order to allow the patient to participate in their chosen activities of life (in their roles as spouse, family member, friend; in sports, leisure activities and work).

Sense of control

A core objective of treatment should be at all times to support patients to develop a sense of control over their pain, or, if this seemingly cannot be achieved easily, as in chronic pain, a sense-of well-being in spite of the pain. The process of developing a sense-of control, and with this working on the self-efficacy and internalizing of locus of control with regards to pain, may be well expressed in the following quote:

> One of the main goals of the infant is to try to gain some control over his or her environment. The attempt to reduce uncertainty and establish control seems to be one of the most fundamental human drives. One of the key aspects of personality is the strength of this drive and the balance between our personal needs for control and the needs of others. These beliefs are probably not innate, but more likely a product of learning and social conditioning ...] In rearing children every parent has to find the right balance between affection and nurturing on the one hand, and the imposition of control on the other.[...] Our self-confidence is related in part to the extent to which we have established sufficient control over our environments to meet our needs[...] As a result of this life experience, we all form beliefs about the extent to which we are able to get control of our lives [...].
>
> [...] Gaining control over back pain means actually mastering the pain and associated disability. The ability to do this is largely dependent upon the individual's own judgement of their capabilities.
>
> Waddell 1998, p. 196

Box 6.2

Scope of practice of physiotherapists specialized in MSK-physiotherapy/manipulative physiotherapy as defined by International Federation of Orthopaedic Manipulative Physiotherapists in relation to the work with patients with NSLBP

Critical and evaluative evidence based practice

- The use of evidence to support the use of exercise, manipulative physiotherapy and movement therapies in the management of low back pain
- Systematic reviews, European guidelines, NICE guidelines.

Critical use of a comprehensive knowledge base of the biomedical sciences

- An understanding of how low back can be classified and identified in relation to it being non-specific, specific, e.g. disc nerve route, spondylolisthesis, stenosis, arthropathy and serious pathology (red flags)
- An understanding of differential diagnosis of low back pain and the clinical features of masqueraders
- Options for orthopaedic and medical management of specific low back pain
- Understanding the process of tissue healing and how this can be enhanced (by movement)
- An understanding of triage outside the scope of practice of physiotherapy.

Critical use of a comprehensive knowledge base of the clinical sciences

- Biomechanics and the physical properties of spinal material (Adams & Dolan 2005, McGill 1997)
- Abdominal muscle function and low back pain (Hides et al. 2010)
- The slump and SLR as a reference standard for neurodynamic sensitivity (Walsh & Hall 2009)
- Pain sciences (Butler & Moseley 2003)
- Recognizing pain patterns to identify the source of symptoms (O'Neill et al. 2002)

Critical use of a comprehensive knowledge base of the behavioural sciences and communication

- Cognitive behavioural therapy and low back pain. (Pincus et al. 2002, Johnson et al. 2007b, Bunzli et al. 2011, Nakao et al. 2012)
- Understanding frame of reference in patients with low back pain
- The broader context of consequences (socioeconomic).

Manipulative physiotherapy and movement therapy principles and practice

- The known and proposed effects of mobilization and manipulation, including their indications and contraindications
- Relating manipulative physiotherapy and movement therapy skills to treatment objectives defined by the levels of disability (WHO 2001), to optimize movement potential.

Clinical reasoning and low back pain

See Chapter 2

Clinical expertise

- Advanced level of practical handling skills (sensitivity and specificity), and communication, enabling effective assessment and management of patients with neuromusculoskeletal disorders.
- Critical understanding and application of the process of research
- Commitment to continuous professional development (CPD)

Data from International Federation of Orthopaedic Manipulative Physiotherapists (2008), Banks (2014)

If patients learn self-management strategies, which they can apply easily in daily life, at initial stages of treatment, the confidence to take on activities that they might have believed to be harmful may be enhanced. Therefore self-management strategies play a central role in the secondary prevention of chronic disability due to low back pain. As this relates to changing movement behaviour, altering movement patterns and thought patterns regarding movement and pain, a cognitive behavioural approach to treatment is essential, in which every action such as communication, education, information and touch are applied in a reflected manner. In this context, Fordyce (1982, 1995) suggests focusing on the question why people develop certain kinds of behaviour, rather than primarily asking which nociceptive processes cause the behaviour. A cognitive behavioural attitude, in which it is acknowledged that behaviour does not change overnight, is important in this process. In the development of these self-management strategies, patients may go through different phases of change (Prochaska & DiClemente 1994) before a desired behaviour may be fully integrated in habitual daily life activities.

It is essential that the strategies are simple enough, that they can be applied or adapted directly to daily life situations and that the patient is guided towards a sense of success

Furthermore, to enhance compliance and a sense of success, it is often useful, to provide patients with the possibilities of (telephone) contact, if any queries or insecurities about the self-management strategies would come up, particularly in those cases of an acute phase of (nociceptive) NSLBP, in which a patient is only seen a single time (see also Chapter 8).

Physiotherapists with their specific professional expertise have numerous possibilities to guide patients towards a sense-of-control over their pain or well-being, as for example:

- Repeated movements, often in contrasting direction to the habitual movement patterns (McKenzie 1981)
- Automobilizations, stretching exercises
- Muscle recruitment exercises
- Relaxation strategies
- Pacing strategies in which active and relaxing cycles in daily life follow each other
- Body awareness, including the awareness of thoughts, emotions and behaviours on bodily reactions and pain
- Proprioceptive awareness
- Physical agents, as hot packs, cold packs.

Optimizing movement capacity

Another important goal of treatment is the optimization of the movement capacity of a person. In order to motivate patients towards the normalization and optimization of movement functions and activity, a process of collaborative goal-setting is essential (see Chapter 3). Within this process it is important to recognize the possible barriers to the restoration of full function and to address them in treatment by implementing self-management strategies, educational interventions about neurophysiological pain mechanisms, the role of movement in pain or stress-physiology in an early phase of treatment. Furthermore, also in this phase of treatment, a cognitive-behavioural approach to physiotherapeutic treatment is essential to enhance continuous and profound changes with the patients concerned.

In order to provide a meaningful rehabilitation towards full activity, the subjective and examination procedures should be directed towards questions about restrictions and possibilities of activities and to the establishment of the conditions required to achieve optimum activity levels. The core sets of ICF (Box 6.3; WHO 2001) may be more comprehensive than the activities as outlined by the Paris Task Force on Low Back Pain (Abenhaim et al. 2000). They may aid in the definition of collaborative outcomes and the fostering and development of a public health framework within the physiotherapist's scope of practice.

Psychosocial aspects in treatment

As stated before, treatment will always have psychosocial effects, in one form or another. They may be a part of the implicit, intuitive process; however, there are clinical situations in which a deliberate multidimensional approach to treatment should be taken. In this approach, goals on cognitive, affective and behavioural levels should be defined explicitly next to objectives on the enhancement of movement behaviour and movement capacity. It seems that these factors are first considered when a pain problem has become chronic. However, it may be of use to consider these factors immediately in a first consultation of acute NSLBP, or when a patient is seen for a second session after approximately 7–10 days.

Vlaeyen & Crombez (1999) postulated that a pain experience may change over time. Within 2–4 weeks after an acute nociceptive situation cognitive and affective factors, for example anxiety, helplessness, different cognitions about causes of the problem, and treatment options for the pain, may become important contributing factors in the maintenance of pain, disability and distress. Therefore any concerns a person has because of the pain need to be addressed in the first consultation and creating a climate in which the patient feels they can ask questions or seek advice, even between treatment sessions, may become central in the process of secondary prevention of chronic pain.

It has been recognized that physiotherapists are aware of the need for a more multidimensional approach to treatment – at the latest in the fourth treatment session, once they notice that the patient's reduction of pain and improvement of activity levels have not improved as expected in the prognosis at the first consultation. In fact, discrepancies between pain, disability and the expected time of functional

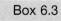

Box 6.3

International Classification of Functioning, Disability and Health (ICF) domains for low back pain

Code	Description	Code	Description
b130	**energy and drive functions**	s1201	spinal nerves
b1300	energy level	**s760**	**structures of the trunk**
b1301	motivation	s7600	structures of the vertebral column
b1302	appetite	s7601	muscles of the trunk
b1303	craving	s7602	ligaments and fascia of the trunk
b1304	impulse control	**s770**	**additional musculoskeletal structures**
b134	**sleep functions**		**related to movement**
b1340	amount of sleep	s7700	bone
b1341	maintenance of sleep	s7701	joints
b1343	quality of sleep	s7702	muscles
b1344	functions involving the sleep cycle	s7703	extraarticular ligaments, retinacula, bursa
b152	**emotional functions**		etc.
b1520	appropriateness of emotions	d240	handling stress and other psychological
b1521	regulation of emotions		demands
b1522	range of emotions	d2400	handling responsibility
b280	**sensation of pain**	d2401	handling stress d2402 handling crisis
b455	**exercise tolerance functions**	**d410**	**changing basic body position**
b4550	general physical endurance	d4100	lying down
b4551	aerobic capacity	d4101	squatting
b4552	fatiguability	d4102	kneeling
b710	**mobility of joint function**	d4103	sitting
b7100	mobility of a single joint	d4104	standing
b7101	mobility of several joints	d4105	bending
b7102	mobility of joints generalized	d4106	shifting body centre of gravity
b715	**stability of joint function**	**d415**	**maintaining a body position**
b7150	stability of a single joint	d4150	maintaining a lying position
b7151	stability of several joints	d4151	maintaining a squatting position
b7152	stability of joints generalized	d4152	maintaining a kneeling position
b730	**muscle power functions**	d4153	maintaining a sitting position
b7300	power of isolated muscles and muscle	d4154	maintaining a standing position
	groups	**d430**	**lifting and carrying objects**
b7301	power of muscles of one limb	d4300	carrying in the hands
b7302	power of muscles of one side of the body	d4301	carrying in the arms
b7303	power of muscles of lower half of body	d4302	carrying on the shoulders, hips, back
b7304	power of muscles of all limbs	d4303	carrying on the head
b7305	power of muscles of trunk	d4304	putting down objects
b7306	power of muscles of the whole body	**d450**	**walking**
b735	**muscle tone functions**	d4500	walking short distances
b7350	tone of isolated muscles and muscle groups	d4501	walking long distances
b7351	tone of muscles of one limb	d4502	walking on different surfaces
b7352	tone of muscles of one side of the body	d4503	walking around obstacles
b7353	tone of muscles of lower half of body	d530	toileting
b7354	tone of muscles of all limbs	d5300	regular urination
b7355	tone of muscles of trunk	d5301	regular defecation
b7356	tone of muscles of the whole body	**d540**	**dressing**
b740	**muscle endurance functions**	d5400	putting on clothes
b7400	endurance of isolated muscles	d5401	taking off clothes
b7401	endurance of muscle groups	d5402	putting on footwear
b7402	endurance of all muscles of the body	d5403	taking off footwear
s120	**spinal cord and related structures**	d5404	choosing appropriate clothing
s1200	structures of the spinal cord	**d640**	**doing housework**

Continued

Box 6.3—cont'd

Code	Description	Code	Description
d6400	washing and drying clothes and garments	**d760**	**family relationships**
d6401	cleaning cooking area and utensils	**d845**	**acquiring and keeping and terminating a job**
d6402	cleaning living area		
d6403	using household appliance	**d850**	**renumerative employment**
d6404	storing daily necessities	**d859**	**work and employment, other specified and unspecified**
d6405	disposing of garbage		

Analysis: The ICF core sets for low back pain (above) have been identified through consensus and form a framework for the assessment, intervention and outcome measurement of patients with low back pain. The categories have been developed as core sets as they reflect the presenting functional difficulties associated with low back pain. Physiotherapist can have confidence that they can assess and measure limitation and restriction of functional capacity of these categories and thus be able to set clear rehabilitation goals in order to restore or maximize physical performance in the life tasks and life areas domains (e.g. independent living, work, recreation, feeling of healthiness and well-being)

b=body functions; s=body structure; d=activity and participation (capacity or performance qualifier).

Stier-Jarmer et al. (2009) identified ICF core sets for low back pain. Personal and environmental mediators for low back pain can be found in the domains of body structure and function (movement impairment), activity limitations and participation (WHO 2001). With permission from World Health Organization.

---

restoration with regard to physiological tissue regeneration appear to be core factors in the determination of a need for a more multidimensional approach to treatment (Hengeveld 2001).

Phases of NSLBP and physiotherapeutic treatment

Maher et al. (1999) suggested physiotherapeutic treatment objectives, which are described in Table 6.2. However, it needs to be noted that defining sub-acute and chronic phases only based on the course of time may be problematic. It is important to know which kind of treatment the patient has received so far. Pain may be persisting because of interventions, which have not been thoroughly reassessed, hence they have not been perceived by the patient as being effective. Some patients may not have had any treatment at all for their problem. Also, generalized exercises, without specific self-management strategies to control pain, may be not effective enough. Furthermore, in some neurogenic pain states, severe pain may last much longer than a more simple nociceptive process. History taking, including exact information on the treatment so far, their immediate effects and a detailed analysis of the self-management strategies (which ones? when are they performed? can they be integrated in daily life? and what are the immediate effects on the pain/well-being?) should be the basis of every physiotherapeutic treatment programme, regardless of the phase in time of the symptoms and signs.

Classifications, subgroups and models

Current best evidence confirms the beneficial effects of movement in the treatment of NSLBP; however, several studies show that no active therapy seems more superior than another. It would be oversimplified to conclude that 'it would not matter what is done'; it appears more likely that different treatment approaches, as for example motor control exercises and graded activity, have similar effects (Macedo et al. 2012). It seems that the quality of, and the therapeutic climate in which, the exercises are implemented is important and that better results are being observed in individualized, supervised exercise programmes (Hayden et al. 2005, O'Sullivan 2011).

In spite of results in favour of individualized, supervised exercises in which therapists may follow their personal preferences, numerous questions should be answered in studies in which a better subgrouping of patients out of the heterogeneous group of NSLBP is undertaken.

Questions that may need to be pursued deeper in systematic study with well-defined subgrouping of the included subjects are:

Table 6.2 Physiotherapeutic activities recommended for the different phases of NSLBP based on an extensive literature review (Maher et al.1999)

Acute (pain< 6/52)	**Advice**
	Encourage normal activity
	Progress activity by time not pain (*or may consider interval activities, in which patients perform self-management strategies to control pain)
	Discourage fear of pain and activity (*by simple educational/information interventions adapted to cognitive level of patient)
	   1. Spinal manipulative therapy
	   2. Repeated (active) movements (McKenzie 1981) (*or other self-management strategies)

Subacute (pain 6/52 – 3/12)	**Supervised exercise programme** Individual, sub-maximal, gradually increased exercise programme to improve the patient's level of function using a cognitive behavioural approach to encourage 'well' behaviours and discourage 'pain' behaviours (* include self-management strategies directly aimed at promotion of well-being) **Advice** Explain benign nature of NSLBP and reassure patient that light activity will not damage their back but will instead enhance recovery Encourage patient to mobilize their spine by light activity and to set their own goals for exercise, encourage gradual return to normal activity (* by giving patient the opportunity to experience these during the therapy sessions, either as an exercise, or in reassessment procedures in which meaningful DLA are being reassessed.) Encourage patient not to be fearful of NSLBP or be over cautious
Chronic (pain > 3/12)	**Supervised exercise programme** Whole body intensive exercise program Quotas of exercise Time and function, not pain contingent (* or, of patient are not willing/capable: interval training with the inclusion of self-management strategies, based on movement and direct bodily relaxation while moving) Reward 'well' behaviours **Functional restoration programme** Comprehensive fitness programme Work stimulation, work hardening (* this includes work in household, garden) Recreational activities e.g. games, swimming Psychological pain management Job acquisition skills
Prevention	**Group fitness classes** Supervised whole body exercise programme including a range of exercises designed to warm up, improve mobility, strengthen muscles and improve cardiovascular fitness. Finish class with 5–10 minutes of relaxation Commitment to do the same at home at least once per week (*include 3–5 ×/week brisk walking for 30 minutes)

*Additional note from the authors of this chapter.

- Which kind of patients react better to individualized, supervised treatment in contrast to group treatment?
- Is it possible that patients with a clear motor deficit respond better to motor control programmes, while persons with higher fear avoidance behaviour and lower fitness levels may react better to a graded activity approach? (Macedo et al. 2012)
- Which group of patients reacts better to spinal manipulative therapy in combination with a certain kind of exercises, or which groups need an approach with repeated movement and which groups would respond more to general bodily awareness and relaxation?
- Which groups of patients may need to be considered more from a perspective of changes in the brain, based on cortical reorganization

and degeneration rather than singled out in subgroups of bio-psychosocial diagnosis and treatment (Wand & O'Connell 2008).

Additionally, with a more complex question into clinicians' attitudes and models: which groups would respond best to an approach in which clinicians apply treatments as usual, but from the perspective of supraspinal (re)learning and reorganization?

Primary research and evaluation of best practice informs physiotherapists about the meaningfulness of their manual examination and intervention methods for low back pain (O'Sullivan 2005, Kamper et al. 2010, Flynn et al. 2002, Smart et al. 2012, Schafer et al. 2011, Slater et al. 2012).Therefore, if treatment based sub-groups could be reliably identified, it would represent an important advance in low back pain treatment and the pursuit of this goal has been identified as a priority for low back pain researchers (Kamper et al. 2010).

The necessity to define subgroups for scientific inquiry and decision-making regarding treatment of low back pain has been increasingly acknowledged in the past two decades. However, Billis et al. (2007) described in a cross-country review in nine countries, that most studies were classified according to patho-anatomic and/or clinical features. Only a few studies utilized a psychosocial and bio-psychosocial approach. They concluded that no internationally established, effective, reliable and valid classification system is available, which incorporates the different subgroups for the definition of valid inclusion-criteria and statistical analysis. McCarthy et al. (2004), based on a literature review with 32 studies, suggest developing an integrated system, which allows for the assessment of NSLBP from biomedical, psychological and social constructs. This viewpoint is shared by Ford and Hahne (2012), who argue that researchers in low back pain need to incorporate both pathobiological and psychosocial perspectives, without emphasizing one model and neglecting the other. Furthermore, they recommend researchers to follow the clinical reasoning of clinician physiotherapists and to develop subgroups, which reflect daily clinical decision-making processes.

Also, various physiotherapists have suggested the development of subgroups based on movement-preferences of patients, with consequences for the selection of active movement therapies based on repeated movements (McKenzie 1981) and motor control exercises (Maluf et al. 2000).

In spite of missing international uniformity, numerous studies have been performed in which different subgroups have been established and which demonstrate the effectiveness of different physiotherapeutic approaches:

In particular, research has investigated sub-groups of patients who are more likely to respond to manual therapy or neural mobilization. The role of motor control strategies based on well developed knowledge have also been shown to influence back pain in many groups of patients (Hodges 2011, Dankaerts & O'Sullivan 2011, Hides et al. 2010, Macedo et al. 2009).

O'Sullivan (2005) has proposed a sub-classification of chronic NSLBP which identifies dysfunction at an impairment level. O'Sullivan is of the opinion that a range of models (Table 6.3), which identify the reasons for chronic low back pain, are needed within a bio-psychosocial framework; however, physiotherapists need to be aware of classifications which link directly to their domain of practice, that is, movement therapies.

Classifying chronic low back pain at an impairment level, O'Sullivan (2005) proposes that particular direction specific provocative spinal postures and

Table 6.3 Models of low back pain classification

Classification model	Clinical application
Patho-anatomical model	Conditions such as protruded intervertebral (IV) disc, spondlolysthesis, stenosis
Neurophysiological model	Cortical disorganization and the pain experience
(Bio)-psychosocial model	The impact of back pain on the individual and in society
Signs and symptoms model	Pain provoked by movement and motion testing
Mechanical loading model	Occupational/postural stresses and ergonomics
Motor control model	Failure in segmental and global motor control
Peripheral pain generator model	Pain generated by the IV disc, facet, sacroiliac joint
Disability model	Movement disorders: impairment, activity andparticipation levels

movement patterns indicate the presence of either movement (restriction) or control impairments. The former being characteristic of restricted movement associated with fear avoidance, anxiety and both peripheral and central neurophysiological sensitization and responding well to manual techniques and active strategies which restore ideal movement and enhance movement conditioning. The latter being characterized by impairment of the motor system such that tissue strain in specific movement directions is not restricted but poorly controlled and responds well to motor control and muscle balance strategies to enhance pain relief and improved function.

In follow-up to these proposals, Dankaerts & O'Sullivan (2011) reviewed randomized control trials evaluating the validity of the motor control impairment sub-classification and note that it is good practice to utilize not only functional activation of the motor system but also cognitive-behaviour strategies to enhance motor control and reduce maladaptive movement.

Slater et al. (2012) carried out a systematic review to investigate the effectiveness of sub-group specific manual therapy for low back pain. Seven studies were identified for their methodological standard, although graded low in quality. The review suggested that there were significant treatment effects when heterogenous sub-groups were identified for intervention using manual therapy compared with pain treatments and activity.

Flynn (2002) provided the clinical prediction rule (CPR; Box 6.4) in the better quality studies (PEDro www.pedro.org.au/) and therefore the basis of the subgroup of patients with low back pain for which manual therapy provides a significant treatment effect.

 Box 6.4

Clinical prediction rule for manual therapy for low back pain

4/5 criteria present to predict a favourable outcome from manual therapy:

- Duration of symptoms ≤16 days
- FABQ work subscale score ≤19
- At least one hip with ≥ 35° of internal rotation
- Hypomobility in the lumbar spine
- No symptoms distal to the knee

(Flynn 2002)

Schafer et al. (2011) carried out an experimental design cohort study on sub-groups of patients with low back pain and leg pain to find out whether pain and disability outcomes differed between these sub-groups following neural mobilization techniques.

Seventy-seven recruited patients were sub-classified following interview and examination by experienced manual therapists. Patients' sub-groups were those classified as:

- Neuropathic sensitization (predominance of parasthesia and dysaesthesia with pin-prick hypo/hyperalgesia)
- Denervation (nerve conduction loss/ neurological deficit)
- Peripheral nerve sensitivity (nerve trunk mechanosensitivity with positive straight leg raise (SLR), PKB and positive nerve palpation)
- Musculoskeletal (the rest with none of the above).

All recruits received seven neural mobilization interventions twice per week that incorporated two passive mobilization techniques. The techniques were a foraminal opening technique (lateral flexion in sidelying), and a neural sliding technique (hip and knee flexion and extension in sidelying).

Outcome measures consisted of a numerical pain rating scale, the Roland Morris disability questionnaire and a global perceived changes scale from 1– 'completely recovered' to 7– 'worse than ever'. Results indicate that patients classified as peripheral nerve sensitivity showed the best outcome scores and a more favourable prognosis.

This study suggests that it is important for physiotherapists to consider the type of presenting neural symptoms in order to apply specific neural mobilization techniques to the most appropriate subgroup of patient for best effect.

Smart et al. (2012), in a cross-sectional trial between subjects, investigated the discriminant validity of a mechanisms-based classification of patients with low back pain (with or without leg pain) by analyzing data on the self-reporting of pain, quality of life, disability and anxiety/depression.

One aim of the study was to improve clinical outcomes by using mechanism-based classifications to help physiotherapists apply appropriate clinical practice approaches. Using interview and examination, patients in the study ($N=464$) were classified into mechanism-based subgroups:

- Nociceptive pain (peripheral receptor terminal activity-tissue based)

- Peripheral neurogenic pain (lesions or dysfunction in peripheral nerves)

- Central sensitization pain (abberent processing and sensitivity within the central nervous system pain neuromatrix).

On analysis of the self-reporting in each subgroup it became clear that patients with nociceptive pain report less severe pain, have fewer quality of life and disability issues and suffer less anxiety and depression. In contrast, patient in the subclass central sensitization pain reported higher scores in each of the areas. Peripheral neurogenic pain classified patients reporting was in between the other two.

The suggestion here is that if physiotherapists can recognize patients in each of these mechanism subgroups they can be confident that, in general, patients with nociceptive pain will respond to tissue based interventions (manual therapy, active strategies) without cognitive behaviour barriers. Patients with peripheral neurogenic pain will respond to neural mobilization with some need to address cognitive behavioural issues. Whereas patient with central sensitization pain will need more interventions directed towards the maladaptive central nervous system processing (i.e. cognitive behavioural strategies) in conjunction with the application of tissue based approaches.

May & Aina (2012) investigated the centralization of symptoms and preference in movement directions in a literature review. It was found that the centralization phenomenon is more prevalent in acute than in sub-acute or chronic symptoms. They found 21 of 23 studies supporting the prognostic validity of centralization, including three high-quality studies. They conclude that findings of centralization or directional preference may be useful indicators of management strategies and prognosis in acute low back pain.

Kent & Kjaer (2012) investigated in a literature review if subgroups of people with particular psychosocial characteristics, such as fear avoidance, anxiety, catastrophizing, could be targeted with different treatment approaches. It appeared that graded activity plus treatment based classification aimed at people with high fear of movement was more effective in reducing this fear than treatment-based classification alone. Also, they describe that active rehabilitation with physical exercise classes based on cognitive behavioural principles was more effective than GP care at reducing activity limitations. However, they conclude that only few studies have investigated targeted psychosocial interventions. Overall they suggest more properly designed and adequately powered trials to find further responses to these queries.

It may be concluded that researchers in low back pain have recognized the necessity of subgroups in classifications for scientific studies. Many of these studies seem to reflect the clinical reasoning processes of physiotherapists, however currently it may be challenging to develop trials, which mirror the complexity of the clinical decision-making processes fully.

Clinical reasoning

The scope of the Maitland Concept, underpinned by open-minded clinical reasoning and patient-centred practice, is within the domain of rehabilitation. A classic example of this scope is evident from the following experience of one of the authors.

Whilst leading a course week on The Maitland Concept in a major European city with 20 students, a patient demonstration was arranged.

The patient, a 17-year-old male handball player, presented with low back pain and left-sided sciatica. He had hurt his back when he threw a ball in mid-air and landed awkwardly, twisting his back. He had had these symptoms for several months without resolution and he was only able to train for handball for half an hour before his symptoms became severe enough for him to have to stop.

He informed the group that he had a spondylolisthesis. His X-ray, in fact, showed a pars defect of congenital origin at L4. The group as a whole then began to think exclusively about the spondylolisthesis as the major factor in his problem and the focus of management.

Clinical examination, however, revealed a restriction in lumbar flexion, which became more so with cervical flexion as an addition but easier when deep abdominal muscles were activated. Lumbar extension was very restricted and reproduced his buttock and calf pain. When he jumped, as in handball, on initiation of the jump he lost control of his trunk lateral flexion. His SLR was restricted on the left and his L5 segment was stiff. He felt most comfortable lying on his right side.

Based on these findings and evidence he began to be able to control his symptoms and increase his exercise tolerance (1 hour training) over 4 days of functional interventions including:

- Restoration of pain-free SLR by the use of neural gliding techniques in right side lying with lumbar rotation and activation of deep abdominal muscles
- Mobilization of L5 whilst activating deep abdominal muscles
- Tonic control of the trunk in gradually loaded positions up to jumping and throwing.

The message here is that independent of pathological defects within the spine, which do not fully explain the onset and nature of the patient's symptoms, functional restoration and conditioning can and does have an effect on movement related symptoms, activity limitations and participation restrictions.

This example demonstrates the complexity of the clinical reasoning processes of physiotherapists, with the different paradigms and theoretical models, which they employ during assessment and treatment. With the 'brick wall model' of clinical reasoning, as developed by Maitland (1986), it is suggested that physiotherapists follow a different decision-making process from that of other professionals (e.g. medical practitioners), as the core of a physiotherapists' work lies in the analysis and treatment of movement functions. With the brick wall model Maitland moved away from the biomedical diagnosis as primary basis for decisions regarding the selection and application of physiotherapy treatments. Furthermore, he accentuated the necessity of independent decision-making processes in order to provide the best MSK-physiotherapy care (manipulative physiotherapy) possible. However, Maitland (1995) emphasized that manipulative physiotherapy should always occur under the umbrella of recognized health-care practice.

Physiotherapists often employ various forms of clinical reasoning, dependent on the particular needs of a situation. Most known is procedural clinical reasoning, with assessment and treatment procedures based on hypotheses generation and testing as well as on clinical pattern recognition (Jones 1995; for example, a physiotherapist examining a patient with sciatica and numbness in the big toe would include neurological examination and SLR as part of the assessment procedure). It has been recognized that therapists employ other forms of clinical reasoning as for example interactive, narrative, conditional or educational reasoning in addition to procedural reasoning strategies (Edwards 2000, Hengeveld 1998). As the subjective examination

follows mostly a semi-structured interview, there is ample opportunity to integrate both procedural and interactive and narrative clinical reasoning, in which patients are enabled to give an account of their experience in sufficient depth.

Sound clinical reasoning is based on a profound and wide clinical knowledge base and cognitive and metacognitive abilities (Jones 1995). Also, theoretical knowledge from varied basic sciences is being applied to clinical situations: for example, the physiotherapist might think that a patient has nociceptive facet joint pain if the patient complains of deep unilateral aching stiffness in the lumbar spine when moving. This analysis is born out of knowledge of structure, mechanics and specific innervations of structures. Therefore, physiotherapists need a reflective and analytical approach to most, if not all, decisions they make in clinical practice and to develop an attitude of lifelong learning, in which they recognize their current specific learning needs.

Hypotheses generation and testing

At the moment a patient registers for treatment with a physiotherapist, the process of hypotheses generation will start, on the one hand by the physiotherapist, on the other hand by patients themselves.

Categorization of hypotheses support clinicians to distinguish relevant information from irrelevant information, to become aware of subtle expressions of the patient indicative of the individual illness experience with the illness-behaviour and to become more comprehensive when summarizing information from assessment procedures (Thomas-Edding 1987, Jensen et al. 1999). These hypotheses categories are described in Chapters 2 and 7.

Patients may focus on questions such as 'what do I have', 'what can be done for it', 'how long will it take'. Their attitude towards treatment will be affected by their thoughts, emotions, belief-system, influences from their social environment and earlier experiences with therapy. For example, a patient may reveal that they are frightened of bending since they hurt their back because they don't want the same experience of pain again. They say 'I do not want you to hurt me'. The analysis here is that the therapist must try to employ mobilization techniques in a way that also helps the patient to regain confidence in movement again. Explanation and inclusion in treatment decisions therefore become crucial. As these factors may be crucial in final treatment outcomes, they need to be considered by the therapist as contributing factors to the (movement) disorder or even determining factors in the individual illness experience of their clients. Therefore, physiotherapists should include hypotheses categories such as 'contributing factors' and 'individual illness-experience' in the reflection and planning of assessment, treatment and the therapeutic relationship.

Overall, the hypotheses and clinical decisions of physiotherapists may pivot around three main issues (Mattingly 1991):

1. What are possible causes and contributing factors to the patient's disorder? This relates to questions and tests regarding:
   a. Possible pathobiological processes, including red flags
   b. Analysis of causes of movement dysfunctions (movement behaviour)
   c. Analysis of (movement-)impairments, activities, participation, contributing factors
   d. Contribution of the individual illness-experience and behaviour, including yellow flags. E. e. Neurophysiological pain mechanisms
   f. Physiological tissue-processes, as for example stages of tissue-healing.
2. Which treatment approaches may be most effective? This is associated with decisions on the current best evidence of therapies, but also with the question whether the current best evidence seems suitable to the patient as an individual. Therapists need to understand the role of passive and active movement, as well as other physical applications in treatment.

   Possible habitually selected treatments based on the notion 'I've always done it this way and it worked' need to be reflected upon; however, it is equally important to remain attentive of following injudiciously the favourite current treatment forms of a clinical and scientific cultural society. For any treatment chosen, clinical proof of its effects need to be given by consequent, comprehensive and well-reflected reassessment procedures (see Box 6.5).
3. How can patients be actively engaged in the therapeutic process?

   There is increasing scientific support for the role of the therapeutic relationship in treatment outcomes and person-centred, multidimensional approaches with a cognitive behavioural perspective (Asenlöf et al. 2005, 2009). Also active engagement of a patient into treatment should support the process of patient-empowerment, as advocated by the World Health Organization (WHO 2008). Hall et al. (2010), in a review on the influence of the therapeutic relationship on treatment outcome, concluded that particularly beneficial effects could be found in treatment compliance, depressive symptoms, treatment satisfaction and physical function.

   The question of active engaging patients in the therapeutic process is related to consideration of:
   a. The roles of both therapist and patient in treatment (e.g. coach, educator, curative role, preventive role) (e.g. is the patient expecting something to be done to them or are they expecting the therapist to inform them on what they can do for themselves)
   b. Expectations of the patients towards therapy (do they expect to be given manipulation or exercises for their back pain; also, do they have positive expectations towards the treatment)
   c. Cognitive factors as belief systems about the causes and treatment options. Also the paradigms and perspectives patients have on their problem. If this differs from that of the physiotherapist, educational strategies at an early stage are necessary (e.g. the patient might think that moving and exercising will cause damage to their back whilst the therapist thinks that movement is necessary for recovery and reducing pain)
   d. Affective factors, as for example gentle guidance towards more confidence in trusting to move (both in reassessment procedures as in explicit movement/exercise experiences)
   e. Influence on, and by, the social environment. In this relationship at times the concept of secondary gain has been brought forward. Secondary gain is described as a social advantage attained by a person as a consequence of an illness; however, tertiary gains may also exist, in which others in the direct environment benefit from the illness of the person. It is warned not to focus

Box 6.5

Reassessment procedures

Reassessment procedures are one of the cornerstones of the Maitland Concept of MSK-physiotherapy. It is essential that physiotherapy clinicians find clinical evidence, in collaboration with the patient, of the effectiveness of the selected treatment-interventions. This procedure may be considered as an art in itself, should be seen as an integral part of treatment and should be considered from a cognitive-behavioural attitude. No treatment should be selected without in-depth assessment; additionally no treatment procedure should be performed without consequently monitoring its outcomes

Reassessment procedures should take place at each treatment session:

- During the initial physical examination phase of the first encounter after the examination of various active and passive movement tests and before investigating the possibility that another movement component is involved
- At the beginning of each subsequent treatment session: pre-treatment assessment to reflect on the reactions to the last treatment and the time before the patient came to the current therapy session
- Immediately after the application of the various treatment interventions: proving the value of the intervention and monitoring, if treatment objectives step-by-step are being achieved. These interventions may include passive mobilization techniques, active movements, application of physical agents as well as information and educational strategies
- At the end of the treatment session

The purposes of reassessment procedures are:

- To allow the physiotherapist and patient to compare treatment results, hence proving the value of selected interventions
- Differential diagnosis: not only examination findings, but also reactions to treatment interventions make a contribution to differential diagnosis of the sources of movement dysfunctions ('differentiation by treatment')
- To enable the physiotherapist to reflect on the decisions made during the diagnostic and therapeutic processes. Through reassessment procedures, hypotheses with regard to sources, contributing factors, and management may be confirmed, modified or rejected. The therapist learns to recognize patterns of clinical presentations, which will aid in future decision-making. Reassessment procedures support the development of the personal experiential knowledge base of the physiotherapist; hence playing a central role in the development of clinical expertise

- To enable the patients in their learning processes. From a cognitive-behavioural perspective, reassessment procedures play a central role in the development of the perception that beneficial changes indeed occur, even if the pain still seems to be lasting. If patients are being guided towards the *experience* of the various changes in the test movement (e.g. quantity, quality of the movement, next to symptom responses), they may learn to perceive changes which they initially did not expect to occur
- Reassessment procedures are one of the crucial aspects of the therapeutic process

Indicators of change

It is essential to bear in mind how symptoms and signs may change, in order to guide the patient comprehensively in reassessment procedures and to monitor even minor beneficial changes. However, it is essential that the starting point is clear: if it is not sufficiently clear from the first assessment which daily life functions are limited due to pain or other reasons, no good comparison will be possible in later sessions. This may often leave the patient in doubt as to whether the therapy has really served its purpose. Furthermore, the definition of clear treatment objectives may be impeded and neither the patient nor physiotherapist is capable of observing in sufficient detail if something is changing beneficially in the patient's situation.

Subjective examination

- Pain: sensory aspects such as intensity of pain (may be expressed in visual analogue scale) quality of symptom, duration, localization, frequency
- Normalization of level of activity and participation
- Confidence in use of body during daily life situations
- Decrease in use of medication
- Increased understanding
- Deliberate employment of coping strategies if discomfort increases again

Physical examination

- Inspection parameter (posture, form, skin, aids, etc.)
- Active testing: range-of-motion (ROM), quality of movement, symptom-reaction
- Passive testing (neurodynamic testing, accessory and physiological intervertebral movements, muscle length): change in behaviour of pain, sense of resistance and motor responses
- Muscle testing: changes in strength, quality of contraction and symptom response
- Palpation findings: quality and symptom response

Continued

Box 6.5—cont'd

- Neurological conduction testing: changes in quantity and quality of the responses

Treatment intensity

Higher intensity of active movements, passive mobilizations (grade, duration, inclination, combinations), exercises, soft-tissue techniques without provoking discomfort

Behavioural parameters

For example, facial expression, non-verbal language, eye contact, use of key-words and key-gestures, habitual integration of extremity with daily life functions.

A balanced approach to reassessment of subjective and physical parameters is necessary. Some physiotherapists focus solely on the observation of physical examination findings and may only employ tests with an acceptable inter- and intra-tester reliability. However, it is argued that a certain degree of scepticism should be retained if tests with a high reliability coefficient are directly claimed to be clinically useful and vice versa: that tests with a relatively low coefficients would not be useful clinically (Keating & Matyas 1998, Bruton et al. 2000). Often the combination of tests of both subjective and movement parameters may provide the clinician with valid reassessment parameters (MacDermid et al. 2009).

Leaving out subjective parameters carries the inherent danger that the therapeutic process becomes rather mechanical, whereby not much space is left for the patient's individual perceptions of change with regard to the disorder. Furthermore, the observation of the more subtle behavioural parameters (e.g. less guarding of the affected arm, changes in facial expression and use of words) may be indicative that changes in the individual's illness experience are taking place

The 'art' of reassessment

- With reassessment procedures it is essential that physiotherapists develop a clear image as to which interventions have an effect on the patient's condition. Some interventions may influence some active parameters, whilst other interventions influence other tests and activities.
- It is necessary to follow consequently multiple parameters in reassessment procedures

- Profound reassessment: the physiotherapist has to monitor the indicators of changes meticulously rather than being satisfied with a more superficial question at the beginning of a session, such as 'how have you been?' without further follow-up of the information
- Balanced approach to reassessment and treatment procedures: if some patients have a condition with a high level of irritability, or have difficulties getting on and off a treatment table, it may be useful to reassess only the subjective experience regularly, and to perform some reassessment test whilst the patient is still lying on the treatment plinth
- Cognitive objectives: in the case of educational treatment strategies, the physiotherapist has to monitor whether the given information has been understood, and whether the patient feels capable of implementing the recommendations in daily-life activities and exercises
- Reassessment procedures need to be recognized as such by the patient. They have to be announced by the therapist. Patients should be guided towards statements of comparison (rather than of fact) during test movements, not only about pain, but also how they personally perceive change in quality and quantity of movement. A brief summary of what the therapist heard what the patient said about the perceived changes may enhance learning from a cognitive-behavioural perspective ('reinforcement')
- In some cases, where pain seems to have become a dominant feature in the individual illness experience, without any changes over time, it may be useful to find metaphors for the experience of the patient (e.g. a wave on the ocean, which may get less high). In other cases it may be helpful to integrate more functional movements as, for example, a 'tennis service' or a working activity – in which the patient learns to observe various parameters other than pain alone as a sensation
- It is essential that the physiotherapist remains in control of the treatment collaboratively with the patient. Given practice and experience, treatment including profound reassessment procedures is not a lengthy procedure

---

solely on secondary gain of a person with pain without asking what may be the secondary losses to the person (Fishbain 1994). (Here the patient and therapist must have the same goals e.g. to return a patient with back pain to a working and productive life or, as in the case of chronic disability, to provide the patient the strategies to master their situation themselves.)

f. Behavioural factors, as for example movement behaviour, expression, guarding, confronting.

It is recommended that within a therapeutic relationship patients need to be treated as equals and experts in their own right, and that their reports on pain need to be believed and acted upon. Opportunities need to be provided to communicate, to talk with and listen to the patients about their problems, needs and experiences. In addition, independence in choosing personal treatment goals and interventions within a process of setting goals with, rather than for, a patient needs to be encouraged (Mead 2000). See also Chapter 3.

Experiential knowledge, clinical patterns

While reassessment-procedures primarily aim at monitoring clinical evidence of treatment-outcomes, they also fulfil an important role in the development of the *experiential knowledge base* of clinicians, as described by Schön (1983). It appears that experts may have more patterns in memory and may be capable of overseeing a situation quickly and are capable to find more comprehensive and effective solutions, faster than novices in a field (De Groot 1946). This is often an intuitive, implicit process. The concept of clinical patterns as a part of the experiential knowledge base has found acceptance in physiotherapy education and practice (Jones 1995). Studies between experts and novices demonstrated differences in 'if … then …' rules as a form of forward reasoning, being more present with experts. These rules may be considered as an expression of clinical pattern recognition and students need to be encouraged to express their 'if … then … rules' explicitly and to engage in consequent, written planning of assessment-procedures and treatment sessions (for example, an expert physiotherapist will have the experiential knowledge and professional knowledge to know quickly whether a patient with back pain will respond to manual therapy or will need cognitive approaches. In this way expert physiotherapists will reach a successful outcome quicker than the novice or move the patient on to self-management more quickly).

The development of clinical patterns cannot occur only by theoretical learning. Direct clinical experiences are necessary, in which clinical presentations and individual stories of patients are being encapsulated in clinical memory (Schmidt & Boshuyzen 1993). The application of theoretical knowledge, direct patient-contact, disciplined

processes of hypotheses-generation and testing with consequent reassessment procedures and structured reflexion are prerequisites to the development of clinical patterns and expertise.

The following groups of clinical patterns may be distinguished:

- *Movement disorders in conjunction with pathobiological processes.* This is related to the question if, in the background of the movement disorder, pathobiological processes are present. Associated issues are:
  - do they provide any contraindications to physiotherapeutic treatment?
  - do they provide any precautions to treatment?

  How do they influence the short term and long term prognosis of the movement disorder?

  In cases of NSLBP: are any movement patterns attributable to nociceptive processes in lumbar spine structures (e.g. disc, facet joint) or clinical syndromes (e.g. lumbar stenosis, neurogenic pain, lumbar structural/functional stability dysfunction), which need a specific approach to treatment?

- *One-component versus multicomponent movement disorder.* Movement disorders where it is more likely that one movement component is involved versus multiple movement components. One-component movement disorders may occur more frequently in younger people, with a single trauma in history (e.g. knee-distortion) with pain-reduction and improvement of activity levels occurring to the expected time of tissue-healing. Multicomponent movement disorders are more likely to occur where there is a degenerative, osteoarthritic background. In the latter case, screening of possible contributing areas to the nociception is important in the first three treatment sessions (e.g. pain in the buttock area often requires assessment of the lumbar spine, sacroiliac joint, hip, neurodynamic functions, possibly thoracic spine, and muscular functions).

- *Approach to treatment: one-dimensional versus multidimensional approach.* A movement disorder, which requires an explicit multidimensional approach to treatment. This means that contributing factors such as cognitive, affective, sociocultural and behavioural factors need to be explicitly defined in treatment-planning and in reassessment-procedures. In this case the quality of the therapeutic relationship, communication (interactive clinical reasoning), education and information may play a crucial role. This multidimensional approach is more likely to be required in chronic pain states or where recuperation of normal function and pain-reduction take much longer than normally expected. This is particularly necessary in those cases, where patients express a sense of helplessness, hopelessness or strong frustration with the provided health-care, with conflicting information; differ in beliefs / paradigms regarding causes and treatment; present avoidance-behaviour which has become maladaptive; perceive their state as highly disabling; demonstrate hypervigilant movement behaviour.

Prognosis and clinical prediction rules

Making a prognosis is an important skill in physiotherapy practice. However, often it is a daunting task (Maitland et al. 2005) as clinicians are more likely to be dealing with probabilities more than with certainties. Making a prognosis is a skill, in which clinicians match the clinical presentation of a patient's problem with theoretical knowledge (e.g. tissue healing) and clinical experiences made with patients who present with similar dysfunctions and resources. Hence, it contains elements of clinical pattern recognition. The years of experience which a clinician has spent with the assessment and treatment of particular disorders of persons will certainly aid in making a more accurate prognosis; however, experienced clinicians probably express themselves carefully while making a prognosis, as more stories may be encapsulated in their clinical memory in which patients' processes of recuperation differed from the initial prognosis made by the therapist.

Nevertheless, a clinician frequently needs to estimate in which way results may be achieved, how long treatment may take and which concrete results may be achieved. Patients often want to know, what is wrong with them, what can be done about it and how long it is going to take? Also, from the viewpoint of insurance companies and referring doctors, a physiotherapeutic prognosis may be essential.

Prognosis takes place in various phases:

1. At the beginning of a treatment series:
   a. What can be achieved on a short-term basis: which results can be expected within the first three or four sessions (for example, the therapist might think, if the patient with acute low back pain improves by 80% within the first 3–4 sessions then there is a high probability that they will return to their normal duties)?
   b. What can be achieved on a long-term basis during the overall process of physiotherapy?
   c. What may not be achieved?

2. During the treatment series, especially during retrospective assessment in every third or fourth session. It is essential to reflect on all the hypotheses formed and rejected thus far in the therapeutic process; especially the reflection on the prognosis may aid the clinician to learn profoundly from each encounter with a patient, and to develop and deepen clinical patterns in memory (for example, the therapist may find that the patients back pain is settling within 2–3 sessions of mobilization but their leg pain is not changing. The therapist may then think that the problem may take longer to sort out and other, additional treatment approaches may need to be considered).

3. At the end, during final analytical assessment – making a prognosis for the time after the therapy has been be completed:
   a. The likely restraints on lifestyle.
   b. The likelihood of recurrences of episodes of the disorder, and the possible early warning signs that the patient must heed in order to minimize the severity of the recurrence, and the steps the patient then needs to take.
   c. The need for specific ongoing exercises, intermittent maintenance treatment, or follow-up assessment (for example, one patient with back pain may feel that they do not need any further advice where as another may be pain free and yet still fear that they will hurt their back again if they go back to work. In the second case it is important for therapy to include graded work hardening to ensure sustainable recovery and a favourable prognosis).

Specific hypothesis categories should also be considered to make a comprehensive prognosis:

1. Disorders that are easy or difficult to help (e.g. complex regional pain syndromes).
2. Nature of the person, including attitudes, beliefs, feelings, values, expectations, (movement) behaviour, and so on.
3. Nature of the disorder (intraarticular and periarticular disorders; mechanical osteoarthritis/inflammatory osteoarthritis; acute injury/chronic degenerative injury, nociception alone/nociception with peripheral neurogenic or central sensitization).
4. The body's capacity to inform and adapt. (The way the patient 'feels' about the disorder often correlates well with other aspects of prognosis. For example: 'I've had back pain for 20 years so I know I'll never totally get rid of it, but I've been able to cope with it so far'.)
5. Contributing factors and other barriers to recovery (structural anomalies, systemic disease, general health problems such as diabetes, ergonomic/socioeconomic environments such as: keyboarding, heavy manual work; repetitive, monotonous activities; little control over work circumstances).
6. Expertise of the physiotherapist, especially in the field of communication and handling.

The bio-psychosocial model of the ICF (WHO 2001) may serve as an aid in considering aspects of a prognosis. If only function impairments are present – as, for example, slight restricted mobility of the hip and muscle imbalance in an otherwise healthy patient who is without great activity limitations, participation restriction and no relevant context factors – the prognosis will be, of course, much more favourable than if disturbances of all elements are present. The physiotherapist has to evaluate whether discrepancies among the elements of the model are present.

In prognosis-making, numerous factors need to be taken into consideration in either short-term or long-term prognosis:

- General health
- General fitness level
- Stage of tissue healing and damage
- Mechanical versus inflammatory presentation of the disorder
- Irritability of the disorder
- Relationship between impairments, activity limitations and participation restrictions

- Onset of the disorder, duration of the history, stability of the disorder and progression/course of the disorder (are attacks more frequent or disabling?)
- Pre-existing disorders and dysfunctions (e.g. the patient has fallen on the shoulder; however, they may have had degenerative changes in the neck with some pain for some years)
- One- or multicomponent movement disorder (e.g. only local movement dysfunction in elbow, or the disorder has more components contributing to it: shoulder, cervical and thoracic spine, neurodynamic dysfunction)
- Contributing factors – 'cause of the source' (e.g. posture, muscle weakness or tightness, discrepancies in mobility of joint complexes, such as spine or wrist)
- Cognitive, affective, sociocultural aspects, learning processes: patient's beliefs, earlier experiences, expectation, personality, life style, learning behaviour, movement behaviour
- Multidimensional approach to treatment: consideration if the cognitive, affective and behavioural dimensions need to be addressed in treatment.

After some years of clinical experience, physiotherapists learn to recognize which kinds of clinical presentation react more or less favourably to treatment (Table 6.4).

At the third or fourth treatment session, and the final analytical assessment, the manipulative physiotherapist should be able to answer the following questions about a patient's disorder in the quest for a prognosis:

- What is the biomedical diagnosis and which pathobiological mechanisms (tissue mechanisms – pathology, healing processes; neurophysiological pain mechanisms)?
- What is the source(s) of the patient's symptoms?
- What are the contributing factors to the source of the symptoms ('cause of the source')
- To what extent is movement impaired and activities/participation restricted by the symptoms?
- To what extent is severity or irritability limiting movement and activity?
- Which predictions can be made about the natural history of the disorder based on its onset, stage of pathological development, and

Table 6.4 Factors in prognosis

Disorders easy to help	Disorders which may be more difficult to help
Strong relationship of patient's symptoms and movement	Weak relationship between the symptoms and movements in the patient's mind
Recognizable/typical syndrome or pathology	Atypical, unclear patterns, syndromes or pathology
Predominantly primary hyperalgesia and tissue-based pain mechanisms (nociception; peripheral neurogenic)	Predominantly secondary hyperalgesia from central nervous system sensitization rather than stimulus-response related tissue responses
Model of patient: helpful thoughts and behaviours ('I can still do some things'; 'I have found ways to get relief')	Maladaptive thoughts and behaviour: ('I don't think I ever get better'; 'I dare not move because always hurts me') and other yellow flags
Familiar symptoms which the patient recognizes as tissue based ('it feels like a bruise')	Unfamiliar symptoms which the patient has difficulty describing in sensory terms
No or minimal barriers to recovery of predictors of chronicity ('yellow flags')	Multifactorial/multicomponent /complex regional pain syndromes
Severity, irritability and nature of the patient's symptoms correspond to the history of the disorder/to injury or strain to the structures of the movement system	Severity, irritability and nature do not fit with the history or stage in the natural history of the disorder
The patient has had a previously favourable sampling experience with manipulative physiotherapy	Previous unfavourable sampling experiences or knowledge of manipulative therapy ('my mate had manipulation of his shoulder and he said it
There are easily identifiable signs of impairment and activity limitations which have a strong relationship with movement	was much worse afterwards')Evidence of movement impairments but with little correspondence to the degree of activity limitation
Patients are touch tolerant (gain relief by touch, rubbing or massage)	Patients are touch intolerant ('I don't like anyone touching my knee')
An internal locus of control ('I just need to know how I can help myself'); locus of control with regard to health and well-being is consistent	An externalized locus of control ('you are the physiotherapist, you sort me out') or inconsistency in locus of control with regards to health and well-being
The patient has realistic expectations for recovery which correspond with the natural history of the disorder	Unrealistic expectations for recovery ('I wish I would wake up and all the pain would be gone')
Patients will resume appropriate activity and exercise at relevant stages of recovery	Ongoing pain states with little changes in symptoms over a long period of time

pathological stability/lability (e.g. healing phases of a lumbar disc)?

- Which predisposing factors are influencing the course of the disorder (pre-existing pathology, comorbidity, weak link, the nature and extent of injury, age-related processes, general health state, physique, occupation, hobbies, life style, genetic predisposition, etc.)?
- Which factors are contributing to a favourable or unfavourable prognosis?

- Is the disorder one that will be easy or difficult to help based on examination and response to treatment)?
- What do we understand about the patient's nature and response to injury and illness (adaptive/maladaptive behaviour; beliefs, thoughts, feelings, attitude, former experiences, values, etc.)?

In summary, prognosis is a forecast of the future history of a patient's disorder based on the probability of physical, psychological and functional recovery of the patient and the disorder. Therefore, consideration should be given to:

1. The natural history of a particular disorder. (Careful: some studies claim that some disorders, e.g. tennis elbow or frozen shoulder, recuperate over 2 years; however, what is the amount of remaining functional impairment?)

2. The response to MSK/manipulative physiotherapy – has the progress been acceptable?

3. What is acceptable to the patient – has the main problem been solved?

4. Possible need for prophylaxis – is a self-management programme needed to complement or maintain recovery? Is the patient capable of implementing elements of this programme at adequate moments? Is 'top up' treatment required periodically?

5. Prognosis, which should at all times be realistic.

It is essential to maintain at all times a self-critical attitude towards prognosis and regularly pose the same questions as in retrospective assessment, if therapy seems to be stagnating:

- Have I compared the subjective and physical parameters ('asterisks') regularly enough and in sufficient detail?

- Did I ensure that the patient would become aware of positive changes in these parameters as well?

- Did I follow up the correct physical asterisks, which reflect the patient's main problem and the goal of the therapeutic intervention?

- Have I performed a review of the therapeutic process with retrospective assessment procedures, collaboratively with the patient?

- Has the right source of the symptoms been treated?

- Have the self-management procedures been pursued profoundly enough? Did these procedures provide the patient with sufficient control over the pain and well-being on all daily life situations? Did I teach them well enough?

- Are any medical or other interventions necessary?

Even if physiotherapists embark on a therapeutic process with a less favourable prognosis, they should bear in mind that a prognosis deals with probabilities and hypotheses, hence still maintain a positive attitude towards treatment. The following quote relating to neurological rehabilitation may serve as a demonstration of this principle:

A positive approach right from the start can contribute greatly to the success of treatment. I find it helpful when I first start treating a patient to picture him walking out of the hospital unaided one day, well-dressed and waving goodbye with a smile, even if things look bleak during the early days following his admission. Should a patient not survive the initial trauma or sadly never regain consciousness, nothing will have been lost by the active intervention, but so much gained. All too often I am told that things went so wrong because everyone thought that the patient would not survive for long. Statistical studies concerning prognosis can also lead to negative attitudes, but statistics are not about individuals, and there have been many surprising exceptions. It has been wisely pointed out that the clinician's attitude may influence the recovery to the extent that cessation of recovery after 6 months, a widely held belief, may possibly in fact be the result of a self-fulfilling prophecy.

Davies 1994 (p. XI)

Clinical prediction rules

Clinical prediction rules have found increasing attention in the field of clinical physiotherapeutic research. These rules are clinical decision making tools designed to aid clinicians in determining a diagnosis, prognosis, or likely response to an intervention. They contain predictor variables obtained from patients' history, examination and diagnostic tests, which have been statistically analyzed and found to be meaningful predictors of a condition or outcome (Glynn & Weisbach 2011). They are not meant to replace individual decision-making processes, but should be considered within the philosophy of evidence-based practice, in which clinicians are encouraged to incorporate the best available evidence in their examination and treatment procedures. Hence they are meant to support the clinical decision making processes (Cleland 2011). Clinical prediction rules should not be blindly incorporated in clinical reasoning processes, as they can only be applied to similar patient populations which are similar to the population in which they have been researched (Huijbregts 2011).

Some clinical prediction rules with regards the lumbar spine and low back pain are listed in Table 6.5 (for further reference: Glynn & Weisbach, 2011).

Table 6.5 Selected clinical prediction rules with regards to the lumbar spine

Diagnostic	Lumbar spinal stenosis (LSS) *(to distinguish from other lower leg symptoms. Scores >7 : LSS is probable; score <2: LSS less probable)*	Age: 60–70 (score 2–3) Symptoms present > 6 months (score 1) Symptom improve when bending forward (score 2) Symptoms improve when bending backward (score –2) Symptoms exacerbating when standing up (score 2) Symptoms with walking, improve with rest (score 1) • (intermittent claudication) • urinary incontinence + (score 1)
	Sacroiliac joint (SIJ) *(three or more tests provoke buttock / leg pain: probable that pain originates from nociceptive processes in SIJ)*	Positive SIJ compression test (SL) Positive supine SIJ traction ('opening innominates') Positive femoral shear test Positive sacral provocation (generalized PA) Positive right Gaenslen's test Positive left Gaenslen's test
	Ankylosing spondylitis	Morning stiffness > 30 minutes Improvement of back pain with exercise, but not with rest Awakening because of back pain in second half of the night only • alternating buttock pain Reference standard: • low back pain • limited lumbar motion • reduced chest expansion • bilateral grade > 2 sacroilitis on X-ray • unilateral grade > 1 sacrolilitis on X-ray Mean age: 35.9; male : female – 64 : 36%
Interventional	Lumbar stabilization for low back pain	Predictor variables of success: • SLR > 90° • < 40 years • aberrant motion to forward bending • positive prone instability test Predictor variables of non-success: • FABQ – physical activity <8 • aberrant movement in flexion absent • no hypermobility during PA-testing • negative prone instability test
	Lumbar manipulation *(4 or more variables: probability of success increased)* *Probability of non-success with scores > 5 points*	Predictor variables of success: • pain does not travel below knee • onset ≤ 16 days ago • Lumbar hypomobility (PA movements) • Both hips > 35° of internal rotation • FABQ – work subscale <19 Predictor variables of failure: • decreased average ROM of total hip rotation • longer duration of symptoms • not having low back pain only • negative Gaenslen's test • absence of lumbar hypomobility (PA-movement) • decreased hip internal rotation – discrepancy between sides

Reflective practice

Clinical reasoning and assessment procedures are twin elements of this concept in NMS-physiotherapy. In order to enhance reflective practice and to develop expertise, it is essential that therapists make their hypotheses and decisions explicit during critical phases of the assessment and therapeutic process, reflect upon them and to plan the following steps of action in therapy.

The structuring of thought processes is best made explicit in the following critical phases of the therapeutic process:

- After referral
- During the initial contact ('welcoming phase')
- First session: during the subjective examination
- First session: planning the physical examination and the first treatment
- Planning of the second (and third) session
- Planning of overall treatment (latest at the end of the third session)
- Planning retrospective assessments (in about every fourth or fifth session)
- Planning the conclusion of therapy.

Simple comprehensive recording is highly relevant in, which should give a quick overview of the most essential details. The recordings should include:

- All relevant information from subjective, physical examination and treatment
- All relevant reflections, hypotheses and planning steps made by the physiotherapist.

Planning steps may be expressed in a flowchart, particularly if several decision options are simultaneously present. An example of written planning to enhance pattern development and reflective practice is included in Figure 6.2.

Examination of the lumbar spine: subjective examination

In the process of examining low back and/or leg pain it is the specific task of the MSK-physiotherapist to systematically investigate whether movement disorders are present. There may be relevant movement-impairments in the lumbar spine, sacroiliac joints, and/or hip. In some cases the other pelvic connections need to be examined as well. Furthermore, neurodynamic dysfunctions may contribute to pain and disability. Also it needs to be investigated whether changes in muscular control are contributing to the movement disorder. Analysis of movement habits in daily life (e.g. sitting habits), the general level of fitness, the impact of the problem on the life of the patient and information about the belief system about causes and treatment-options may also be part of the assessment procedures of the therapist.

Using semi-structured interviews, facilitating collaborative responses, listening for key words or phrases and following up with questions that qualify misunderstandings and ambiguities supports an attention to detail in the collecting of subjective data as a measure of the patients experience of their low back pain

The clinical reasoning model of the 'symbolic permeable brick wall' helps the clinician to categorize information into clinical evidence and theoretical knowledge.

Hypotheses categories can then be established, which help to shape and design physical examination and intervention based on the patient's individual needs.

When a person presents with low back and/or leg pain, during the subjective examination, the therapist may decide to pursue the procedures of the interview along a more strict protocol; to use paralleling techniques, in which the line of thought of the patient is guiding the interview; or to engage in narrative clinical reasoning, with active listening, in which patients can give a full account of the history of the problem and treatment. In any form of interviewing, it is essential that the therapist is aware of the hypotheses generated and modulated during the information-process and asks clarifying questions if necessary. Novices in the field, practising the art and skill of interviewing, may prefer to use a more strict protocol; however, also in this case it is essential to pursue clarifying and deepening questions, in order to confirm, modify or reject hypotheses generated during the discussion with the patient. A well-balanced approach between procedural and interactive reasoning will always be necessary (see also Chapter 2).

The subjective examination is an essential part of the overall assessment. Due to time restrictions, therapists may decide to shorten the interview or to start to control the interview with strict sets of (closed) procedural questions. However, important information may be missed, resulting in

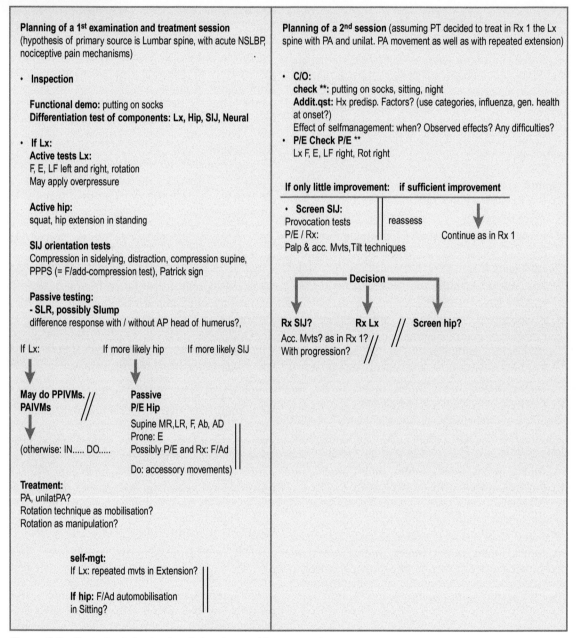

Figure 6.2 • Example of planning in a first and second therapy session.

superficial clinical decisions. It is recommended that physiotherapists engage in other forms of clinical reasoning, as for example narrative or interactive reasoning next to procedural reasoning. This allows the therapist:

> ... to get an account of the patient's individual story rather than controlling the patient with strict

assessment criteria in which the patient may only be allowed to talk about those aspects which are relevant to physiotherapeutic diagnosis and treatment-planning from the perspective of the physiotherapist.

(Thomson, 1998, p. 90)

By shortening the necessary time interviewing, conclusions about causes and treatment may be based on first sight information, which should have been refined during the subjective examination. Frequently this leads to disappointing results, as parameters to compare treatment outcomes are not detailed enough to allow for thorough comparison of changes in later sessions.

Subjective examination may be considered as a first phase of a learning process, in which not only the therapist learns about patients' problems and the impact on their life, but also patients may learn to see relationships between their pain, disability, activities and life-style. Furthermore it may set the tone for a person-centred agenda of treatment (Greenhalgh & Hurwitz, 1998). Hence the subjective examination is intrinsically therapeutic and should be allocated sufficient time in the encounters with a patient.

The procedures of the subjective examination may be grouped into five main categories:

1. Establishing the main problem from the perspective of the patient
2. Localization of symptoms
3. Behaviour of symptoms in relation to activities
4. History (current, previous)
5. Medical and health screening questions ('special questions').

Particularly for novices in the field it is useful to follow these groups in sequence, but especially in cases of a recent, traumatic incident leading to the patient's symptoms, therapists may decide to follow up the history of the problem immediately after the establishment of the main problem. If a long lasting or recurrent history is present, at times it is better to wait with collection of the information regarding history, but to get a clear picture what is bothering the patient in the 'here and now'. On the other hand, if patients with persistent symptoms and disability appear to be frustrated with the provided health care, telling their full story from their perspective may be intrinsically therapeutic, as they learn to make more sense of their experience and learn to cope better with a situation (Kleinmann 1988, Heath 1998, Main & Spanswick 2000). However, within this process of engaging in narrative reasoning the therapist should attempt to keep an overview of the basic procedures and of the planning of next steps of assessment and treatment. Otherwise it may be better to follow more procedural steps of interviewing and to seek support from a more experienced peer.

Introduction to the assessment process

It may be difficult for a patient to understand that each member in a multidisciplinary team follows a unique frame of reference, which in a sense is exclusive to their profession (Kleinmann 1988). Therefore, it is essential to inform the patient about the specific role of the physiotherapist in the diagnosis and treatment of movement dysfunctions, being complementary to medical diagnosis. This information needs to be given at an early phase of the encounter, before embarking on the examination and treatment process.

Furthermore, explanations need to be given about the setting and the steps that will be followed in the first session (interview, physical examination/ movement testing, first probationary treatment, reassessment). It may be necessary to explain that this examination is highly important to individualize the treatment to the specific problem and needs of the patient.

Additionally, it is necessary to find out whether or not the patients/clients have been expecting physiotherapy as a treatment option for their problems (particularly in those cases where a patient has been referred by another medical practitioner). Also, it is useful to grasp if the patient understands that physiotherapy encompasses many various methods of movement therapy (hence, not only gymnastics), touching (e.g. passive mobilizations, manipulations, soft-tissue techniques) and other modalities.

In this introductory phase, by means of careful listening and observing, the therapist may become aware of some sensitivities of the patient with regard to therapy, setting and therapist, which can also be addressed (Main & Spanswick 2000).

Main problem

It is essential to establish the current main problem from the patient's perspective. Allowing the patient to express in their own terms what is bothering them provides the therapist with several hypotheses, as for example:

• Does patient's problem seem to be a movement disorder, or does it give an impression of another, pathobiological problem, which may need the attention of another primary clinician?

- Does it seem that the movement disorder can be treated from a one-dimensional approach, or does it need a multidimensional approach, in which extra care is given to the communication with the style of questioning and information processes during the overall examination and treatment? Also more time often needs to be allocated for the interview and the therapist should remain aware not only to ask questions about pain, but also about the current movement capacity and activity limitations. Central questions, at a later stage in the interview, will relate to how the patient is able to cope with the problem in daily life.

- Does it appear to be a movement disorder with severe or irritable symptoms, which needs extra caution during initial examination and treatment procedures?

People with lumbar movement disorders frequently present with low back, buttock and/or leg pain. Other symptoms may be, for example, stiffness or a sense of tiredness in the back and/or legs, numbness or paraesthesia in defined areas of the leg.

This may be expressed in different terms, which at times provide a therapist with first hypotheses about possible structures, clinical syndromes or movement components involved. For example:

- A sense of tiredness in the back, particularly if it spreads in a small line across the spine may be indicative of a stability disorder with discrepancies between more mobile and stiff intervertebral segments in the lumbar spine

- A band-like sensation of stiffness across the area of lower back may hint towards a movement disorder with discogenic features, particularly if these symptoms occur when rising from bed in the morning or rising from a chair after a prolonged period of sitting

- Sensation of muscle tiredness, cramp-like sensations may support hypotheses on neurogenic pain mechanisms and neurodynamic dysfunction.

Perceived disability

Next to the establishment of the main problem from the perspective of the patient, at this stage it is important to seek information in general terms about how patients perceive their disability and current movement capacities with their symptoms. First hypotheses will be developed about the question if the level of disability appears to be adaptive to the current process of nociception, or does it seem that the patient has developed maladaptive avoidance behaviour? For example: a man presents with a localized area of pain on the right unilateral side of L4–5, and reports that this pain has severely limited him in several daily life functions for the past few days only. The patient has learned to avoid the activities concerned, but has remained as active as the pain allows. Furthermore, the patient says that it seems that the pain has reduced somewhat already and he feels slightly more capable of using his body. This problem may be classified as severe (nociceptive) pain, with adaptive movement behaviour. On the other hand, if, for example, 4 months later the same patient reports that he still cannot carry out many daily life activities, it is possible that the protective behaviour has become maladaptive and may be labelled as 'fear avoidance behaviour' (provided that no other pathobiological processes can explain the pain and disability).

Also based on this information, the therapist can decide if a multidimensional approach to the examination and treatment needs to be adopted.

Localization and quality of symptoms

Precise description of the perceived symptoms on a body chart is essential in assessment. It will serve the therapist and patient in reassessment procedures in consecutive treatment-sessions and in the development of clinical patterns in the physiotherapist's memory. By comparing body charts with the symptom areas, therapists will develop hypotheses if typical, recognizable pain-patterns are present (i.e. end organ-dysfunction related to a recognizable incident in recent history or nociceptive or peripheral neurogenic patterns or at times, autonomic nervous system patterns). If the symptom distribution is atypical, caution should be given if a pathology is present, which needs further investigation (e.g. multiple sclerosis), or if a generalized tenderness has developed based on central nervous system sensitization processes. In this case the question should be followed up why central nervous system modulation seems to have taken place: are any pathophysiological processes present, which may be contributing cognitive, affective and /or behavioural factors?

Examples of body charts of patients with a lumbar movement disorder

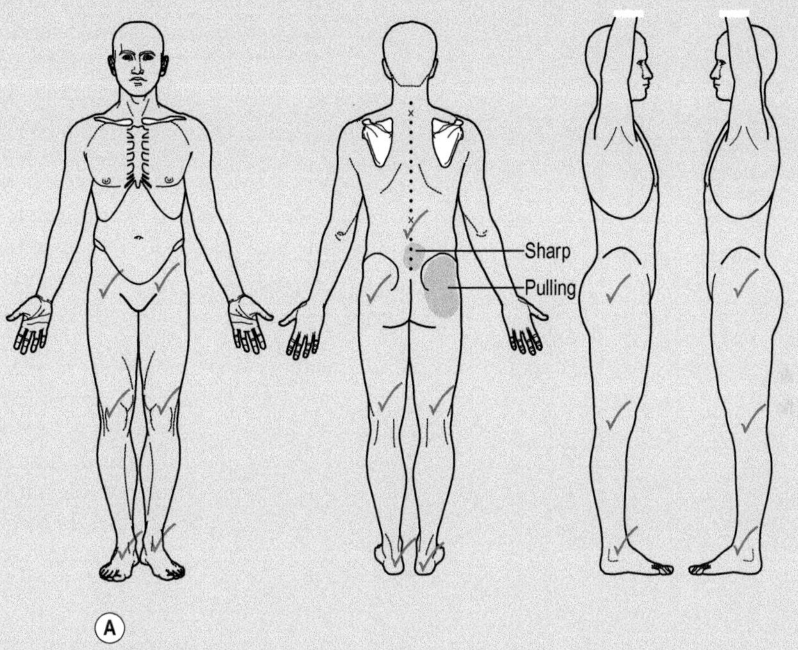

Sharp
Pulling

(A)

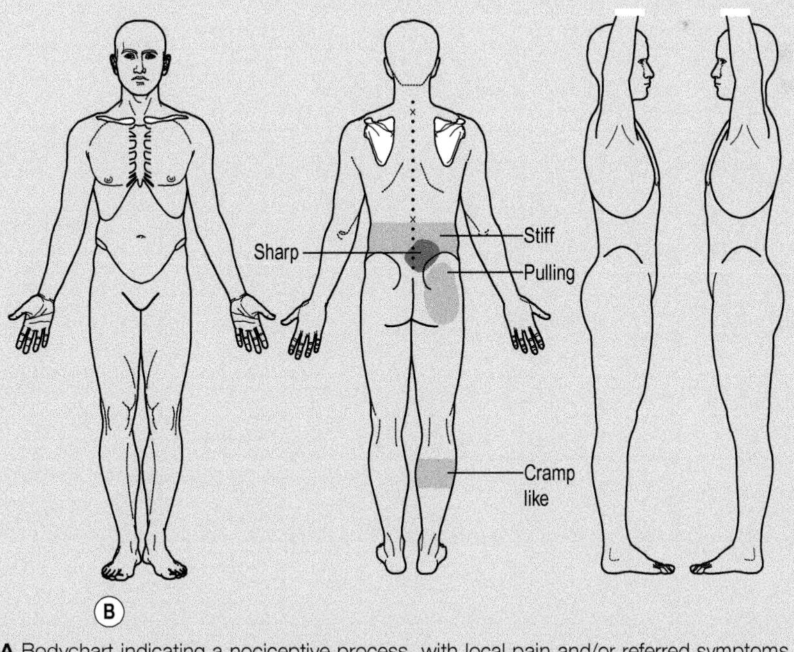

Stiff
Sharp
Pulling

Cramp
like

(B)

Figure 6.3 • A Bodychart indicating a nociceptive process, with local pain and/or referred symptoms of lumbar spine, SIJ and/or soft tissues. The sharp area in the back may be due to a small facet joint disorder; **B** Bodychart indicating a nociceptive process, with local pain and/or referred symptoms of lumbar spine, neurodynamic system, SIJ and/or soft tissues (e.g. triggerpoints). The stiff area in the back may be due to a discogenic movement disorder;

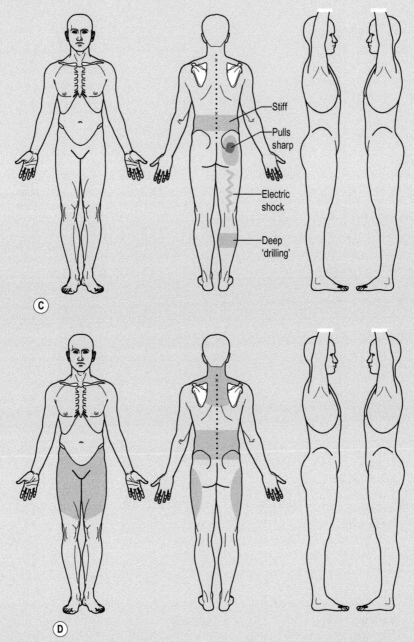

Figure 6.3 • cont'd C Bodychart indicating nociceptive and peripheral neurogenic processes, possibly due to a lumbar spine disorder and radiculopathy; **D** Body chart indicating various areas of symptoms. These may be local nociceptive processes; however, hypotheses reg. central nervous system sensitization may be generated as well.

Note: some patients may have a movement disorder in various movement components, contributing to the same area of symptoms (e.g. nociceptive processes rising from the lumbar spine and the hip. Also mixed nociceptive and central nervous system processing may be present).

With sufficient attention to detail clinicians may start to subgroup clinical patterns in their memory, which may serve in the research of the development of scientific subgroups and clinical prediction rules. The following text from Maitland (1986, p 259–260) demonstrates this principle:

> Yet with all the programmes that have been published (and there are many), none of the authors seem to realize that a patient who feels pain as a very localized spot between the spinous processes of L4 and L5 (say), does not have the same problem as the patient who has pain spreading in a line across his back at the L4/5 interspinous space. Nor do they seem to realize that a patient who has a band of pain across his back, which may extend superiorly to L3 or L4 and inferiorly to S1, is different again, as is the patient who has a band of pain spreading across his back at the middle or lower sacral level is yet another different group. These areas of pain that have been mentioned do not take into account the differences that exist if the patient has pain that spreads across his back but is greater on one side than on the other, or if his pain is only felt on one side of his back. Similarly, these are all different from the patient who feels his pain in the area of the sacroiliac joint or in his gluteal area, yet these are still frequently classed in the (non-specific) back pain grouping for survey purposes. It is my belief that for any project to determine usefully the effect of manipulative treatment, the groupings of patients must be made much more specific. And this is relating the problems to 'site-of-pain' only. The behaviour of the pains then needs to be classified into separate groups.

As neurophysiological pain mechanisms seem to play a growing role in clinical decision-making processes and appear to become increasingly relevant inclusion criteria to research projects, Bogduk (2009) discusses the necessity to make a clear distinction between nociceptive back pain, somatic referred pain, radicular pain and radiculopathy. If radicular pain is not distinguished from somatic referred pain, diagnostic errors may occur and patients may be allocated to faulty (sub-) groups in scientific research leading to erroneous results (Table 6.6). Bogduk postulates that nociceptive back pain and somatic referred pain occur more frequently than radicular

Table 6.6 Distinction between common types of pain (combinations are possible) (Bogduk 2009)

Description	Cause	Remarks	Type of pain
Nociceptive back pain	Noxious stimuli of lumbar structures		'Dull, aching pain in back' Stimulus-response related occurrence of symptoms
Somatic referred pain	Noxious stimuli of lumbar structures – no stimulation of lumbar root structures. Explanation: convergence of nociceptive afferent impulse on the secondary afferent neuron	Distinguish this type of symptoms from visceral referred pain and radicular pain	Normally this type of pain is perceived in those areas, which shared segmental innervation. 'Dull, aching, gnawing', at times: 'expanding pressure'. Tends to be fixed in location, difficult to define boundaries of the area – pattern of presentation does not necessarily share dermatomal patterns
Radicular pain	Pain caused by ectopic salvos in dorsal root or spinal ganglion. May occur, but not necessarily always, in conjunction with disc protrusions. Inflammation of the nerve may be the critical pathophysiological mechanism	A nerve root does not react on compression, unless an inflammation is present. A spinal ganglion on the contrary is highly sensitive on compression and may react with heterospecific impulse 'salvos' within the whole nerve	Lancinating pain quality, Shocking, burning, electric quality. (the term sciatica should be replaced by radicular pain)
Radiculopathy	Neurological condition with a nerve block	Radiculopathy is not defined by pain, but by motor and sensory changes	Numbness (dermatomal), weakness, reduced reflex activity

pain and radicular pain may be investigated with MRI or X-ray procedures, while somatic referred pain often gives inconclusive MRI and X-ray results.

Behaviour of symptoms

Information of the behaviour of symptoms during the day, week or even a month, provides information regarding:

- Parameters for reassessment procedures in consecutive sessions
- Precautions: information about the intensity of the perceived pain and concomitant level of activity will often be a decisive factor in the determination of the dosage of examination and treatment techniques
- Functional capabilities (capacity, performance, mediators) as well as confidence to move
- Coping strategies: deliberate (physiotherapeutic /movement, relaxation, heat/cold applications; medical advice, advice from complementary medicine, e.g acupuncture), intuitive (guarding postures, rubbing, movements)
- Neurophysiological symptom-mechanisms, sources of dysfunction
- Defining treatment objectives: rehabilitation of activity limitations and participation restriction, coping strategies to control pain and well-being, contributing factors as for example information from lifestyle as for example, average activity levels during a week, stress.

Next to the behaviour of symptoms, information about the general activity levels and preferences need to be sought, in order to develop hypotheses about the current movement capacity and resources of a patient.

Particular activities and postures in which lumbar spine movement dysfunctions may be (co-)involved are, for example:

- Sitting, rising up from sitting – note differences if sitting in a high chair, low chair, with legs crossed influences the symptoms
- Bending over as, for example, lifting something from the floor, putting on socks in standing, cleaning a kitchen cupboard
- Getting dressed
- Standing for longer periods
- Walking vigorously or slowly

- Activities in half-flexion as for example washing hair over a bathtub, shaving in standing over a faucet, cleaning /polishing surfaces.

Other activities related to lumbar spine disorders haven been described in the ICF-domains (see p. 232).

It is important not only to find aggravating factors but also easing factors, for example when a patient having lower back pain in sitting, shifts his weight to the other buttock and the pain reduces, it is possible that the lumbar spine is involved with a lateral flexion disorder or preference, respectively. Also, this may be indicative of a sacroiliac involvement. If the patient additionally stretches the leg forward and pushes himself slightly up on the arm rests of the chair to ease the pain, an associated hip disorder next to a lumbar spine dysfunction may be suspected.

In pursuing information regarding coping strategies it is important to seek detailed information about the deliberate or intuitive strategies a person has developed.

Deliberate, explicit strategies may encompass:

- Suggestions from a physiotherapist (which ones, and to which effect)
- Suggestions from the medical doctor
- Suggestions from alternative health practitioners

Other strategies, as for example prescription-free medication.

With intuitive strategies, patients may describe that they feel helpless when the pain increases. However, most patients will somehow intuitively grasp or move the area, without being conscious of this. Often exactly these strategies may be suitable to employ in treatment and as self-management strategies. It needs detailed observation of the patient's movement behaviour and careful communication in guiding the patient towards an increased bodily-awareness, with meaningful self-management strategies. This process may start at times already during the subjective examination (see Box 6.6).

'Making features fit'

'Making features fit' as a principle has been described by Maitland (1986), meaning that at all times during the subjective examination, physical examination as well as during treatment and reassessment, all information needs to be reflected upon, to judge if the information would fit in with a certain clinical

Box 6.6

Communication example to establish intuitive coping strategies if patients feel helpless to control their pain

PT: If your pain has increased, is there anything you have discovered or learned that may help you to reduce this?

Pat: I do know anything to control the pain!

PT: If your pain would increase, right now, as you are sitting here next to me – what would you feel you would do?

Pat: Well, I certainly have to stand up

PT: Could you please show me that right now? Let's assume the pain indeed has increased, what would your body need now/what would you do?

Patient stands up, bends slightly forward and away from the painful side, while guarding the back with his hands and holding his breath somewhat

PT: I see that you have bent over and away and that you are holding your breath a bit and are supporting your back?

Pat: Yes the pain makes me do this!

PT: Do you feel that it eases off the pain somewhat?

Pat: Oh yes, but it will not last

PT: At least it is a strategy with which you instinctively seem to do the right thing from my perspective as a physiotherapist. Often we can use exactly these strategies in treatment, for example by me moving your back very gently or making it a repeated movement with control of breathing. What do you think about that?

Authors' note: in this case, initial treatment techniques consisted of combined passive mobilizations in F/LF in side lying; as self-management strategies to control pain/well-being, the patient was encouraged to perform the guarding movement of F/LF as a repeated movement, while trying to remain relaxed in movement and breathing patterns. At a later stage other active movement procedures were added to the treatment (e.g. muscular control, cardiovascular training)

---

pattern. For example, from the body-chart a therapist may develop different hypotheses about different sources of the nociceptive process (e.g. lumbar spine, hip, sacroiliac joint); during the phase of '24h behaviour of symptoms' it appears that some activities in which the pain occurs may be linked to movements of the hip and others may be related to movements of the lumbar spine.

If the physiotherapist is confronted with a situation in which features do *not* fit, meaning that no known clinical pattern can be recognized, further questioning is essential. In some cases, when the symptoms and signs, and at times the treatment-reactions, do not develop into a picture where the features would fit, the patient may need to be referred to a medical practitioner or a second opinion with another physiotherapist may need to be sought.

Features of some typical activities and postures related to the lumbar spine fitting to hypotheses structural involvement of discs, facets joints, neurodynamic functions (possibly minor end-organ dysfunction leading to nociceptive and/or peripheral neurogenic processes):

- Pain or a sense of stiffness when getting up from sitting, as well as activities in semi-flexed positions such as shaving or washing hair, may be indicative of a discogenic disorder being part of the movement dysfunction
- Facet joints frequently, but not exclusively, may provoke more localized, unilateral/bilateral symptoms while stretching the joint structures towards flexion and contralateral sideflexion and/or compressing the structures towards extension and ipsilateral sideflexion
- Pain provoking activities, as for example using the gas pedal while driving a car, may give a hint towards a neurodynamic dysfunction.

History of symptoms

The history of the symptoms and disability is an important phase of the subjective examination. Particularly details about the onset of the problem may give worthwhile information about risk factors, movement behaviours as well as mediators of pain and, particularly in cases of recent traumatic onset of pain and disability, possible structures involved.

Recent history

This relates to questions such as:

- When did the symptoms occur for the first time (when did ongoing symptoms increase)?
- Which circumstances have led to the onset/increase of the symptoms (traumatic, spontaneous onset)?
- Course of symptoms and activity levels since onset/increase?

- Current symptoms and disability compared with the period on onset/increase (e.g. 'how is it now compared with 2 weeks ago, when it got worse')?

In cases of spontaneous onset, questions about the use of the body, the capability of the structures to bear stress and the general stress levels/stress capacity of a person will be very informative for the selection of therapies regarding self-management strategies and prevention (e.g. long unilateral movements in awkward positions without interruption may need regular interruption with repeated movements in contralateral directions or light bracing with motor control actions). Particularly challenging for patient and therapist are work situation in which a high concentration is asked of the person, as particularly in these circumstances it may be challenging to change habitual patterns of movement behaviour and general tension. For example: a puppeteer in a theatre is standing for a long time with puppets held high above her head with the lumbar spine in extension, right rotation and left sideflexion. She is advised to change the position of the puppets used in the show from her left side to the right side on the floor, in order to achieve flexion and sideflexion during the show; during breaks as a first thing to do, she is encouraged to perform repeated movements in flexion, rotation left and/or sideflexion right and to relax physically and mentally with breathing exercises, combined with a visualization technique).

Especially in cases of recurrent symptoms of acute low back pain the history of the problem, the kind of treatment received and its immediate and long-term effects may provide highly relevant information about the first actions in therapy to take. It is essential to be thorough with follow-up questions. Patients may state that physiotherapy or medication have not helped 'at all'; however, with some clarifying questions, the patient may say that the interventions have helped for a certain period of time, but that the symptoms returned. A central question will be why this may have occurred:

- Certain techniques may have been helpful, but effects did not remain. This, for example, may be because progression of treatment techniques should have been followed up (e.g. treatment of accessory movements of the spine in an end-of-range position).
- Quality of the self-management strategies. It is possible that the patient has not developed an awareness of the specific objectives of the exercises/interventions concerned, as for example knowing which strategies to *select* when increase of pain occurs and which exercises are meant to optimize motor control or general fitness. Often patients are provided with a list of exercises, with a consequence that they perceive that the list has to be worked off (mechanically) at a regular basis. Also, they may not have gained a sense of success regarding self-management to control pain, as the exercise may have been taught once and not been reassessed on its effectiveness in consecutive session or during final analytical assessment procedures (see Chapter 1).
- Stage and stability of the disorder. In some cases, as for example neurogenic pain mechanisms with radicular symptoms, recurrence may occur because the disorder was not stable enough. Patients may have resumed higher levels of activities, including work, but the pain was still quite severe. Particularly radicular symptoms in contrast to simple nociceptive processes, frequently need more time to resume (Bogduk 2009) and therefore a more cautious progression towards higher levels of activity.

Previous history

In long lasting or recurrent episodes, information on the historical context of a problem establishes mediators and risk factors, which may needs to be followed up in treatment planning. Question about the previous history should encompass questions as:

- Episodes of symptoms and activity limitations: which episodes and when did they occur?
- How did the episodes usually start (habitual time patterns and patterns of movement behaviour, e.g. lumbar symptoms in periods of high stress and concentration in the office; yearly recurring activities as for example potato harvest on the farm)?
- How did they improve?
- How were the symptoms and activity levels between episodes (some patients, especially after a large trauma, with subclinical or clinical nerve trauma, may state that the pain recurs at times, but that the overall activity levels have improved over the course of years)?

- How did the symptoms and particularly activity levels change over the course of time?
- How is the current episode in comparison with former episode? (It is possible that a more 'discy', degenerative movement-disorder changes towards a presentation of lumbar stenosis; other may state that the current episode of low back pain is better than before, as they walk more regularly since they have retired from sedentary work.)

Medical and health screening questions

Several questions must be asked so that the physiotherapist is aware of any inherent dangers from treatment or should limit treatment in general. In certain circumstances, as for example osteoporosis, dizziness based on possible vertebrobasilar insufficiency (VBI), treatments such as manipulations with high velocity thrust will not be indicated, but gentle passive movement may be the treatment of choice as long as possible side-effects are monitored.

Special or screening questions encompass the following:

- General health, medication (which, to which effect), involuntary weight loss, medical imaging (incl. results)
- 'Red flags' (see p. 235)

- Information regarding osteoporosis, long-term steroid and anti-coagulant use, diabetes, neurogenic disorders (polyneuropathy)
- Questions regarding bodily systems as cardiac, pulmonary, gastrointestinal, genito-urinary, vascular and musculoskeletal functions, which are part of the screening process of possible biomedical disease. These questions are particularly important in cases of direct contact/self- referral of the patient; however, also, the questions may also be relevant in cases of medical referral as the clinical presentation may have changed since contact with the medical doctor (see pp. 28 and 53 in Chapter 2).
- Additional questions concerning yellow flags, provided the information has not been gained yet during previous questions of the subjective examination (see p. 233 of this chapter).

Typical patterns of clinical presentation

Table 6.7 provides information about some typical clinical presentations in which the lumbar spine may be involved. Clinical patterns may contain clinical prediction rules, but, as they are normally a result from a theoretical and individual experiential knowledge base, they may differ in details from person to person.

Table 6.7 Typical clinical presentations involving the lumbar spine

Clinical syndrome	Clinical presentation	Consequence for physical examination / treatment
Specific low back pain – indicating serious pathology. Also hypotheses about pathologies, which have not been medically assessed yet (e.g. self-referral with a history of back-pain, which developed after a fall on the buttock)	Severe pain, particularly at night interfering with sleep and no effective strategies to reduce symptoms (medication, rest and/or, gentle movements). Minor incident in onset of symptoms resulting in severe pain and large activity limitation. History of cancer. Overall general health reduced (drug abuse, HIV). Involuntary weight loss. Symptom development after traumatic incident (self-referral to therapist)	Refer to medical doctor

Continued

Table 6.7 Typical clinical presentations involving the lumbar spine—cont'd

Clinical syndrome	Clinical presentation	Consequence for physical examination / treatment
Specific low back pain – lumbar spinal stenosis	Pain in lumbar spine area, may radiate to one/both legs Pain may be aggravated particularly during walking and extending activities of the spine Sitting or assuming half flexed positions may reduce the symptoms may be particularly present in patients over 55 years of age (Watters et al. 2008) Physical examination presentation Extension provokes symptoms. Sideflexion (directed towards the painful side) provoking symptoms may be indicative of a lateral stenosis Movements of neighboring joints (hip, thorax) need to be analyzed for any restricted ROM, particularly in extension. Prone lying may be very painful, especially if the ROM in extension is restricted, therefore examination of accessory movements may need to be performed in sidelying or in prone with a flexed position of the spine PAIVMs, PPIVM – may be restricted and tender over various segments	Lumbar spine – accessory movements, with the lumbar spine in pain-free flexed position If accessory movements may be too painful flexion or rotation techniques may need to be considered Mobilizations of the hip, thoracic spine, particularly in extension direction – to reduce impact of restricted hip and/or thoracic movements on the lumbar spine movements, particularly in extension Automobilization of the lumbar spine, thorax and hip Pain control by little lumbar rotation or sideflexion/flexion movements to be integrated in daily life situations, when symptoms are increasing
NSLBP – general	NSLBP is characterized by a variety of descriptions of pain in the low back associated with positional or activity aggravation. There may be or not symptoms referring into the lower extremity (Burton et al, 2009). The individual experience relates to an unknown or innocuous onset or a history of sprain or strain often as a recurrence. The patient is worried, distressed and concerned about their future. Symptoms may persist because of these worries or because of the continuation of adaptive /protective responses. Other issues within work or family or economics may mediate the patients experience or eventual outcome Patients usually identify positions, activities or participating recreation where their capacity is restricted or limited. There are usually no specific health impacts or evidence of serious pathology apart from the patient feeling that their general well-being is being affected because of pain, worry and incapacity The patient considers a successful outcome to be such that they can return to their normal everyday life and recreation without pain.	See pp. 228-254

Table 6.7 Typical clinical presentations involving the lumbar spine—cont'd

Clinical syndrome	Clinical presentation	Consequence for physical examination / treatment
Lumbar discogenic dysfunction (may be more or less specific; frequently attributed to NSLBP)	Recurrent episodes of deep, central lumbar pain; over time may increasingly refer into one buttock and leg frequently related to overuse and misuse of the body in repeated or prolonged flexed positions without altering/repeated movements into other directions Furthermore, it is possible that general fitness levels will have been reduced Physical examination presentation: inspection. May present with an antalgic posture (pelvis shift / lumbar list; hyperextension lumbar spine) Active tests, particularly flexion and rotation may provoke the symptoms Neurological conduction testing may or may not be changed Neurodynamic testing may be symptom-provoking and restricted in range (indicative of neural involvement) PAIVM, PPIVMs may be restricted and tender over various segments	Treatment of the involved lumbar segments with e.g. rotation techniques, accessory movements If neural involvement is present see below (radicular syndrome) Early intervention with self-management strategies as for example repeated movement into extension or sideflexion; ergonomic advice for bending and sitting. Development of programs to enhance motor control for segmental and global stabilization of the lumbar spine / trunk Information-strategies on regenerative potential of discs and the role of movement in this process
NSLBP, nociceptive mechanisms	More likely localized symptoms, referred symptoms more proximally stimulus response-related symptoms, activity and posture related history related: over a course a few days after onset pain is reducing and activity levels are improving may or may not be related to an end organ-dysfunction (Apkarian & Robinson 2010)	See recommendations for treatment of NSLBP (see pp. 228-254) Be aware of multicomponent movement disorders (e.g lumbar spine involvement as well as SIJ and hip involvement) Construct of severity/irritability may be applicable (i.e. adapting P/E and Rx directly to P1)
Peripheral neurogenic syndrome radicular pain (maybe more like attributed as 'non specific' radiculopathy (frequently attributed as 'specific'	Tingling, numbness in dermatomal areas loss of motor control (e.g. walking on heels, on toes) Quality symptoms may be superficial burning or deep throbbing in the leg Hx: symptoms in distal parts over the leg have become more severe, at times more than in the proximal part Latency of symptoms may be present Physical examination presentation: may present with an antalgic posture with the lumbar spine in slightly flexed/sideflexed position away from the painful side; furthermore slight knee flexion may be present Neurological testing of reflexes, muscle contractions and/ or sensation may show differences compared with the unaffected leg Nerve palpation may be sensitive in the buttock or upper thigh area (hamstrings area) Neurodynamic testing may be restricted and pain provoking	Distinguish radicular pain from radiculopathy (Bogduk 2009) Neurological conduction testing in P/E necessary Treat the primary sources of the neurogenic dysfunction (e.g. movement impairments of lumbar spine and or hip movements disorders; muscular control), while regularly monitoring reflex activities, motor control and skin sensation may include neurodynamic treatment if neurological conduction tests remain unchanged. For example gentle 'slider' techniques within a pain-free range to the nervous systems may be considered (Coppieters & Butler 2008) Medication at initial stages when pain is severe recommended

Continued

Table 6.7 Typical clinical presentations involving the lumbar spine—cont'd

Clinical syndrome	Clinical presentation	Consequence for physical examination / treatment
NSLBP, indication of facet joint involvement in movement disorder	Relatively localized pain area over the joint, may refer proximally in leg Opening movement patterns in flexion, closing movement patterns in extension may provoke the pain	Treatment of symptoms and signs, prevention of recurrences by addressing movement behaviour leading to symptoms Passive mobilizations, e.g. unilateral PA movements; may consider localized or generalized HVT-manipulation Automobilizations, repeated movements, muscular control exercises Bodily awareness about movement behaviour, use of body during daily life If persistent: may consider joint block (infiltration)
NSLBP – multi-factorial, persistent	Patient may express a sense of helplessness on control of pain, in spite of numerous therapies with different clinicians History and course of symptoms and disability do not match with expected time of tissue regeneration and functional recuperation Protective behaviour of initial episode has maintained, although higher levels of activity seem to be /should have been possible	Multidimensional approach to treatment, if possible in an interdisciplinary team Note: ensure that sufficient assessment of pathobiological investigation has taken place, before (prematurely) considering the problem as multifactorial because symptoms and disabilities seem to last longer than would be expected (Hancock et al. 2011) Constructs of severity/irritability need to be considered from a behavioural perspective as an expression of maladaptive movement-behaviour
Stability dysfunction (structural with discrepancies between hypomobile and hypermobile intervertebral segments; functional: altered motor control patterns)	Local pain in lumbar area, may present as a small line crossing the lumbar spine. symptoms may be aggravated with activities as bending over, while holding heavier loads; standing for longer periods of time; sleeping-in during the weekend, various episodes of symptoms, of spontaneous onset. Frequently no clear incident why symptoms recur. *Physical examination presentation:* flexion – may occur with a lordotic posture, patient needs the hands as support coming up from flexion. Supporting the lower abdomen during the movement may reduce the pain Pain may be provoked during extension and/ or sideflexion. Note if any local muscle protective reactions occur during the test movements PAIVM and PPIVM may indicate one segment more mobile than the neighbouring segments. Furthermore, pain may be provoked with central and/or unilateral PA-movement on the segment involved Muscle tests in supine, sitting, standing, active movements indicate loss of / altered motor control patterns	May consider treating the nociceptive active joints with gentle passive mobilization: flexion or rotation techniques or accessory movements – short before P1, not too far into R. May need to mobilize the neighbouring segments if they have reduced joint mobility (e.g. L1–3 area, hip) – however, care needs to be given not to irritate the painful segments further, as they may be moved as well during the treatment Enhance segmental muscular control; first by addressing the local stabilizing muscle system, then by addressing the global stabilizing system It is essential to integrate the training of muscular control in functional positions and activities

Physical examination

At the end of the subjective examination it is often important to first summarize the main information of the interview, to clarify open questions and to find agreement with the patient on activity limitations which need to be rehabilitated and coping strategies regarding pain control.

The subsequent physical examination should be considered and communicated as the examination of movement impairments which often, but not always, are prerequisites to the restoration of optimum functional capacity. From a clinical reasoning perspective the physical examination is one of the stages in the therapeutic process in which hypotheses may be confirmed and/or modified.

Planning the physical examination procedures

As already stated, regular planning in critical phases of the therapeutic process is essential to comprehensive clinical practice. Regular planning may have become an automatic, implicit process for the more experienced MSK-physiotherapist, as they will be able to 'reflect in action' more frequently (Schön 1983). However, novices may actively enhance their path to professional expertise if they explicitly go through reflection and planning phases after having performed certain procedures of the physiotherapy process ('reflection on action'). In this learning process it is essential not only to document the results of examination procedures and therapeutic interventions, but also to record the reflections and the planned procedures.

After completion of the subjective examination, it is often useful to summarize its main points and the goals of treatment agreed with the patient so far. It may also be necessary to explain to the patient the objectives of the next stage of the initial assessment – the physical examination.

Planning after the subjective examination as a preparation for the physical examination has three phases:

- Reflection on the subjective examination process – the physiotherapist needs to verify that the subjective examination is sufficiently complete in order to be able to perform a comprehensive physical examination, respecting precautions and contraindications, as well as performing subjective reassessment procedures in subsequent sessions (see Reflection on the subjective examination process, below).
- Expressing hypotheses which will influence the physical examination process. Hypotheses regarding pathobiological mechanisms, sources, contributing factors, precautions and contraindications and management in particular need to be made explicit (see Hypotheses, below).
- Planning the procedures of examination, including anticipation on possible findings, the kind of examination (dosage or extent of examination procedures), sequence of testing and reassessment procedures (see Planning of the physical examination procedures, below).

Precautions to examination procedures

Hypotheses with regard to precautions and contraindications to physical examination and treatment procedures serve to determine the extent of the physical examination that can be safely undertaken. Furthermore, they aid in the decision if contraindications to examination procedures or treatment interventions are present.

The precautions and contraindications are mostly determined by hypotheses with regard to pathobiological processes and neurophysiological pain mechanisms and may include the following factors:

- Pathobiological processes – tissue mechanisms, stages of tissue healing, neurophysiological pain mechanisms
- Irritability of the disorder (see Box 6.7)
- Severity of the disorder (see Table 6.7)
- Stage and stability of the disorder
- General health
- Patient's movement behaviour, perspectives and expectations.

Physical examination and the lumbar spine

Physical examination procedures should follow a structured, integrated format, but they should be flexible enough to be individualized to the patient's needs. This includes precautions to the test-procedures as well as the patient's preferences to move. Sometimes a phenomenological perspective

Box 6.7

Constructs of severity and irritability of the pain: a cognitive-behavioural perspective

Irritability has been defined as 'a little activity causing severe pain, discomfort, paraesthesia or numbness, which takes relatively long to subside' and that of severity as 'the activity that causes the symptoms has to be stopped, because of the intensity of the pain' (Maitland et al. 2005).

A comparatively minor activity (e.g. ironing for half an hour) that causes pain of a severity that forces the patient to stop ironing, but subsides within 10 minutes such that another half hour of ironing can be carried out, indicates minor irritability of the disorder. This, therefore, frequently permits a full examination plus some treatment on the first day, without the likelihood of exacerbation. If, however, the pain did not subside until the patient had had a full night's sleep, the disorder would be considered to be highly irritable and the examinations and treatment would have to be tailored to avoid exacerbation (Maitland et al. 2005).

It is argued that the word 'irritability' may have been misunderstood and misused by physiotherapists (Sayres 1997). Irritability and severity need to be considered from various perspectives. On the one hand it describes the reported pain sensation; on the other hand it reports the activity provoking the symptoms, including the patient's reaction to it.

- If the symptoms appear to be due to dominant nociceptive or peripheral neurogenic input mechanisms, a direct stimulus response and historical relationship may be present, in which the intensity of the symptoms may be interpreted as a direct result of end-organ dysfunction provoking nociceptive processes (e.g. ischaemia). In these cases the extent of the examination strategies will usually be taken to the point in movements when pain commences or increases (P1). Frequently only a few tests need to be performed in order to find comparable signs which may serve as parameters in subsequent reassessment procedures.

- Central nervous system processing and (neurophysiological) output mechanisms (Gifford 1998) may also contribute to ongoing tenderness and sensitivity to touch or movement, which may distort the direct stimulus–response relationship. This may lead to misinterpretations of severity and irritability with regard to the extent of examination and treatment procedures as well as the education of and instructions to the patient.

- In this example the constructs of irritability and severity may be considered as a form of avoidance behaviour, as the person having the pain will often interrupt the activity causing the pain (Hengeveld 2002).

- In order to make a differentiated hypothesis with regard to 'irritability' or 'severity' it needs to be determined if the behaviour is adaptive to acute nociceptive or peripheral neurogenic processes or if the behaviour has become maladaptive over time due to learning processes and central nervous system mechanisms. Asking the patients when it was the last time that they have performed the activity concerned will give a good indication.

- Some patients may tell during the subjective examination that they are not capable of, for example, carrying a bag or putting on socks because it is too painful. Based on this information the symptoms of these patients may be classified as 'severe' or 'irritable'. However, on further questioning it may become clear that it was months ago that such activities were tried for the last time. In this case it may be a form of avoidance behaviour due to learning processes with affective, cognitive and sociocultural variables rather than a direct result of abnormal nociceptive or peripheral neurogenic input alone.

It has been acknowledged that the clinician's behaviour during the performance of examination procedures may reinforce the illness behaviour and experience of the patient (Hadler 1996, Pilowsky 1997). In such a situation it may be possible that the careful testing only until the onset of pain (P1) and immediately away from the point of pain in fact may reinforce the maladaptive avoidance behaviour of the patient further.

As the decision on severity/irritability in this stage of the examination will determine the extent of the examination procedures, it is important to be aware of these possible reinforcing effects due to interactions and behaviour during the examination procedures.

In the above-mentioned situation it is possible to plan the extent of the physical examination as recommended for those patients with severity or irritability, i.e. to perform a few tests or the standard procedures without overpressure.

Test movements may be taken slightly 'beyond the onset of pain', rather than only 'until the onset of pain'. A point in the movement may occur where the patient indicates that the pain increases. The therapist then gently moves back in the movement to check if the pain subsides quickly enough, then moves on to the onset of the pain again, at the same time enquiring if the patient has the trust to move a bit further. For example, if the patient is able to bend forward to 20° of inclination before the pain starts, but still has trust to move on until about 40°, the physiotherapist has found two important variables in the test movement:

Box 6.7—cont'd

- P_1 at 20° of inclination (lumbar flexion)
- 'Confidence$_1$' at 40° of inclination, indicating the point in the movement at which the patient 'trusted to move' to in spite of the pain

The following communication example may explain some of the subtleties of the examination process in these circumstances:

(ET: Examiner's thoughts; Q: question; A: answer)

Q 'I would like to examine the movements of your back – how far you may be able to move your back, and if some movements are okay but others provoke discomfort. However, I would not like to push you into any movements that you are not confident of doing yourself. Will you give me a sign if that happens?'

A 'Oh yes.'

Q 'Could you bend forward, as far as you trust yourself to do?'

A (moves until c. 20° of inclination) 'Oh no, not further than this.'

Q (guides the patient back to a straight position) 'And if I move it like this?'

A 'Now it is alright again.'

Q *(gently guides the patient again until 20° of inclination)* 'If you do this again, how is it now, here again?'

A (grimaces) 'Oh, there it hurts again.'

Q (back to upright position) 'Now, okay again?'

A 'Yes.'

Q 'Was the pain the second time the same as the first time? Or did it get worse the second time?'

A 'No, it was the same.'

ET *If the pain had increased the second time I would stop the testing now. However, it seems to have more of an 'on–off' character than I initially thought. I want him to move the arm gently 'beyond P1'.*

Q 'Okay, could I gently take you back to that point of pain?'

A 'Okay.'

Q 'Now it hurts again?'

A 'Yes.'

Q 'Would you trust yourself to move a bit further in spite of the pain? Only as far as what you trust to move!'

A (*grimaces and moves until c. 40°*) 'Until here.'

Q 'Okay, and back again. How are you now?'

A 'It's alright again.'

Q 'I would like you to remember this movement, as we will check it later in therapy again – maybe your pain has changed after the treatment or maybe you will trust to lift your arm a bit higher.'

Performance of an examination in such a manner requires an awareness of the subtleties of communication and the effects of touch during the examination process. In fact the patient may learn various aspects from the examination procedures, for example:

- The pain may be more movement dependent (stimulus-response related) than initially believed
- There may be movements which provoke more discomfort and there may be movements which are less discomforting instead of believing that 'everything hurts all the time' in the same manner
- It is not dangerous to move *carefully* beyond the point where a pain has commenced
- The patient may learn to trust the physiotherapist, as the questioning and testing indicated that the patient would not be forced to move in ways, which he did not trust himself.

A procedure performed in such a manner may be seen as an expression of a bio-psychosocial approach to initial treatment of fear avoidance behaviour with regard to movements and activities. **Hence, the gradual exposure to activities may start with the first physical examination procedures**

with salutogenic approach to examination may be more beneficial than a therapist-directed approach to testing (see Chapters 1 and 2 of Volume 2 and Chapter 8 of this volume).

The scope of practice of a physiotherapist is reflected in the examination procedures. Making a movement diagnosis is a key issue, rather than making a structural diagnosis (although this hypothesis of pathobiological is an important element in clinical reasoning) and to design examination around safety, interventions and outcomes. In cases where the pain and disability are based on peripheral nociceptive and/or neurogenic processes, one of the goals of examination procedures will be reproduction of the patient's symptoms. However, other information regarding motor control patterns, habitual movement patterns, joint-position sense and proprioceptive feedback, as well as neurological conduction tests, may also be integrated into the examination procedures.

During the physical examination process, it needs regular phases of 'brief appraisal', in which the therapist reflects on the findings so far and if the examination procedures can be carried on as planned, or if they have to be adjusted and adapted to the patient's situation.

The physical examination should aim to confirm the hypotheses established through clinical evidence gathering in the subjective examination.

The main aim therefore, using movement analysis and manual examination, is to establish:

- The level of functioning of the movement system, including an impression of the movement potential
- The movement impairments and evidence for the need for movement therapy interventions
- Measures of the effectiveness of such interventions [P/E ASTERISKS***]
- Patient's confidence to move, at times in spite of the pain.

Specific aims of the physical examination should include (Higgs et al. 2008):

- Test the C/O hypotheses
- Reproduce the patient's symptoms
- Find comparable signs-adaptive, protective, restrictive
- Find the source/cause of the source/ contributing factors
- Establish components, mechanisms, dimensions for each symptom area
- Identify movement impairments (range, symptom response, quality of movement)
- Establish functional activity limitations
- Examine relative to the severity, irritability and nature of the symptoms (movement to P_1 or limit with overpressure if necessary)
- Screen other potential components, predisposing factors
- Carry out special testing where appropriate
- Establish the role and desired effects of mobilization/manipulation.

Physical examination procedures place an emphasis on range, symptom response and quality of movements. They are mainly, but not exclusively, impairments based. However, functional demonstration tests may encompass all activities from daily life, which patients have been avoiding.

It is essential to link the therapeutic interventions to the physical examination findings, expressed in reassessment procedures after the application of the intervention. Furthermore, they need to be linked to the results from the subjective examination, which usually are compared at the beginning of subsequent sessions.

Table 6.8 provides an overview of the general test procedures related to the examination of the lumbar spine and related structures. It should be noted that reassessment procedures are part of the overall physical examination, even if not all planned tests may have been performed. If there is a pain sensation at the beginning of the physical examination ('present pain'), this needs to be reassessed regularly to ascertain whether this present pain is changing as a result of, for example, active tests. Furthermore, it is possible that examination procedures, e.g. for accessory movements of the spine, may have a therapeutic effect, which has to be evaluated before, for example, hip movements are passively examined.

Observation

Observing the patient in a variety of positions and a variety of views while standing, sitting and/or lying will enable the clinician to start to identify structural faults, signs of impairment such as wasting or bruising, adaptive and protective mechanisms resulting in postural asymmetry, balance and alignment of body parts, including common faults associated with the risk of developing low back pain (such as sway back, flat back and kypholordosis).

- Furthermore, the therapist gains an impression about the willingness and confidence to move.
- The therapist's in-depth knowledge of alignment, pelvis neutral position, neutral zone, tone etc. will enhance an ability to recognize motor control faults, which could be contributing to deficits in movement (Sahrmann 2011)
- *Present pain:* any symptoms at resting postures need to be established before embarking on active examination procedures
- Correction of faults will clarify whether or not these faults are related to the current patient's symptoms. With the reproduction of symptoms on correction, the posture can be considered as an antalgic posture or protective deformity. See pelvic shift correction in Figure 6.4.

Table 6.8 Possible physical examination procedures of the lumbar spine and associated movement components

Basic procedures	Additional tests, if appropriate or indicated

Observation

Spontaneous movement behaviour (e.g. when undressing), willingness and confidence to move

Alignment, postural faults, asymmetry, e.g. shift correction

Present pain (PP)?

Protective deformities – antalgic postures. Effect on symptoms of correction?

Functional demonstration

Including differentiation tests if possible (e.g. bending and lifting to pick up boxes at work)

Active tests lumbar spine	Screening:

Flexion

Extension

Sideflexion to right, left

Rotation to right, left

Adding overpressure to active test movements if full active movement is pain-free

Local overpressure may be applied to extension, sideflexion

All movements may be performed from caudad–cephadad

May apply 'if necessary testing, if active movements, including overpressure are pain-free
- sustained positions, repeated movements, quicker movements, from one extreme range to opposite extreme
- combined movements
  a) 2 movement directions combined (e.g. LF & E; Rot Ⓡ & F etc.)
  b) 3 movements directions combined (incl. lumbar quadrant)

May need to do active testing in sitting, lying positions

Screening:

Hip: squat, standing on one leg, extension/MR/Add

Knee: squat, bouncing in hyperextension in standing

Thoracic spine F, E, LF, Rot

Sacroiliac joint/pelvic girdle: provocation tests, orientation tests:
- spreading innominates ('traction')
- compressing innominates ('compression')
- Patrick sign
- F/Ad & femur shaft compression (posterior shear/thigh thrust technique)
- MR & LR of hip
- active SLR
- compression pelvis

Neurological conduction testing

Reflexes: patella, achilles jerk

Muscles

Sensation

Neurodynamic testing

SLR, including differentiation (sensitizing) movements in DF, MR/Add hip, neck flexion

Slump, including variations

Prone knee bend

Slump tests in sidelying

Nerve palpation

Palpation T10–L5/S1

Skin temperature, sweating, tone

Muscle tone, thickness

Bony alignment (particularly spinous processes)

Interspinous space, laminae: soft / leathery thickness

Continued

Table 6.8 Possible physical examination procedures of the lumbar spine and associated movement components—cont'd

Basic procedures	Additional tests, if appropriate or indicated
PAIVMS T10–L5, followed by reassessment procedures: central PA, unilateral PA movements May include: transverse movements	AP-movements Continue screening: passive testing, followed by reassessment • Thorax: accessory movements • Hip: F/Add or accessory movements • SIJ (symphysis pubis, ox coccygeus): • AP, PA tilts of innominate in sidelying • Accessory movements of sacrum and/or ilium
PPIVM T10– L5-S1 F E Sideflexion right, left Rotation right, left	AP–PA gliding added at end-of-range of segmental flexion/extension movement as an indication of enlarged neutral zone (Panjabi 1992)
Examination of motor control impairment – observe patterns of F, E and/or rotation control In supine, prone, side-lying, quadruped position In functional positions, e.g. sitting, standing, bending over During functional movements	

Functional demonstration

Functional demonstration testing may serve different purposes:

- The patient will often be able to demonstrate a movement or activity, involving the lumbar spine, which reproduces his symptoms. This may be a daily activity that he knows hurts his back, such as bending forwards to tie his shoelaces. He may also be able to demonstrate the movement he was doing when his back was strained – for instance, a backhand at tennis. By asking the patient to demonstrate such an activity to the onset on pain (P1), or to the limit, the therapist can analyze the range of movement, symptom response and quality of movement. This test movement may serve as a parameter ('asterisk') for reassessment procedures.
- Differentiation at this stage may help to confirm the movement components at fault if there is any doubt. For example, the patient may be able to reproduce his left buttock pain by demonstrating the backhand tennis shot that injured him. This movement principally involves rotation of the spine and hip. By using the lumbar spine/ hip differentiation test involvement of the spine rather than the hip may be revealed (or vice versa) (Fig. 6.5).
- Further brief appraisal of the spine with active movements and hip with for example the observation of squatting and one-leg hip extension will confirm the need to examine the spine or hip in more detail. Treatment should then reinforce the initial hypothesis.

Further differentiation of the functional demonstration or injuring movement may be of value when improvement has slowed or stopped. For example, after several sessions of treatment, the patient may have to stretch a lot further into the backhand shot to reproduce his pain. Further differentiation may reveal that lumbar extension and lateral flexion to the painful side adds to the buttock pain being

Pelvic shift correction

Patient starting position: patient presents with pelvic shift to right / trunk list to left

Therapist starting position: standing at patient's left side

Localization of forces: both forearms dorsally and ventrally of pelvis with hands on patient's right iliac crest; therapist's shoulder/ clavicle supports patient's left arm in patient's side

Application of forces:

Correction a. Therapist pulls patient's pelvis towards herself. Observe range, quality of movement and symptom-response (Fig. 6.4A).

Correction b. Therapist pushes patient's trunk away from herself. Observe range, quality of movement and symptom-response (Fig. 6.4B)

Correction c. As a progression of testing: combination of (a) and (b) (Fig. 6.4C).

Remarks: the therapist ensures that with each hand an equal force is applied. The trunk/pelvis have to move in a horizontal line (avoid sideflexion to the right).

Note: range of movement, quality and/or symptom-response.

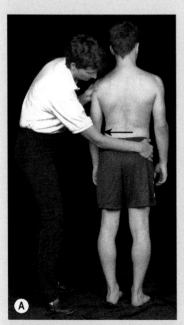
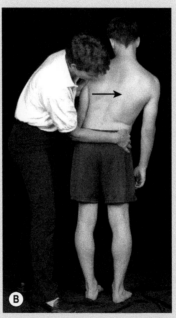
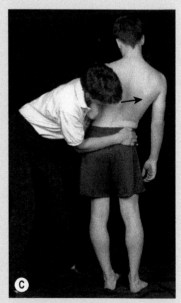

Figure 6.4 • A Pelvic shift correction to the left; **B** Trunk list correction to the right; **C** Combination of pelvic shift to the left and trunk list to the right.

Lumbar spine/hip differentiation test: rotation

Patient starting position: standing, twisting the trunk to right until the onset of pain (symptom reproduction), then – if possible – balances on the right leg (refer to Fig. 6.5A and B)

Therapist starting position: in front of patient.

Localization of forces:

- Patient places both hands on both shoulders of therapist for balance (refer to Fig. 6.5C)
- Therapist stabilizes patient's pelvis with both hands (refer to Fig. 6.5D).

Application of forces:

Step 1: Patient derotates lumbar spine, by moving right hand from the left shoulder to the right shoulder of the therapist (refer to Fig. 6.5E) – therapist maintains pelvis in position to prevent rotation

Step 2: Patient's hands again on both shoulders of therapist: patient is asked to move the right hand further into right trunk rotation (therapist stabilizes pelvis)

Step 3: Patient's hands again on both shoulders – ensure that the pain is still reproduced. Therapist moves patient's pelvis into further right rotation: this increases hip rotation, decreases lumbar rotation (refer to Fig. 6.5F)

Step 4: As step 3, therapist moves patient's pelvis towards left rotation – thus releasing hip rotation and increasing lumbar rotation.

Remarks:

- If the buttock symptoms are provoked by a hip movement disorder, it may be expected that symptoms increase with step 3 and decrease with step 4
- If they are provoked by a lumbar rotational disorder it may be expected that symptoms increase in step 2 and possibly step 4; decrease of symptoms in steps 1 and 3.

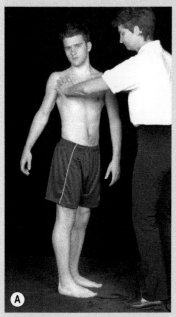

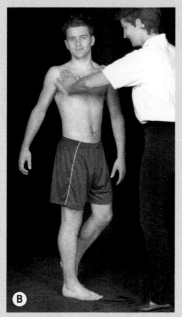

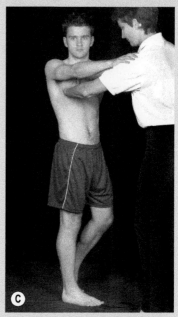

Figure 6.5 • **A** Differentiation test, spinal and peripheral joint pain, part 1. **A** Rotation to the right. **B** Patient balancing on right leg and over-pressure added;

Lumbar spine/hip differentiation test: rotation—cont'd

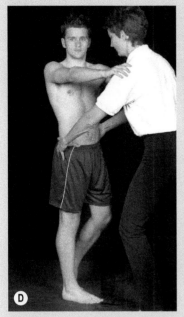
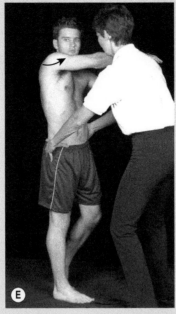
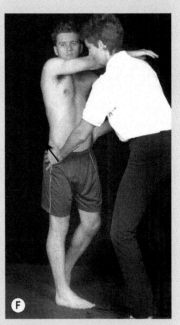

Figure 6.5 • cont'd C Patient balanced; **D** Stabilizing the pelvis; **E** Retaining hip rotation and releasing lumbar rotation; **F** Part 2: retaining released lumbar rotation and increasing hip rotation.

reproduced by rotation of the spine during the backhand shot. Therefore a lumbar rotation treatment technique in lumbar extension and ipsilateral lateral flexion will be a valuable technique as a progression of treatment.

Active tests lumbar spine

Active testing of the lumbar spine includes flexion, extension, rotation and sideflexion of the trunk.

Initially the gross spinal range and pain response to the movement should be noted. Furthermore it is important to notice the quality of the local intervertebral movement and the pain response. These three aspects serve as parameter for reassessment-procedures ('asterisks').

If, for example lateral flexion is limited, the statement may be recorded that the limitation occurs mainly from L3 downwards. Watching the movements from these two aspects (i.e. the gross movements and the local movements) can be likened to taking a photograph with a wide-angle lens for the gross movement, and a second movement using a telephoto lens to highlight the localized limited movement.

However, if these movements do not reproduce any symptoms of the patient, additional stress may be added to the movement, as for example:

- Applying overpressure at the end of the available active ROM. Frequently more range will be gained, when the structures are moved further into the movement in a passive or assisted active way. Overpressure should be applied in a light oscillatory manner, while progressing further into the end of the range of the movement. Any symptom-response by the patient as well as the quality of the resistance perceived by the therapist has to be noted:
  - overpressure may be applied to the overall movement
  - overpressure may be applied locally to the intervertebral segments in E, LF and/or rotation.
- Application of the movements F, E, LF or Rot:
  - faster
  - repeated: do the symptoms increase? Then the movement serves as a parameter for reassessment procedures

○ do the symptoms decrease with the repetition of the movement? Then the movement may be adapted to serve as a self-management exercise to control the pain

○ moving from one extreme position to the other. This is frequently useful in later treatment sessions, to check if the structures have been cleared sufficiently

○ sustained: maintaining the movement into end-of-range position, with a slight overpressure. This test variation may be particularly helpful in those cases, where symptoms occur only in sustained daily life positions.

• Most movements of the trunk in lumbar spine testing occur from a cephadad to caudad direction. However, at times it is more informative to test the movements from caudad to cephadad upwards

• Combination of movement directions. These combinations may give almost endless variations, as two directions, three movement directions may be combined. In some exceptional cases even an accessory movement has to be applied to the movement combination, before symptoms may be reproduces.

• Changing position of the patient: some symptoms may only be reproduced if the tests are being performed while the patient is sitting or lying.

The active tests, including a selection of test variations, are described below.

Neurological conduction testing

Neurological conduction testing is the manual testing of reflexes, muscle reactivity and skin sensation to support in clinical decision-making processes.

Text continued on p. 288

Lumbar flexion and variations

Patient starting position: standing.
  Therapist starting position: therapist stands at the right side of patient.
  Localization of forces

• Overpressure (Fig. 6.6): left forearm of therapist stabilizes patient' pelvis, therapist's right hand is positioned between patient's scapulae

• Test combinations: patient folds arms in front of chest; therapist supports patient's pelvis with legs, trunk and right arm to control flexion position. Therapist's left arm assists the patient's movement.

  Application of forces: active movement

• Observe active test: normal movement should be unrolling smoothly during downward

• Movement and during recovery from flexion (Fig. 6.7)

• Observe any deviations in the movement, e.g. during flexion sideflexion to the right

• Correction of the deviation may lead to a more limited range of movement and pain reproduction

• Overpressure (Fig. 6.6): therapist's right hand pushes patient's trunk towards stabilizing forearm at the patient's pelvis.

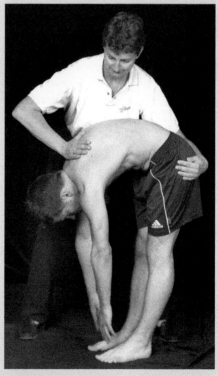

Figure 6.6 • Lumbar flexion with over-pressure at upper thorax directed towards the pelvis.

Lumbar flexion and variations—cont'd

Test combinations: therapist keeps the patient in end of range flexion, any added movement as e.g. LF or rotation is done in an assisted active way: patient is asked to rotate the head and trunk up (Fig. 6.8AB) or to move the trunk sideways towards lateral flexion (Fig. 6.9A). Also combinations of three directions is at time possible (Fig. 6.9B & C)

Variations:

- Application of neck flexion at the end of range of lumbar flexion (Fig. 6.10)
- Active flexion from caudad to cephadad upwards (Fig. 6.11)
- Test combinations e.g. flexion + LF ; flexion + rotation (Fig. 6.8AB)
- Test combinations are also possible in ½ flexed position (depending on the daily life activity which provokes the symptoms e.g. pain occurs while brushing teeth)

Note: test combinations in flexion should only be performed in stable clinical situations, in which the pain is recuperating quickly after being provoked.

Change position of patient to sitting, sidelying, supine if necessary

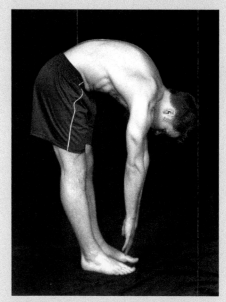

Figure 6.7 • Lumbar spine flexion from above downwards.

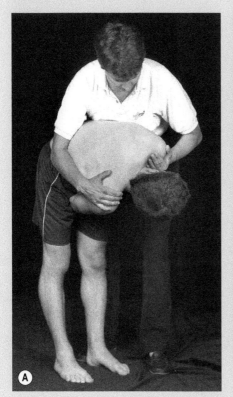

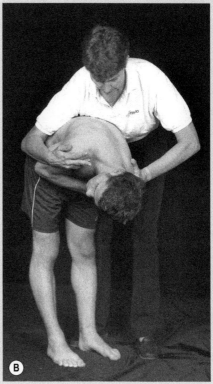

Figure 6.8 • Lumbar flexion over-pressure adding rotation with over-pressure. **A** Rotation left; **B** Rotation right.

Continued

Lumbar flexion and variations—cont'd

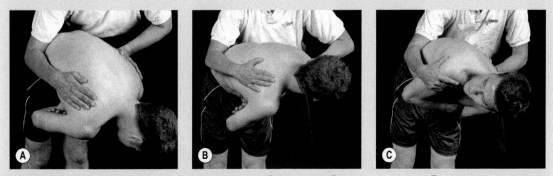

Figure 6.9 • Combined movements in flexion. **A** F + LF Ⓛ; **B** F + LF Ⓛ + Rot L; **C** F + LF Ⓛ + Rot R.

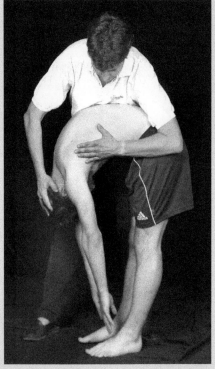

Figure 6.10 • Lumbar flexion: superimposed over-pressure to neck flexion.

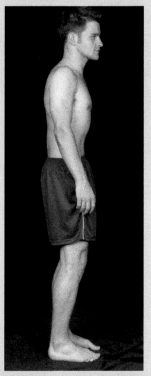

Figure 6.11 • Lumbar spine flexion from below upwards.

Lumbar extension and variations

Patient starting position: standing

Therapist starting position

- Most tests: at the side of the patient
- In some test combinations: therapist may stand behind patient (as in lumbar quadrant)

Localization of forces

- Overpressure generalized movement: therapist's left hand grasps around patient's chest and contralateral should; therapist's right hand is placed on patient's sacrum (Fig. 6.12)
- Localized overpressure: instead of placing the right hand on the sacrum, the therapist's thumb-pad and bent index fingers are gently placed around the spinous process of L5, L4, L3, L2 subsequently (Fig. 6.13)
- Combined movements, incl. lumbar quadrant (e.g. quadrant left: extension/sideflexion left/ rotation left):

Application of forces

- Overpressure: therapist's right hand on the sacrum stabilizes patient's pelvis; left hand moves gently towards the stabilizing hand (Fig. 6.12)
- Before applying overpressure, encourage the patient to arch the back further. It is important that the patient maintains *his own balance*
- Localized overpressure: the therapist moves the patient's trunk gently around the stabilizing fingers at the patient's spinous process (Fig. 6.13)
- Combined test movements: is possible in numerous directions.
- Localization of forces is the same as in extension & overpressure (Fig. 6.14); Extension + Rot (r): therapist pushes patient's left shoulder forward and right shoulder backwards with her left hand. Therapist's right index finger supplies counter pressure to the movement (Fig. 6.15).

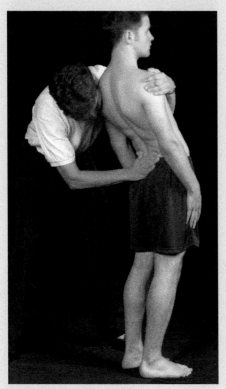

Figure 6.12 • Assessing lumbar extension by over-pressure.

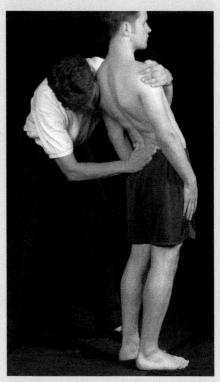

Figure 6.13 • Localized overpressure in extension.

Lumbar extension and variations—cont'd

Lumbar quadrant:

a. lumbar quadrant may be build up as in normal extension: first apply extension, add left sideflexion, then left rotation (as in Fig. 6.14)

b. While standing behind the patient therapist's hands placed on patient's shoulder for control, *after* patient moved towards extension. Through her hands the therapist applies some pressure to the extension. By using the hands on patient's shoulders, the therapist guides the patient's trunk into the corner by laterally flexing and rotating his trunk away from her. Move until the limit of range (Fig. 6.16)

Variations:

a. Extension from caudad-cephadad upwards; particularly if the extension while arching backwards is pain-free and a lumbosacral movement disorder is suspected (Fig. 6.17AB)

b. Change position of patient to sitting, sidelying, supine/prone if necessary

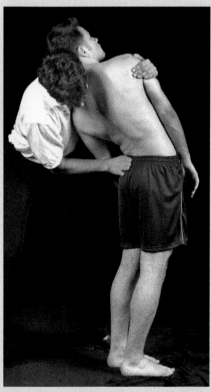

Figure 6.14 • Combined movement in E + Rot left + sideflexion left.

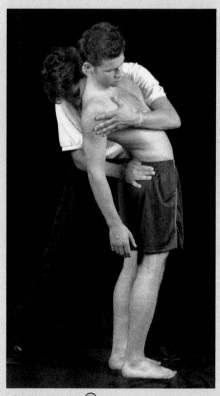

Figure 6.15 • E + Rot Ⓡ.

Lumbar sideflexion and variations—cont'd

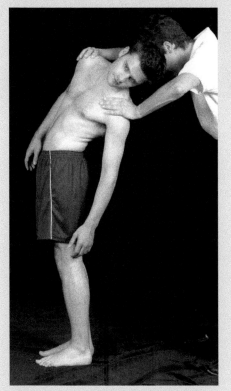

Figure 6.16 • Quadrant test for lumbar spine.

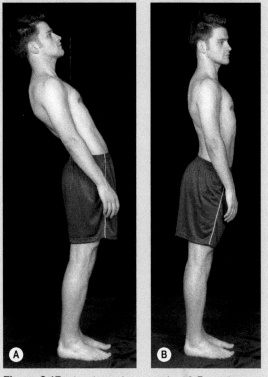

Figure 6.17 • Lumbar spine extension. **A** From above downwards; **B** from below upwards.

Lumbar sideflexion and variations

Patient starting position: standing.

Therapist starting position: at the side of the patient.

Localization of forces:

- Overpressure generalized movement: therapist's left axilla rests on patient's left shoulder; therapist's left arm grasps around patient's trunk towards patient's left upper arm. Therapist's right hand stabilizes patient's left crista iliaca (Fig. 6.18)
- Localized overpressure: therapist's left arm is position as in generalized overpressure, therapist's right thumb, supported by index finger is place laterally against spinous process of L5, L4, L3, L2 subsequently.
- Combined movements: as in generalized overpressure (Figs 6.19–6.22).

Application of forces:

- Overpressure of generalized and localized movement: hand at patient's crista /spinous process stabilizes the movement, which is initiated by the therapist's pressure on the patient's left shoulder towards the stabilizing hand at the pelvis. Overpressure is only applied after the patient moved actively towards the limit of the movement
- Combined movements: as in generalized overpressure. Therapist's hand at crista iliace may change anteriorly or posteriorly on the crista to stabilize the movements (Figs 6.19–6.22).

Variations:

a. Sideflexion from caudad–cephalad upwards (Fig. 6.23ABC)
b. Change position of patient to sitting, sidelying, supine if necessary.

Continued

Lumbar sideflexion and variations—cont'd

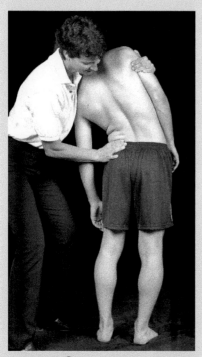

Figure 6.18 • LF Ⓛ generalized overpressure.

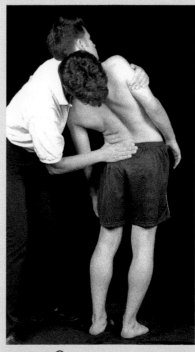

Figure 6.19 • LF Ⓛ + E

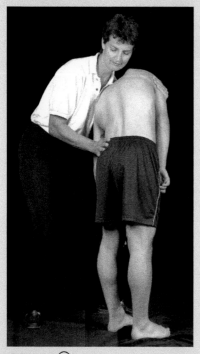

Figure 6.20 • LF Ⓛ + F.

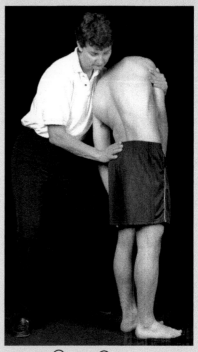

Figure 6.21 • LF Ⓛ + Rot Ⓛ.

Lumbar sideflexion and variations—cont'd

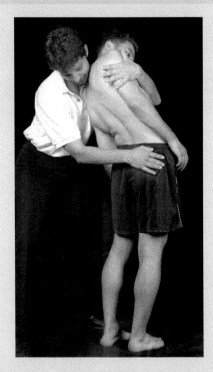

Figure 6.22 • LF Ⓛ + Rot Ⓡ.

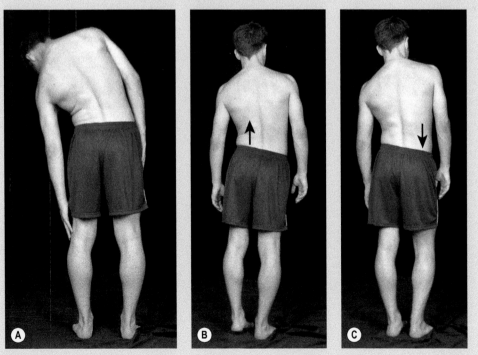

Figure 6.23 • Lumbar spine lateral flexion left. **A** From above downwards; **B** from below upwards, hitching left hip; **C** dropping the right hip.

Lumbar rotation and variations

Patient starting position: standing

Therapist starting position: standing on patient's left side

Localization of forces:

- Generalized overpressure: therapist grasps patient's right shoulder posteriorly, and gently grasps left shoulder anteriorly (Fig. 6.24A)
- Combined movements: after taking patient's trunk into full rotation, therapist changes her grasp to hold full range of rotation with her left axilla and hand (Fig. 6.24B)

Application of forces:

- Generalized overpressure: ensure that the thorax remains straight, gently rotate the trunk until full range of movement, then oscillating overpressure is applied towards the whole movement

- Combined movement, depending on the additional movement directions, the therapist's right hand changes position on the patient's pelvis to stabilize the overall movement at the lumbar spine (Figs 6.25–6.29)

Remarks/variations:

a. If generalized overpressure provokes symptoms in the buttock area, differentiation testing may be considered (see Fig. 6.5 differentiation testing)
b. Rotation from caudad–cephadad upwards (Fig. 6.30AB)
c. Change position of patient to sitting, sidelying, supine if necessary

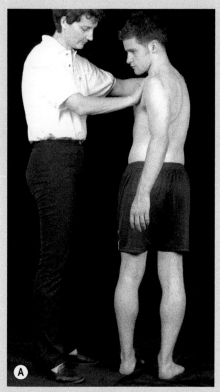
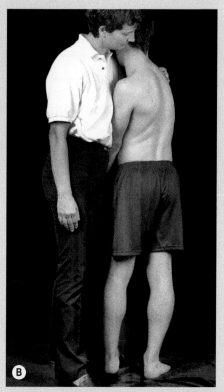

Figure 6.24 • Combined movements in rotation left. **A** Initial adopting position; **B** End-position before adding other movements.

Lumbar rotation and variations—cont'd

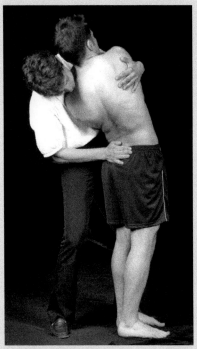

Figure 6.25 • Rot Ⓛ + E.

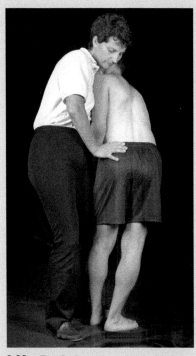

Figure 6.26 • The flexion component added.

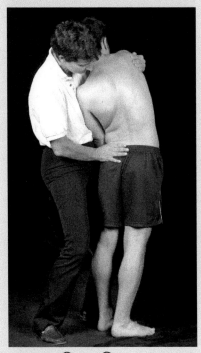

Figure 6.27 • Rot Ⓛ + LF Ⓛ.

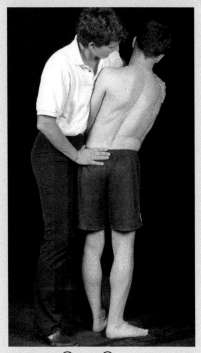

Figure 6.28 • Rot Ⓛ + LF Ⓡ.

Continued

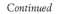

Lumbar rotation and variations—cont'd

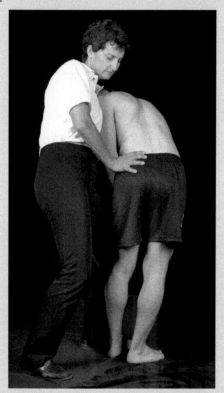

Figure 6.29 • Lateral flexion right added. Rot ⓛ + F + LF Ⓡ.

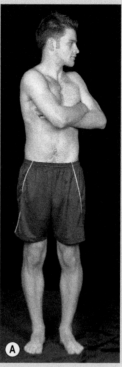
Ⓐ

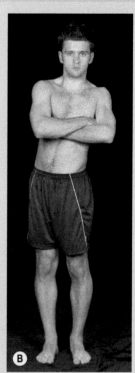
Ⓑ

Figure 6.30 • Lumbar spine rotation, commonly referred to as rotation to the left. **A** From above downwards; **B** from below upwards.

If recent changes occur, the tests should be monitored regularly during the therapeutic process.

They are indicative of numerous processes in the nervous system (Butler 2000), but they may be particularly helpful in hypothesis generation regarding precautions to examination and treatment procedures and sources of the movement dysfunction, provided that the tests are placed within the overall context of subjective and physical examination findings.

Neurodynamic testing

See Table 6.9 for neurological conduction tests of the lower extremity.

Text continued on p. 292

Table 6.9 Neurological conduction tests of the lower extremity (Banks & Hengeveld 2010)

Reflexes	Muscles	Skin sensation
Patellar reflex	Iliopsoas (L1–2)	Check ventral/medial side of thigh (L3)
Achilles reflex	Quadriceps, vastus medialis (L3)	Medial border of foot (L4)
	Tibialis anterior (L4)	Dorsum of foot (L5)
	Extensor hallucis longus	Lateral border of foot (S1)
	Flexor digitorum	Medial side of heel (S2)
	Triceps surae	Check upper leg, lower leg, foot using a circular movement to detect any area with a change in sensation
	Hamstrings	

SLR (sciatic nerve)

Patient starting position: supine

Therapist starting position: standing next to the patient's knee, facing the leg

Localization of forces

One hand controls the knee extension, the other hand controls the lower leg (holding around the distal part of the tibia) (Fig. 6.31)

Application of forces

In midposition between MR/LR and Ab/Ad of the hip the leg is raised until the onset of pain /resistance. Depending on the symptom localization, differentiation may take place by adding dorsiflexion of the foot, neckflexion, hip adduction or medial rotation of the hip (Fig. 6.32)

Remarks/variations: may add inversion or eversion of the foot

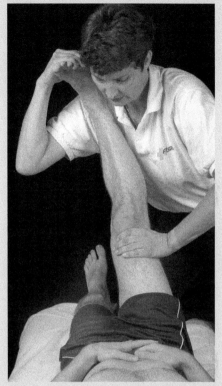

Figure 6.31 • Straight leg raising (SLR Ⓛ). Reproduced with permission from Banks & Hengeveld (2010).

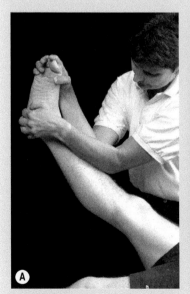 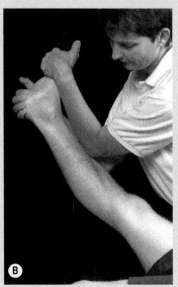 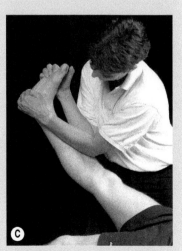

Figure 6.32 • Straight leg raise: **A** inclined to the deep and superficial peroneal nerve; **B** inclined to the tibial nerve; **C** inclined to the sural nerve. Reproduced with permission from Banks & Hengeveld (2010).

Slump test

Patient starting position: patient is sitting, well back at the short side of the bed (Fig. 6.33)

   Therapist starting position: standing at the patient's side

Localization of forces

Application of forces

- Whilst controlling the patient's neck, the patient flexes the trunk fully (Fig. 6.34)
- The sacrum is placed in a vertical position whilst maintaining the flexed position of the trunk
- Neck flexion is added with *gentle* overpressure (Figs 6.35, 6.36)
- Knee extension is added whilst gently controlling the patient's trunk flexion and neck position (Fig. 6.37)
  - alternative grip: therapist's elbow at the upper part of the patient's thorax and the web of the hand is placed under the patient's occiput to control the flexion position of the neck)

- If necessary dorsiflexion may be added to the procedure (Fig. 6.38)
- To differentiate any symptoms in the lumbar area or the leg, the neck will be raised from flexion to neutral position (Fig. 6.39)

Remarks/variations

- A pain-free lack of 30° knee extension can be normal, as can pain be felt at the T9–10 level of the spine (Maitland 1980)
- When firmer overpressure may be required the test may be performed in long-sitting position (Fig. 6.40)

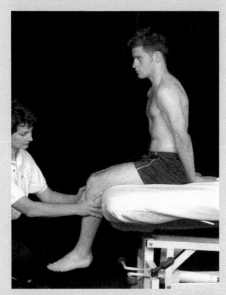

Figure 6.33 • The slump test: pain response while sitting well back.

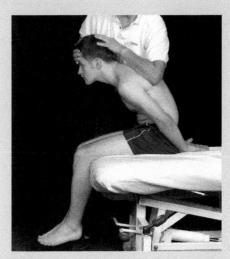

Figure 6.34 • Fully flexed spine, from T1 to sacrum.

Slump test—cont'd

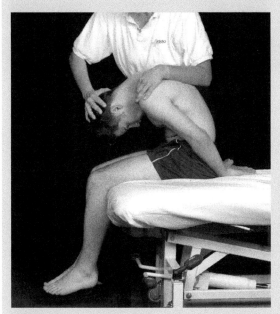

Figure 6.35 • Fully flexed spine, from head to sacrum.

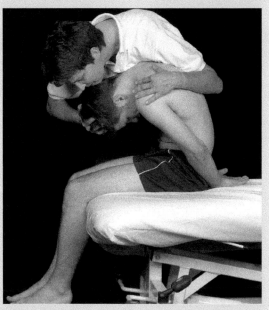

Figure 6.36 • Maintenance of over-pressure with physiotherapist's chin.

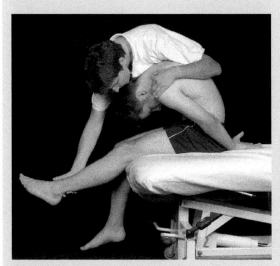

Figure 6.37 • Knee extension with entire spine under over-pressure during slump test.

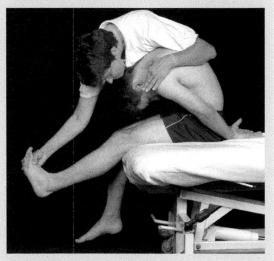

Figure 6.38 • Active dorsiflexion of ankle, with knee extension and spine over-pressure.

Continued

Slump test—cont'd

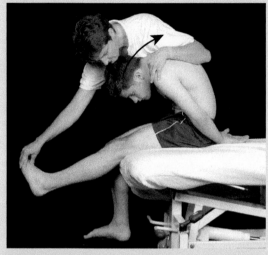

Figure 6.39 • Raising of neck to neutral position in slump test.

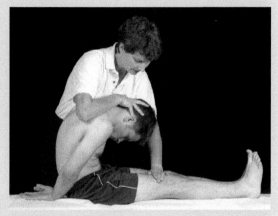

Figure 6.40 • The slump test in the long-sitting position.

Prone knee bend (femoral nerve)

Patient starting position: prone, hip in neutral position between abduction and adduction

   Therapist starting position: standing at the patient's side

   Localization of forces: gently stabilize patient's pelvis, other hand distally at tibia

   Application of forces: Knee flexion

   Remarks/variations: Strong pulling or burning sensation at the front of the thigh may be indicative of a neurodynamic movement disorder of the femoral nerve. In case of low back pain, the PKB needs to be repeated whilst the therapist counteracts the lumbar extension by pressing the sacral apex in caudad direction. Reduction of pain is indicative of a lumbar extension problem.

   In order to differentiate symptoms, the test needs to be performed as the slump test in side lying

Slump test

The slump test is an accumulating test, adding increasingly movement and tension to the neural system. Hence, extreme care needs to be taken if pathophysiological changes of the neural system are suspected.

Palpation

Manual diagnosis of the spine, including soft tissue palpation and passive intervertebral testing, has been found to be a reliable means in identifying symptomatic lumbar segmental levels. This is the case when manual diagnosis is compared with spinal anaesthetic block procedures (Jull et al. 1988, Phillips & Twomey 1996). Studies like these demonstrate that inter-tester reliability coefficients may be very high if a reference standard other than the comparison between individual therapist's palpating is chosen. Furthermore, it shows that training enhances the discriminative qualities of palpation skills (Jull et al.1997).

It is suggested to perform palpation examination as follows:

A. Tissue palpation

   1. Skin palpation (temperature, sweating, skin tone by gently lifting a skin fold)

   2. Muscle (tone and texture)

   3. Bony alignment

   4. Interspinous space and lamina areas (Figs 6.43–6.46).

Small differences in temperature can be detected by the skilled therapist (Lando 1994). A small increase in temperature, sweating and skin tone may be indicating the spinal level at fault. All lumbar

Slump in sidelying (femoral nerve)

Patient starting position

Sidelying, pelvis at the side of the bed; lower leg in hip flexion. Patient stabilizes the knee of the lower leg with the hands (Fig. 6.41). Trunk is fully flexed, head in neutral position

Therapist starting position: standing behind patient, at the level of the pelvis.

Localization of forces

One hand stabilizes the pelvis; the other hand supports the knee. Patient's foot may be placed on the side of the therapist's trunk (Fig. 6.41) or the lower leg may be carried by the therapist's forearm (Fig. 6.42)

Application of forces: The hip is extended until the onset of symptom /end of available range. Knee is kept in 90° F. Differentiation by neck flexion

Remarks/variations: Variation: patient may start in full neck flexion – differentiation will take place by moving out of the neck flexion

Test variations:

- In case of lateral thigh pain, adduction and medial rotation of the hip may be added to emphasize the lateral cutaneous femoral nerve
- Knee extension and eversion of the foot may emphasize the saphenous nerve

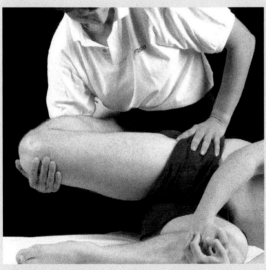

Figure 6.41 • Slump in sidelying. Reproduced with permission from Banks & Hengeveld (2010).

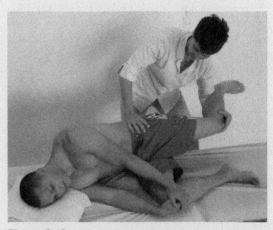

Figure 6.42 • Prone knee bend, leg free. Reproduced with permission from Banks & Hengeveld (2010).

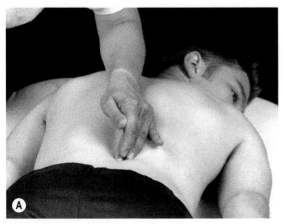

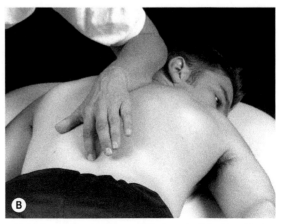

Figure 6.43 • **A** Palpating medially into the right side with the middle finger; **B** palpating medially into the left side with the index finger.

interspinous processes should be palpated with discernment, as should the lateral surface of the spinous processes. Thickening can occur on one or both sides of the process or in the space, event to the extent where the interspinous process can be completely obliterated by thickened hard tissue.

Figure 6.43 shows how this can be performed without the examiner having to move her position. She stands alongside the patient facing his feet, and uses her middle fingertip to probe into the right space and her index finger to dig medially into the left space. She can change rapidly from side to side, and equally rapidly from one level to the next, upwards or downwards.

It is also necessary to use the index and middle fingers to palpate into the interspinous space. When doing so, the fingers are held tightly together and oscillated back and forth sideways in an attempt to sink deeply into the space (Fig. 6.44).

Deeper palpations of the interspinous area are illustrated in Figure 6.45. By using the tip of the thumb a greater depth, even as deep as the lamina, can be reached. An assessment of this depth should be carried out if the more superficial area is normal.

Palpation of the paravertebral soft-tissue structures is illustrated in Figure 6.46. Both thumb tips are utilized, and the probing deep palpation should be carried out in many different directions – medially, lateral, caudally and cephalad. Also, the palpation should not be limited to the interlaminar area but should be extended to the adjacent upper and lower borders of the lamina and over the lamina itself.

B. Passive movement testing, as passive intervertebral movement (PAIVMs), and if needed, passive physiological intervertebral movements (PPIVMs). See below.

C. Nerve palpation

Nerve palpation may be a diagnostic aid in the assessment of mechanosensitivity of the neural system (Butler 2000). Under normal circumstances peripheral nerves are painless to non-noxious stimuli. However, in cases such as nerve inflammation, gentle provocation, e.g. palpation, can cause pain, protective muscles responses or abnormal tingling-responses (Hall & Quintner 1996).

A comparative study investigating reliability of nerve palpation clinical examination in comparison to pain pressure threshold demonstrated excellent validity, reliability and diagnostic accuracy of nerve palpation in clinical examination at three different sites in the leg (Walsh & Hall, 2009).

Nerves can be palpated at various sites of the buttock and leg, as for example (Butler 2000):

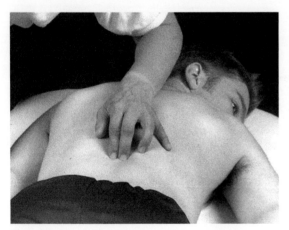

Figure 6.44 • Palpating posteroanteriorly in depth.

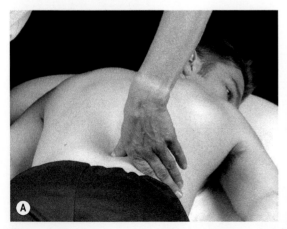 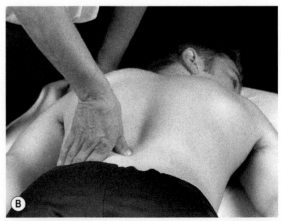

Figure 6.45 • Deeper palpation of the interspinous area. **A** Right side. **B** Left side.

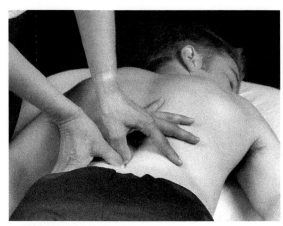

Figure 6.46 • Palpation of the paravertebral soft-tissue structures

- Sciatic nerve in buttock area
- Tibial:
  - in fossa of knee
  - at tarsal tunnel (dorsal and caudad of the medial malleolus)
- Peroneal nerve:
  - communal peroneal nerve at caput fibulae
  - superficial peroneal nerve at dorsal site of foot
  - deep peroneal nerve between head of ossae metatarsale I and II
- Sural nerve at lateral border of foot and dorsocaudad of the lateral malleolus
- Femoral nerve in groin-area
- Saphenous nerve medially at knee-joint.

Passive testing

Passive physiological intervertebral movements (PPIVMs)

Passive physiological intervertebral movements are performed to examine the intervertebral mobility of one segment of the spine in relation to the neighbouring segment in more detail. Particularly discrepancies in mobility between mobile and stiff neighbouring segments are of interest, which may be indicative of a stability dysfunction of the motion segment.

Other purposes of PPIVMs:

- They may serve in reassessment procedures after joint manipulation
- At times PPIVMs may be adapted to treatment techniques.

Over many years it has been debated that the reliability coefficients of intervertebral movement examination may be insufficient; however, it is essential to consider the results from these tests within the overall information of subjective examination findings and other physical examination tests. There are various studies available which demonstrate an increase in reliability values if combinations of test procedures are being used in physical examination (Cibulka et al. 1988). It has been suggested not to condemn examination procedures without offering meaningful clinical alternatives and research from different perspectives with different reference standards (Bullock-Saxton 2002).

PPIVMs T10–L5/S1: flexion–extension

Patient starting position: sidelying, hips and knee flexed. A little pillow may be positioned under the lower waist, if the lumbar spine would sag into sideflexion
  Therapist starting position: in front of the patient
  Localization of forces
  Therapist supports both lower legs of the patient with both legs in the groin area (Fig. 6.47); the other hand palpates the interspinous space from below (Fig. 6.48)
    Application of forces
    Movement is performed either in flexion or extension direction by movement of the patient's pelvis (in a circular manner around the palpating finger).

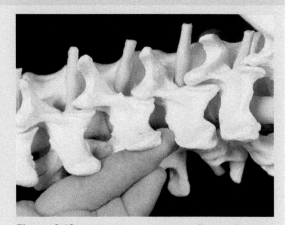

Figure 6.48 • Intervertebral movement T11–L5/S1. Position of palpating finger for lumbar spine.

Continued

PPIVMs T10–L5/S1: flexion–extension—cont'd

Remarks/variations

- Single leg technique: as an alternative the test may be performed with one leg (Fig. 6.49)
- PA–AP shunt: if a movement seems more mobile at one segment in comparison to the neighbouring segment, a gentle PA glide may be added at the

end of range of flexion by pulling at the thighs; or a gentle AP movement at the end of range of extension by pushing through the thighs. A normal feeling is that a sense of tissue-resistance should be perceived immediately at the application of the AP or PA movement.

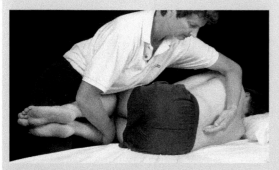

Figure 6.47 ● Intervertebral movement. T11–S1 (flexion/extension).

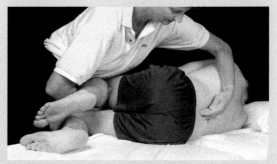

Figure 6.49 ● Intervertebral movement. T11–S1 (flexion/extension). Single leg technique.

PPIVMs T10–L5/S1: rotation

Patient starting position: patient is positioned on the couch

Therapist starting position: in front of the patient

Localization of forces

Palpating finger as above (Fig. 6.48), lower arm is positioned paravertebral; other hand is positioned on crista iliaca an anterior spinous process of the ilium

Application of forces

Rotation is performed by gently rocking the pelvis posteriorly towards the palpating finger (Fig. 6.50AB)

Remarks/variations: in order to test the other direction, the patient is positioned on the other side

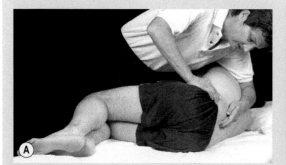

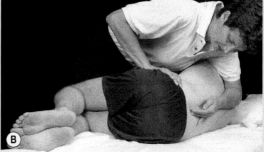

Figure 6.50 ● **A, B** Intervertebral movement. T11–S1 (rotation).

PPIVMs T10 – L5/S1: sideflexion

Patient starting position: patient is positioned on the couch

   Therapist starting position: in front of the patient
   Localization of forces

   Palpating finger as above (Fig. 6.48), lower arm is positioned paravertebral; other arm grasps around the upper pelvis/tuber pelvis

Application of forces
Remarks/variations

   In order to test the other direction, the patient is positioned on the other side

   Alternative grip: the therapist grasps around the pelvis, by holding the lower large trochanter and stabilizing the patient's pelvis between the arm and shoulder (Fig. 6.51AB)

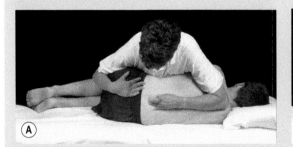 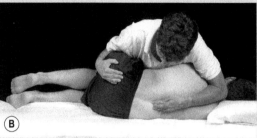

Figure 6.51 • A, B Intervertebral movement. T11–S1 (lateral flexion).

Passive accessory intervertebral movements (PAIVMs)

Movement testing with intervertebral accessory movements should be carried out in the posteroanterior, unilateral posteroanterior and transverse directions of the spine. Additionally, anteroposterior movement of the lumbar spine may be performed.

On the one hand accessory movements are essential test procedures in physical examination, but on the other hand all accessory movements may be performed as a treatment technique as well.

 Central PA movement ↕ ⌐

Patient starting position: prone lying, arms by the side

   Therapist starting position: at the side of the plinth, facing the patient's lumbar spine. Hands or thumbs are used as the contact points; elbows relaxed, but stable. Sternum is over the hands
   Localization of forces

- Unilateral PA: both thumbs are placed in direct contact with each other adjacent to the spinous process in the intervertebral lamina (Fig. 6.52)
- Central PA: soft pad distally of hamate bone of the wrist is placed on the spinous process, hand is in a more or less vertical position; the soft pad of the other wrist is placed on top of the lower hand in the area of the anatomical snuffbox, 2nd and 3rd fingers grasp around the fingers of the lower hand

to maintain the vertical position. Sternum of therapist is over the hand, elbows are relaxed (Figs 6.53–6.55)

- Gentler central PA movements may be produced by using the thumbs, as in unilateral PA techniques (Fig. 6.56)

   Application of forces: movement is produced by the therapist's body
   Remarks/variations

- In supine, do PA or unilateral PA movement (with pads of middle fingers; Fig. 6.57)
- In sideflexion right, do PA or unilateral PA movement (Fig. 6.58)
- In flexion, do PA, or unilateral PA movement (Fig. 6.59)

Continued

Central PA movement—cont'd

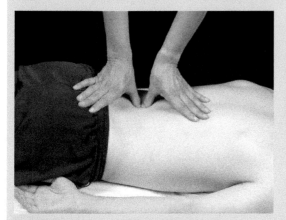

Figure 6.52 • Posteroanterior unilateral vertebral movement ⌐↓.

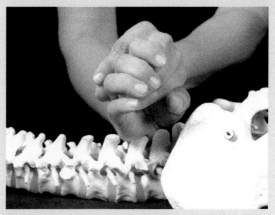

Figure 6.53 • Posteroanterior central vertebral movement ↕.

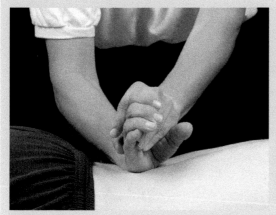

Figure 6.54 • Posteroanterior central vertebral movement ↕.

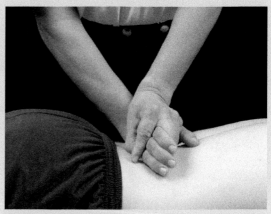

Figure 6.55 • Posteroanterior vertebral movement ↕.

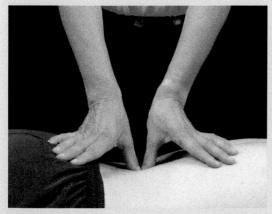

Figure 6.56 • Posteroanterior vertebral movement ↕.

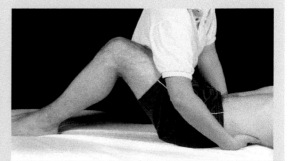

Figure 6.57 • Posteroanterior movement.

Transverse movements—cont'd

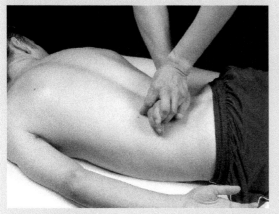

Figure 6.58 • Posteroanterior central vertebral movement as a combined movement, in lateral flexion right (in LF Ⓡ Do ↕).

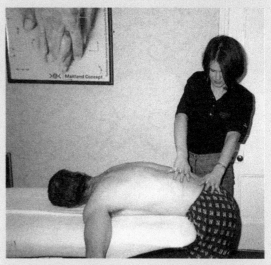

Figure 6.59 • Accessory movement in flexion.

Transverse movements ←•→

Patient starting position: prone lying, arms by the side

Therapist starting position: at the side of the table; height about at level of therapist's thorax

Localization of forces: therapist stands with one leg in front of the other, the pads of both thumbs are placed laterally against the spinous process; fingers are spread over the contralateral side of the thorax. Elbows are relaxed

Application of forces

Movement is produced by the therapist's body, transferring the weight back and forth over both legs (Fig. 6.60A)

Remarks/variations

The technique may be intensified by holding the leg of the patient in abduction, resulting in sideflexion of the lumbar spine.

1. in sideflexion: do transverse movements
2. in transverse movement: do sideflexion of lumbar spine (by moving the leg into more / less abduction (Fig. 6.60B)

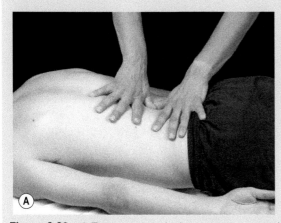

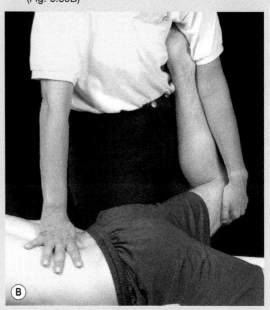

Figure 6.60 • A Transverse vertebral movement←•→, starting position; **B** ←•→, strong technique.

Anteroposterior movement ↕

Patient starting position: supine, legs resting on a pillow in a flexed position

Therapist starting position: at patient's side, facing the patient's abdomen

Localization of forces

Pads of the second to fourth fingers are placed on top of each other and gently placed into the abdominal area, caudad of the umbilical area for L4 (Fig. 6.61)

Application of forces

Movement is produced by the therapist's body

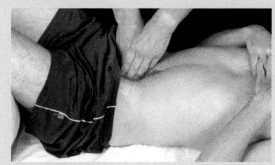

Figure 6.61 • Anteroposterior central vertebral movement ↕.

Examination of motor control impairment

Comprehensive strategies for motor control of the lumbar spine are widely available in companion texts and supporting references: Sahrmann (2011), O'Sullivan (2005), Richardson et al. (2004). Furthermore, examples of techniques integrating motor control strategies with mobilization techniques are detailed on page 313 of this chapter in the subsection entitled 'integrated treatment techniques'.

Mobilization and manipulation treatment techniques

As stated before, accessory movements of the spine can be used as treatment techniques. It is a special feature of the clinical reasoning processes of this concept of NMS-physiotherapy that the techniques may be applied in any physiological position of the spine, depending on the symptoms of patient. Also, physiological movements may be applied as a treatment technique. Furthermore, both accessory movements and physiological movements may be combined in an active of passive manner.

For example if the objective of treatment is the mobilization of sideflexion, it is possible to position the patient in sideflexion and then to apply accessory movement techniques and vice versa.

In this way a clinical rehabilitative approach to the normalization of movement impairments may be pursued. Next to the variations of active and passive arthrogenic techniques, integrated approaches of joint oriented techniques with neurodynamic treatment or motor control strategies often aid in the optimization of treatment results.

In this way almost endless variations of the treatment are possible. Hence the selection, the progression and adaption of treatment techniques must be based upon thorough examination procedures and the effects need to be monitored with disciplined reassessment procedures (see Box 6.5).

More details regarding selection and progression of treatment techniques can be found in Chapter 8 Management of knee disorders (Hengeveld & Banks 2014).

Accessory movements and variations

See p. 303 of this chapter.

Physiological movements and variations: mobilizations, manipulations

Text continued on p. 305

Flexion techniques

Patient starting position

- Supine
- Prone
- Sidelying

Therapist starting position: as displayed in Figures 6.62–6.66

Localization of forces

- Supine/prone. Contact is taken with the SIAS of the pelvis
- Sidelying: both hands have contact with the lumbar spine

Application of forces

Movement is produced by the therapist's body

Adaptation of techniques towards E, SF

The technique may be adapted towards different directions:

- Supine lying: extension (Fig. 6.67)
- Supine lying, legs of patient over legs of therapist: sideflexion and/or rotation (Fig. 6.65)

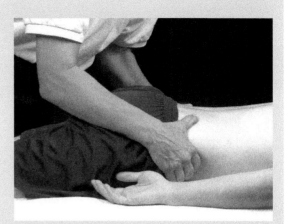

Figure 6.62 • Flexion: first starting position (F).

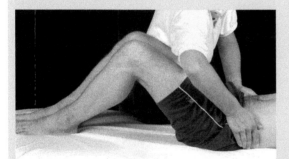

Figure 6.63 • Flexion.

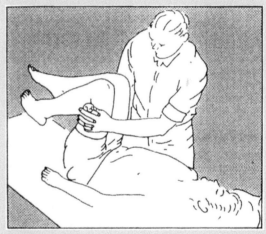

Figure 6.64 • Flexion: second starting position (F).

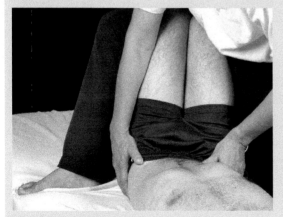

Figure 6.65 • Starting position for flexion, extension, lateral flexion, rotation from below upwards and 'coupled' by using the femur and pelvis.

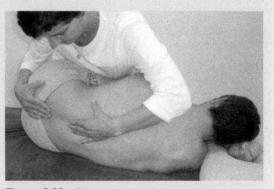

Figure 6.66 • Flexion in sidelying. Reproduced with permission from Banks & Hengeveld (2010).

Continued

Flexion techniques—cont'd

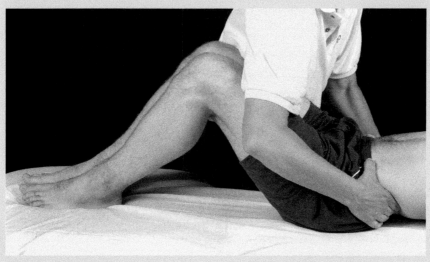

Figure 6.67 • Extension.

Rotation mobilization

Patient starting position: Sidelying, knees on top of each other, about 5–10 cm over side of plinth

- Grade I: upperlying forearm is gently placed in front of trunk (Fig. 6.69A)
- Grade II. Arm is placed on side (Fig. 6.69B)

- Positioning Grade IV, III (Fig. 6.69C):
  a. pelvic rotation: maintain upper leg in neutral position between F/E for the treated segment; lower leg is extended, while palpating the lumbar , foot of the upper leg may be placed behind the knee fold of the patient

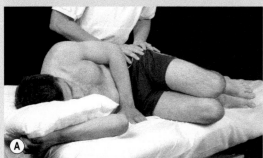

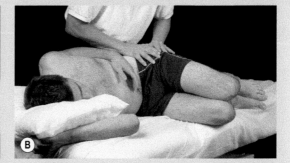

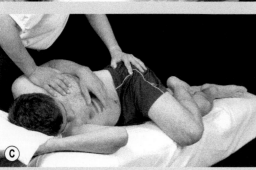

Figure 6.69 • Rotation. **A** Grades I and II; **B, C** Grade III.

Rotation mobilization—cont'd

b. Rotation of the trunk until the onset of movement of the lumbar segment. To achieve this, the patient places the hand of the upper arm lightly on the therapist's shoulder. Therapist hold the patient in the interscapular area while gently turning the patient's trunk into rotation

Therapist starting position

Standing at back of the patient, level with the pelvis
For grades III, IV: may place lower leg on plinth, behind patient's pelvis

Localization of forces

Grade I, II: both hands are placed over the ilium, next to each other/behind each other

Grade III, IV: one hand grasps around the pelvis, ensuring the control of the forward and backward movements of the pelvis during the application of the technique; other hand is placed gently over the pectoralis major area to stabilize the trunk rotation (gently holding – no pressure of the hand)

Application of forces: movement is produced by the therapist's body, towards the pelvis

Variations

- As a gentle grade I, II technique: see Figs 6.65 & 6.70.
- Localized rotation as end of range mobilization: as in IV (manipulation); however, performed in an oscillatory manner as a grade IV or III technique (refer to the figure of localized rotation manipulation (Fig. 6.71AB)

- Combined rotations as a progression of treatment in stable movement disorders (Figs 6.72–6.74)

Often the movement combination which provokes the patient's symptoms may be selected as a treatment technique, provided the problem is of a stable, nociceptive nature.

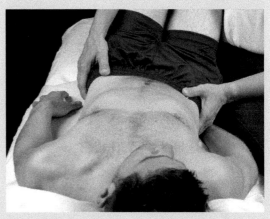

Figure 6.70 • Rotation.

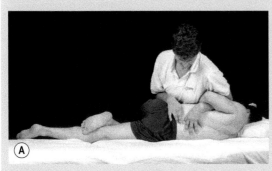

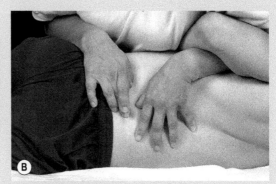

Figure 6.71 • **A** Intervertebral joints, T10–S1 (rotation) localized manipulation; **B** close up on hands.

Continued

Rotation mobilization—cont'd

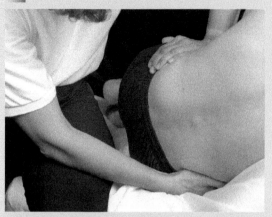

Figure 6.72 ● Rotation in flexion, and lateral flexion left, from below upwards with vertebral axis (in F + LF Ⓛ, do Ⓛₓ axis).

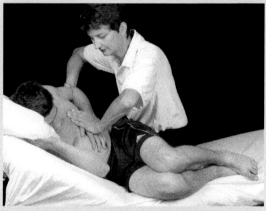

Figure 6.73 ● Rotation in flexion and lateral flexion left from above downwards (in F + LF Ⓛ, do Th).

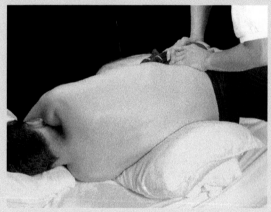

Figure 6.74 ● Rotation in flexion and lateral flexion, and lateral flexion left, from below upwards (in F + LF Ⓛ, do ↻)

Localized rotation manipulation

Premanipulative screening
   Particularly screen for:

- Cauda equina and cord signs
- Lower limb nerve conduction loss
- Osteoporosis and other bone pathologies

   Patient starting position: sidelying with the stiff/painful side (the side to be manipulated) uppermost. Preposition the patient so that they do not fear rolling off the bed and so their lower foot does not inhibit the effects of rotation.

   Therapist starting position: stand in front of the patient at the level of the lumbar spine, thread one arm through the patient's arm and place the other forearm over the patients greater trochanter

   Localization of forces
   Localize the forces to L4–5 by placing the upper thumb firmly against the upper side of the L4 spinous

process and the index/middle fingers of the lower hand firmly against the lower side of the spinous process of L5 (see Fig. 6.71A,B)

   Application of forces

- Adjust the position so that L4–5 is neutral, take up the slack, let the patient's upper leg drop off the bed. Roll the patient over to a balance point so that the thrust will affect the pelvis and thorax equally
- Secure the thumb and finger contact
- Thrust along the joint plane by a drop/twist of the body using the forearm against the greater trochanter and the sternum against the ribcage as leverage

   Uses: simple mechanical low back pain in the absence of any risk factors

Neurodynamic techniques

The neurodynamic system can be treated in different ways. On the one hand the direct surroundings of the nerves may be treated, for example with passive mobilizations or soft tissue techniques, or directly in which it is distinguished between 'slider' and 'tensioner' techniques (Butler 2000, Coppieters & Butler 2008, Shacklock 2005)

Combination of arthrogenic techniques and neurodynamic mobilizations (example)

Lumbar rotation mobilization with neurodynamic emphasis

Patient starting position: (left) sidelying, same position as for lumbar rotation mobilization, grades III and IV

1. Patient's upper leg is hanging loosely over the side of the treatment table (Fig. 6.75)
2. As in (a) (Fig. 6.76)

Therapist starting position

1. Same position as for lumbar rotation mobilization, grades III and IV.
2. As a progression of (a). Therapist is standing in front of the patient; stabilizes the patient's leg between the knee

Localization of forces

1. Same as for lumbar rotation mobilization, grades III and IV.

2. Therapist's (left) hand stabilizes patient's shoulder in the pectoral area, therapist's right hand is placed posteriorly at patient's left pelvis

Application of forces

1. Same as for lumbar rotation mobilization, grades III and IV
2. Therapist stabilizes the patient's leg in the chosen position of SLR, stabilizes the patient's shoulder and performs the rotation movement at the pelvis

Remark

These techniques are possible as a progression of treatment. It is crucial to consider the stability of the (neurogenic) pain mechanisms: the pain should be stable and behave in a more 'on-off' character during daily life activities.

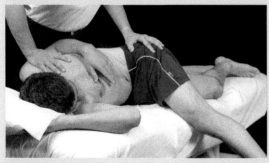

Figure 6.75 • Rotation. Grade IV, with neural emphasis.

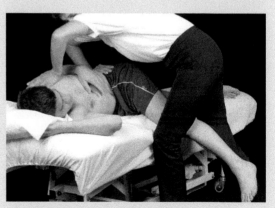

Figure 6.76 • Rotation with straight leg raising ⤵.

Direct neurodynamic mobilization techniques

 'Slider' techniques for the sciatic nerve (example)

Patient starting position: side lying, hipflexion (evt. adduction) short of onset of pain (P1)

Therapist starting position: standing next to the patient, on the level of the hip. Facing the patient's thigh

a. Therapist teaches patient to extend cervical spine (ensuring that this is possible without pain provocation)

b. Therapist extends the patient's knee, establishing the point of onset of pain in buttock or leg. The therapist's thigh block the patient's lower leg in a position of knee F/E shortly before P1

Localization of forces

One hand stabilizes the pelvis, the other hand holds the patient's tibia

Application of forces

While the therapist gently moves the patient's knee back and forth into extension, short of P_1, the patient extends and flexes the cervical spine in the rhythm of the knee movements. In this way a 'slider' technique to the neurodynamic system may be applied (Fig. 6.77)

Variations

• The technique may carefully be progressed into a 'tensioner' technique in which the patient stops moving the cervical spine, especially if the SLR is limited by resistance and the pain behaves in an 'on-off' manner

• Similar techniques as described above may be performed in supine lying, and sitting as well

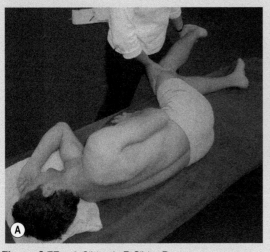
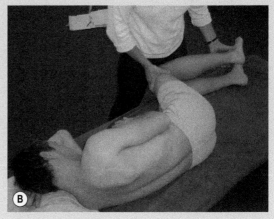

Figure 6.77 • A Slider A; **B** Slider B.

Lumbar spine mobilization and manipulation techniques linked to clinical and supporting research evidence

In a number of studies it has been demonstrated that the grade, rhythm and direction of movement in which treatment techniques are being performed have an important influence on treatment outcomes. This has been demonstrated in a number of studies with treatment techniques in other joints such as the shoulder (Johnson et al. 2007a, Vermeulen et al. 2006), knee (Moss et al, 2007), elbow (Paungmali et al. 2003), ankle (Yeo & Wright 2011) or hip (Makofsky et al. 2007)

An increasing number of studies demonstrate physiological effects of lumbar mobilization techniques, such as accessory movements or rotation mobilization techniques:

• Perry and Green (2008), in a randomized controlled trial on normal male subjects, found that a grade III oscillatory mobilization applied at 2Hz to the left L4/5 facet joint had an effect on sympathetic activity in the left lower extremity over and above the effects produced in a control and placebo group (see Fig. 6.52).

- Krouwel et al. (2010), in a single blind randomized within subject repeated measurement study design, found in 30 asymptomatic subjects that a posteroanterior mobilization applied to L3 using a force platform to regulate force and frequency of oscillation (1.5Hz) had a significant (p= 0.013) effect on raising measured pressure pain threshold but this was independent of whether the amplitude of the mobilization was large (50–200N) or small (150–200N) (see Figs 6.55 & 6.56).

- Adams et al. (2010), in a review of intervertebral disc healing, suggest that a rotational mobilization might facilitate inter-lamella movements and prevent extensive scarring. In clinical practice, controlled mobilization of a recently-injured spinal level can be difficult due to pain and muscle spasm, but manual therapy can help to reduce pain and normalize muscle tone (Boal & Gillette 2004) and thereby decrease stress concentrations in the disc. Gentle early mobilization could also benefit the bony endplate, because repetitive micromovement stimulates fracture healing in adult long bones (Kenwright et al. 1991; see Fig. 6.69).

- Perry et al. (2011) in a quasi-experimental random design on 50 healthy participants, found that there was a significant (0.0005) increase in lower extremity sympathetic activity after grade V rotation manipulation, compared with extension exercises (see Fig. 6.71A).

Integrated treatment

In clinical practice, physiotherapists have established competencies and skills to deal with impairments of segmental mobility (arthrogenic), motor control and postural stability (myogenic) and nerve mechanosensitivity.

Physiotherapists should design individualized treatment programmes, collaboratively with the patient, based on the contemporary scope of practice, including an understanding of contextual mediators of the pain and disability and a comprehension of whether they would be modifiable or not. All impairment oriented treatments should follow up with an emphasis on restoring functional capacity,

and guiding patients in the transition from health care needs to healthy life-styles/healthy living.

It is important that the treatment interventions, being arthrogenic, myogenic and/or neurodynamic oriented, are linked to examination findings. If possible clinical predictor rules may be applied to the selection of low back pain interventions and validated outcome measures such as Measure Yourself Medical Outcome Profile[†] (MYMOP; Paterson 1996) may be incorporated in the reassessment processes. Assessment during the application of an intervention and retrospective assessment are outlined in Box 6.8.

Research and best practice clinical guidelines have demonstrated that segmental mobilization and manipulation have a role to play in the treatment of patients with low back pain originating from the lumbar spine (NICE 2009).

Advances in knowledge in neuromuscular function have informed therapists how to fine tune movement, activate muscles and utilize motor control strategies to help patients recover from episodes of back pain (Macedo et al. 2009).

Clinical studies have demonstrated that restoration of ideal nerve gliding and tensioning after nerve injury or entrapment are important therapeutic considerations (Schafer et al. 2011).

What is not well known is the impact on recovery and outcome if these strategies are used in combinations and integrated into functional activities. The following example may illustrate this principle:

What if an SLR is mobilized whilst activating transverse abdominus muscles (TrAb).Will functional recovery be enhanced? The answers to such questions are beyond the scope of this text and the domain of the researcher. The next logical step, however, in selection of manual and movement therapy interventions for movement related NMS

---

†MYMOP is a patient-generated, or individualized, outcome questionnaire. It is problem-specific but includes general wellbeing. It is applicable to all patients who present with symptoms, and these can be physical, emotional or social. On the first occasion the questionnaire is completed within the consultation, or with some confidential help. The patient chooses one or two symptoms that they are seeking help with, and that they consider to be the most important. They also choose an activity of daily living that is limited or prevented by this problem. These choices are written down in the patient's own words and the patient scores them for severity over the past week on a seven-point scale. Lastly, wellbeing is scored on a similar scale. On follow-up questionnaires the wording of the previously chosen items is unchanged, and follow-up questionnaires may be administered by post if required. (Source: www.sites.pcmd.ac.uk/mymop/)

Box 6.8

Reassessment, assessment whilst performing a treatment procedure and retrospective assessment are necessary in the continuous evaluation process of monitoring changes in the patient's clinical presentation

- Reassessment: see Box 6.5.
- Assessment whilst performing a treatment procedure

Assessment during the application of treatment procedures needs to be distinguished from reassessment procedures.

Whilst performing a passive movement, exercises, educational session or other therapeutic procedures with a patient, the physiotherapist has to pursue the following questions:

- Are the objectives of the treatment procedure being achieved?
- Do any undesirable side-effects occur?

Particularly during the application of passive mobilizations, changes in the behaviour of pain and sense of tissue resistance should be monitored. If pain or the sense of resistance changes, immediate adaptation of the techniques will then be possible. As long as these changes are favourable, the technique may be continued. Also, when the changes cease to take place after a period of treatment, it is often useful to perform a reassessment-procedure of the main parameters of physical examinations to evaluate the direct effect of the technique applied. Hence, assessment whilst applying a treatment technique is a decisive factor in the determination of the duration of a technique being performed.

On the other hand, the physiotherapist needs to consider possible undesired side effects. In some cases, whilst monitoring the desired results of a therapeutic intervention, simultaneously the physiotherapist may need to observe the following aspects by noting 'Nothing at price of…':

- Inflammatory signs (alertness to swelling, redness, temperature)
- Increase of pain (particularly in cases of acute, irritable nociceptive and peripheral neurogenic pain states)
- Neurological conductivity (monitoring reflexes, muscle function, sensation)
- Healing processes in soft tissues or bones (in relation to the phases of physiological healing processes)
- Autonomic reactions, such as redness of skin, sweating, coldness (e.g. during palpation of the spine)
- General tension with increased muscle-guarding and breathing patterns (particularly in those patients, whose contributing factor to their disorder may be lack of relaxation or autonomic imbalances)

- Self-efficacy beliefs / externalization of locus of control/development of passive coping strategies (in cases where the patients seems to attribute the effects of treatment only to the hands of the therapist, without applying the suggested self-management strategies)
- Fear to move (e.g. increase in fear avoidance behaviour)
- Confusion (e.g. in educational sessions, where much information is given without reassessment and consideration of the cognitive level, previous knowledge and beliefs of the patient).

Retrospective assessment

One of the most essential, but often neglected, forms of reassessment is retrospective assessment in combination with skilled communication (Maitland 1986). Retrospective assessment should take place at regular intervals in the overall process, in which the physiotherapist reflects on all the decisions and hypotheses made so far, and patients are encouraged to compare changes in their condition over a longer period than from session to session.

The following need to be pursued:

- Assessment of the overall well-being of the patient in comparison to the first sessions
- Which subjective and physical parameters ('asterisks') have improved so far? Which ones have remained unchanged?
- Are agreed treatment goals being achieved?
- What has the patient learned so far? What was especially important to the patient in the learning process?
- Monitoring the effects of the various treatment interventions (patient's information as well as checking of treatment records)

Prospective assessment: (re)determination of the treatment objectives for the next period of therapy:

- Does the therapy need to be adapted to newly defined goals? It may be useful to 'think from the end': which treatment objectives should be followed in order to optimize the 'individual sense of well-being' with regard to activities in daily life (see Chapter 8)
- Determine whether other therapeutic or medical measures may be necessary

Box 6.8—cont'd

- Does the therapist need to undertake more compliance enhancement strategies in order to support the patient in the behavioural change with regard to suggestion, exercises and recommendation
- (Re)determination of the parameters to monitor the agreed goals of treatment (may become more functional movement parameter, as for example tennis service, bending activities as performed at work).

The therapy seems to be stagnating

Retrospective assessment is also useful if the therapy seems to be stagnating or does not seem to bring the desired results. The following reflections need to be considered:

- Have I compared the subjective and physical parameters ('asterisks') regularly enough and in sufficient detail?

- Did I ensure that the patient would become aware of positive changes in these parameters as well?
- Did I follow up the correct physical asterisks, which reflect the patient's main problem and the goal of the therapeutic intervention?
- Have I performed a review of the therapeutic process with retrospective assessment procedures, collaboratively with the patient?
- Has the right source of the symptoms been treated?
- Have the self-management procedures been pursued profoundly enough? Did these procedures provide the patient with sufficient control over the pain and well-being in all daily life situations?
- Are any medical or other interventions necessary?

---

disorders of the lumbar spine is the merging of examination findings with treatment. For example, a patient may feel low back pain and neurogenic type symptoms in the back of the leg when bending forwards. The leg symptoms increase when the patient is asked to flex his cervical spine, in addition a posteroanterior glide on L4 reduces the leg pain and with a further addition of abdominal bracing the pain is less still, allowing greater range of cervical flexion. The logical treatment technique must be based on these findings, given that there is no nerve conduction loss and the leg symptoms settle quickly after provocation. The treatment technique is designed around the clinical evidence (supported by C/O evidence that the patient is troubled by leg pain when sitting or bending, the back feels stiff and the whole trunk feels weak).

A possible treatment technique in this case is:

In forward bending to pain + a posteroanterior pressure to L4 + activation of TAb
Active cervical flexion from neutral to full flexion (Fig. 6.78)

The challenge for the therapist is to take manual therapy and movement therapy interventions for low back pain into the domain of impairment interrelationships. Recovery may be enhanced by a lumbar accessory movement in PA-direction, abdominal activation or neural gliders alone; however, the challenge to clinical reasoning and handling skills is to merge integrated examination

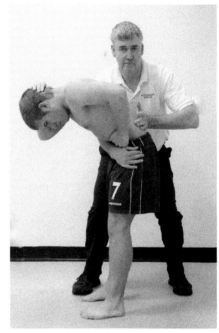

Figure 6.78 • Postero-anterior pressure to L4 + activation of TAb

findings with treatment and design treatment techniques which address the relationship between movement impairments.

Below is a selection of such techniques. The reader is encouraged to reason how and why such techniques have been designed.

Text continued on p. 320

Where there is evidence of neurogenic and myogenic impairments coexisting

Position: standing+SLR+ TAb activation
  Method

A. Cervical flexion with ankle PF

B. Cervical extension with ankle DF

  Purpose: sciatic-type leg symptoms restricting bending (pain and protection) when putting on socks; pain provoked with cervical flexion. Provocation less when abdominals activated to enhance neutral zone (Panjabi 1992) of lumbar segments
  Starting position of patient
  Standing with left heel resting on a stool and bending to point of leg symptom onset. Abdominals activated
  Starting position of therapist
  Standing by the left side of the patient facing forward.
  Localization of forces
  Therapist's left hand stabilizing and monitoring patient knee. Right hand spread over the crown of the patient's head with the right forearm resting along the patients thoracic spine
  Application of forces
  Whilst monitoring the patient's knee in extension, the therapist flexes the patient's cervical spine at the same time as the patient performs active ankle plantarflexion [P/F]. Grade II+ or III- for both ankle P/F and cervical flexion
  As the therapist brings the patient's head back to neutral, the patient's ankle is actively dorsiflexed
  Uses
  Where bending is impaired by painful protected sciatic-type leg symptoms without major conduction block
  Where there is evidence of a need for restoring neural gliding supported by activation of stabilizing muscles to enhance postural stability

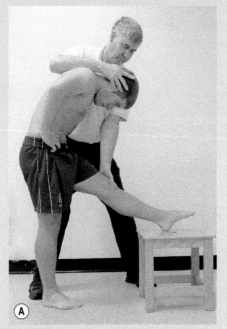
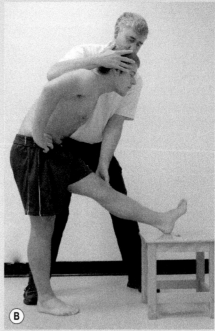

Figure 6.79 • A Cervical flexion with ankle PF; **B** cervical extension with ankle DF. Reproduced with permission from Banks & Hengeveld (2010).

Position: sidelying+ TAb activation
Method

1. Cervical flexion with knee flexion
2. Cervical extension with knee extension

Purpose: if the patient has sciatic-type leg symptoms, is comfortable in side lying, and needs neural gliding techniques to reduce neural mechanosensititvity. In addition, if the gliding techniques are facilitated by abdominal bracing and a greater pain free range of neural mobility is possible

Starting position of patient: side lying in the middle of the bed, painful leg uppermost (on most occasions). Spine parallel with the edge of the bed, hips flexed, knees together

Starting position of therapist: standing in front of the patient facing across the bed at the level of the pelvis

Localization of forces: therapist's right hand stabilizes the pelvis behind the iliac crest. Left hand holds the patients foot and ankle. Therapist's left thigh stabilizes the patient's knee

Application of forces

The patient is asked to activate transverse abdominus, and then actively flex the head. As the patient's head returns to neutral, the therapist extends the patient's knee and dorsiflexes [DF] the ankle. This rhythmical slider is continued

Uses: grade II or III to effect neural gliding supported by postural control of the spine with the desired effect of reducing sciatic nerve sensitivity to movement and increase movement capacity supported by motor control strategies

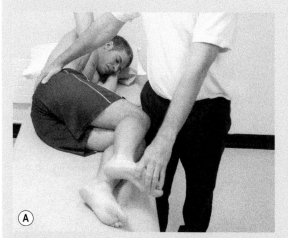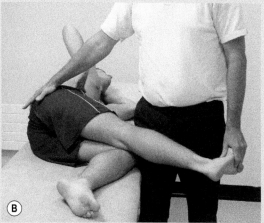

Figure 6.80 • A Cervical flexion with knee flexion; **B** Cervical extension with knee extension.

Position: supine lying+ TAb activation

Method: SLR+ DF

Purpose: where a patient has sciatic-type symptoms and needs neural mobilization to reduce nerve mechanosensitivity and where the SLR+ DF has a greater available range when the abdominal muscles are activated to effect improved foraminal dynamic roominess (hypothesis)

Starting position of patient: Supine lying in the middle of the bed

Starting position of therapist: Standing by the patients right side (for right leg symptoms), right knee on the bed facing the patients opposite shoulder

Localization of forces: therapist supports the patient's heel on the therapist's right shoulder in a position of SLR for treatment. The therapist holds the patient's foot at the toes with the right hand and stabilizes the knee in SLR with the left hand

Application of forces:
With abdominal muscles activated the patient's ankle is dorsiflexed through a range of movement to effect reduction in neurodynamic mechanosensitivity

Uses:
Grade III to IV where there is a need for increase in range of SLR and where a component of lumbar segmental stability is inhibiting recovery of nerve mobility

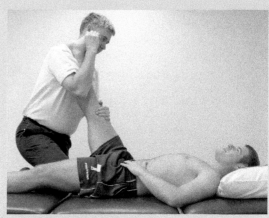

Figure 6.81 • In supine lying+ TAb activation: SLR+ DF.

Position: supine lying+ SLR + ankle DF + cervical flexion

Method: TAb activation exercises

Purpose: activation in neural loading where capacity to activate is impaired at the limit of neural mobility

Starting position of patient: Supine lying

Starting position of therapist: Sitting on the side of the bed facing the patient's head at the level of the patient's pelvis

Localization of forces: both of the therapist's hands facilitate activation of abdominals

Application of forces
Abdominals activated in progressive amounts of neural loading (left knee flexed to 90°, foot on bed), right leg resting on left flexed knee and relaxed foot, in SLR, in SLR+ DF, neck flexed chin to chest

Uses
Activation of abdominals for motor control acquisition in progressive amounts of neural loading so that the patient has the capacity to activate muscles selectively (dissociation) in neural loaded positions. Activation should be pain-free in all instances

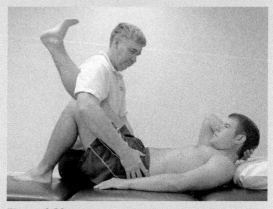

Figure 6.82 • In supine lying+ SLR+ankle DF + cervical flexion: TAb activation exercises.

Where there is evidence of arthrogenic and neurogenic impairments coexisting

Position: sidelying + SLR

Method: lumbar rotation

Purpose: to regain end of range lumbar rotation in a neural loaded position – maximize segmental and neurodynamic capacity

Starting position of patient: Sidelying and maximum rotation of the trunk, neurodynamic restricted leg uppermost. Upper leg in tolerable extreme of SLR position, resting on the edge of the bed, left forearm resting on the lower rib cage

Starting position of therapist: standing behind the patient at the level of the pelvis

Localization of forces: therapist's left hand (for right rotation and right SLR) is spread over the patient's left greater trochanter and iliac crest. The therapist's right hand stabilizes the trunk over the anterior pectoral area adjacent to the left shoulder

Application of forces

Whilst the therapist's right hand stabilizes the trunk, the left hand and body working together produce rotation of the pelvis to the right in relation to the stabilized trunk

Uses

Grade IV in a direction localized to a specific spinal segment (e.g. L4/5) where there is segmental restriction in rotation and this restriction is increased when the leg is in an end of range SLR+DF position

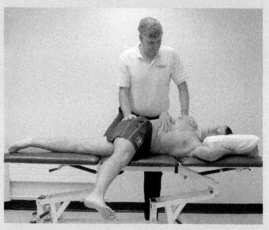

Figure 6.83 • In side lying + SLR: lumbar rotation.

Position: side lying + lumbar rotation

Method:

A. Cervical flexion with knee flexion

B. Cervical extension with knee extension

Purpose: to create a position of dynamic roominess and an ideal interface environment for the neural tissues to be 'flossed' (Butler 2000)

Starting position of patient: side lying in lumbar rotation

Starting position of therapist: standing in front of the patient facing across the bed at the level of the patients pelvis

Localization of forces

Therapist's left hand (for patient in right side lying in lumbar rotation to the left) cradles the patient's occipital area. The therapist's right hand holds the patient's right foot. The therapist's right thigh stabilizes the patient's right thigh just above the knee

Application of forces

Whilst the patient's lumbar spine is in rotation the therapist flexes the patient's cervical spine at the same time as flexing the patient's right knee. The therapist then extends the patient's cervical spine at the same time as extending the patient's right knee. This sliding action is repeated at a smooth rhythm

Uses

As a grade II or III – where the patient has sciatic type symptoms restricting SLR with end of range segmental stiffness

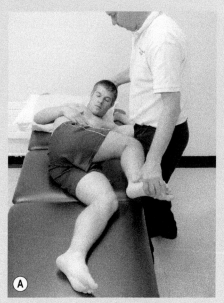 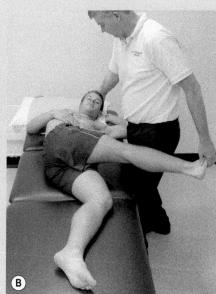

Figure 6.84 • In side lying: **A** cervical flexion with knee flexion; **B** cervical extension with knee extension.

Position: supine lying + PA L4
   Method: SLR + DF[active]
   Purpose: where a PA on L4 is shown to enhance the range of SLR and dorsiflexion (neural tensioning) (right)
   Starting position of patient: supine lying, left knee bent and right leg (back of the knee) resting on the left knee
   Starting position of therapist: standing on the patient's right side facing the patient head at the level of the pelvis
   Localization of forces: therapist's index fingers make contact with the spinous process of L4, hands resting on the patient's back adjacent to the spine

Application of forces
   Therapist applies a PA pressure on L4 with the index fingers at the same time as the patient actively extends the right knee and dorsiflexes the ankle. As the PA pressure is released, the patient relaxes the right leg
   Uses
   Grade II, III – range of active SLR and DF with grade III– PA where back and leg symptoms are quite painful and the patient is comfortable lying supine

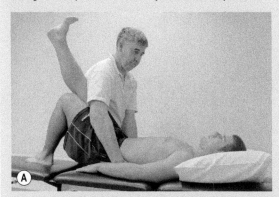 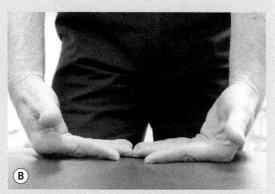

Figure 6.85 • A, B In supine lying + posteroanterior L4: SLR + DF (active).

Where there is evidence of arthrogenic and myogenic impairments coexisting

Position: prone lying + TrAb activation
   Method: PA L4
   Purpose: if activation of TAb reduces pain responses and helps modulate pain effects of PA mobilization in acute LBP
   Starting position of patient: prone lying, neutral pain-free
   Starting position of therapist: standing by the side of the patient at the level of L4, leaning over so that the therapist's sternum is over L4 segmental level
   Localization of forces: therapist's hands are interlocked so that the area between the pisiform and hook of hamate of the therapist's contact hand is against the L4 spinous process. Therapist's elbows slightly bent
   Application of forces
   Whilst asking the patient to activate TAb to 20%, the therapist performs a PA mobilization on L4
   Uses
   Grade I and II for episode of LBP where pain and protection with movement are the predominant features

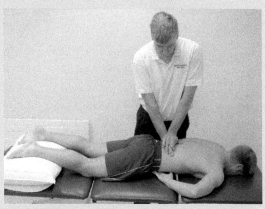

Figure 6.86 • In prone lying + TrAb activation: posteroanterior L4.

Position: prone lying + PA pressure on L4 +TrAb activation

Method: active control of hip medial rotation in 90° of knee flexion (dissociation activity)

Purpose: PA pressure on L4 to reduce pain inhibition of activation and maximize motor control strategy

Starting position of patient: prone lying with one knee bent to 90°

Starting position of therapist: standing by the side of the patient at the level of L4, leaning over so that the therapist's sternum is over L4 segmental level

Localization of forces: therapist's hands are interlocked so that the area between the pisiform and hook of hamate of the therapist's contact hand is against the L4 spinous process. Therapist elbows slightly bent

Application of forces

Whilst the therapist applies a PA pressure grade II, III to L4 the patient is asked to activate abdominals and at the same time dissociate hip rotation from pelvic movement

Uses

Where segmental mobilization reduces pain inhibition of activated muscles to support effective dissociation strategies

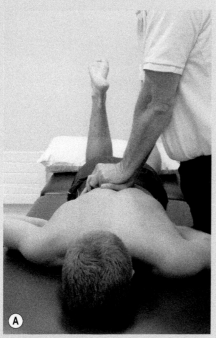
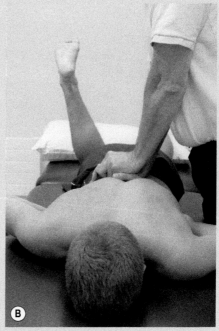

Figure 6.87 • A In prone lying + posteroanterior pressure on L4 +TrAb activation: active control of hip medial rotation in 90° of knee flexion (dissociation activity); **B** in prone lying + posteroanterior pressure on L4 +TrAb activation: active control of hip medial rotation in 90° of knee flexion (dissociation activity).

Position: standing + TrAb activation

Method: PA L4 with lumbar FF (MWM – mobilization with movement)

Purpose: when bending forwards or sustained bending is painful due to segmental restriction and motor control impairment

Starting position of patient: standing

Starting position of therapist: standing behind the patient and just to one side

Localization of forces: the therapist's left hand stabilizes the patient's trunk using the forearm against the patient's abdomen below the segmental level to be mobilized. The heel of the therapist's right hand is placed over the spinous process of L4 (for example) and directed upwards slightly

Application of forces

Whilst the patient bends forwards to P1 or limit with the abdominal muscles activated, the therapist, whilst stabilizing the patient's trunk, applies a posteroanterior pressure directed cephalad to the spinous process of L4

Uses

To improve pain free range and restriction of forward bending where the patients feels more stable with abdominal activation and can move further with PA pressure grade III, IV therefore allowing the patient to stretch further into range to increase forward flexion range

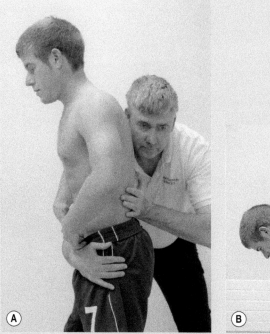
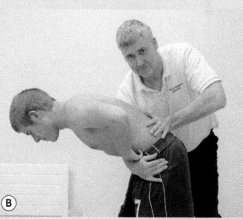

(A) (B)

Figure 6.88 • A, B in standing + TrAb activation: posteroanterior L4 with lumbar FF (MWM – mobilization with movement).

Where there is evidence of arthrogenic, myogenic and neurogenic impairments coexisting

Position: lumbar machine traction (supine, prone, sidelying)
Method:

A. SLR+ ankle DF
B. Hip ABD/LR with TrAb activation
C. Lumbar rotation
D. PA mobilization of L4

Purpose: using machine traction as an interface mobilization, an enhancer of muscle activation or as a segmental mobilization

Starting position of patient: supine, prone, sidelying

Starting position of therapist: standing by the side of the traction bed

Localization of forces

Traction harnesses applied to thorax and pelvis

Application of forces

Apply appropriate traction force to effect symptom reduction along with:

A. The therapist mobilized ankle dorsiflexion in SLR
B. In crook lying, the patient activates abdominals and then dissociates hip abduction and lateral rotation for trunk rotation or extension
C. The therapist performs lumbar rotation mobilization by holding onto each iliac crest
D. The therapist performs a posteroanterior mobilization of L4 with the patient in supine lying and the therapist's index fingers applying a mobilization pressure against the spinous process of L4

Uses

A. Where traction allows further remobilization of SLR grade III, IV
B. Where traction supports dissociated motor control
C. Where traction reduces pain to support pain relieving effects of lumbar rotation grade I, II
D. Where traction supports segmental mobilization grades I–IV

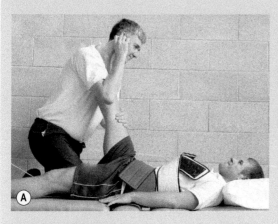
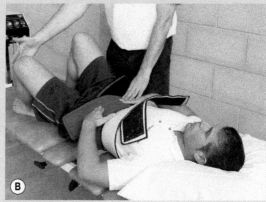
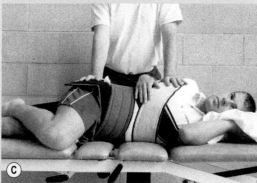
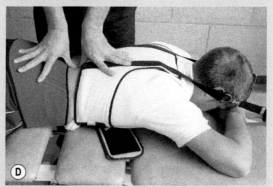

Figure 6.89 • A In machine traction: SLR+ ankle DF; **B** in machine traction + TAb activation: hip AB and LR control; **C** in machine traction: lumbar rotation; D in machine traction: posteroanterior pressure.

Where there is protective muscle spasm coexisting with arthrogenic, other myogenic and neurogenic impairments

Position: flexion over the bed

Method:

A. Traction with sustained unilateral PA mobilization of L4

B. Traction with TAb activation

C. Traction with TAb activation and knee extension as a neural mobilization

Purpose: where protective spasm is inhibiting effects of mobilization, co-contraction or nerve gliding and where the flexed position over the bed allows sustained stretching to reduce protective spasm

Starting position of patient: flexed over the bed with knees bent under the bed and feet resting on the floor

Starting position of therapist: standing by the side of the patient

Localization of forces: therapist places one hand over the mid-thoracic area and the other over the sacrum or L4

Application of forces

The patient is asked to flex their knee under the bed to allow the pelvis to flex thus producing a traction effect on the lumbar spine and a sustained stretch to the erector spinae muscles in particular.

A. The therapist uses one hand to apply a unilateral PA mobilization to L4

B. The patient is asked to activate the abdominal muscles and extend each hip in turn to facilitate dissociation and trunk stability

C. The patient is asked to activate the trunk muscles and at the same time rhythmically extend one knee to produce a neural gliding effect

Uses

Where this starting position effects a relief of protective spasm to allow more effective mobilization, more effective activation and more effective neural gliding

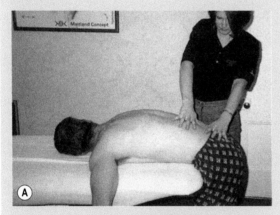

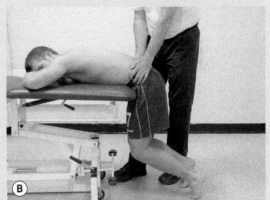

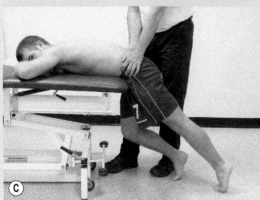

Figure 6.90 • A In flexion over the bed; **B** in flexion with traction: TAb activation; **C** in flexion with traction + TAb activation: knee extension.

Case studies

The following two case examples are included in this chapter to demonstrate:

- The gathering and analysis of patient reported problems and information
- The use of clinical reasoning strategies to enable open-minded and effective sorting out of the clinical information

- Linking patient problems to examination and interventions driven by the patient's functional and cognitive needs
- Evidence informed selection of the most appropriate interventions and treatment techniques
- The use of evaluation to drive progression of treatment towards patient reported outcomes.

Case study 6.1

The 45-year-old joiner with a stiff back

Question 1. My back feels stiff after I have been *sitting for a while* and then I get up. It's uncomfortable ① if I have walked for half an hour so I have to sit down

Successful outcome? To be able to *move around without discomfort* and to be able to *do my job without stiffness*.

Areas of symptoms. ① An area from just above the iliac crests to the mid-sacral area, in the middle of the spine, deep, intermittent stiff and aching. Radiating both sides but more to the left (Fig. 6.91).

Behaviour of symptoms. I am a bit stiff in the morning when I get up but this eases after 5 minutes moving around. I do struggle to put my socks on ① when I have to *bend and twist when sitting*. I am a bit worried about going back to work because I have to do a lot of bending and twisting.

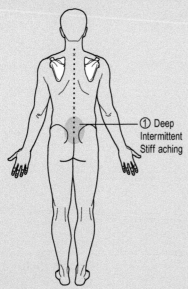

- ① Deep Intermittent Stiff aching

Figure 6.91 • Body chart, 45-year-old joiner with a stiff back.

When I am sitting down, I am fine, just a bit achy, but if I have been sitting for an hour or so and I come to get up I move slowly because of stiffness in my back.

If I have been *walking round the shops* with my wife, after an hour, I start to stiffen up and my back gradually aches ① more and more. If I sit down for a while, I am ok after 10 minutes.

Sometimes I wake up at night if *I roll over* awkwardly and it just gets my back in the wrong position, usually turning over onto my right side [pain and stiff] ①

History of symptoms. I pulled my back at work 4 weeks ago ①. It is a lot better now but still not fully better, so the Doctor has sent me here. I was lifting a plank of wood and it slipped in my hand. This jarred my back ① as I bent and twisted to catch it before it fell on my leg.

I have had twinges and a stiff back in the past but it always goes off in a day or so. It comes with the work.

I have had a few knee and ankle injuries playing football on the right side but nothing major.

Special questions/medical and health screening. My general health is fine, I just get tired if I am working away from home and I have to *drive a long way*. I do not think this helps my back. I do get acid reflux and I take medication for this. I had a back X-ray and it just came back as slight wear and tear in the lower back. I try not to take any tablets although the doctor gave me some anti-inflammatory tablets. They did not help much.

Hypotheses from subjective examination

- Likely to be segmental hypomobility related to strain
- Possible P/E findings: dysfunction in combined movements at end of range (flexion and rotation causing pain)
- There will be some motor control issues after 4 weeks, so screen for this

Case study 6.1—cont'd

- No evidence of maladaptive protective mechanisms or central sensitization
- Nature of work may be a factor in risk and injury reduction/recurrence
- Check for contributing factors in lower extremity related to old injuries (hip, knee and ankle)
- Being clear regarding outcome measures for return to work and daily activities.

Physical examination

Sway back, over activity in left erector spinae (T8–L2) [protective response], contralateral protective shift [correct, stiff ① increased in intensity].

Functional demonstrations

*Sitting, reach forward as to put sock on left ① when stretches [lumbar flexion and rotation, hip flexion 90° and lateral rotation 30°, reaches ankle]. ① ISQ with activation of abdominal muscles, lateral glide of the hip and neural loading [cervical flexion in lumbar flexion and left lateral flexion].

**FF 40' + LLF 20' ①. ISQ with activation of abdominals and neural loading.

E ✓✓.

E 30+ LLF 20+ LR 20 ①. ISQ with activation of abdominal and neural loading.

*PPIVMs and PAIVMs reveal hypomobility at L3/4 more on the left (lateral flexion, rotation and ULPA). Local pain provoked at end range.

*Stiff hip flexion /adduction on left and weak gluteus medius.

Slump test full range of knee extension in slump position.

Plan of treatment

- Restore pain-free, resistance free segmental mobility at site of injury at L3/4
- Mobilize stiff hip and activate gluteus medius in the functional positions that reproduce ①
- Recondition for work including self-management strategies with repeated movements towards extension and contralateral rotation/LF
- Main outcome measure- FF + LLF + LOAD (PAIN FREE): to enable restoration of functional performance (sitting without stiffness, carry out job related tasks without pain and stiffness).

Supporting evidence for plan

- Clues from subjective examination and from knowledge of clinical, functional and behavioural sciences support the use of mobilization and physical activity in health and well-being (CSAG 1994)
- There is evidence for the effectiveness of hip mobilization for early osteoarthritis along with exercises (Sims 1999, Van Baar et al. 2000)

- PPIVMs help to localize segmental impairment (Cook & Hegedus 2010)
- PAIVMs – posteroanterior segmental stiffness is a prediction rule for the effectiveness of lumbar manipulation (Flynn et al. 2002)
- Loss of motor control is known to contribute to hip and back pain (Macedo et al. 2012)
- Behavioural and physical conditioning are key to sustainable physical and mental performance (Main & Spanswick 2000)
- NICE guidelines recommend mobilization and manipulation to enhance recovery from NSLBP (NICE 2009)
- Yeris et al. (2002) and Makofsky et al. (2007) noted that passive hip mobilizations demonstrated immediate effect on gluteus maximus contraction force.

Treatment

D1

Thinking: start by trying to reduce segmental stiffness and pain with mobilization techniques as movement related pain and stiffness are most evident and there seems little influence on symptoms with neural loading or trunk motor control in functional positions.

Treatment: in lumbar extension+ left lateral flexion+ left rotation mobilize L3/4 with a Ⓛ unilateral posteroanterior pressure grade III+ for 3 minutes, repeated twice. Grade III+: with slight pain in rhythm of the movement. The aim is to reduce the pain and restriction in a compression pattern which is occurring through the active range of movement. Assessment during treatment. After 2–3 minutes sense of resistance changing ('freer') and patient felt less pain.

Effects: reaching forward in sitting, FF+ LLF isq, hip F/ADD isq, gluteus medius control isq. Lumbar E+ LLF+ ROT better.

Home automobilization: sent home with a self-mobilization of L3/4 unilaterally on the left into lumbar extension/left lateral flexion and left rotation in standing as per treatment dosage. With instructions to do the exercise every 4 hours 10 × 3 and ensure symptoms reduce with repeated movements.

Follow up appointment 1 week later

Therapist's thinking: mobilization of L3/4 in combined movements in extension eased an old facet restriction and compression pattern but did not change the more recent pain and restriction into flexion. This is qualified by the fact that the patient felt better standing for longer and was less stiff after sitting but still had problems with bending and twisting and putting his socks on. The hip and gluteus medius impairments are likely to be separate components, as they did not change with lumbar mobilization.

Continued

Case study 6.1—cont'd

Repeat the first treatment to clear the extension pattern and confirm this has little effect on flexion and hip components then add in mobilization in flexion to reduce aching and stiffness with bending and twisting (standing and sitting).

Treatment: in lumbar extension+ left lateral flexion+ left rotation mobilize L3/4 with a Ⓛ unilateral posteroanterior pressure inclined medially grade IV+ for as a progression of treatment 3 minutes, repeated twice. The aim is to reduce the pain and restriction compression pattern. During treatment pain was provoked with the stiffness at end of range. The pain reduced as the stiffness reduced and full range was achieved.

Effects: reaching forward in sitting, FF+ LLF isq., hip F/ADD isq., gluteus medius control isq. Lumbar E+ LLF+ ROT no pain or restriction.

Therapist's thinking: it is clear now that the old extension pattern has cleared up sufficiently with mobilization but the flexion and hip components will need other interventions. Flexion and sideflexion is the painful stiff functional movement so use this as a treatment technique incorporating lumbar rotation

Treatment: in lumbar flexion and left lateral flexion: did right pelvis rotation grade III to L3/4 stretching into discomfort ① for 3 minutes repeated once. Effects during treatment – after 2 minutes each time discomfort settled, resistance improved.

Effects: improvement in flexion and lateral flexion and reaching in sitting to put socks on but hip flexion/adduction and gluteus medius control remain unchanged.

Home programme: as extension is now pain-free, automobilization can be stopped but advised patient to restart if stiffness and aching with sitting and standing starts to creep back in.

Advised to try to maintain the gains from mobilization into flexion combined movements using the functional activities that remain stiff and painful. Instructions given were to move into the functional direction until slight sense of pulling during every functional opportunity to maintain treatment gains.

2 weeks later

Therapist's thinking: the patient feels as though his mobility has improved but he still gets sore after repeated bending and twisting so he is wary about returning to work, as he feels weak still. He is not as stiff after sitting or standing but still feels restricted putting his socks on.

This information suggests that the segmental pain and stiffness is settling but motor control has not fully recovered. The hip is still stiff so will need mobilizing to ensure contributing factors are addressed effectively.

On examination of unilateral posteroanterior pressure of L3/4 there is no loss of range just a deep soreness when pushing at the limit of the range. When asked to contract gluteal muscles actively the soreness on palpation diminishes significantly. When asked to flex and left side flex the lumbar spine there is a feeling of discomfort and weakness in this position that needs to be discomfort free and strong for work. When asked to contract the gluteal muscles in lumbar flexion and lateral flexion the discomfort reduced significantly. The same response to gluteal activation occurred in the functional position of reaching to put socks on as in sitting.

The important intervention now is to work towards sustainable functional capacity and return to work. To mobilize the hip and see if this reduces pain inhibition of gluteus medius and improve its stabilizing capacity.

Treatment: hip flexion/add grade III mobilization for 3 minutes repeated twice. During treatment the stiffness and discomfort gradually reduced over the 3 minutes of treatment time.

Effects: this helped the range of hip flexion when reaching to put socks on but did not improve the activation ability of gluteus medius.

Treatment: active exercises to activate gluteus medius in side lying 3 × 10 daily

Home programme: patient shown automobilization of hip flexion/add as per treatment and, as well as gluteus medius exercises, activation of gluteal muscles when performing functional tasks such as bending and twisting or putting socks on.

1 week later

Thinking: the patient has mastered the gluteus medius activation. This has also improved forward bending, as the hamstrings are less tight. The hip is more flexible and the bending and twisting with loads equivalent to work is pain-free. Use this last session as an information session to explain to the patient: the importance of regular physical activity: the need to maintain strength and mobility to reduce risk of injury again at work: the role of pain in protection but also how pain can lead to maladaptive and chronic deconditioning.

Treatment: advice and information on physical activity. Review exercises and functional capability.

Effects: patient has better understanding of the importance of physical activity, maintaining functional capability for his job and understanding pain and its role in protecting and ensuring recovery from injury.

Home programme: staged return to work, hand over to occupational health staff and discharge from health care to return to healthy living.

Case study 6.2

It is useful to include here an example of how the manipulative physiotherapist thinks her way through a patient's difficulty and atypical spinal problem. This particular example demonstrates how to link the theory with the clinical presentation. It also demonstrates the different components a patient's problem may have, and how one component may improve and another not. This patient's disorder demonstrates how the therapist must adapt her techniques to the expected and unexpected changes in the symptoms and signs. The example also demonstrates how open-minded she must be, and how detailed and inquiring her mind must be in making assessments of changes and interpreting them.

Mr L

Eighteen months ago, a 34-year-old fit, well-built man (Mr L) with no history of previous back problems, wakened with pain in his left buttock area. Over the previous 2 days he had suffered very bad low lumbar backache, which his doctor had diagnosed as being viral because he also had general aching in other parts of his body. Mr L did say that, although he had 'flu-like aches all over', his lower back was the worst area. He had been on holiday during the previous week and had done a lot of lifting and been wind-surfing (a new experience for him). Two days after the onset of his buttock pain it spread, overnight, down the left leg with tingling into the big toe area of his left foot (? L5 radicular symptom). Some days later, the big toe tingling alternated with tingling along the lateral border of his foot and into the lateral two toes (? S1 radicular symptom). At no time prior to 18 months ago had he ever had any back symptoms, and there was no familial component. He had undergone numerous forms of treatment (orthodox and unorthodox) over 6 months, but without success. Over a period of time the symptoms eased, but he did not become symptom free.

Following a fall 3 weeks ago, which exacerbated his disorder, he had a lumbar puncture (which proved negative) and hospital traction for a week. Following this, his low back pain increased. When he first went for physiotherapy his symptoms were as follows (Fig. 6.92):

1. He would waken in the morning with back pain and back stiffness, and the stiffness would last for a few hours. (Unusual for a non-inflammatory musculoskeletal disorder.)
2. Coughing caused both back pain and left calf pain.
3. He was using indomethacin (Indocid) suppositories every night, and he felt that these were essential to lessen the level of his pain. (Perhaps this means there must be an inflammatory component.)
4. Bending caused him severe back and leg pain, both of which eased immediately on standing upright.

(This latter fact indicates that a treatment technique that provokes leg pain may not be a contraindication to its use; the technique, to be effective, may in fact need to provoke leg pain.)

5. On standing for 1 minute, the pain would increase in his back and would spread down his leg. (This indicates that a sustained technique may be required.)
6. The only neurological change present was calf weakness.

The initial physiotherapy treatment, which he had undergone elsewhere, had improved all of his symptoms marginally. The first three of these treatments consisted of PAs on L5 and unilateral PAs to the left of L4. The latter, he said, provoked calf pain in rhythm with the technique. On the third treatment intermittent traction had been introduced, but this did not help him.

Assessment

I saw him for the first time 5 days later.

1. On more positive questioning to determine his area of pain, it was interesting to note that, although his main lower leg pain was posterior, he had what he described as 'a different pain' in the upper posterolateral calf. These two pains were sometimes present at the same time, but were more frequently felt separately. (This tends to indicate that they may arise from two different sources – two components.)
2. Standing (and he could not stand erect, in fact he had a lumbar kyphosis) provoked pain in his left leg, and he was unable to bend backwards because of increased leg pain.
3. He had an ipsilateral list on flexion. (Items (2) and (3) seem to indicate that he has a disc disorder, which is provoking possible radicular pain. The offending part of the disc is probably medial to the nerve root and its sleeve, and will therefore be harder to help by passive movement techniques.) Neck flexion while he was flexed was limited by increased leg pain. (There must be a canal component in his disorder.) It did not increase his back pain. (The cause of his back pain is probably not causing his leg pain. Two aspects of the one structure perhaps? The disc?)
4. While still in the flexed position, rotation to the left increased his leg pain by about 100%. Rotation to the right in flexion decreased the leg symptoms, slightly but definitely. (It is very helpful from a treatment point of view to have different responses with the different directions of rotation.) In this man's circumstances it is wise, when considering the selection of technique, to choose

Continued

Case study 6.2—cont'd

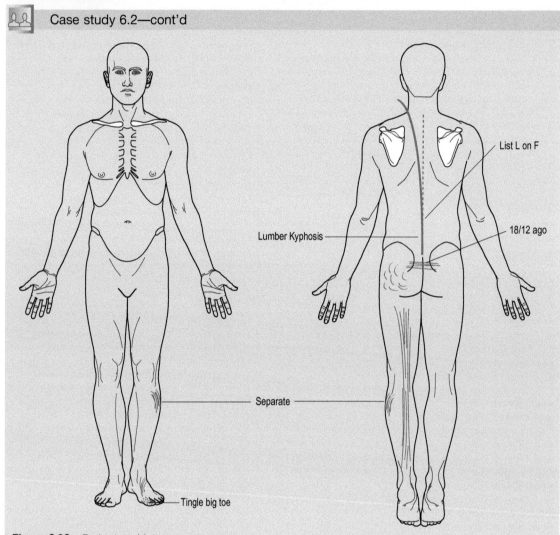

List L on F

Lumber Kyphosis

18/12 ago

Separate

Tingle big toe

Figure 6.92 • Body chart, Mr L.

the relieving position while performing the relieving direction for the rotation.

5. In the upright position, performing a lateral shift of his trunk towards the left decreased his pain; shift to the right slightly increased the symptoms. (Because of this pain response, the list must be directly related to his disorder.)

6. Straight leg raise on the left was 35°, causing posterior leg pain. On the *right* it was 70°, and he said it caused an uncomfortable tight feeling, plus tingling, in the *left* foot laterally. (Crossed SLR response – treatment may need to include mobilizing the right SLR.)

7. Testing the power of his calf in standing demonstrated some weakness, which may have been a neurological weakness but may also have been a pain inhibition reaction.

8. Attempting to stand, from sitting only a short time (half a minute), he had back pain and a severe lumbar kyphosis, which took some 15 seconds or more (a long time) to dissipate. (Because the kyphosis developed so quickly, this meant that the disorder causing his back pain was *very mobile*.)

9. His leg pain was minimal on first standing but then gradually increased in intensity and also in the length of the pain referral down his leg. (This meant that the disorder causing his leg pain had a *latent component*.)

10. His leg pain and his back pain could be provoked separately. (This meant that there were *at least two components to his disorder*. With the added information in number (1) above, he has at least three components. Number (4) above makes it four components.)

Case study 6.2—cont'd

11. Tingling was felt either in the big toe or the lateral border of his foot. (This indicated the *possibility* of two nerve roots being involved. This could mean that two intervertebral discs may be involved, or the patient may have an anatomically abnormal formation of the nerve roots.)

12. He also had canal movement abnormalities as well as intervertebral joint movement abnormalities.

Mr L's disorder was obviously atypical. The disc component seemed to be causing him more disability than the radicular aspect, but obviously the radicular aspect took higher priority. Being atypical means that one has to be very quick to notice the changes in the examination signs of the separate components, and to react with appropriate technique changes.

Treatment

Because it seemed to be discogenic (getting up from sitting) with a nerve-root irritation:

1. The choice of technique would be rotation, as the symptoms and signs are clearly unilateral

2. The rotation would be performed in the 'symptom-relieving' position and direction to avoid provoking pain

3. Thinking ahead to further treatment techniques, it seemed possible that the canal signs would not improve in parallel with the joint signs, and that therefore SLR stretching may be required later.

Mr L was positioned lying on his left side with a support (folded towel) under his iliac crest to gain a lateral shift to the left position (his comfortable shift position, *see* item (5) above). He was also positioned in a degree of flexion to keep his lumbar spine away from the painful and markedly limited extension position. A rotation of this thorax to the right in relation to the pelvis was also adopted, and his right leg was kept up on the couch to avoid any canal tensioning (which would occur if his right leg were allowed to hang over the edge). The technique was to rotate his pelvis to the left (that is, the same direction as thoracic rotation to the right, but performed from below upwards) as a sustained (sustained because of the latent component) grade IV.

- During the performing of the technique he felt an easing of his leg symptoms, which was a favourable indication.

- On reassessing his movements after the technique, the joint movements were improved but SLR was unchanged.

- The technique was repeated, but more firmly and for a longer sustained period. During the performing of

this technique all tingling in his foot disappeared. Following the technique movements had further improved, but

- SLR was still unchanged

- Symptomatically, he felt more comfortable and felt he could stand straighter.

After four such treatments Mr L was greatly improved, but SLR, although improved, was nowhere near as much improved as were the joint movements. Sitting was also improved. His calf power was normal. During this stage of treatment, a scan revealed posterior disc protrusions slightly lateral to the left of the posterior longitudinal ligament at both the L4/5 and L5/S1 levels.

Because the, ?discogenic?, component was improved, and also the radicular symptoms were less (plus calf power improvement), left SLR was used as a technique and after four treatment sessions of this his left SLR became full range and pain free. However, the right SLR still felt tight and did provoke minimal left leg symptoms. It was decided to do right SLR as the treatment technique. The tightness cleared and remained clear for 4 hours.

The next treatment session consisted of performing SLR on each leg and ending the session with a repeat of the previous positioning and rotation technique. It was decided to stop treatment (unless he had an exacerbation) and review all aspects in a month.

The assessment after a month revealed that he had not only retained all of the improvement from treatment but also found he could sit, stand and be much more active. His movements were full and almost free of any discomfort. He was reviewed again after 2 months and discharged. Aspects of 'back care', especially in relation to the 'weak link', the capacity for harm to accumulate painlessly and the need to be aware of predisposing factors (*see* Appendix 4) were forcibly emphasized.

This presentation emphasizes that the manipulative physiotherapist must understand the pathology that may be involved in such a patient's disorder, yet she must take most notice of the changes in symptoms and signs. For example, the fact that his disorder may have been progressing towards a nerve-root compression did not prevent SLR being used as treatment, because the possible nerve condition signs were improving and the possible radicular symptoms were also improving. Nevertheless, the first SLR mobilization had to be done only once, and that once was a mild stretch. The 24-hour assessment indicated that it should be continued with care.

References

Adams MA, Dolan P: Spine biomechanics, (Perspective) *J Biomech* 38(10):1972–1983, 2005.

Adams MA, Stefanakis M, Dolan P: Healing of a painful intervertebral dis should not be confused with reversing disc degeneration: Implications for physical therapies for discogenic pain, *Clin Biomech* 2010. doi: 10.1016/j.clinbiomech.2010.07.016.

Airaksinen O, Hildebrandt J, Mannion AF, et al: European guidelines for the management of chronic nonspecific low back pain, *Eur Spine J* 15(Suppl 2):S192–S300. 2004.

Abenhaim L, et al: The role of activity in the treatment of low back pain, *Spine* 25(4):1S–31S, 2000.

Apkarian AV, Robinson JP: Low back pain, *IASP Pain Clinical Updates* VXIII(Issue 6), 2010.

Asenlöf P, Denison E, Lindberg P: Individually tailored treatment targeting activity, motor behaviour and cognition reduces pain-related disability: a randomised controlled trial in patients with musculoskeletal pain, *J Pain* 6:588–603, 2005.

Asenlöf P, Denison E, Lindberg P: Long-term follow-up of tailored behavioural treatment and exercise based physical therapy in persistent musculoskeletal pain: a randomised clinical trial in primary care, *Eur J Pain* 13:1080–1088, 2009.

Banks K: The Maitland Concept as a clinical practice framework of NMS disorders. In Hengeveld E, Banks K, editors: Maitland's Peripheral Manipulation (vol 2), ed 5, Ch 1. Edinburgh, 2014, Elsevier.

Banks K, Hengeveld E: *Maitland's Clinical Companion: An Essential Guide for Students*, 2010, Churchill Livingstone.

Billis EV, McCarthy CJ, Oldham J: Subclassification of low back pain: a cross-country comparison, *Eur Spine J* 16:865–879, 2007.

Boal RW, Gillette RG: Central Neuronal Plasticity, Low Back Pain and Spinal Manipulative Therapy, *J Manipulative Physiol Ther* 27(5):314–326, 2004.

Bogduk N: On the definitions and physiology of pain, referred pain and radicular pain, *Pain* 147:17–19, 2009.

Borkan JM, Koes B, Reis J, et al: A report from the second international forum for primary care research on low back pain, *Spine* 23:1992–1996, 1998.

Briggs AM, Buchbinder R: Back pain; a national health priority area in Australia, *Med J Aust* 190:499–502, 2009.

Bruton A, Conway JH, Holgate ST: Reliability: what is it and how is it measured? *Physiotherapy* 86(2): 94–99, 2000.

Bullock-Saxton J: The palpation reliability debate – the experts respond, *J Bodyw Mov Ther* 6(1):19–21, 2002.

Bunzli S, Gillham D, Esterman A: Physiotherapy-provided operant conditioning in the management of low back pain disability: a systematic review, *Physiother Res Int* 16(2011): 4–19, 2011.

Burton K, Muller G, Balagne F, et al: Chapter 2: European Guidelines for the prevention of low back pain November 2004, *Eur Spine J* (2006) 15(Suppl. 2):S136–S168, 2009.

Butler D: *The sensitive nervous system*, Adelaide, 2000, NOI-Group publications.

Butler D, Moseley L: *Explain pain*, Adelaide, Australia, 2003, Noi Group Publications.

Chartered Society of Physiotherapy: Scope of Practice, *CSP* 1–17, 2008.

Cibulka M, Delitto A, Koldehoff R: Changes in innominate tilt after manipulation of the sacroiliac joint in patients with low back pain, *Phys Ther* 68:1359–1363, 1988.

Cleland JA: Foreword. In Glyn PE, Weisbach PC, editors: *Clinical Prediction Rules. A Physical Therapy Reference Manual*, Massachusetts, 2011, Jones and Bartlett Publisher Sudbury.

Coaz W: Paradigmenwechsel – auch in der Physiotherapie? *Physiother Bull* 33:1–12, 1993.

Cook C, Hegedus E: Systematic review. Diagnostic utility of clinical tests for spinal dysfunction, *Man Ther* doi:10.1016/j.math.2010.07.004, 2010.

Coppieters M, Butler DS: Do 'sliders' slide and 'tensioners' tension? *Man Ther* 13:213–221. 2008.

Cott CA, Finch E, Gasner D, et al: The movement continuum theory for physiotherapy, *Physiother Can* 47:87–95, 1995.

CSAG: *Report on Back Pain*, London, 1994, Clinical Standards Advisory Group. HMSO.

Dankaerts W, O'Sullivan P: The validity of O'Sullivan classification system (CS) for a subgroup of NS-CLBP with motor control impairment (MCI): Overview of a series of studies and review of the literature, *Man Ther* 16:9–14. 2011.

Davies P: *Starting again: early rehabilitation after traumatic brain injury*, Berlin, 1994, Springer Verlag.

De Groot AD: *Het denken van den schaker. Eenexperimenteelpsychologischestudie*, Amsterdam, 1946, Noord-Hollandse Uitgeversmaatschappij.

Edwards I. *Clinical Reasoning in three different fields of physical therapy - A qualitative case study*. PhD-Thesis, Adelaidem, 2000, School of Physiotherapy, Division of Health Sciences, University of South Australia.

Fishbain DA: Secondary gain concept. Definition problems and its abuse in medical practice, *APS Journal* 3:264–273, 1994.

Flynn T, Fritz J, Whitman J, et al: A Clinical Prediction Rule for Classifying Patients with Low Back Pain Who Demonstrate Short-Term Improvement With Spinal Manipulation, *Spine* 27(24): 2835–2843, 2002.

Ford JJ, Hahne J: Pathoanatomy and classification of low back disorders, *Man Ther* doi:10.1016/j.math.2012.05.007, 2012.

Fordyce WE: A behavioural perspective on pain, *Br J Clin Psychol* 21: 313–320, 1982.

Fordyce WE: On pain, illness and disability, *J Back Musculoskeletal Res* 5:259–264, 1995.

Gifford L: Pain, the tissues and the nervous system: a conceptual model, *Physiotherapy* 84:27–36, 1998.

Glynn PE, Weisbach PC: *Clinical prediction rules.a physical therapy reference manual*, Massachusetts, 2011, Jones and Bartlett Publishers Sudbury.

Gowers WR: Lumbago: Its lessons and analogues, *Br Med J* 1:117–121. 1904.

Greenhalgh T, Hurwitz B: Why study narratives. In Greenhalgh T, Hurwitz

B, editors: *Narrative Based Medicine*, London, 1998, British Medical Journal Press.

Hadler NM: If you have to prove you are ill, you can't get well, *Spine* 20:2397–2400, 1996.

Hall T, Quintner J: Responses to mechanical stimulation of the upper limb in painful cervical radiculopathy, *Aust J Physiother* 42(4):277–285, 1996.

Hall AM, Ferreira PH, Maher CC, et al: The Influence of the Therapist-Patient Relationship on Treatment Outcome in Physical Rehabilitation: A Systematic Review, *Phys Ther* 90:1099–1110, 2010.

Hancock MJ, Maher CG, Laslett M, et al: Discussionpaper: what happened to the 'bio' in the bio-psycho-social model of low back pain? *Eur Spine J* 20:2105–2110. 2011.

Hayden JA, van Tulder MW, Tomlinson G: Systematic review: strategies for using exercise therapy to improve outcomes in chronic low back pain, *Ann Intern Med* 142:776–785, 2005.

Heath J: Following the story: continuity of care in general practice. In Greenhalgh T, Hurwitz B, editors: *Narrative Based Medicine*, London, 1998, British Medical Journal Press.

Hengeveld E: Clinical Reasoning in Manueller Therapie – eine klinische Fallstudie, *Manuelle Therapie* 2:42–49, 1998.

Hengeveld E: Gedanken zum Indikationsbereich der Manuallen Therapie. Teil 1, Teil 2, *Manuelle Therapie* 2(3):176–181, 2–7, 1998, 1999.

Hengeveld E: *Psychosocial issues in physiotherapy in Switzerland: manual therapists' perspectives and observations*. MSc-Thesis. London, 2001, University of East London.

Hengeveld E: A behavioural perspective on severity and irritability, *IMTA Newsletter* 7:5–6, 2002.

Hengeveld E, Banks K: *Maitland's Peripheral manipulation (vol 2)*, ed 5, Edinburgh, UK, 2014, Elsevier.

Hides J, Stanton WR, Wilson J, et al: 2010. Retraining motor control of abdominal muscles among elite cricketers with low back pain, *Scand J Med Sci Sports* 20:834–842, 2010.

Higgs J, Jones M, Loftus S, et al: *Clinical Reasoning in the Health Professions*, ed 3, Amsterdam, 2008, Elsevier Butterworth Heinemann.

Hodges PW: Pain and motor control: from laboratory to rehabilitation,

J Electromyogr Kinesiol 21:220–228, 2011.

Huijbregts PA: Introduction. In Glyn PE, Weisbach PC, editors: *Clinical Prediction Rules. A Physical Therapy Reference Manual*, Massachusetts, 2011, Jones and Bartlett Publishes Sudbury.

IFOMPT (International Federation of Orthopaedic Manipulative Physiotherapists): Educational Standards in Orthopaedic Manipulative Physical Therapy. www.ifompt.com, 2008.

Jensen GM, Gwyer J, et al: *Expertise in Physical Therapy Practice*, Boston, 1999, Butterworth-Heinemann.

Johnson AJ, Godges JJ, Zimmerman GJ, et al: The effect of anterior versus posterio glide joint mobilization on external rotation range of motion in patients with shoulder adhesive capsulitis, *J Orthop Sports Phys Ther* 37(3): 88–99, 2007a.

Johnson RE, Jones GT, Wiles NJ, et al: Active exercise, education and cognitive behavioral therapy for persistent disabling low back pain. A randomised clinical trial, *Spine* 32(15):1578–1585. 2007b.

Jones M: Clinical reasoning and pain, *Man Ther* 1:17–24. 1995.

Jull G, Bogduk N, Marsland A: The accuracy of manual diagnosis for cervical zygapophysial joint pain syndromes, *Med J Aust* 148:233–236, 1988.

Jull G, Zito G, Trott P, et al: Inter-examiner reliability to detect painful upper cervical joint dysfunction, *Aust J Physiother* 43:125–129, 1997.

Kamper SJ, Maher CG, Hancock MJ, et al: Treatment-based subgroups of low back pain: A guide to appraisal of research studies and a summary of current evidence, *Best Pract Res Clin Rheumatol* 24:181–191, 2010.

Keating J, Matyas T: Unreliable inferences from reliable measurements, *Aust J Physiother* 44:5–10. 1998.

Kendall NAS, Linton SJ, Main CJ, et al: *Guide to assessing psychosocial yellow flags in acute low back pain: risk factors for long-term disability and work loss*, Wellington, New Zealand, 1997, Accident Rehabilitation & Compensation Insurance Corporation of New Zealand and the National Health Committee.

Kent PM, Keating J: Do primary-care clinicians think that nonspecific low

back pain is one condition? *Spine* 29:9, 1022–1031, 2004.

Kent PM, Kjaer P: The efficacy of targeted interventions for modifiable psychosocial risk factors of persistent nonspecific low back pain. A systematic review, *Man Ther* doi:10.1016/j.math.2012.02.008, 2012.

Kent PM, Keating JL, Buchbinder R: Searching for a conceptual framework for nonspecific low back pain, *Man Ther* 14:387–396, 2009a.

Kent PM, Keating JL, Taylor NF: Primary care clinicians use variable methods to assess acute nonspecific low back pain and usually focus on impairments, *Man Ther* 14:88–100, 2009b.

Kenwright J, Richardson JB, Cunningham JL, et al: Axial movement and tibial fractures – a controlled randomized trial of treatment, *J Bone Joint Surg* 73-B:654–659. 1991.

Kleinmann A: *The illness narratives: suffering, healing and the human condition*, New York, 1988, Basic Books Harpers.

Krouwel O, Hebron C, Willett E: An investigation into the potential hypoalgesic effects of different amplitudes of PA mobilisations on the lumbar spine as measured by pressure pain thresholds (PPT), *Man Ther* 15:7–12, 2010.

Lando A: Temperature testing by manipulative physiotherapists in spinal examination. In Boyling JD, Palastanga N, editors: *Grieve's Modern Manual Therapy*, ed 2, Edinburgh, 1994, Churchill-Livingstone.

MacDermid JC, Walton D, Avery S, et al: Measurement properties of the neck disability index: a systematic review, *J Orthop Sports Phys Ther* 39(5):400–417, 2009.

Macedo LG, Maher CG, Latimer J, et al: Motor control exercises for persistent, nonspecific low back pain: a systematic review, *Phys Ther* 89(1):9–25. 2009.

Macedo LG, Latimer J, Maher CG, et al: Effect of motor control exercises versus graded activity in patients with chronic nonspecific low back pain: A randomiszed controlled trial, *Phys Ther* 92(3):363–377, 2012.

Makofsky H, Panicker S, Abbruzzese J, et al: Immediate effect of Grade IV inferior hip joint mobilisation on hip abductor torque: a pilot study,

J Man Manipulative Ther 15(2):103–111, 2007.

Maher C, Latimer J, Refshauge K: Prescription of activity for low back pain: what works? *Aust J Physiother* 45:121–132, 1999.

Main CJ, Spanswick CS: *Pain management – a multidisciplinary approach*, Edinburgh, 2000, Churchill Livingstone.

Maitland GD: Movement of pain-sensitive structures in the vertebral canal in a group of physiotherapy students, *S Afr J Physiother* 36:4–12, 1980.

Maitland GD: *Vertebral Manipulation*, ed 5, Oxford, 1986, Butterworth-Heinemann.

Maitland GD: The development of manipulative physiotherapy, *SVMP-Bulletin* 10:3–5, 1995.

Maitland GD, Hengeveld E, Banks K, et al: *Maitland's Vertebral manipulation*, ed 7, Edinburgh, 2005, Elsevier. Butterworth-Heinemann.

Maluf KS, Sahrmann SA, Van Dillen LR: Use of a classification system to guide nonsurgical management of a patient with chronic low back pain, *Phys Ther* 80:1097–1111. 2000.

Mattingly C: What is clinical reasoning? *Am J Occup Ther* 45:998–1005, 1991.

McGill SM: The biomechanics of low back injury: implications on current practice in industry and in the clinic, *J Biomech* 30:5, 465–475, 1997.

May S, Aina A: Centralization and directional preference: a systematic review, *Man Ther* doi:10.1016/j. math.2012.05.003, 2012.

McCarthy CJ, Arnall FA, Strimpakos N, et al: The biopsychosocial classification of nonspecific low back pain: a systematic review, *Phys Ther Rev* 9:17–30, 2004.

McKenzie R: *The lumbar spine. Mechanical diagnosis and therapy*, New Zealand, 1981, Spinal Publications.

Mead J: Patient partnership, *Physiotherapy* 86:282–284, 2000.

Moseley L: Evidence for the direct relationship(between cognitive and physical change during an education intervention in people with chronic low back pain, *Eur J Pain* 8(1): 39–45, 2004.

Moss P, Sluka K, Wright A: The initial effects of knee joint mobilisation on oateoarthritic hyperalgesia, *Man Ther* 12:109–118, 2007.

Nachemson AL, Jonsonn E, editors: *Back and neck pain: Scientific evidence of Cause, diagnosis and treatment. Swedish Council of technology assessment and health care (SBU)*, Philidelphia, 2000, Lippincott Willams and Wilkins.

Nakao M, Shinozaki Y, Nolido N, et al: Responsiveness of hypochondriacal patients with chronic low-back pain to cognitive-behavioral therapy, *Psychosomatics* 53:139–147, 2012.

NICE: Low back pain: early management of persistent non-specific low back pain, *National Institute for Health and Clinical Excellence (UK)* 1–10, 2009.

O'Neill CW, Kurgansky ME, Derby R, et al: Disc stimulation and patterns of referred pain, *Spine* 27:4 2776–2781, 2002.

O'Sullivan P: 2005. Diagnosis and classification of chronic low back pain disorders: maladaptive movement and motor control impairments as underlying mechanisms, *Man Ther* 10(4):242–255, 2005.

O'Sullivan P: It's time for change with the management of non-specific chronic low back pain. Editorial, *Br J Sports Med* 4–6, doi:10.1136/bjsm.2010.081638, 2011.

Paterson C: 1996. Measuring outcomes in primary care: a patient generated measure, MYMOP, compared with the SF-36 health survey, *BMJ* 312:1016–1020, 1996.

Panjabi M: The stabilising system of the spine: Part II Neutral zone and instability hypothesis, *J Spinal Disord* 5(4):390–396, 1992.

Paungmali A, O'Leary S, Souvlis T, et al: Hypoalgesic and sympathoexcitatory effects of mobilisation with movement for lateral epicondylalgia, *Phys Ther* 83:374–383. 2003.

Perry J, Green A: An investigation into the effects of a unilateral mobilisation techniques on peripheral sympathetic nervous system activity in the lower limbs, *Man Ther* 13:492–499, 2008.

Perry J, Green A, Watson P: A preliminary investigation into the magnitude of effect of lumbar extension exercises and a segmental rotatory manipulation on sympathetic nervous system activity, *Man Ther* 16(2):190–195, 2011.

Phillips DR, Twomey LT: A comparison of manual diagnosis with a diagnosis established with a lumbar block procedure, *Man Ther* 2:82–87, 1996.

Pilowsky I: *Abnormal illness behaviour*, Chichester, 1997, John Wiley.

Pincus T, Vlaeyen JWS, Kenall NAS, et al: Cognitive behavioral therapy and psychosocial factors in low back pain – directions for the future, *Spine* 27(5):E133–E138, 2002.

Prochaska J, DiClemente C: Stages of change and decisional balance for twelve problem behaviours, *Health Psychol* 13(1):39–46. 1994.

Quebec Task Force on Spinal Disorders: Scientific approach to the assessment and management of activity-related spinal disorders. A monograph for clinicians. Report of the Quebec Task Force on Spinal Disorders, *Spine* 12(Suppl 7): S1–S59, 1987.

RCGP: *Clinical Guidelines for the Management of Acute Low Back Pain*, London, 1999, Royal College of General Practitioners.

Richardson C, Hodges P, Hides J: *Therapeutic exercise for motor control and lumbopelvic stabilisation: a motor control approach for the treatment and prevention of low back pain*, Edinburgh, 2004, Elsevier Churchill Livingstone.

Sahrmann S: *Movement system impairment syndromes of the extremities, Cervial and Thoracic Spine*, ed 2, St Louis, 2011, Elsevier Mosby.

Sayres LR: Defining irritability: the measure of easily aggravated symptoms, *Br J Ther Rehabil* 4:18–20, 37, 1997.

Schafer A, Hall T, Muller G, et al: Outcomes differ between subgroups of patients with low back and leg pain following neural manual therapy: a prospective cohort study, *Eur Spine J* 20:482–490. 2011.

Schön DA: *The reflective practitioner. How professionals think in action*, Aldershurt, 1983, Arena.

Schmidt H, Boshuyzen H: On acquiring expertise in medicine, *Educ Psych Rev* 5(3):205–221, 1993.

Shacklock M: *Clinical neurodynamics: a new system of musculoskeletal treatment*, Edinburgh, 2005, Elsevier. Churchill Livingstone.

Sheehan NJ: Magnetic resonance imaging for low back pain: indications and limitations, *Ann Rheum Dis* 69:7–11, 2010.

Sims K: Assessment and treatment of hip osteoarthritis, *Man Ther* 4(3):136–114, 1999.

Slater SL, Ford JJ, Richards MC, et al: The effectiveness of sub-group specific manual therapy for low back pain: a systematic review, *Man Ther* 17(2012):201–212, 2012.

Smart K, Blake C, Staines A, et al: Self-reporting pain severity, quality of life, disability, anxiety and depression in patients classified with 'nociceptive', 'peripheral neurogenic' and 'central sensitisation' pain. The discriminant validity of mechanism-based classification of low back (+/– leg) pain, *Man Ther* 17: 119–125. 2012.

Stier-Jarmer M, Cieza A, Borchers M, et al: How to apply the ICF and ICF core sets for low back pain, *Clin J Pain* 25:29–38, 2009.

Thomas-Edding D: Clinical problem solving in physical therapy and its implications for curriculum development. Proceedings of the 10th International Congress of the World Confederation of Physical Therapy, Sydney, 1987.

Thomson D: Counseling and clinical reasoning: the meaning of practice. *Br J of Therapy and Rehabilitation* 5:88–94, 1998.

Turner JA, LeResche L, Korff Von M, et al: Backpain in primary care – patient characteristics, content of initial visit and short-term outcome, *Spine* 23:463–469. 1998.

Van Baar ME, Assendelft WJ, Dekker J, et al: Effectiveness of exercise therapy in patients with osteoarthritis of the hip or knee. A systematic review of randomized clinical trials, *Arthritis Rheum* 42:1361–1369. 2000.

Van Tulder M, Becker A, Bekkering T, et al: European Guidelines for the management of acute low back pain, *Eur Spine J* (Suppl 15):131–300, 2006.

Vermeulen HM, Rozing PM, Obermann WR, et al: Comparison of high-grade and low grade mobilisation techniques in the managemnt of adhesive capsulitis of the shoulder: randomized controlled trial, *Phys Ther* 86(3):355–368, 2006.

Vlaeyen JWS, Crombez G: Fear of movement/(re)injury, avoidance and pain disability in chronic low back pain patients, *Man Ther* 4:187–195. 1999.

Vleeming A, Albert HB, Östgaard HC, et al: European Guidelines for the diagnosis and treatment of pelvic girdle pain, *Eur Spine J* 17:794–819, 2008.

Waddell G: A new clinical model for the treatment of low back pain, *Spine* 12:632–644, 1987.

Waddell G: *The Back Pain Revolution*, Edinburgh, 1998, Elsevier. Churchill Livingstone.

Waddell G: *The back pain revolution*, ed 2, Edinburgh, 2004, Elsevier. Churchill-Livingstone.

Walsh J, Hall T: Reliability, validity and diagnostic accuracy of palpation of the sciatic, tibial and common peroneal nerves in the examination of low back related leg pain, *Man Ther* 14(2006):623–629, 2009.

Wand BM, O'Connell NE: Chronic non-specific low back pain – subgroups or a single mechanism? *MBC Musculoskelet Disord* 9:11, 2008. doi:10.1186/1471-2474-9-11.

Watson P, Kendall N: Assessing psychosocial yellow flags. In Gifford LS, editor: *Topical Issues in Pain*, ed 2, Swanpool, UK, 2000, CNS Press.

Watters W, Baisdenn J, et al: Degenerative lumbar spinal stenosis: an evidence-based clinical guideline for the diagnosis and treatment of degenerative lumbar pinal stenosis, *Spine J* 8:305–310. 2008.

WHO: *ICF – International Classification of Functioning, Disability and Health*, Geneva, 2001, WHO.

WHO: *WHO global strategy on diet, physical activity and health – A framework to monitor and evaluate implementation*, Geneva, 2008, World Health Organization.

WHO/EUROPE: *What is the best way to treat low back pain?* Health Evidence Network/Publications, p 1. Online. Available from: www.euro.who.int 2000.

Yeris S, Makofsky H, Byrd C, et al: Effect of mobilisation of the anterior hip capsule on gluteus maximus strength, *J Man Manipulative Ther* 10(4):218–224, 2002.

Yeo H, Wright A: Effects of performing a passive accessory mobilization technique in patients with lateral ankle pain, *Man Ther* 16:373–377, 2011.

7

Management of sacroiliac and pelvic disorders

Elaine Maheu   Elly Hengeveld

CHAPTER CONTENTS

Pelvic girdle pain (PGP) as a clinical
entity 330

Relating clinical practice to current
scientific evidence 332

Clinical reasoning and PGP 337

Subjective examinaton 341

Physical Examination 345

The role of motor control in PGP 365

Common clinical presentations 366

Key words

Pelvic girdle pain (PGP), sacroiliac joint (SIJ), force closure, form closure, lumbopelvic–hip complex, functional tests of load transfer, pain provocation tests, self-locking mechanism of the SIJ, nutation/counter-nutation of the sacrum, motor control, local and global muscle systems, excessive/insufficient compression of the SIJ, mobilizations/manipulations of the SIJ

Introduction

Low back and leg pain may have various causes and contributing factors. These include biomedical elements as pathobiological processes as well as movement impairments of the lumbopelvic–hip complex.

Over the past two decades numerous research efforts have contributed to the knowledge of the role of the pelvic girdle in movement disorders leading to pelvic, low back and leg pain.

Clinical note

It has become accepted that pelvic girdle pain (PGP) needs to be treated as a clinical entity distinct from low back pain.

PGP has been defined as follows:

> Pelvic girdle pain generally arises in relation to pregnancy, trauma, arthritis and osteoarthritis. Pain is experienced between the posterior iliac crest and the gluteal fold, particularly in the vicinity of the SIJ. The pain may radiate in the posterior thigh and can also occur in conjunction with/or separately in the symphysis.
>
> The endurance capacity for standing, walking and sitting is diminished.
>
> The diagnosis of PGP can be reached after exclusion of lumbar causes. The pain or functional disturbances in relation to PGP must be reproducible by specific clinical tests.

(Vleeming et al. 2008, p. 797)

It is proposed that the definition for pelvic musculoskeletal pain should be under the title 'pelvic girdle pain' in order to exclude gynaecological and/urological disorders (Vleeming et al. 2008).

Symptoms associated with the sacroiliac joints (SIJ) represent a subgroup of pelvic girdle disorders (O'Sullivan & Beales 2007a, 2007b). Based on a study including joint-infiltrations, Maigne et al. (1996) conclude that the prevalence of sacroiliac disorders may be approximately 18.5% in a general population. Vleeming et al. (2008), after a review of four prospective studies, conclude that there is strong evidence of a point prevalence of close to 20% of women during pregnancy. These results show that it is necessary for clinicians to routinely consider the pelvic girdle and particularly the SIJ as a possible cause or contributing factor to a patient's low back and leg pain.

Numerous studies have been undertaken to test the validity and reliability of clinical sacroiliac tests with inconclusive results particularly with regards to mobility testing. However, there does appear to be agreement that pain provocation tests are supportive in clinical decision making regarding the role of the SIJ if composite tests of pain provocation procedures reproduce the patient's symptoms consistently (van der Wurff et al. 2000, Laslett et al. 2005, Vleeming et al. 2008).

With regards to treatment, the European Guidelines for the diagnosis and treatment of PGP recommend specific individualized motor control exercise programs for pregnant women and individualized multimodal treatment for other patients (Vleeming et al. 2008).

The choice of the best treatment for each patient is based on a thorough subjective and physical physiotherapy assessment; an essential feature of the Maitland Concept. The primary focus of the examination of lumbopelvic and leg symptoms frequently needs to be placed on the reproduction of the patient's symptoms. The signs and symptoms found on assessment then need to be related to the functional limitations of the patient. The treatment objectives are first defined and then priorities are set.

Note

Treatment objectives will be based on the movement impairments, activity limitations, resources and participation restrictions, as defined in the International Classification of Functioning Disabilities and Health (WHO 2001).

Although musculoskeletal manual physiotherapists adhere increasingly to the concept of evidence based practice, it is essential to bear in mind that:

> ... external clinical evidence can inform, but can never replace individual expertise, and it is this expertise that decides whether the external evidence applies to the patient at all, and if so, how it should be integrated into a clinical solution.
>
> (Sackett et al. 1998, p. 3)

Physiotherapists should therefore constantly reflect upon their clinical reasoning in decision-making throughout the process of assessment and treatment.

When symptoms are suspected to be of pelvic girdle origin, physiotherapists need to incorporate in their assessment, the examinations of the sacroiliac joints and when indicated that of the symphysis pubis and coccyx. Furthermore the assessment of motor control patterns needs to be included.

Clinical note

Coexisting dysfunctions in the areas adjacent to the pelvis, such as movement disorders of the hip, lumbar spine and neurodynamics, are very common.

Clinical note

The primary function of the lumbopelvic – hip complex is to transfer loads safely while fulfilling the movement and control requirements of a task (Lee & Lee 2010). The pelvic girdle is part of a functional unit as it moves with the lumbar spine and the hips.

Clinical note

As there is limited motion in the SIJ (Sturesson et al. 2000a), it is of utmost importance for the therapist to include a thorough evaluation of the lumbar spine, the hips and the neurodynamic system before concluding that the sacroiliac joint is one of the sources of the symptoms.

Applied theory and evidence supporting practice

The pelvic girdle is a very stable structure, which as a unit supports the abdomen and the organs of the lower pelvis. Furthermore it provides a dynamic link between the spine and the lower extremities (Fig. 7.1).

Form closure, force closure, mobility

The pelvic girdle receives its stability from the interconnection between the symphysis pubis and the sacroiliac joints, a strong ligamentous system and the wedge shape of the sacrum, fitting vertically between the innominates. These elements build a self-locking system (Kapandji 2008) and contribute to the form closure of the pelvic girdle (Vleeming et al. 1997).

Furthermore, various muscle groups and fasciae cross over the pelvic girdle. Their function adds to the dynamic stability of the system, which relates to the dynamic force closure.

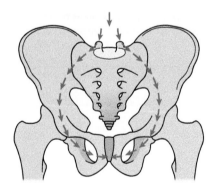

Figure 7.1 • Transference of forces between the trunk, pelvis and femur. Reproduced from Palastanga et al. (1994) with kind permission from Elsevier.

Clinical note

Form closure refers to a stable situation with closely fitting joint surfaces, in which no extra forces are needed to maintain the state of the system, once it is under a certain load (Vleeming et al. 1997).

The wedge-shaped sacrum is suspended between the innominates and contributes to the stability in the transverse plane because of its irregular semilunar joint formation and the connection to the (short) dorsal sacroiliac and sacrotuberous ligaments (Kapandji 2008, Vleeming et al. 1997). Furthermore, the symphysis pubis contributes to the stability of the pelvic girdle (Kapandji 2008). In this self-locking mechanism, nutation of the sacrum plays an essential role, as it winds up most of the sacroiliac ligaments (Vleeming et al. 1997).

However, if the sacrum were to fit perfectly between the innominates, practically no movement would be possible. Some degree of movement in the sacroiliac joints has been described and up to 1.6 mm of translation and about 4° of rotation has been measured in radiostereometric analysis of the sacroiliac movements (Sturesson et al. 2000b). In order to withstand vertical loads, such as in standing positions, and to prevent shear forces, a lateral force and friction are needed to maintain stability. This occurs by the nutation movement of the sacrum in relation to the innominates and by compression generated by the myofascial structures (*force closure*; see Fig. 7.2).

Numerous studies demonstrate poor interexaminer reliability values with regard to the mobility of the sacroiliac joints (van Deursen et al. 1990, Laslett et al. 2005, van der Wurff et al. 2000). A reason for this phenomenon is offered by Sturesson et al. (2000a) who observed, in radiostereometric

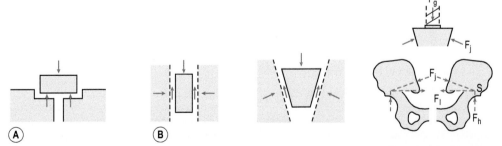

Figure 7.2 • A combination of form closure **A** and force closure **B** allow for the strong stability of the pelvic girdle. Reproduced with permission from Vleeming et al. (1997).

analyses of the movements of the sacroiliac joints during weight bearing positions, a further decrease in the already small mobility, which adds to the difficulty to detecting movement during manual examination procedures.

In symptomatic patients, the mobility may be marginally increased (Kissling & Jacob 1997), which may also be a challenge to detect with manual testing.

Local and global stabilizing muscle system

Based on widespread publications regarding lumbopelvic stabilization, the following aspects need to be taken into consideration:

Clinical note

It has become increasingly accepted that improvement of motor control patterns should be included in the treatment of PGP, in order to enhance joint compression and improve force closure (O'Sullivan & Beales 2007a, 2007b, Vleeming et al. 2008, Laslett 2008, Lee & Lee 2010).

• Panjabi (1992) discussed that effective load transfer and stability is achieved when passive, active and neural control systems work together in harmony. As part of the passive sub-system, form closure with its osteoarticular and ligamentous structures plays a central role. The structures making up the passive system give feedback and have a direct link to the neural control system. In the active system, force closure with its myofascial elements are just as important, give feedback and are influenced by the neural control system.

Clinical note

The **local muscle system**, with the (tonic activity of) transversus abdominis (TA) muscle, lumbosacral multifidi (MF), diaphragm and pelvic floor (PF) muscles, is considered to play a primary role in (active) lumbopelvic stabilization (primary stabilizers; Richardson et al. 2004, Lee 2004).

See Figure 7.3 for a diagrammatic representation of the abdominal-pelvic cavity surrounded by muscles contributing to lumbopelvic stability, intra-abdominal pressure and continence.

Clinical note

This notion finds support in various clinical studies:

• Hungerford et al. (2003) observed in a group of 14 men with the clinical diagnosis of SIJ pain, delayed electromyography (EMG)-reaction patterns of the internal oblique, multifidus and gluteus maximus muscles during hip flexion in standing, while the biceps femoris showed an earlier recruitment pattern in comparison to healthy control subjects. EMG onsets were also found to be different between the symptomatic and asymptomatic sides in the men with SIJ pain.

• In another study with motion analysis and video observation with markers, Hungerford et al. (2004) observed that symptomatic males showed significant alterations to the motion of the innominates during single leg support while performing hip flexion with the other leg. The weight bearing innominate rotated posteriorly and translated superiorly in the healthy controls, while in the symptomatic subjects the weight bearing innominate rotated anteriorly and translated inferiorly in relation to the sacrum. It was

concluded that anterior rotation of the innominate during one-leg weight-bearing and contralateral hip flexion is indicative of failure of the self-bracing mechanism and load transfer through the pelvis with a resultant decrease in the ability to oppose vertical shear loads during weight bearing.

• An additional study investigated the reliability of the one leg weight bearing–hip flexion test ('Stork test'). Three physiotherapists were asked to detect the altered movement patterns of the weight bearing innominates. It was concluded that the ability to distinguish between no relative movement and anterior rotation was good when a 2-point scale was used. It was emphasized that this test does not assess the relative mobility of the SIJ and is not suited to be a pain provocation procedure. Instead this test assesses the ability of a subject to maintain a stable alignment of the innominate bone relative to the sacrum during a functional load transfer task. A positive test is indicative of a failure to activate the self-bracing mechanism to maintain the self-locking system of the sacroiliac joints (Hungerford et al. 2007).

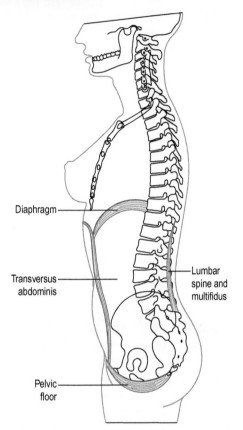

Figure 7.3 • Diagrammatic representation of the abdominal-pelvic cavity surrounded by muscles contributing to lumbopelvic stability, intra-abdominal pressure and continence. From Sapsford (2001a).

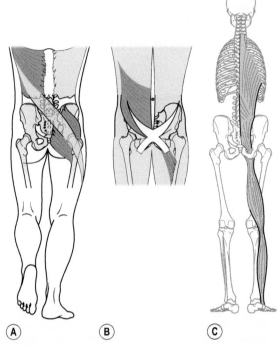

Figure 7.4 • Posterior, anterior and longitudinal slings of the global stabilizing muscle system. (**A** from Vleeming et al. 1995; **B** and **C** from Lee 2004, with permission.)

TA has been shown to impact stiffness of the pelvis through its direct attachment to the innominate, to the middle layer and to the deep lamina of the posterior layer of the thoracolumbar fascia (TLF). The pelvic floor muscles should be given sufficient attention as their importance is not negligible (next to the function of transverse abdominal and multifidi) in enhancing increased stiffness of the pelvic ring and proper load transfer in the lumbopelvic region, particularly in the treatment of PGP in women (Pool-Goudzwaard et al. 2004). Based on a study with needle EMG, Sapsford and colleagues (Sapsford 2001, 2004, Sapsford & Hodges 2001) conclude that the abdominal muscles contract in response to pelvic floor contraction and vice versa: the pelvic floor muscles contract in response to both a 'hollowing' and 'bracing' visualization exercise of the lower abdominal wall. Richardson et al. (2002) have reported that co-contraction of TA and MF increases the stiffness of the SIJ. Pel et al. (2008) showed that shear forces through the SIJ could be significantly reduced by simulated activity of TA and PF muscles. It is therefore obvious that local muscles work in synergy and tend to co-contract to stabilize the pelvic girdle.

The timing of contraction of local muscles appears to be important for force closure of the pelvis. Intramuscular EMG analysis suggests that TA exhibits contraction prior to perturbation of the trunk and before rapid limb movements are initiated (Hodges & Richardson 1998). Hungerford et al. (2003) have also found that during one leg standing (OLS), the onset of TA and internal oblique (IO) precede a weight shift in healthy individuals.

The global (stabilizing) muscle system is made up of four slings of muscles groups which have been described as stabilizing the pelvis regionally (Fig. 7.4; Lee 2004):

- Posterior oblique sling, containing connections between the latissimus dorsi and the contralateral gluteus maximus through the thoracodorsal fascia (Vleeming et al. 1995)
- Anterior oblique sling, containing connections between the external oblique muscles, the anterior abdominal fascia, contralateral internal oblique muscles and the adductors of the hip

- Longitudinal sling, connecting the peroneal muscles, biceps femoris, sacrotuberous ligament, the deep layer of the thoracodorsal fascia and the erector spinae
- Lateral sling, containing the primary stabilizers of the hip – gluteus medius, minimus, tensor fascia latae, contralateral adductors and the lateral stabilizers of the thoracopelvic region.

These four global muscle slings do not function in isolation, but they interconnect, partially overlap and function together (Lee 2004). Although the global muscle slings may not directly control intervertebral motion, as does the local stabilizing system, the global muscles can generate tension in the thoracolumbar fascia which can produce compression on the posterior pelvis, which assists in the control of shear and rotation forces to which the lumbopelvic region is submitted (Vleeming et al. 1995, Hodges 2004, Barker et al. 2004). The slings are assumed to play a role in the capacity to use our legs and trunk for energizing the body (Vleeming & Stoeckart 2007).

The posterior oblique sling

- The posterior oblique sling has been shown to affect the force closure at the SIJ.
- Gluteus maximus (GM) has the greatest capacity for force closure via the posterior layer of the TLF and has been noted to transmit tension directly behind the SIJ as low as S3 (Barker et al. 2004, Barker 2005).
- van Wingerden et al. (2004) report that GM contraction causes an increase in stiffness at the SIJ ×2–3 that noted with contraction of latissimus dorsi during gait.
- Rotation against resistance has been found to activate the posterior oblique sling (Vleeming & Stoeckart 2007).
- GM creates a muscle link between the tensor fascia lata and the TLF. Contraction of the GM increases stiffness in both fascia that span the lumbar spine, SIJ and hips.
- Hungerford et al. (2003) have found that the onset of contraction of gluteus maximus is altered with SIJ dysfunction.

The deep longitudinal sling

- ES and MF are part of the deep longitudinal sling that simultaneously contribute to compression of the lumbar segments and provide a dynamic restraint to A/P shear stresses in the lumbar spine.
- The muscles making up this sling increase tension in the TLF and compress the SIJ.
- Biceps femoris can influence sacral nutation through its connection to the sacrotuberous ligament and plays a role in the intrinsic and extrinsic stability of the pelvis in relation to the leg (Vleeming et al. 1997).

The anterior oblique sling

Muscles of the anterior sling with the anterior abdominal fascia create compression across the pubic symphysis (Snijders et al. 1993).

Optimal strategy in motor control will vary between individuals and for different tasks. Multiple strategies are needed to ensure stability during both static and dynamic tasks. Optimal force closure is just the right amount of force being applied at just the right time. Situations of high load and low predictability will require a stiffening strategy whereas many other low load tasks of high predictability, such as walking, will require a dynamic strategy through phasic muscle activity (Hodges et al. 2003).

Patients with failed load transfer present with inappropriate force closure in that certain muscles become overactive while others, known to stabilize the pelvis (such as IO, MF and GM) remain inactive, delayed or asymmetric in their recruitment (Richardson et al. 2002, Hungerford et al. 2003, 2004). Maladaptive motor control strategies can minimize the function of muscles such as the IO and TA and thereby impede the bracing mechanism of the pelvic joints (Beales et al. 2009). Changes in motor control can occur in situations when pain is anticipated but not present and when there is a real or a perceived risk of injury or pain (Hodges & Cholewicki 2007).

Some common maladaptive compensation strategies around the pelvis:

- Women with stress incontinence may have increased EO activity which may overcome the activity of the PF muscles and lead to incontinence
- Deficits in respiration and continence may lead to compromised spinal control (Hodges & Cholewicki 2007)
- Hyperactivity of global muscles such as the obliques, erector spinae and external rotators of

the hip can lead to chest gripping (hyperactivity of obliques), back gripping (overactivity of erector spinae), butt gripping (hyperactivity of hip external rotators – piriformis and obturator internus). These strategies are often seen in patients who lack segmental spinal, intrapelvic and/or hip motion control (Lee 2004). If any of these strategies are noted, releasing the hypertonic muscles should be addressed prior to assessing and training the local muscles.

Healthy integrated neuromyofascial system ensures that loads are effectively transferred through the joints while mobility is maintained, continence preserved and respiration supported (Lee & Vleeming 2007). According to Lee & Lee (2010), it is not enough to know which muscles have the capacity of increasing force closure; there is also a need to understand how the CNS controls and directs synergistic activity in function. Emotional states, influenced by past experiences, beliefs, fears and attitudes should be taken into account as they can impact motor control and affect strategies in function (Lee & Vleeming 2007).

Classification model

O'Sullivan and Beales (2007a) propose a broad classification model for the management of chronic PGP disorders, in which, among others, the following issues need to be taken into consideration to direct appropriate management of a patient's problem:

- Considering chronic PGP within a bio-psychosocial framework, in which attention needs to be given to potential physical, patho-anatomical, psychosocial, hormonal and neurophysiological factors
- Questioning if the PGP disorder is related to a specific or a non-specific pain disorder (see Fig. 7.5)
- In cases of non-specific pain disorders, with nociceptive pain mechanisms, reflecting on the cause of the disorder whether it is associated with an excessive force closure due to muscle hyperactivity of the pelvic muscles or to a reduced force closure due to a motor control deficit.

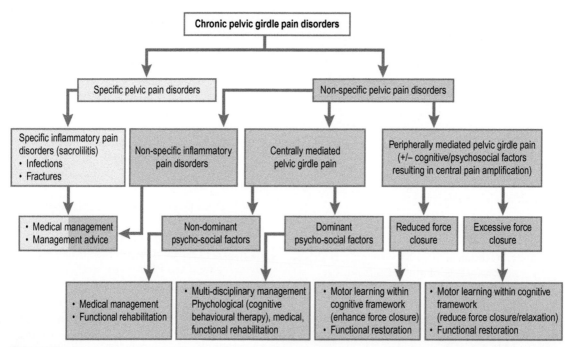

Figure 7.5 • Mechanism based classification of chronic pelvic pain disorders. (From O'Sullivan & Beales (2007a) with permission.)

Treatment

Based on the best available current evidence, the European Guidelines for the Diagnosis and Treatment of Pelvic Girdle Pain (Vleeming et al. 2008) provide various recommendations for treatment.

The aims of treatment are to relieve pain, improve functional stability and prevent recurrences and chronic disability due to pain.

Clinical note

Management should include:
- Adequate information and reassurance of the patient
- Individualized exercises for pregnant women
- Individualized multimodal treatment for other patients
- Pain medication, if necessary, for pain relief (except for pregnant women)

Recommendations for specific treatment interventions are described in Table 7.1.

There is evidence that passive mobilization and manipulation can be effective for the relief of pain and restoration of mobility in the short term (Koes et al. 1996, AAMPGG 2003). However, in order to maintain long-term results, motor control, education and self-management strategies are essential (O'Sullivan et al. 1997, Richardson et al. 1999, AAMPGG 2003). Manipulation has also been suggested for treatment of both acute and chronic low back pain patients (van Tulder & Koes 2010). This could be extended to the SIJ in cases where there is excessive force closure, as long as it is only part of a multimodal approach to treatment.

Consideration of other factors leading to PGP

In the presentation of non-mechanical or unclear symptoms, which do not respond to adequate treatment, clinicians need to bear in mind that different pathobiological processes may cause or contribute to PGP, which may require medical attention (Table 7.2).

Table 7.1 Recommendations of the European Guidelines for the diagnosis and treatment of PGP (adapted from Vleeming et al. 2008)

Information, reassurance	Although there is no evidence to recommend information as a single treatment, information as part of a multimodal treatment should reduce fear and encourage patients to take an active part in their rehabilitation
Stabilizing exercises	… the use of an individualized treatment programme focusing on specific stabilizing exercises as part of a multimodal treatment. (Vleeming et al. 2008, p. 808), in which individualized treatments have been demonstrated to be more effective than general group training or no treatment. The stabilizing exercises should focus on normalization of control and stability of force closure
Joint mobilization, manipulation	Joint mobilization and manipulation may be used to test for symptomatic relief, but should only be applied for a few treatments
Pelvic belt	A pelvic belt may be fitted to test for symptomatic relief, but should only be applied for short periods
Pain medication	May be given, if necessary, for pain relief. First choice: paracetamol; second choice: NSAIDs
Intra-articular injections	May be recommended for ankylosing spondylitis (under imaging guidance)

Clinical reasoning

As stated before, it is essential that physiotherapists are aware of all decisions they make during the whole therapeutic process. The clinical reasoning processes are complex. Hence, in order to guide clinical practice, it is essential to make the hypotheses that have been generated during assessment and treatment explicit at regular intervals during treatment sessions and to reflect upon them.

To optimize efficiency, categorization of the hypotheses is recommended (Jones 1995, Thomas-Edding 1987). The possible hypotheses are listed in Table 7.3.

Table 7.2 Pathobiological conditions leading to PGP (adapted from Hansen & Helm 2003; Huijbregts 2004)

Musculoskeletal	Inflammatory	Malignancy	Medical/metabolic
Ankylosing spondylitis	Inflammatory bowel disease	Lymphoma	Osteoporosis
Fracture dislocation, stress fracture	Pyogenic sacroiliitis	Ovarian cancer	Abdominal aneurysm
Juvenile rheumatoid arthritis	Sickle cell anemia	Intraspinal neoplasms	Paget's disease
Osteochondroma	Reiter's syndrome	Carcinoma of colon, prostate	Osteomalacia
	Psoriatic spondylitis	Multiple myeloma	Acromegaly
	Diffuse idiopathic skeletal hyperostosis (DISH)		Hyperparathyroidism
			Retroperitoneal fibrosis
			Gynaecological disorders
			Urogenital disorders

Table 7.3 Hypotheses categories which guide the decisions in the overall clinical process

Hypotheses category		Remarks
Pathobiological processes Tissue pathology	It is essential to ask screening questions related to different bodily systems, indicative of possible contraindications, which need the attention of a medical practitioner	This is guided by the question: *'is there any pathobiological process on the background of this movement disorder?'* If they are no contraindications, they determine a precaution to treatment or may guide the selection of treatment techniques
Neurophysiological symptom mechanisms	Nociceptive mechanisms Peripheral neurogenic mechanisms Central nervous system Modulation Autonomic nervous system processes	Nociceptive mechanisms, as well as certain peripheral neurogenic mechanisms may be considered part of 'end-organ dysfunction' (Apkarian & Robinson 2010) in which the patient feels pain because of nociceptive processes in the spine, SIJ etc. Normally the pain occurs in a 'stimulus-response relationship' and appears in relation to the history of the problem: over time the pain reduces and the levels of activity are normalizing again. In cases of larger peripheral neurogenic lesions, central nervous system modulation and ongoing autonomic nervous system processes, altered nervous system processes appear to be occurring. Pain and activity intolerance do not occur in a stimulus response relationship and seem to last longer than could be expected if normal healing/recuperative processes occur
Sources of nociceptive processes and movement dysfunction	Possible sources of symptoms and movement dysfunction in relation to PGP: Sacroiliac joint Symphysis pubis Coccyx Lumbar spine Hip Thoracic spine Neurodynamic system Muscles, e.g. trigger points in m.piriformis Soft tissues	This relates to movement impairments and structures, which may be responsible for the (nociceptive and/or peripheral neurogenic) pain It is possible that different sources are simultaneously responsible for the pain (e.g. SIJ and lumbar spine) which need to be addressed in treatment. In cases of non-mechanical presentation or insufficient reaction to adequate treatment, other causes as for example visceral dysfunctions need to be considered

Table 7.3 Hypotheses categories which guide the decisions in the overall clinical process—cont'd

Hypotheses category		Remarks
Contributing factors	This may include any physical, biomechanical, emotional, cognitive and behavioural factors which may contribute to or maintain the problem	Motor control patterns frequently play an essential role in the maintenance and recurrence of PGP symptoms (Hodges 2004, Lee 2004, O'Sullivan & Beales 2007a, 2007b)
Individual illness experience	This may be influenced by earlier experiences, thoughts, feelings, beliefs, values and social environment. The individual illness experience has a core influence on the illness behaviour, incl. the employment of coping strategies of a patient. From a phenomenological perspective physiotherapists guide patients towards an individual sense of health and health promoting behaviour with regards to movements functions (Hengeveld 2000)	Patient with PGP may have been told that their pelvis is 'displaced' or 'unstable' leading to beliefs that no active control can be achieved, thus becoming dependent on someone to fix their problem. Educational and motivational strategies may be needed to explain contemporary viewpoints on the role of muscular recruitment and rehabilitation.
Precautions and contraindications	Defined by the severity and irritability of the nociceptive processes, stability of the disorder, as well as by underlying pathobiological processes, stages of tissue healing, other pathologies and the patient's confidence to move	
Management	Determined by the activities and participation restrictions as described in the subjective examinations, by the movement impairments found in physical examinations and the contributing factors as well as the individual illness experience	In cases of nociceptive pain, first priorities may be put on pain reduction with passive mobilization and automobilization techniques. Motor control exercises need to be incorporated in an early phase of treatment. In cases of ongoing pain and disability, possible pathobiological processes need to be ruled out. Furthermore neuropathic processes need to be considered as well as 'yellow flags', for example, beliefs regarding treatment, lack of sense-of-control over the pain, fear, habitual movement patterns and non-helpful thoughts as contributing factors to the problem

Continued

Table 7.3 Hypotheses categories which guide the decisions in the overall clinical process—cont'd

Hypotheses category		Remarks
Prognosis	Which results may be expected from treatment on a short term basis, after e.g. four sessions? Which results may be expected as an end-result of treatment? Which results may not be achieved? If after four sessions the results do not mirror the short term prognosis, the physiotherapist has to reconsider all hypotheses and check if certain aspects of treatment need to be followed up more	The following factors may determine a favourable prognosis (Banks & Hengeveld, 2010): Strong relationship of patient's symptoms and movement Recognizable syndrome (clinical pattern) Predominantly primary hyperalgesia and tissue-based pain mechanisms Model of patient: helpful thoughts and behaviours ('I can still do some things', 'I have found ways to get relief') Familiar symptoms, which the patient recognize as tissue based ('It feels like a bruise') No or minimal barriers to recovery or predictors of chronicity ('yellow flags') Severity, irritability and nature of the patient's symptoms correspond to the history of the disorder/to injury or strain to the structures of the movement system Previous, favourable experiences with manipulative physiotherapy Patients are touch tolerant Internalized locus-of-control with regards to health and well-being Realistic expectations of the patient towards recovery which correspond to the natural history of the disorder Patients resume appropriate activity and exercise at relevant stages of recovery

Clinical reasoning and assessment procedures

Assessment procedures and clinical reasoning are inseparable elements in the therapeutic process. Ongoing assessment takes place at the beginning of each treatment session, during treatment and after the application of therapeutic techniques. Hypotheses are continuously being confirmed, discarded or modified.

At times it may be challenging to determine if the SIJ is contributing to the movement disorder of the patient. It is possible that only one (highly sensitive) sacroiliac test, for example the Posterior Pelvic Pain Provocation Test (P4-test), consistently reproduces the patient's symptoms. If this test is the most comparable sign in the examination, the SIJ should then be treated first.

The therapists can then use the principle of 'differentiation by treatment', another feature of the Maitland Concept to validate their decision.

Clinical note

Maitland recognized the challenges involved in diagnosing SIJ dysfunctions. He recommended a balanced approach between the interview of the patient and the detailed, comprehensive physical examination, on which the first treatments should be based:

> … by encountering subtle clinical clues, the manipulative physiotherapist may build a case to implicate the sacroiliac joint. More often than not, retrospective assessment will be the final determinant. Therefore she should seek to establish a series of relevant findings that build into a case implicating the joint.
>
> (Maitland et al. 2005, pp. 401–2).

Evidence based practice

Evidence based practice is defined by Sackett et al. (1998, pp. 2 & 3) as:

The conscientious, explicit and judicious use of current best evidence in making decisions about the care of individual patients. The practice of evidence-based medicine means integrating individual clinical expertise with the best available external clinical evidence from systematic research.

Although compliance with evidence based practice is highly recommended, physiotherapists may face dilemmas in making decisions with regards to the choice of best management, including communication, educational strategies and selection of treatments. It is well known that there is not enough research evidence for every clinical situation so clinicians need to be informed of what is known and make their own clinical decisions accordingly (Lee & Lee 2010). Physiotherapists need a balanced and pragmatic approach towards clinical and evidence-based-practice. Not only will physiotherapists need a 'mastery of patient interviewing and physical examination skills' (Sackett et al. 1998, p. IX), they will also need 'a proficiency in the application of various treatments, including communication abilities and clinical reasoning skills' (Hengeveld & Banks 2005, p. 81).

Subjective examination

An important feature of the Maitland Concept is a detailed interview of the patient, which includes the patient's perspective on the pain, concomitant disability, coping strategies and beliefs regarding pain, causes of the problem and necessary treatment strategies.

Various forms of clinical reasoning may be employed during the process of subjective examination. Within the diagnostic process and the determination of treatment *procedural reasoning* with hypotheses generation and pattern recognition frequently plays a central role (Payton 1987). The other forms of clinical reasoning frequently used include *interactive, conditional and narrative clinical reasoning* (Edwards 2000, Jones & Rivett 2004). It is considered that the various strategies of clinical reasoning are in an intrinsic relation in clinical practice, in which the physiotherapist moves between the various forms of clinical reasoning to shape an optimum examination and treatment process collaboratively with the patient (Edwards et al. 2004). Procedural reasoning aids the diagnostic process and treatment planning. Forms of narrative and interactive clinical reasoning are frequently employed to develop a deeper understanding of the patient's

individual experience regarding pain and disability, including beliefs, thoughts, feelings and sociocultural influences.

It may be concluded that well-developed communication skills are essential elements of the physiotherapy process. They serve several purposes (Hengeveld & Banks 2005):

- They aid in the process of information gathering with regard to physiotherapy diagnosis, treatment planning and reassessment of results
- They may serve to develop a deeper understanding of the patient's thoughts, beliefs and feelings with regard to the problem. This information assists in the assessment of psychosocial aspects which may hinder or enhance full recovery of movement functions
- Empathic communication also enhances the development of a therapeutic relationship
- They serve in the process of collaborative goal formulation, in which in cooperation with the patient therapeutic objectives, parameter for reassessment procedures and selection of therapeutic interventions are being determined.

Detailed information on communication and the therapeutic relationship is included in Chapter 3.

Specific objectives of subjective examination

The overall process of examination aims to determine the physiotherapy diagnosis, precautions and contraindications to treatment procedures, the development of a treatment plan and the definition of parameters to monitor the results of treatment and to initiate treatment.

Additionally, subjective examination follows several specific objectives to support decisions regarding physical examination and initial treatment:

- *Determination of the problem from the patient's perspective.* This includes assessment of pain or other symptoms as well as the assessment of movement and movement control (dys) functions. Furthermore, the beliefs of the patient regarding causes and best treatment procedures, as well his sense of control on pain including chosen coping strategies, should be established.
- Defining *subjective parameters* which serve reassessment procedures. These parameters

include information regarding pain sensation, activity limitations and participation restrictions, behavioural aspects such as coping strategies, use of medication and indication of psychosocial factors, which may hinder a recovery to full function.

- Determination of *precautions and contraindications* to physical examination and treatment procedures. The pain experience and the concomitant disability are indicative of specific precautions to examination procedures. Frequently this will be described within the constructs of irritability and severity.
- *Generation of multiple hypotheses*, to be tested during physical examination procedures and treatment interventions. The hypotheses categories have been listed in Table 7.3.

Information phase

In this phase the patient is informed about the scope of physiotherapy, as a specialty in the analysis and treatment of movement disorders, about the course of the first sessions, including the role of the assessment procedures employed. In this phase it is investigated if the patient is expecting physiotherapy as the treatment of his choice for his problem, if the patient understands the movement perspective of physiotherapists in problem solving processes and if certain reservations may exist regarding the therapy and the treatment setting, or if there is a lack of confidence about the treatment.

Subjective examination

The physiotherapist may decide to follow a more procedural approach to the interview, and/or to follow the line of thought of the patient ('parallelling') on the one hand or, on the other hand, to follow a more narrative approach to the interview, in which the patient is encouraged to tell the story of his illness from his perspective. Regardless of the style of interviewing, it is essential that the therapist keeps an overview of the information and organizes these accordingly into five groups as listed below.

1.   Main problem

It is vital to establish the current main problem from the perspective of the patient, expressed in the patient's words. In the case of a sacroiliac disorder the patient may complain about pain, a sense of tiredness in the leg, particularly during weight bearing activities.

As the pain may be of a sudden, sharp quality, some patients feel strongly restricted in their daily life activities. However, many patients complain of a pain that may not interfere strongly with the tasks of daily living as they are able to make compensatory movements.

2.   Area of symptoms

A precise drawing of the areas of symptoms, as indicated by the patient, helps in the hypotheses-generation of the possible sources of symptoms and, at times, of the precautions and contraindications and neurophysiological pain mechanisms.

Symptoms arising from the SIJ are unlikely to cross the midline. The most frequently reported symptoms overlay the posterior aspect of the SIJ; symptoms may be referred into the buttock, groin, posterior thigh and even in the calf and foot (Fortin et al. 1994, Schwartzer et al. 1995, Mens et al. 1996). Figure 7.6 illustrates typical areas of symptoms.

It is well known that lumbar structures as well as hip tissues may produce similar pain and symptom distribution as the SIJ. Therefore the area of symptoms should never be relied on solely for diagnosis.

3.   Behaviour of symptoms and activity-levels

This phase of the subjective examination needs to be followed up with great care, as it is essential for the definition of precautions of physical examination and monitoring of treatment results in subsequent sessions. The following aspects need to be determined:

- Which activities are restricted due to the pain? These activities serve as parameter to monitor changes in the patient's complaint over the course of therapy. Furthermore it provides the therapist with information on deficits and resources of activities and participation in daily life.
- Often it is useful to know how the pain behaves over a course of 24 hours or even during a 7-day period. The patient and the therapist have an opportunity to learn if and how the symptoms are directly related to certain activities of the patient in the previous days before the symptoms occur.

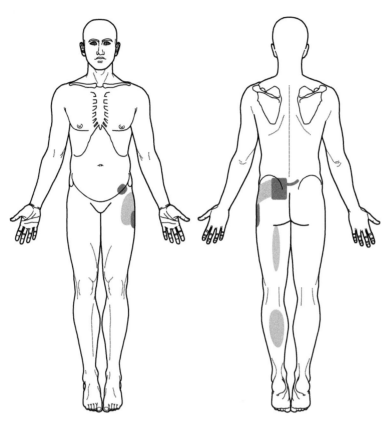

Figure 7.6 • Typical areas of symptoms related to the sacroiliac joint. Note the overlap with symptoms that may be referred from the lumbar spine.

- The most common aggravating factors for patients with PGP are related to unilateral weight bearing such as walking, climbing stairs, stepping off a curb, standing on one leg while dressing, as well as sitting, bending forward, lifting, turning in bed, lying supine with extended legs and getting up from a chair. This observation has been confirmed in a study of 394 women with peripartum pain (Mens et al. 1996; see Table 7.4).

- How does the patient cope with the pain? Is the patient taking an active or a more passive role in managing his symptoms? Even if patients seem to take a more passive role, they may intuitively choose useful strategies to diminish the symptoms. Often, even when patients state that they cannot influence the pain, they may instinctively choose certain positions, rub or hold certain areas or move the structure concerned in a certain way. Careful observation of the patient during the subjective and physical examination may demonstrate these unconscious behavioural patterns. They may become decisive in selecting directions of passive mobilization techniques and enhance self-management strategies.

Typically for sacroiliac disorders, patients may brace the pelvis by crossing their legs in sitting, by shifting the weight to the other buttock in sitting, by gently pushing the knees together in standing, by holding the pelvis with one or two hands while pressing the innominate anteriorly.

- It is essential to collect information in such detail that the therapist can almost visualize the way the patient moves once the pain occurs and what he or she does to reduce to pain.

- Furthermore, this phase of subjective examination may be useful to establish the general levels of activity of the patient during the day and during the week.

4. History (Hx)

As the symptom distribution and the activities related to the pain may be provoked by structures other than the SIJ, the history can be most useful in indicating whether or not a sacroiliac disorder is a dominant contributing factor to the patient's pain and disability.

Table 7.4 Activity restriction due to pain arising from the SIJ (Mens et al. 1996)

ADL	% of patients
Standing for 30 min	90
Carrying a full shopping bag	86
Standing on one leg	81
Walking for 30 min	81
Climbing stairs	79
Turning over in bed	74
Having sexual intercourse	68
Riding a bicycle for 30 min	63
Bending forward	62
Getting into and out of bed	62
Driving a car for 30 min	52
Swimming	51
Sitting on a favourite chair for 30 min	49
Travelling by public transport	46
Lying in bed for 30 min	8

PGP is most commonly associated with pregnancy, trauma or inflammatory disorders (Vleeming et al. 2008):

- Questions regarding onset of the symptoms are essential. Symptoms related to pregnancy, the first few months post-delivery or increased symptoms with the second of third pregnancy strongly indicate the presence of a PGP disorder, possibly due to a lack of motor control mechanisms and, possibly, increased mobility of the SIJ.
- Details about a traumatic incident may give indications of the structures that may possibly be involved in the disorder. Trauma can include macro-trauma such as a car accident, a fracture of the pelvis or a fall on the buttocks. Microtrauma may occur with repeated strains or overuse, often associated with faulty postures, faulty movements and/or motor control impairments within the lumbopelvic –hip complex.

Restricted hip or lumbar spine movements may contribute to excessive strain and compensation of the sacroiliac joints. Repeated strains to the adductor muscle groups or hamstrings can also influence the pelvis and may lead to added strain on the symphysis pubis or sacroiliac joints.

Long standing morning stiffness (lasting longer than 2–3 hours) may be indicative of an inflammatory disorder.

5. Special questions (SQ)

Special questions need to include information regarding general health status of the patient, unexpected weight loss, use of medication, results from possible laboratory findings and imaging findings as for example X-ray, MRI or CT-scans.

A medical history of family members may be useful, especially when suspecting arthritic/inflammatory disorders (e.g. rheumatoid arthritis, ankylosing spondylitis).

Specific screening questions regarding possible dysfunctions of the gastrointestinal, urogenital, cardiovascular, pulmonary, endocrine and nervous systems need to be incorporated in to the interview, particularly in cases of direct referral of the patient to the physiotherapist (Boissonault 2011, Goodman & Snyder 2007). Particularly fever, unexplained weight change, general fatigue, nausea/vomiting, bowel dysfunction, numbness, weakness, syncope, dizziness, night pain, dyspnea, dysuria, urinary frequency changes and sexual dysfunction may need further medical investigation (Boissonault 2011).

Questions regarding urinary incontinence should not be neglected as there is indication that incontinence is associated with increased risk of low back and PGP (Smith et al. 2006). Urinary incontinence may occur for various reasons. If the changes develop over a relatively short period of time, they may be indicative of a cauda equina lesion. If they develop over a longer period of time, gynaecological or urological investigations may be necessary. Stress incontinence is most often associated to insufficient control of the muscles of the pelvic floor.

Planning of the physical examination ('structured reflection')

Before embarking in the physical examination, a process of 'structured reflection' needs to take place to allow for a comprehensive examination. The following steps need to be considered and, preferably, recorded:

- Summary of the subjective examination:
  - have sufficient parameters to guide reassessment procedures been collected?
  - is there enough information to make clear statements regarding contraindications and/or precautions to examination and treatment procedures?
- Have hypotheses regarding sources, contributing factors, pathobiological processes, precautions and contraindications been made explicit to help guide the dosage of examination procedures (which symptoms should be reproduced/avoided during physical examination; extent of test procedures – only until the onset of pain/testing into pain provocation; making use of only a few tests to prevent exacerbation/using complete examination procedures or even specific test combinations) and the exact course of the steps of examination procedures?

Physical examination

Refer to Box 7.1 for an overview of the physical examination.

Clinical note

In clinical practice, it is common to find combinations of impairments (either mobility or motor control) in all three regions of the lumbopelvic–hip complex in the same patient.

Although the lumbopelvic–hip complex works as a functional unit and the pelvis cannot be studied in isolation during active/functional movements, the lumbar spine, hip and pelvis should be assessed individually with passive movements to correlate findings.

A thorough physical assessment helps identify the various impairments in the lumbopelvic–hip

 Box 7.1

Overview of the physical examination

Observation
- Gait
- Posture

Active movements
Trunk
- Forward bending
- Backward bending
- Side-bending
- Rotation
- Movements from below upwards

Hip
- Squatting
- Lunging
- Weight bearing tests on one leg
- Active movements in non-weight-bearing

Functional tests of load transfer
- Stork test
- Active straight leg raise

SIJ pain provocation tests
- Posterior pelvic pain provocation test (P4)
- Distraction test
- Compression test

- Gaenslen's test
- Sacral thrust test
- Patrick's Faber test
- Long dorsal SI ligament test
- Palpation of the symphysis pubis

Passive testing of SIJ
Positional tests
Passive mobility tests
Passive physiological movements:
- Posterior rotation of the innominate
- Anterior rotation of the innominate
Passive accessory movements:
- Oscillatory movements on the innominate, sacrum and coccyx
- Passive mobility of the SIJ in the anteroposterior plane
- Passive mobility of the SIJ in the craniocaudal plane

Form closure /force closure

Palpation

Motor control
1. Local muscles
2. Global muscles – slings
3. Assessment of local muscles

complex and the functional restrictions presented by a patient. Differentiation between lumbar pain and PGP is important in order to plan treatment accordingly.

Clinical note

Current evidence suggests that a single test is not reliable for diagnosis of SIJ pain or dysfunction, whereas a cluster of tests is more acceptable (Laslett et al. 2005, Robinson et al. 2007).

Hypotheses should be generated based on the results of multiple tests as to what region/joint may be the source of pain and what the causes of the symptoms may be.

Observation

Gait

Analyzing gait can give valuable information about how the patient is transferring load through his pelvis and lower extremities. Here are some key elements to note:

- Minimal deviations of the head and body vertically and laterally (about 5 cm)
- No sign of Trendelenburg or compensated Trendelenburg
- Maintenance of good motor control and joint alignment of the lumbar spine, pelvis, hip, knee and foot
- Minimal rotation of the pelvis in the transverse plane.

Common manifestations of poor motor control are:

- Trunk deviations
- Hip drop
- Excessive foot pronation
- Medial rotation of the femur
- Excessive rotation of the lumbar spine/pelvis
- Sway-back.

Clinical note

If failed load transfer is observed, correction of alignment should be attempted to modify the biomechanics and see the impact of the correction on the symptoms and on gait. This is very helpful in identifying the primary area of failed load transfer.

Posture

Observation of the pelvic girdle should include:

- Orientation of the sacrum about the horizontal and sagittal axes, and the sacrum's relationship to the lumbar lordosis in both standing and sitting
- Bony landmarks such as iliac crests, anterior and posterior superior iliac spines, greater trochanters and prominence of the femoral heads in the groin
- Position of the innominates relative to each other – no rotation should be observed (intrapelvic torsion)
- Position of the sacrum – should be slightly nutated (sacral base anterior) and should not be rotated (in both sitting and standing)
- Femoral heads should be centered in the acetabulum and should be symmetrical in standing and sitting
- Alignment of the femur, tibia and ankle/foot
- Differences in muscle bulk in the trunk, buttock and lower extremities
- Position of the thorax relative to the pelvis is also assessed for neutral spine position. The manubriosternal junction should be in the same coronal plane as the pubic symphysis and the anterior superior iliac spine of the innominates (Lee & Lee 2010). Postural alignment is illustrated in Figure 7.7.

Positional faults, on their own, are not necessarily related to the patient's symptoms and no conclusion can be drawn from these findings alone. The effect of correcting a positional fault may be more informative as to its link to the patient's symptoms. If, on correction, the patient's symptoms are reproduced, the posture can be considered to be antalgic, adaptive to the patient's condition. If, on correction, symptoms are improved then the posture may be maladaptive and attempts will be made to change it.

It is common for patients to adopt passive postures such as a sway-back position in standing (maximum nutation of sacrum), where the symphysis pubis sits anterior to the manubriosternal junction, and a slumped sitting position (counter-nutation of sacrum). Adopting these extreme postures for any length of time can lead to tissue overload and can cause symptoms. These patients will have to be shown and trained to adopt more neutral spine positions as these faulty postures may be a factor in perpetuating their symptoms.

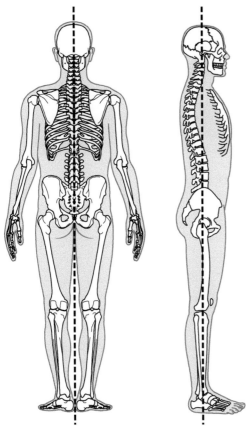

Figure 7.7 • Reference point to observe postural alignment. (From Kendall, F.P, Kendall McCreary, E., Provance, P.G. (1993) Muscles Testing and Function, 4ᵗʰ edition, Williams & Wilkins.)

Active movements of the trunk

Functional movements of the trunk will incorporate movement of the lumbar spine, hip as well as the pelvic girdle. The patient is first asked to demonstrate a movement or position that aggravates or reproduces his symptoms. The therapist then analyzes the strategies used by the patient when performing his specific movement.

Clinical note

An attempt will be made by the therapist to correct faulty strategies to see if symptoms can be modified. This differentiation can guide the therapist in deciding which tests should be done or which region should be evaluated in more detail to further clarify the source of symptoms.

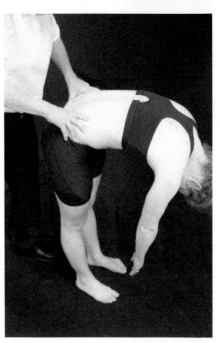

Figure 7.8 • Palpation of the innominates during forward bending.

Special attention should be given to the quality of movements and the apex of the curves as it is common to observe excessive range of motion (ROM) at one lumbar segment in the presence of a stiff hip or poor motor control and compensation of the pelvic girdle due to stiffness of the lumbar spine.

Forward bending

During forward bending, hip flexion should occur concurrently with lumbar flexion. The ilia should anteriorly tilt symmetrically over the hips with no relative rotation between them. The sacrum should remain in a nutated position throughout the range so relatively, both innominates should stay posteriorly rotated (Lee & Lee 2010). If failed load transfer occurs, where there is loss of optimal alignment/ movement/control of one of the innominates, that innominate has been shown to anteriorly rotate relative to that side of the sacrum (Hungerford et al. 2004, 2007). The erector spinae muscle should be symmetrically active in the first part of the range and should relax in the latter part as more strain is taken up by the inert structures (Fig. 7.8).

Backward bending

During backward bending, there should be reversal of the thoracic kyphosis, controlled segmental extension of the lumbar spine (no hinges) and the innominates should posteriorly rotate symmetrically over the hips causing the hips to extend (Lee & Lee 2010). The sacrum should remain nutated and the innominates should stay posteriorly rotated. Again, if there is failed load transfer, the innominate on the affected side is often seen to anteriorly rotate relative to the sacrum (Fig. 7.9).

Side-bending

During side-bending of the trunk, the body should stay in the frontal plane. A small amount of movement of both innominates is expected as a physiological intrapelvic torsion occurs during side-bending. On side-bending to the left, the left innominate will anteriorly rotate slightly as the right innominate will posteriorly rotate. The sacrum will rotate to the right as it moves congruently with the lumbar spine which side-bends to the left and rotates to the right. The lumbar spine should show a smooth curve with no kinking (Fig. 7.10).

Rotation

During rotation of the trunk to the right, the sacrum should follow the lumbar spine and rotate to the right as the left innominate rotates anteriorly and the right innominate rotates posteriorly. The left leg should internally rotate in space and the left foot should pronate while the right leg should externally rotate in space and the right foot should supinate.

Movements from below upwards

As mentioned in Chapter 6, movements of the pelvis and lower lumbar spine can be assessed in standing by asking the patient to initiate movement through the pelvis first (from below upwards). The patient is asked to perform a posterior tilt, anterior tilt, lateral tilt (hip drop Fig. 7.11) and rotation of the pelvis relative to the lumbar spine. Some restrictions may be more obvious when the movements are tested this way and the pain response elicited may also be different.

Active movements of the hip

Quick screening tests involving the hip can be done in weight bearing to evaluate the presence of any restriction or reproduction of symptoms.

- Squatting can be done with the heels off and on the ground. This will assess full hip flexion in weight bearing. Note the amount of flexion in the lumbar spine as there might be excessive lumbar flexion if one hip has a flexion restriction.

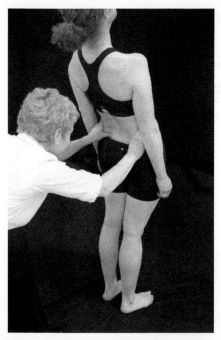

Figure 7.9 • Palpation of the innominates during backward bending.

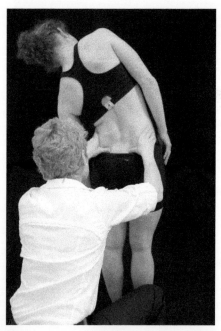

Figure 7.10 • Palpation of the innominates during left side-bending.

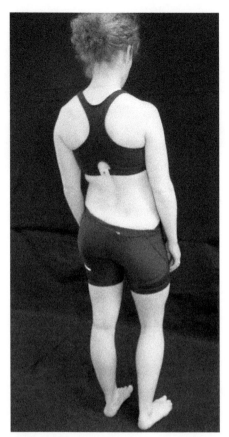

Figure 7.11 • Right hip drop which creates a left side-bending of the lumbar spine.

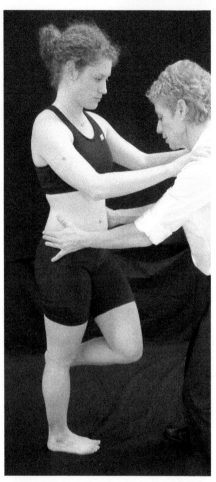

Figure 7.12 • Rotation of the pelvis to the right creating a medial rotation of the right hip.

- Lunging with one foot on the edge of a chair or low plinth will test for hip flexion and extension. Note for any compensation in the spine or innominate.
- Weight bearing tests on one leg are more functional tests and may be more useful in determining restrictions or reproduction of symptoms at the hip.

  Patient starting position: standing on the affected leg, holding the physiotherapist's shoulder to maintain balance (Fig. 7.12).

  Therapist starting position: standing in front of the patient.

  Localization of forces: physiotherapist holds onto both innominates of the patient's pelvis

  Application of forces: therapist guides the patient's pelvis in F/E direction, Ad/Ad direction and MR/LR direction.

- Active/passive movements in non-weight-bearing should also be assessed (refer to

Chapter 7 in Hengeveld & Banks 2014 for more detailed information).

Functional tests of load transfer

> **Clinical note**
>
> The focus of clinical assessment procedures for PG function has shifted in the last decade from SIJ mobility testing to functional assessment procedures that test the ability of the pelvis to maintain stability during load transfer between the spine and the lower extremity (Hungerford et al. 2007).

These tests have evolved from the increased understanding of the role of the pelvis in load transfer and poor reliability and validity of many SIJ mobility tests. The stork test and the active straight leg raise test (ASLR) will be described here as they have both shown acceptable inter-tester reliability. Other tests for load transfer have also been described in the literature. O'Sullivan and Beales (2007a, 2007b) use the prone leg lift test and Lee and Lee (2010) also look at the squat test, stepping forward/backward, prone knee bend and prone hip extension. Lee and Lee (2010) also assess lateral tilts of the pelvis in both supine and standing to test load transfer through the symphysis pubis.

Stork test

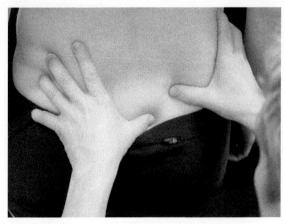

Figure 7.13 • Position of the thumbs during the Stork test – left thumb inferior to the right inferior lateral angle (ILA) of the sacrum, right thumb inferior to the right PSIS.

Clinical note

The Stork test, also known as the Gillet test or one leg standing (OLS) test, assesses the ability of the patient to transfer load through the pelvis in standing and to maintain a stable alignment of the innominate relative to the sacrum (self-braced alignment of the pelvic bones). This is a motion control test where both form and force closure mechanisms interplay.

This test has also been described as the modified Trendelenburg test (Albert et al. 2000), a provocative test for the symphysis pubis. The test is positive when the pain is experienced in the area of the symphysis pubis.

Patient starting position: standing

Therapist starting position: kneeling behind the patient

Localization of forces: one hand on the innominate on the side of weight bearing with the thumb inferior to the posterior superior iliac spine (PSIS); the thumb of the other hand palpates the sacrum at either S2 or the ipsilateral inferior lateral angle (ILA) of the sacrum (Figs 7.13 and 7.14).

Movement: the patient is asked to stand on one leg and to flex the contralateral hip and knee towards the waist. This test is done on both sides and the ability and effort required to do the test is observed. The transfer of weight should be done smoothly and the pelvis should remain in its original position.

Hungerford et al. (2007) noted that the pattern of intrapelvic motion is altered during the single-leg support in subjects with PGP. No relative movement should occur within the pelvis during

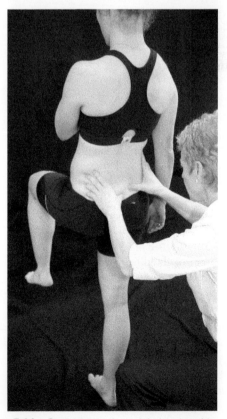

Figure 7.14 • Stork test on the weight bearing side

load transfer whereas anterior rotation of the innominate relative to the sacrum occurs during weight bearing in the presence of PGP. These authors noted that the test showed good inter-tester reliability. They also suggest that the test is repeated ×3 to make sure the same pattern is observed each time.

Variations: The ability of the non-bearing innominate to rotate posteriorly relative to the ipsilateral sacrum can also be assessed by this test (Fig. 7.15; Hungerford et al. 2004). Lee & Lee (2010) suggest to assess the pattern of motion between the innominate and sacrum and to look for symmetry between both sides. Positioning for this test is done in exactly the same way as described above except the palpation is done on the non-weight bearing side. This test assesses active movement of the innominate relative to the sacrum and the results of this test must be correlated to the passive mobility tests.

Active straight leg raise test

Clinical note

The ASLR test assesses the ability of the patient to transfer load through the pelvis in supine. This test has shown reliability, sensitivity and specificity for patients with PGP after pregnancy (Mens et al. 1999, 2001, 2002).

Patient starting position: supine, legs extended

Therapist starting position: standing next to the patient to observe the strategy that the patient will use to perform the test and to be in a good position to add compression to various parts of the pelvis

Movement: the patient is asked to lift one leg 20 cm from the bed and to note the degree of effort difference between each leg. The effort can be scored on a scale from 0 to 5 (Mens et al. 1999). The leg should raise effortlessly from the table and the pelvis should not move in any direction relative to the thorax or lower extremity. To be able to perform this test effortlessly, proper recruitment of both local and global muscles is necessary (Fig. 7.16).

Application of compression to the pelvis (bringing the two innominates together anteriorly) has been shown to reduce the effort necessary to lift the leg for peripartum patients (Mens et al. 1999). Varying the compression can assist the therapist to determine where more compression is needed functionally to help load transfer through the pelvic girdle (Lee & Lee 2010). Lee & Lee (2010) hypothesize that compression of different parts of the pelvis

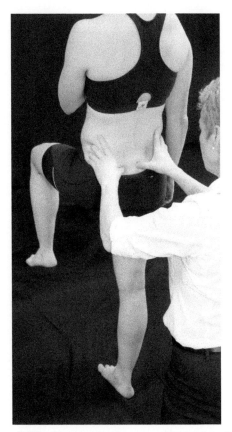

Figure 7.15 • Stork test on the non-weight bearing side

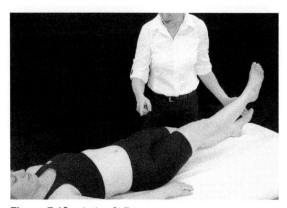

Figure 7.16 • Active SLR test.

(ex. anterior compression, Figs 7.17 and 7.18, posterior compression, Fig. 7.19, or anterior compression on one side and posterior compression on the other side, Fig. 7.20) can simulate the work of various local muscles. The compression that is noted to be most helpful for the patient during the ASLR test should be kept in mind when planning treatment. On the other hand, the pelvic girdle is sometimes under too much compression and the patient will not do well or may find the task of lifting the leg even more difficult with increased pelvic compression.

Pain provocation tests

Several studies have looked at the interexaminer reliability of pain provocation, position and mobility tests for the pelvic girdle. Only pain provocation tests have shown reliability individually and particularly when clustered (Laslett et al. 1994, van der Wurff et al. 2000, Laslett et al. 2005, Robinson et al. 2007).

Clinical note

Szadek et al. (2009) mention that the best evidence shows that at least three SIJ pain provocation tests must reproduce the patient's pain to be regarded as being of SIJ origin.

Laslett et al. (2005) have found that when any two of the four non-specific provocation tests (distraction, compression, thigh thrust, sacral thrust) are positive, the SIJ may be considered to be the source

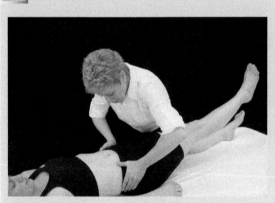

Figure 7.17 • Anterior compression added to the pelvis, bringing both ASIS closer together, thought to simulate the action of the transversus abdominis muscles.

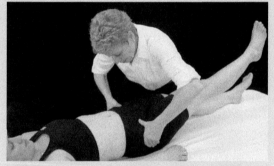

Figure 7.18 • Anterior compression added above the greater trochanters of the hips, thought to simulate the action of the anterior pelvic floor muscles.

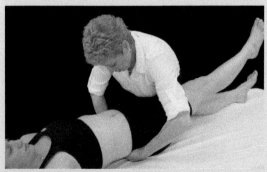

Figure 7.19 • Posterior compression added to the pelvis, bringing both PSIS closer together, thought to simulate the action of the multifidi muscles.

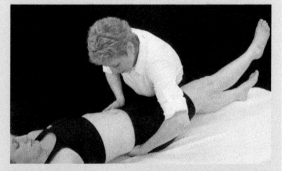

Figure 7.20 • Anterior compression of the left anterior side of the pelvis (ASIS) and the right posterior side of the pelvis (PSIS) towards each other; thought to simulate the action of the left transversus abdominis and the right multifidus muscles.

of pain. When all tests are negative, symptomatic SIJ pathology can be ruled out (Laslett 2007).

Numerous provocation tests have been described in the literature. Laslett et al. (2003) suggested the use of the following tests:

- Thigh thrust or P4 (posterior pelvic pain provocation) test
- Distraction
- Compression
- Gaenslen's SIJ provocation test
- Sacral thrust test.

Albert et al. (2000) suggested:

- P4 test
- Patrick's Faber test
- Palpation of the symphysis pubis.

Vleeming et al. (1996) and Ostgaard (2007) also suggested:

- Palpation of the long dorsal sacroiliac (SI) ligament.

Clinical note

SIJ pain provocation tests are not specific to any structure and are intended to stress the joint, its surrounding ligaments and myofascial structures to provoke the patient's symptoms (Cyriax 1975, Laslett et al. 2003). Note that many of these pain provocation tests will also stress the pubic symphysis and could produce symptoms locally at this joint.

The posterior pelvic pain provocation test (P4 test; Ostgaard 2007)

This test has been shown to have the highest sensitivity (Laslett et al. 2005). See Figure 7.21.

Patient starting position: supine, hip at 90° flexion, knee flexed.

Therapist starting position: standing on the side to be tested, holding on to the patient's knee, stabilizing through the contralateral innominate by pressing down on the anterior superior iliac spine (ASIS; Fig. 7.21) or stabilizing the sacrum posteriorly with the other hand (Fig. 7.22; Laslett 2008).

Application of forces: a posterior force is applied through the femur.

This test is interpreted as being positive when pain is provoked in the SIJ area on the ipsilateral side.

Distraction test (anterior distraction and posterior compression test)

This test has been shown to be most specific (Fig. 7.23; Laslett et al. 2005).

Patient starting position: supine, a small pillow under the knees to keep the lumbar spine more neutral.

Therapist starting position: standing at the level of the patient's thighs, facing the patient's head; heel of the hands on the medial aspect of the ASIS with hands crossed, forearms parallel.

Application of forces: a slow, steady, posterolateral force is applied through the ASIS thus distracting the anterior part of the SIJ and compressing the posterior part. The force should

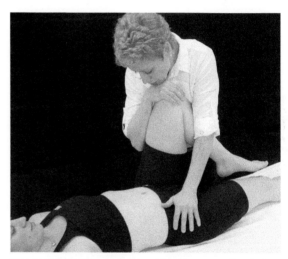

Figure 7.21 • The posterior pelvic pain provocation test (P4 test), stabilizing the contralateral innominate.

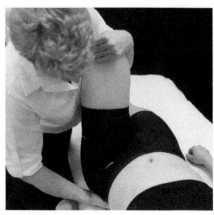

Figure 7.22 • The posterior pelvic pain provocation test (P4 test), stabilizing the sacrum posteriorly.

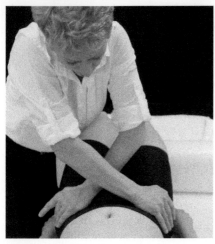

Figure 7.23 • Distraction test.

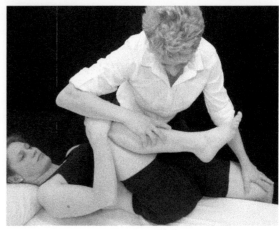

Figure 7.25 • Gaenslen's test.

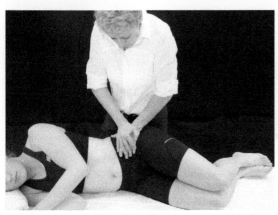

Figure 7.24 • Compression test.

be maintained as the patient is asked about reproduction and localization of pain. It is important to apply enough force during this test.

Compression test (anterior compression and posterior distraction; Fig. 7.24)

Patient starting position: sidelying, hips and knees flexed.

Therapist starting position: standing behind the patient at the level of the patient's pelvis, both hands over the anterolateral iliac crest.

Application of forces: a slow, steady, medial force is applied through the innominate thus compressing the anterior part of the SIJ and distracting the posterior part. The force should be maintained as the patient is asked about

reproduction and localization of pain. The test should be done on both sides. It is also important to apply enough force when doing this test.

Variations: this test can also be done in supine as per the distraction test. The therapist places her hands on the lateral aspect of both iliac crests and a medial force is applied to both innominates.

Gaenslen's test (Fig. 7.25)

Patient starting position: supine, near the edge of the bed, flexion of the hip and knee on the side to be tested.

Therapist starting position: standing on the side where the hip is extended.

Application of forces: the patient's hip is fully flexed onto their abdomen and held there by the patient as the therapist adds overpressure while the opposite thigh is slowly hyperextended by the examiner over the edge of the bed with overpressure over the knee.

This test is positive when it reproduces pain on the tested side (the flexed side).

Sacral thrust test (Fig. 7.26)

Patient starting position: prone.

Therapist starting position: standing, both hands over the dorsal aspect of the sacrum.

Application of forces: a pure posteroanterior pressure is applied to the sacrum. The force should be maintained as the patient is asked about reproduction and localization of pain.

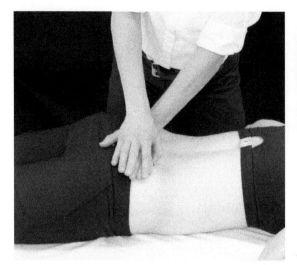

Figure 7.26 • Sacral thrust test.

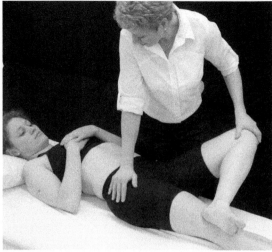

Figure 7.27 • Patrick's Faber test.

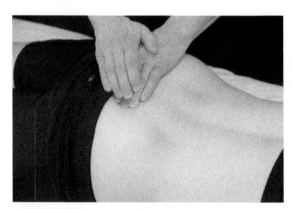

Figure 7.28 • Long dorsal SI ligament test.

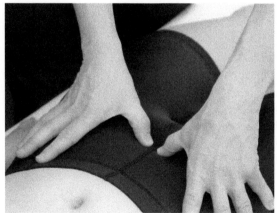

Figure 7.29 • Palpation of the symphysis pubis.

Patrick's Faber test (Fig. 7.27)

Patient starting position: supine.

Therapist starting position: standing on the side of the pelvis to be tested, stabilizes the opposite ASIS.

Application of forces: the heel of the patient's leg is placed on top of their opposite knee so the hip is flexed, abducted and externally rotated (f/ab/er) and gentle overpressure is applied to the knee.

The test is positive when it reproduces pain either in the SIJ or the symphysis pubis as stress is placed on both joints during this test.

Long dorsal SI ligament test (Fig. 7.28; Vleeming et al. 1996, 2002)

Patient starting position: prone (sidelying in pregnancy).

Therapist starting position: standing.

Application of forces: the long dorsal SI ligaments are palpated directly under the caudal part of the PSIS.

The test is positive when pain or tenderness is reproduced on palpation.

Variations: Lee & Lee (2010) have suggested palpation of the ligament as a counter-nutation force is applied to the sacrum (P/A movement on the apex of the sacrum) as this increases the stress put on the long dorsal SI ligament.

Palpation of the symphysis pubis (Fig. 7.29)

Patient starting position: supine, legs straight.

Therapist starting position: standing, palpates the anterior, superior and inferior aspects of the symphysis pubis for any sign of tenderness or pain

Passive tests

> **Clinical note**
>
> Although the reliability of positional and mobility tests have yet to be ascertained, the SIJ is known to move and therefore these passive tests are still very useful and make up an essential part of the assessment of the pelvic girdle.

According to Albert et al. (2000), the low reliability of the mobility tests may be related to the skills of the examiners and the lack of standardization of the tests. Hopefully some of these tests will eventually become more refined and more reliable. In the meantime, the therapist must continue to use these passive tests and reason through the findings of multiple tests before drawing any conclusion from the examination as no single test should be interpreted in isolation.

Positional tests

Positional analysis of the pelvic girdle should be evaluated prior to assessing joint mobility as a difference in mobility may just be a reflection of a different bony starting position. The pelvis is subjected to multiple force vectors from the muscles that attach to it and these can impact on its position. Positional tests should be done in supine and prone. It is suggested by Lee & Lee (2010) that the entire hand is used to more accurately assess the position of the innominates rather than only visualizing one point of the bone. Again it is important to note that positional faults on their own are not necessarily related to the patient's symptoms and that no conclusion can be drawn from these findings alone.

Position of the innominates in supine (Figs 7.30 and 7.31)

Patient starting position: supine, legs extended.

Therapist starting position: standing, palpates the anterior aspect of both innominates with the heels of the hands, the rest of the hand resting on the lateral aspect of the innominates. Note any difference in positioning of the innominates, any torsion or shear of one innominate relative to the other. The position can be confirmed by placing the thumbs on the inferior aspect of the ASIS.

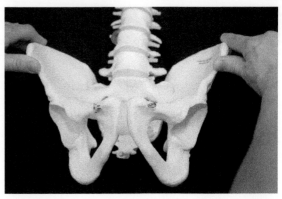

Figure 7.30 • Positional test of the innominate – palpation of the inferior aspect of the ASIS.

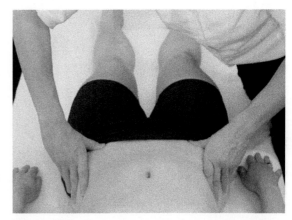

Figure 7.31 • Positional test of the innominate using the thumbs inferior to the ASIS.

Position of the pubic tubercles

Patient starting position: supine, legs extended.

Therapist starting position: standing, the heel of one hand is used to palpate the cranial aspect of the left and right superior pubic rami, noting any difference in the height of one pubic ramus relative to the other, in either a craniocaudal or an anteroposterior direction. The position can be confirmed by placing the thumbs above each pubic ramus.

Position of the innominates in prone (Fig. 7.32)

Patient starting position: prone, legs extended

Therapist starting position: standing, palpates the posterior aspect of both innominates with the heels of the hands on the inferior aspect of the PSIS and the rest of the hand on the back of the innominates. Note any difference in

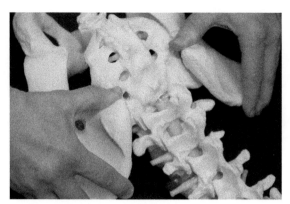

Figure 7.32 • Positional test of the innominate – palpation of the inferior aspect of the PSIS.

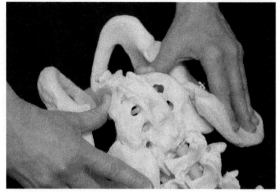

Figure 7.33 • Positional test of the inferior lateral angles of the sacrum.

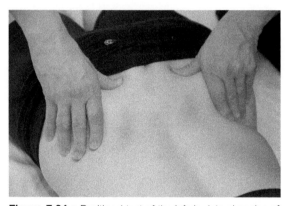

Figure 7.34 • Positional test of the inferior lateral angles of the sacrum using the thumbs.

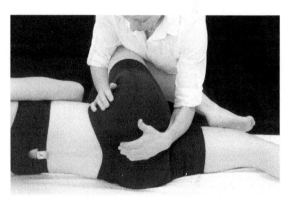

Figure 7.35 • Posterior rotation of the right innominate in sidelying.

positioning. The position can be confirmed by placing the thumbs on the inferior aspect of the PSIS.

The ischial tuberosities can also be used to confirm any vertical shear of one innominate relative to the other. The most inferior aspect of the ischial tuberosities is palpated bilaterally with the thumbs.

Position of the sacrum in prone (Figs 7.33 and 7.34)

Patient starting position: prone, legs extended.

Therapist starting position: standing, palpates the dorsal aspect of the inferior lateral angles of the sacrum (lateral edge of the sacrum at the level of S5) with the thumbs to assess for any rotation of the sacrum. According to Lee and Lee (2010), this bony point appears to be more reliable for assessing the position of the sacrum as the sacral base depth can be influenced by the size and tone of the sacral multifidus.

Passive mobility tests

Clinical note

When testing the passive mobility at the SIJ, both passive physiological movements of the innominate (anterior and posterior rotations) and passive accessory movements of the innominate, sacrum and coccyx are assessed.

Passive physiological movements of the innominate

A. Posterior rotation of the innominate (Fig. 7.35):

Patient starting position: sidelying, the bottom leg is extended (to keep the lumbar spine more neutral) and the top leg is flexed.

Therapist starting position: standing in front of the patient's hips, supports the bent leg, one hand

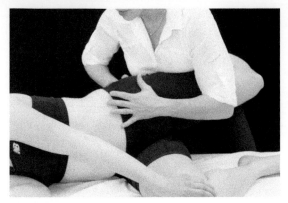

Figure 7.36 • Anterior rotation of the left innominate in sidelying.

is placed on the posterior surface of the ischeal tuberosity and the heel of the other hand is placed over the anterior iliac spine.

Application of forces: by using both arms simultaneously, the posterior rotation of the innominate is assessed by pushing the anterior iliac spine posteriorly and superiorly as the ischeal tuberosity is pulled down and forward.

The quality of the movement, the resistance through range, the end-feel as well as any pain provocation are noted and compared to the same movement on the other side.

B. Anterior rotation of the innominate (Fig. 7.36):

Patient starting position: sidelying, the bottom leg is flexed to 90° (to keep the lumbar spine more neutral) and the top leg is only slightly flexed, closer to extension.

Therapist starting position: standing behind the patient, one hand is placed on the anterolateral margin of the iliac crest and ASIS of the top leg, and the heel of the other hand is placed under the PSIS and buttocks of the same leg.

Application of forces: by using both arms simultaneously, the anterior rotation of the innominate is assessed by pushing the PSIS superiorly and posteriorly as the anterolateral margin of the iliac crest and ASIS is pulled forward and down.

The quality of the movement, the resistance through range, the end-feel as well as any pain provocation are noted and compared to the same movement on the other side.

Passive accessory movement tests

Clinical note

Accessory movement testing includes tests for articular mobility/stability of the SIJ. When testing accessory joint play, the therapist must assess the resistance of the tissues throughout the movement, as well as any presence of pain or motor responses ('spasm').

When testing movement, Maitland (1986) always emphasized the importance of relating range with the symptom response and vice versa. On testing accessory movement, emphasis is placed on picking up R1 (1st barrier of resistance) at the end of the neutral zone (Panjabi 1992), and the resistance through range from R1 to R2, the elastic zone. The behaviour of the resistance and where the resistance starts in the range will be compared for each SIJ. Buyruk et al. (1995a, 1995b) and Damen et al. (2002) used Doppler imaging of vibration (DIV) to measure stiffness of the SIJ and noted that the joint stiffness is variable and therefore the ROM between individuals is likely to be variable. They found that the stiffness values were symmetrical in healthy subjects but not in those with PGP.

Clinical note

Research suggests that ROM is not an indicator of function or dysfunction in the PG. Emphasis of manual motion testing should focus less on how much the SIJ is moving and more on the symmetry or asymmetry of the motion palpated.

A. Oscillatory movements on the innominate and sacrum:

Patient starting position: prone or supine, legs straight.

Therapist starting position: hands on different parts of the sacrum or innominate.

Application of forces:

○ central oscillatory P/A movement over the sacrum at S1 (base), S3 (middle), S5 (apex) (Fig. 7.37)

○ unilateral oscillatory P/A movement over the base of the sacrum at S1 on each side (Fig. 7.38)

○ unilateral oscillatory P/A movement over the inferior lateral angles (level of S5) on each side (Fig. 7.39)

○ P/A movements can also be applied to the PSIS (Fig. 7.40)

○ lateral movement of the PSIS (Fig. 7.41).

• P/A, A/P and lateral movements of the coccyx

• craniocaudal movement innominate relative to sacrum – one hand on the base of the sacrum and the other on the ischeal tuberosity; one hand on the iliac crest and on the apex of the sacrum

• unilateral A/P movement on the pubic ramus adjacent to the symphysis pubis (Figs 7.42 and 7.43)

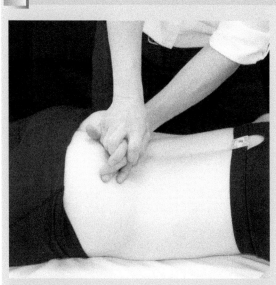

Figure 7.37 • Central P/A movement on the base of the sacrum.

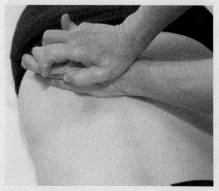

Figure 7.38 • Unilateral P/A movement on S1 on the right.

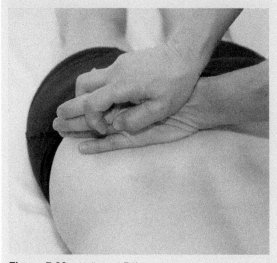

Figure 7.39 • Unilateral P/A movement over the right ILA of the sacrum.

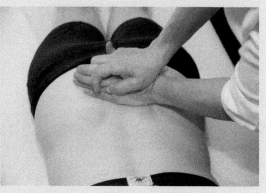

Figure 7.40 • P/A movement on the left PSIS.

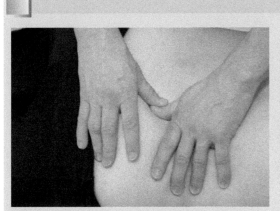

Figure 7.41 • Lateral movement on the right PSIS.

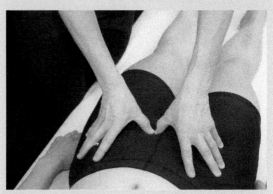

Figure 7.42 • Unilateral A/P movement on the left pubic ramus using the thumbs.

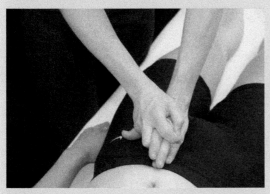

Figure 7.43 • Unilateral A/P movement on the left pubic ramus using the hands.

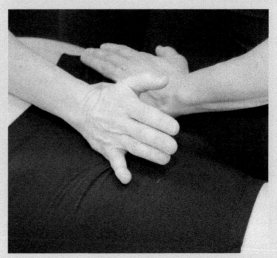

Figure 7.44 • Craniocaudal movement on the pubic rami.

- Craniocaudal movement of one pubic ramus adjacent to the symphysis pubis (Fig. 7.44).

For all of the above, varying angles of the accessory movements can also be assessed. The quality of the resistance as well as any pain provocation are noted and compared with the same movement on the other side.

B. Passive mobility/stability of the SIJ in the anteroposterior plane (Fig. 7.45; Hungerford et al. 2004, Lee & Lee 2010):

Patient starting position: crook lying, legs supported (in this position, the sacrum is in counter-nutation so the joint is in a loose-packed position), arms by the side to decrease the influence of myofascial tensions and to ensure maximum relaxation of the superficial muscles which can influence joint play motion.

Therapist starting position: the tips of the fingers of one hand are placed posteriorly in the sacral sulcus just above and medial to the PSIS; the heel of the other hand is placed over the ipsilateral ASIS (Fig. 7.46).

Localization of forces: the therapist must first find the plane of the joint as this is very variable between individuals; a gentle oscillatory force

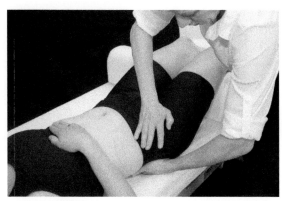

Figure 7.45 • Passive mobility/stability test of the right SIJ in the A/P plane.

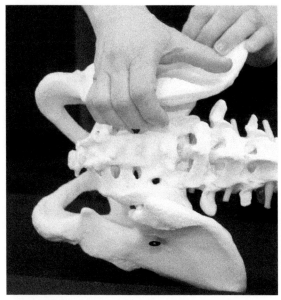

Figure 7.46 • Position of the tips of the fingers in the sacral sulcus.

is applied to the ASIS in an A/P direction with slight medial/lateral inclinations until the plane of least resistance is found.

Application of the forces: Once the plane is found, a *gentle* A/P translation force (a parallel movement) is applied to the innominate relative to the sacrum and attention is paid to when R1 starts, to determine the neutral zone. The quality of the resistance from R1 to R2, the elastic zone, is then assessed as well as the end-feel to the movement. The symmetry of the quantity and quality of the movement is compared between both sides. It is important to apply a gentle

pressure when doing this test in order to pick up R1 and to feel the resistance through range. If the movement is done too hard, only R2 will be felt and no comparison of the symmetry of the resistance through range will be possible.

Variations: The muscular system can increase compression across the SIJ (Richardson et al. 2002, van Wingerden et al. 2004). Lee and Lee (2010) suggest that hypertonicity of certain muscles can compress parts of the SIJ and prevent a parallel glide only at that part of the joint. On testing the A/P translation at the SIJ, they divide their movement into superior, middle and inferior to test the movement at different parts of the joint. According to these authors, the superior part of the SIJ can be compressed by hypertonicity of the superficial fibres of multifidus; the inferior part can be compressed by ischiococcygeus and piriformis can compress all three parts of the joint. Specific palpation of those muscles will help in confirming clinical hypotheses as to why there may be asymmetry when testing movement in this plane.

Interpretation of findings:

Stiff/fibrotic SIJ: very little neutral zone may be felt as R1 will be felt early. The resistance between R1 and R2 will increase rapidly so the elastic zone will be decreased and the end-feel will be quite firm.

Lax/loose SIJ: R1 will start later than expected (increased neutral zone), the distance between R1–R2 will be increased and possibly a softer end-feel will be felt. This may imply that there is lack of form or force closure of the joint. Panjabi (1992) describes that the neutral zone may be increased due to injury, articular degeneration and/ or weakness of the stabilizing musculature. He also states that this is a more sensitive indicator than angular ROM for detecting instability.

C. *Passive mobility/stability of the SIJ in the craniocaudal plane* (Fig. 7.47; Hungerford et al. 2004, Lee & Lee 2010):

Patient starting position: crook lying, leg supported by the therapist.

Therapist starting position: the tips of the fingers of one hand are placed posteriorly in the sacral sulcus just above and medial to the PSIS, the other hand is placed on the patient's ipsilateral knee.

Localization of forces: the therapist must first find the plane of the joint as stipulated in the

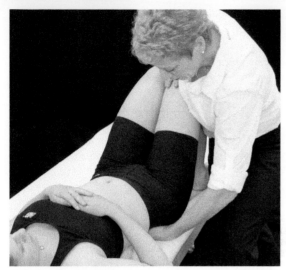

Figure 7.47 • Passive mobility/stability of the right SIJ in the craniocaudal plane.

previous technique; a gentle oscillatory force is applied to the patient's knee in a cranial direction with slight medial/lateral inclinations of the leg until the plane of least resistance is found.

Application of the forces: Once the plane is found, a *gentle* cranial translation force is applied to the innominate relative to the sacrum via the knee. Attention is paid to when R1 starts, to determine the neutral zone, and to the quality of the resistance from R1 to R2, the elastic zone. The symmetry of the quantity and quality of the movement is compared between both sides. It is important to apply a gentle pressure when doing this test in order to pick up R1 and to feel the resistance through range. If the movement is done too hard, only R2 will be felt and no comparison of the symmetry of the resistance through range will be possible.

Interpretation of findings:

Stiff/fibrotic SIJ: very little neutral zone may be felt as R1 will be felt early. The resistance between R1 and R2 will increase rapidly so the elastic zone will be decreased and the end-feel will be quite firm.

Lax/loose SIJ: R1 will start later than expected (increased neutral zone), the distance between R1–R2 will be increased and possibly a softer end-feel will be felt. This may imply that there is lack of form or force closure of the joint. Panjabi (1992) describes that the neutral zone may be

increased due to injury, articular degeneration and/or weakness of the stabilizing musculature. He also states that this is a more sensitive indicator than angular ROM for detecting instability.

The above two tests have yet to be evaluated for validity, sensitivity and specificity for impaired function of the lumbopelvic complex (Lee & Vleeming 2007) but are very useful clinically and help in clinical reasoning when directing treatment.

Form closure/force closure testing

> **Clinical note**
>
> Shear in the SIJ is prevented by the combination of specific anatomical features (form closure) and compression generated by myofascial structures surrounding the SIJ and pelvis (force closure; Vleeming et al. 1990).

Form closure of the joint (bones, joints, capsules, ligaments) is also assessed when testing passive mobility at the SIJ. Lee & Lee (2010) suggest that if the SIJ is felt to have an excessive neutral zone, the joint can be closed-packed by gently pushing the sacrum into full nutation by applying an anterior force with the fingers of the hand on the sacrum while simultaneously rotating the innominate posteriorly. The A/P translation is then reassessed and no movement should occur when the articular system restraints are intact. If there is increased laxity in neutral but stability in the closed-pack position, a motor control impairment may be present. Force closure (the myofascial system) should then be assessed by asking the patient to co-contract the local muscles of the trunk and the translation is retested.

> **Clinical note**
>
> van Wingerden et al. (2004) found that even a slight muscle activation can compress the SIJ, increase its stiffness and resist shear forces.

If there is still increased laxity in the closed-pack position of the SIJ (full nutation), this indicates that form closure is not intact. Force closure can then be assessed as stated above. If there is increased stiffness of the joint with co-contraction of the local muscles, emphasis of treatment will be placed on motor control and the patient may also benefit from wearing a SI belt until his stability has improved. If there is no change in the joint stiffness with muscle activation, this means that there is loss of integrity of the articular restraints and the deep muscles cannot compensate and control motion in the neutral zone. In this case, the prognosis is not as good, the patient will have to be referred for a medical consult as he could possibly benefit from prolotherapy (Cusi et al. 2010, Dorman 1997).

Palpation

The objectives of palpation are to assess for:

- Changes in temperature or evidence of sweating
- Any soft tissue changes (superficial to deep; general to localized)
- Any bony abnormalities
- Any movement anomalies on passive accessory movements (relating them to the findings on passive physiological movement testing)
- Any painful response to soft tissue palpation and passive accessory movements.

Palpation should include:

- Skin temperature, sweating, skin rolling
- The different layers of muscles for soft tissue changes such as thickening, hypotonicity and hypertonicity
- Posterior muscles such as the glutei, piriformis, ischiococcygeus, external rotators of the hip, hamstrings, erector spine, and multifidi
- Anterior muscles such as adductors, rectus abdominis, internal oblique, external oblique, rectus femoris, tensor fascia lata, psoas
- The sacrotuberous ligament, the long dorsal SI ligament, the sacrococcygeal area, the symphysis pubis and groin
- The neural structures such as the sciatic nerve, the femoral nerve, and the lateral cutaneous nerve of the thigh
- The linea alba for its integrity and tension – especially in postpartum women who present with PGP and/or urinary incontinence.

All areas of increased tenderness should be noted and correlated with other examination findings. These can also be used in re-assessment.

Motor control (force closure)

In many low back and pelvic problems, a lack of motor control can play a major role in the maintenance of symptoms.

Clinical note

When assessing for any deficiency in motor control, it is important to note the various strategies used by the patient when asked to recruit specific muscles. It is common to see patients who are unable to recruit the local muscles because the global muscles are too dominant and overactive. In those cases, the global muscle dysfunction has to be addressed first as it can be a source of inhibition of the local muscles. Research suggests that a key impairment in the muscle system is one of motor control rather than strength (Richardson et al. 1999).

Bergmark (1989) classified muscles as being either local or global muscles. The local muscles are deep, segmental, are suited to apply compression across joints and are referred to as stabilizers. The global muscles span many segments or regions of the body and have a dual function of being movers and general stabilizers.

Clinical note

The main group of local muscles that generate tension to stabilize the lumbar spine and pelvic girdle include the transversus abdominis (TA), the deep fibres of the multifidus (dMF), the pelvic floor (PF), the diaphragm (Richardson et al. 1999) and possibly the posterior fibres of psoas major (Gibbons 2007).

Dysfunction of the local muscle system can present as:
- Delayed timing of contraction
- Atrophy
- Loss of tonic function
- Loss of coordination with other local muscles.

Dysfunction of the global muscle system:
- Hypertonicity, co-contraction, dominance
- Non-recruitment, delayed activation, weakness
- Loss of synergistic activity between global muscles
- Loss of flexibility.

Assessment of local muscles

A. Transversus abdominis (TA)

Patient starting position: supine, hips and knees bent.

Therapist starting position: standing, using both thumbs palpate medial and slightly inferior to the ASIS. Sink the thumbs into the abdomen to palpate TA at the deepest layer. Feel for difference in basic tone between sides. This may indicate excessive tone in the internal oblique muscle at rest.

Application of forces: different cues and images can be used to isolate contraction of TA. The effective cue will vary depending on the patient's specific presentation and substitution patterns. Here are some examples:

1. Gently and slowly contract the lower abdomen, trying to draw both ASIS together
2. Gently and slowly contract the pelvic floor muscles as if trying to stop urinating
3. Feel the pressure of my thumbs in your abdomen and try to create the same tension.

Responses:

○ A deep tensioning of the lower abdomen should be felt bilaterally with a flattening of the lower abdomen
○ No bulging should be felt as this is evidence of contraction of the internal oblique muscle
○ No movement of the rib cage, pelvis or lumbar spine should take place
○ No breath holding should occur and there should be no bracing of the rib cage as this indicates global muscle activation.

B. Deep fibres of multifidus (dMF)

Patient starting position: prone, legs straight.

Therapist starting position: standing, using two fingers palpate laterally to the spinous process of the lumbar segment from L1 down to S2 (lateral to the median sacral crest) on both sides at the same time.

Application of forces: apply a gentle, firm pressure into the tissue and compare the tone in the muscle between each side as well as with the segments above and below; also palpate the erector spinae to see if there is hypertonicity as it may prevent you from feeling the dMF muscle. Areas where the fingers sink more easily may correspond to levels of atrophy or decreased resting tone.

Different cues can be used to recruit dMF, such as:

1. Gently and slowly contract, trying to draw both PSIS together
2. Gently and slowly contract the pelvic floor muscles as if trying to stop urinating
3. Imagine that you want to pull your sacrum up towards the spine without moving it.

Reponses:

○ The muscle should swell symmetrically under the palpating fingers (Richardson et al. 2002) and there should be more resistance under the fingers
○ No evidence of substitution of the global muscles – no pelvic or lumbar movement
○ Neutral lumbar spine should be maintained
○ Normal lateral costal breathing should still be possible.

C. Pelvic floor (PF).
Palpation of the abdominal wall can be a useful indicator of PF function but, of course, the PF muscles can be assessed more accurately with ultrasound via abdominal imaging of the bladder or perineal ultrasound techniques.

Patient starting position: supine, hips and knees bent.

Therapist starting position: standing, using both thumbs palpate medial and slightly inferior to the ASIS. Sink the thumbs into the abdomen to palpate TA at the deepest layer.

Application of forces: as mentioned above under recruitment of TA, different cues and images can be used to isolate contraction of TA but in order to assess the pelvic floor, the patient should be asked to gently and slowly contract the pelvic floor muscles as if trying to stop urinating.

D. The diaphragm:

Patient starting position: supine, legs straight or bent.

Therapist starting position: standing, observe the patient's breathing pattern and note where there is greatest expansion on inspiration (upper chest (apical), lateral lower rib cage (lateral costal) or abdominal. Then observe expiration to see if the patient is doing this passively or actively using his abdominal muscles.

Application of forces: the therapist places her hands on the lateral aspect of the rib cage and feels for movement and symmetry of the lower ribs.

The ideal pattern is costolateral breathing on inspiration and expiration should be relaxed. *Variations*: The ability of the diaphragm to expand the lower ribs can be assessed in various positions. The symmetry of lateral chest expansion is then compared and correlated with any hypertonicity in the global muscles that may limit costolateral breathing.

Treatment

Refer to Box 7.2 for an overview of the content of the treatment section.

Clinical note

All patients with failed load transfer through the lumbopelvic–hip complex demonstrate non-optimal strategies during specific tasks.

The reasons for the non-optimal strategy are variable and clinical reasoning is essential for differentiating the causes (Lee & Lee 2010). It is important to reflect on the findings of both the subjective and the physical examinations to see if features fit and to generate the most probable hypotheses that could explain the patient's presentation.

Box 7.2

Overview of the content of the treatment section

Introduction

Common clinical presentations

Insufficient compression of the SIJ
- Management of insufficient compression of the SIJ
- Specific exercise programme
- Motor control retraining
- Sacroiliac belts or taping

Excessive compression of the SIJ
- Management of excessive compression of the SIJ
- Mobilizations/manipulations of the SIJ
  - Anterior rotation of the innominate
  - Posterior rotation of the innominate
  - Gapping of the SIJ

Clinical note

Reproducing the patient's symptoms is only one aspect of the Maitland Concept and pain should always be correlated to movement or resistance felt during the movement and vice versa.

Reproducing pain with a test only tells the therapist that symptomatic structures are being stressed and that they are related to the patient's complaint (provided that no hypersensitization due to central nervous system processes occurs). It is not necessarily an indication for using that technique in treatment.

Clinical note

In deciding what best techniques and what grades of passive movement should be used in treatment, the therapist must reflect on the severity, irritability and nature of the condition (SIN), the stage of healing of the tissues, the pain mechanisms involved and if the SIJ is felt to be responsible for the patient's symptoms or is only the victim of issues elsewhere.

When treatment is directed to the most relevant impairments (physical, cognitive and emotional), successful resolution of the pain and disability, along with attainment of functional goals, usually follows (Lee & Lee 2010).

Clinical note

Re-assessment during treatment is of utmost importance and serves to validate or negate the therapist's original hypotheses about the source of the patient's symptoms (Maitland et al. 2005, Lee & Lee 2010).

Management of PGP patients is much more than using passive movement as these techniques should rarely be used in isolation.

Clinical note

Current evidence demonstrates that a multimodal approach to treatment is most efficient.

Common clinical presentations involving the SIJs are described in the literature as the joint either having too much or too little compression by both the articular and myofascial systems (O'Sullivan et al. 2002, Hungerford et al. 2003, O'Sullivan & Beales 2007a, 2007b, Lee & Vleeming 2007).

Common clinical presentations

Insufficient compression of the SIJ (reduced force closure)

- May have a history of significant trauma or microtrauma over prolonged periods of time which can lead to patho-anatomical changes and passive instability of SIJ or symphysis pubis (loss of form closure; Lee & Lee 2010).
- Excessive strain on pain sensitive structures around the SIJ coupled with motor control deficits of muscles that control force closure at the SIJ is a common finding (Hungerford et al. 2003, O'Sullivan & Beales 2007a, 2007b).
- Decreased force closure can be due to loss of co-contraction of the local muscles and compensation with the global muscles (O'Sullivan & Beales 2007a, 2007b).
- Insufficient compression often occurs postpartum.
- Patients often present with a positive ASLR (O'Sullivan et al. 2002, Stuge et al. 2004).
- ASLR can be improved with compression of the pelvis (Mens et al. 1999, 2001, 2002); location of compression is helpful in prescribing exercises to restore motor control (Lee & Lee 2010).
- Compression just below the ASIS increases stiffness/compression of the SIJ (Damen et al. 2002); compression just above the greater trochanters increases the stiffness/compression of the symphysis pubis (Vleeming et al. 1992).
- Pain is often reproduced on weight-bearing postures such as sitting, standing and walking or loaded activity (O'Sullivan & Beales 2007a, 2007b).
- Positive one leg standing (OLS) test – patient has difficulty transferring weight in standing.
- Poor postures are associated with lack of local muscle activity – sway back, slumped sitting – these patients have a hard time

dissociating pelvic and thoracic movements (O'Sullivan & Beales 2007a, 2007b).
- Increased neutral zone is felt on passive mobility/stability testing.

Management when there is insufficient compression

- Education about the condition and the various factors involved.
- Correction of maladaptive postures – maintaining a neutral spine.
- Advice concerning activities of daily living and avoiding maladaptive movement patterns.
- Assessment/treatment of the hips and lumbar spine are of particular importance as these. adjacent areas may be hypomobile which can cause compensation or excessive strain on the SIJ structures.
- A specific individualized motor control exercise programme to control pain and restore functional capacity. There is good evidence to support this approach (Stuge et al. 2004, O'Sullivan & Beales 2007a, 2007b).
- The use of a belt can be a good temporary measure to increase force closure (Damen et al. 2002).
- General activities such as walking, running and swimming incorporate contraction of gluteus maximus and controlateral latissimus dorsi, thereby increasing tension on the thoracolumbar fascia (TLF).
- Training of muscles such as the gluteus maximus, latissimus dorsi, erector spinae and multifidus can assist in force closure by strengthening the posterior layer of the TLF (Vleeming & Stoeckart 2007).

Specific exercise programme

1. Optimal breathing patterns must be maintained with all exercises.
2. Decrease global muscle activity – including breathing prior to starting on local muscle recruitment.
3. Local muscle recruitment – choose the best position for the patient enhancing global muscle relaxation – find the best cue to isolate contraction of local muscles.
4. Find and maintain neutral spine in different positions (supine, sitting, standing, on

all fours) – moving away from maladaptive postures.

5. Maintain neutral spine with increasing load – add leg/arm loading.

6. Control spinal movement out of neutral.

7. Add proprioceptive challenge – e.g. sitting, standing on a sit-fit or balance board, lying on a half roll.

In their study, measuring after 20 weeks and at 1 year postpartum, Stuge et al. (2004) report that a treatment programme containing specific stabilizing exercises was considered to be more effective in reducing pain, improving functional status and health-related quality of life compared with an intervention without specific stability exercises.

Clinical note

In setting up an exercise programme, individualization of the exercises, supervision and correction are most important. The patient must understand why he is doing the exercises, and not just how to do them, and he must be committed to his exercise programme (Stuge et al. 2004).

Motor control retraining

Many authors suggest three stages of treatment when reeducating motor control:

1. Isolation: isolating the local muscles
2. Integration: stabilizing with the local muscles and adding limb movements
3. Functional integration: stabilizing with the local muscles and adding trunk movements; using functional tasks that are meaningful for the patient or tasks where failed load transfer was noted on assessment (Lee & Lee 2010, Stuge & Vøllestad 2007).

Prioritizing restoration of function in local muscles (Richardson et al. 2004) might lead to better outcomes, as supported by clinical trials in women with postpartum PGP (Stuge et al. 2004).

In training local muscles, the following should be considered:

- Low load exercises
- Low effort
- Slow, gentle contraction
- Isolated contraction without global muscle activation – avoiding rigidity.

In training global muscles, the following must be considered:

- Can the muscle be recruited?
- Can it maintain a contraction (endurance)?
- Can it produce enough force (strength)?
- Can it lengthen?
- Can it stabilize the spine during functional movement without being dominant?

Sacroiliac belts or taping

Clinical note

Although the mechanisms as to how belts or taping work is still unclear, it is known that the stiffness of the SIJ is enhanced when a generic belt is worn just below the ASIS (Damen et al. 2002).

A belt worn just above the greater trochanters has been shown to compress the pubic symphysis (Vleeming et al. 1992). Use of a belt can normalize the ASLR test (Mens et al. 1999) and influence the amount of laxity in the SIJ (Buyruk et al. 1995a, 1995b, Damen et al. 2002).

If ASLR is improved with compression, an SI belt or taping could be used whenever the patient is vertical. This should be seen as a temporary measure and as force closure improves, the patient should be able to reduce the amount of time in the brace until it is no longer needed.

Excessive compression of the SIJ (too much force closure)

- Intrinsic factors such as fibrosis post-trauma or post-inflammation (in inflammatory disorders such as ankylosing spondylitis) can cause excessive compression.
- Extrinsic factors such as overactivity of global muscles in the lumbopelvic region can also compress the SIJ (Lee & Lee 2010).
- Excessive loading of sensitized pelvic structures can cause localized pain of the joint, periarticular tissues and myofascial tissues (O'Sullivan & Beales 2007a, 2007b).

- Pain provocation tests can be positive as the joint is already under a lot of compression.
- OLS is usually negative as the patient does not have a force closure issue.
- ASLR may be negative or poor control may be seen. Some patients may be unable to lift the leg off the table as it is usually more effort to lift the leg on the compressed side; worse or no change with added compression (Lee & Vleeming 2007).
- Decreased neutral zone to passive mobility tests is reported (Lee & Lee 2010).
- Active postures in standing or sitting may become provocative (too much compression from global muscle activation) (O'Sullivan & Beales 2007a, 2007b).

Management when there is excessive compression

- Education – about the condition and the various factors involved.
- Manual therapy (mobilizations, manipulations, muscle energy techniques) is often helpful to increase joint mobility by stretching the connective tissues around the joint and by having a reflex neurophysiological effect on the surrounding tissues.
- Decreasing force closure by downtraining global muscle activity (O'Sullivan & Beales 2007a, 2007b, Lee & Lee 2010), this can be done through:
  - a cognitive approach – teaching the patient to become aware of releasing his muscles
  - breathing
  - relaxation
  - pacing
  - relaxed postures
  - muscle inhibition techniques
  - exercises that release the global muscles.
- Cessation of stabilization exercise training until the global muscles have been downtrained.
- Restoring breathing patterns.
- Teaching new strategies to isolate local stabilizers.
- Postural training – sitting and standing in a neutral spine.
- Correcting maladaptive movement strategies.
- Mobility exercises to maintain range gained with manual therapy techniques.

- Cardiovascular exercises.
- Assessment of the hips and lumbar spine as a stiff SIJ can create compensation elsewhere in the functional unit and create pain in the lumbopelvic–hip complex.

Clinical note

Rigidity is often an issue when the global muscles are dominant.

Here are some suggestions to download the global system (Lee & Lee 2010):

- With chest grippers where the EO are overactive (and possibly IO), the diaphragm must be retrained by encouraging costolateral breathing – this can be done in sidelying with the restricted side up
- With back grippers where the erector spinae (ES) and superficial multifidi (sMF) are overactive, costolateral breathing can also be used to release hypertonicity – this can be done in prone over a ball or in the prayer position
- Therapist encourages breathing in the restricted area by using manual pressure with her hands
- When there is presence of active expiration (more EO activation), the patient must be shown to sigh and to breathe out passively; it is important to address this issue as it may inhibit proper activation of the local muscles
- With butt grippers where the external rotators of the hip are too dominant, release techniques as well as active stretching can be used
- The therapist must help the patient recognize the areas where global muscles are dominant and teach them how to release those areas with awareness.

Mobilizations/manipulations of the SIJ

Accessory movements

Most passive examination techniques can be used as treatment techniques. This applies particularly to accessory movements that are very specific to the Maitland Concept.

Clinical note

The choice of accessory movements (e.g. direction, grade, rhythm) as a treatment technique is mainly based on symptom reproduction and the resistance encountered rather than on biomechanical considerations.

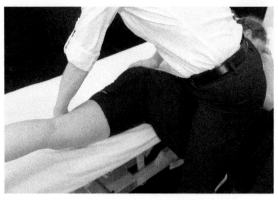

Figure 7.48 • Anterior rotation of the left innominate with the left knee in extension.

There is a variety of accessory movements that can be applied to the pelvic area and these have been previously described in the examination section of this chapter.

Passive joint mobilizations (grades I–IV) are used to decrease pain, increase joint mobility and release hypertonic muscles.

Manipulation

Manipulation (grade V technique) can be used to decrease joint stiffness, release joint adhesions and joint fixations, and when a plateau has been reached with passive joint mobilizations with regards to the treatment of pain.

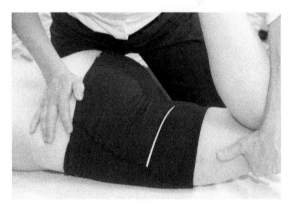

Figure 7.49 • Anterior rotation of the left innominate with the left knee flexed.

Anterior rotation of the left innominate

A. Patient starting position: prone, close to the right side of the bed, right foot on the floor, patient's leg supported by the therapist (Figs 7.48 & 7.49).

Therapist starting position: standing on right side (on the opposite side to the joint to be treated)

Localization of forces: the therapist places the heel of her right hand on the patient's left PSIS and the rest of the hand on the posterior innominate while her left hand grasps under the patient's thigh.

Application of the forces: extend the hip while simultaneously applying an anterosuperior force to the PSIS in the plane of the joint (must vary the direction of the push until the plane of least resistance is found). A muscle energy technique

can be used (contract–relax or hold–relax technique) to reach the limit of the physiological movement and a mobilization technique is then applied to the left innominate using both hands to regain anterior rotation with either grades III or IV mobilizations.

Variation: if indicated, a high velocity, low amplitude thrust (grade V) to the left innominate can be applied in an anterior superior direction.

B. Patient starting position: sidelying, bottom hip and knee flexed at 90°, top hip in extension, knee at 90° supported by the therapist (Fig. 7.50).

Therapist starting position: standing behind the patient.

Localization of forces: the therapist places the heel of her right hand on the patient's left PSIS and posterior innominate while her left hand is placed anteriorly around the ASIS and iliac crest.

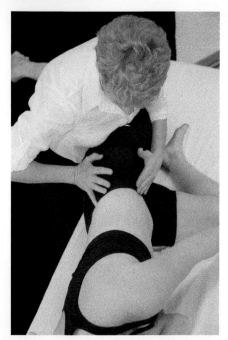

Figure 7.50 • Anterior rotation of the left innominate with the left knee flexed in right side-lying.

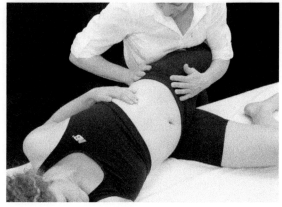

Figure 7.51 • Anterior rotation of the left innominate with the lumbar spine in left rotation – this tightens up the lumbar spine and makes the technique more specific.

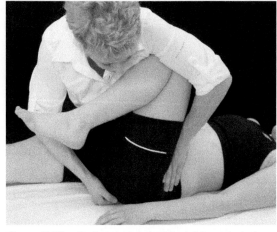

Figure 7.52 • Posterior rotation of the left innominate in supine.

Application of the forces: the thoracolumbar spine is placed into full left rotation down to and including L5/S1 (Fig. 7.51). The therapist extends the left hip and anteriorly rotates the left innominate. A muscle energy technique can be used (contract–relax or hold–relax technique) to reach the limit of the physiological movement and a mobilization technique is then applied to the left

innominate with both hands to regain anterior rotation with either grades III or IV mobilizations. *Variation*: if indicated, a high velocity, low amplitude thrust (grade V) to the left innominate can be applied in an anterior superior direction in the plane of the joint making sure not to extend L5/S1. Note that position A, as described above, is more stable for a grade V technique.

Posterior rotation of the left innominate

A. *Patient starting position:* supine, legs straight, close to the right side of the bed (Fig. 7.52).

Therapist starting position: standing on right side (on the opposite side to the joint to be treated).

Localization of forces: the therapist flexes the patient's left hip at 90° and places the heel of her left hand on the patient's left ASIS while her right hand grasps the patient's posterior innominate and ischeal tuberosity.

Application of the forces: the patient's hip is flexed slightly more than 90° while simultaneously applying a posterior inferior pressure on the ASIS and an anterior superior pressure on the ischeal tuberosity to pick up the posterior rotation of the innominate. A muscle energy technique can be used (contract–relax or hold–relax technique) to reach the limit of the physiological movement and a mobilization technique is then applied to

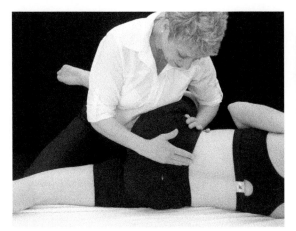

Figure 7.53 • Posterior rotation of the left innominate in right sidelying.

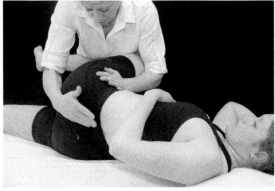

Figure 7.54 • Posterior rotation of the left innominate in right sidelying with the lumbar spine in left rotation – this tightens up the lumbar spine and makes the technique more specific.

the left innominate with both hands to regain posterior rotation with either grades III or IV mobilizations.

Variation: if indicated, a high velocity, low amplitude thrust (grade V) to the left innominate can be applied in a posterior inferior direction

B. *Patient starting position*: right sidelying, right leg straight, left hip and knee flexed at 90°, the left leg is supported by the therapist (Fig. 7.53)

Therapist starting position: standing facing the patient.

Localization of forces: the therapist places the heel of her right hand on the patient's left PSIS and posterior innominate while her left hand is placed anteriorly on the ASIS and anterior innominate.

Application of the forces: the thoracolumbar spine is placed into either full left or right rotation down to and including L5/S1 (Figs 7.54 & 7.55). The choice of the rotation will depend on which direction better stabilizes the lumbar spine. The therapist flexes the left hip slightly more than 90° as she posteriorly rotates the left innominate. A muscle energy technique can be used (contract–relax or hold–relax technique) to reach the limit of the physiological movement and a mobilization technique is then applied to the left innominate to regain posterior rotation with either grades IIIs or IVs.

Variation: if indicated, a high velocity, low amplitude thrust (grade V) to the left innominate can be applied in a posterior inferior direction

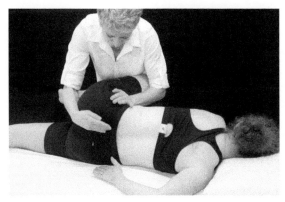

Figure 7.55 • Posterior rotation of the left innominate in right sidelying with the lumbar spine in right rotation –this tightens up the lumbar spine and makes the technique more specific.

Gapping manipulation of the left SIJ (Orthopaedic Division of the Canadian Physiotherapy Association 2006)

A. *Patient starting position*: supine, close to the edge of the bed on the left (Fig. 7.56).

Therapist starting position: standing on left side, place a small rolled towel under the sacrum medial to the left SIJ.

Localization of forces: the therapist takes up the barrier of left hip flexion/adduction.

Application of the forces: place both hands on the patient's left knee and apply an oscillating pressure towards the table along the line of the femur. If

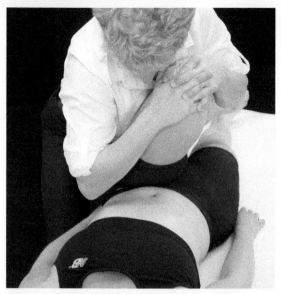

Figure 7.56 • Gapping manipulation of the left SIJ in supine.

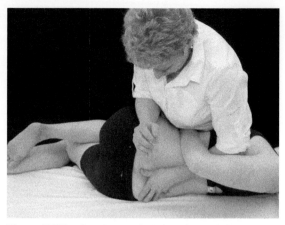

Figure 7.57 • Gapping manipulation of the left SIJ in right sidelying.

the pressure is well tolerated by the patient and no pain is elicited, a high velocity, low amplitude thrust movement (a grade V) is applied at the end of the range.

B. Patient starting position: sidelying on the right close to the edge of the bed (Fig. 7.57)

Therapist starting position: standing facing the patient.

Localization of forces: the thoracolumbar spine is placed into full left rotation down to and including L5/S1. The therapist fixes the sacrum (S2) and right innominate with her left thumb and hand.

The medial aspect of her right forearm is placed on the left innominate, halfway between the greater trochanter and the iliac crest.

Application of the forces: pressure is applied into axial rotation by pushing the innominate forward and down. If the pressure is well tolerated by the patient and no pain is elicited, a high velocity, low amplitude thrust movement (grade V) is applied, gapping the left innominate relative to the sacrum.

Uses:

• Joint stiffness
• Joint adhesions
• Joint fixation
• Treatment has reached a plateau with passive mobilizations.

 Case study 7.1

Subjective examination

Mrs B, a 32-year-old physiotherapist, presents with right groin pain (P1), pain over the symphysis pubis (P2), pain over the right SIJ area (P3) and right anterior knee pain (P4). There was a gradual onset of (P1), (P2) and (P3) which started 10 months ago when walking more than 30 minutes. At that time, she was 7 months pregnant with her first baby. Shortly after delivery, she noticed the right knee pain (P4) when she would attempt to squat with the baby in her arms. She was quite sedentary until 2 years ago when she started aerobic classes twice weekly. As a youth, she participated in gymnastics for 5 years and was noted to have good flexibility. Six months ago, she started a cardio class which involved quick walking with

the stroller and general exercises. She avoids all jumps as she experiences stress incontinence which started during the latter part of her pregnancy.

Mrs B had an uncomplicated pregnancy, gaining 15.5 kg (34 lbs) and delivered a 4.5 kg (10 lbs) baby. At delivery, she sustained a grade II tear of her pelvic floor. She felt that her pelvis was unstable after delivery – this feeling has improved 40% by trying to retrain her core. Functionally, she has trouble lifting her baby out of the crib, out of the car seat and picking her up from the floor. Walking is now less of a problem. Her score on the Lower Extremity Functional Scale is 65/80 (0 indicates inability to function and 80 is full function).

Case study 7.1—cont'd

Behaviour of symptoms

The body chart in Figure 7.58 illustrates the location of symptoms.

(P1) = Intermittent pain in the right groin, intensity 3/10; pain is brought on by standing on the right leg >5 min, going up three steps, standing up from sitting and lying on the right side for 5 min. Pain eases rapidly (within 1 min) by changing position, avoiding aggravating factors and resting.

(P2) = Intermittent pain in the area of the symphysis pubis, intensity 3/10; pain brought on by going up three steps, weight bearing on the right leg > 5 min, standing up from a crouched position, lifting her baby and putting the baby in the car seat. Pain eases rapidly (within 1 min) by sitting down, taking weight off the right leg or avoiding aggravating factors; (P2) is directly related to (P1).

(P3) = Intermittent pain in the right SI area, intensity 2/10; pain brought on by weight bearing on the right leg for >5 min. Pain eases rapidly (within 30 sec) by sitting down or taking weight off the right leg; (P3) is directly related to (P2).

(P4) = Intermittent pain anterior knee; intensity 3/10; pain brought on by coming up from the squat position, worse when she has the baby in her arms; and when going downstairs. Pain eases rapidly depending on how much knee bending she has done.

Over a 24 hour period:

• Night – (P1) with lying on the right side; eases rapidly if changes position
• AM – no morning stiffness, (P1), (P2) and (P3) occur with dressing when weight bearing on the right leg
• PM – symptoms will vary depending on whether she has done any activity that aggravates her symptoms.

Special questions and past history

Mrs B reports no past history of lower quadrant symptoms. She is in good health. She tends to be slightly overweight and currently weighs 4.5 kg (10 lbs) more than before her pregnancy. She is no longer breastfeeding. She has had no surgeries. She has never taken any corticosteroids or anabolic steroids and is not taking any medication. She has good

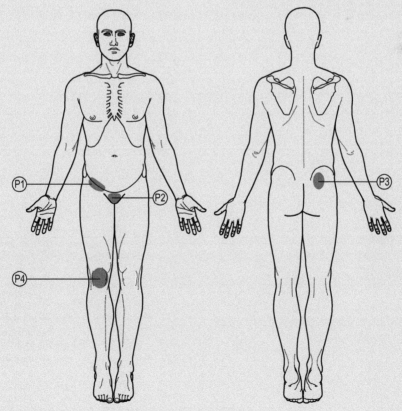

Figure 7.58 • Body chart showing the location of Mrs B's symptoms.

Continued

Case study 7.1—cont'd

control over her bowels but jumping, coughing and sneezing induce stress incontinence. She has no complaints of any numbness or paresthesia in the limbs. She has not had any X-rays.

Physical examination

Posture

- Sway-back, poor tone in her abdominals and buttocks
- R femur in medial rotation, R patella turned medially
- R innominate in slight anterior rotation

Gait

- Medial rotation of the right femur, right patella turned medially
- Lumbar rotation with right hip flexion
- Increased sway-back

Functional tests

- OLS on the right – unlocking of right SIJ (anterior rotation of the R innominate); increased medial rotation of the femur; poor control of the right foot; produces (P1) and (P2)
- ½ squat on the right – unlocking of the right SIJ; increased medial rotation of the right femur; poor control of the right foot; produces (P1), (P2) and (P4)

Active lumbar movements

- Flexion ✓✓ + Cx flex ✓ + 2 SF✓✓
- Extension ¾✓ + OP = R Lx discomfort + (P3); adding RSF, increases R Lx discomfort
- RSF ✓, slight resistance on OP + ext., increased resistance
- LSF ¾, pulls R Lx + ext. = ¾, pulls more in R Lx
- L Rot ✓, slight resistance with OP
- R Rot ✓✓
- Anterior pelvic tilt – some R Lx discomfort
- L hip drop (RSF from below) – slightly more resistance

Neurological examination

- Normal for dermatomes, myotomes and reflexes; negative for clonus and Babinski

Neurodynamic testing

- SLR, slump, PKB – all negative with normal mobility

R hip
- R femoral head position slightly anterior in relation to the left
- F/Add – slight (P1) at end of range, increased (P1) on adding lateral rotation
- Ext ¾, tight capsular/muscular end-feel
- Patrick's Faber test ¾, (P1) and (P2) reproduced
- Muscle flexibility testing – tight TFL and RF – slight (P1) reproduced
- Muscle testing – abductors 4+/5; lateral rotators 4+/5

SIJ/symphysis pubis
- Posterior pelvic pain provocation (P4) test
- Distraction test: ✓
- Compression test in R sidelying = (P1), (P2) and (P3)
- Sacral thrust test: ✓
- Long dorsal SI lig. test on the R: (P3)
- Decreased posterior rotation of the R innominate
- Palpation and caudal mvt R symp. pubis: (P2)
- Passive testing R SIJ in A/P plane: decreased mvt cf. L SIJ

R knee
- Tension R ITB + VL
- Decreased medial glide of the R patella

Lx PPIVMs
- Flex on L at T12/L1, L1/2 = ¾
- Ext. on the R at T12/L1, L1/2, L2/3, L5/S1 = ½
- Ext. on the L at T10/11, T11/12, T12/L1, L1/2 = ¾
- RSF T12/L1, L1/2, L5/S1 = ¾
- LSF T12/L1, L1/2 = ¾

Passive stability testing Lx: ✓

Dynamic stability testing

- ASLR on L and R – both positive, leg felt heavier on the right; better on the L with active recruitment of TA; better on the R with compression of the trochanters
- Active PKB on R – poor control of the Lx spine which goes into extension and right Lx rotation; tight anterior hip structures; control improved with attempt to recruit TA
- Active R hip extension – poor tone in right gluteus maximus; control improved with attempt to recruit TA

Local muscle testing

- TA – difficulty recruiting the TA using the pelvic floor muscles as a cue; weak recruitment of TA, particularly on the R, tends to recruit the IO more than the TA
- PF – hardly any tension generated in TA when trying to recruit the pelvic floor muscles
- Multifidus – good recruitment and good tone on the L, poor tone on the R over the sacral sulcus and L4 and L5, difficulty recruiting

Palpation and accessory mvt testing

- Unilat. P/A on R S1 = softer end-feel, produces (P3) and slight (P1)
- Unilat. P/A mvt on R on L5, T10–L1 = stiff
- Unilat. P/A mvt on L from L5–T10 = stiff

Case study 7.1—cont'd

- Palpation of symp pubis = P2
- Atrophy of multifidus on the R of L4, L5, S1, S2
- Hypertonicity of longissimus and iliocostalis bilaterally from T11–L2

Clinical hypotheses

Based on the findings of both the subjective and the physical examinations, the following physical impairments were identified and helped to define treatment goals:

1. *Right SIJ dysfunction (irritability/hypomobility):*
   - Symptoms on weight bearing on the right leg that started during the latter stage of pregnancy
   - Presence of a cluster of positive SIJ provocation tests
   - Anterior position of the R innominate observed in standing and decreased posterior rotation of the R innominate
   - Decreased give of the R SIJ in the A/P plane on passive mobility testing
   - Anterior position of the R innominate could be a compensation to decreased hip extension on the R
   - Dysfunction of the R SIJ can produce symptoms locally at the SIJ (P3) as well as refer pain into the R groin (P1). Concurrently, a SIJ dysfunction can affect the symphysis pubis (P2) which is seen in this case. Palpation of the symphysis pubis and caudal glide on the R reproduces (P2)

2. *Poor dynamic control of the lumbar spine and pelvis:*
   - Positive load transfer tests with unlocking at the SIJ felt on OLS and on ASLR (R > L)
   - Unable to stabilize the lumbar spine and pelvis on active PKB and hip extension in prone
   - Poor abdominal tone in standing, sway-back posture, poor tone of buttocks
   - Atrophy of multifidus on the R from L4–S2
   - Poor tone in buttocks – lack of force closure at the SIJ
   - Difficulty recruiting the pelvic floor (probably related to her stress incontinence and the grade II tear of her pelvic floor), her R multifidus and her R TA; R ASLR helped by compression of the trochanters which possibly simulate the work of the pelvic floor muscles

3. *Muscle imbalance around the R hip with poor control of the R femur on weight bearing:*
   - Medial rotation of the femur on OLS and on ½ squat on the R – can lead to unlocking of the SIJ, increased stress on the knee (P4) and lack of foot control on weight bearing

   - Tight anterior muscles – RF, TFL, ITB, VL – possibly related to the anterior femoral head position (could also contribute to (P1) on weight bearing) and the anterior position of the R innominate; the tight ITB and VL can create a lateral force on the patella thereby also contributing to (P4)
   - Weakness of abductors and lateral rotators of the hip – can contribute to poor control of medial rotation of the femur
   - Poor tone in buttocks

4. *Lumbar dysfunction (hypomobility):*
   - Decreased active range into the right extension quadrant – decreased ext. + RSF, RSF + ext., anterior pelvic tilt
   - Most restrictions felt in the thoracolumbar segments bilaterally as well as at L5/S1; stiffer segments in the left Lx spine and sacral base; hypertonicity of the global muscles (longissimus) in the thoracolumbar area; probably an area of compensation for her faulty posture and her lack of motor control in the lower lumbar spine and pelvis

Treatment

The patient was seen on treatment once a week over an 8-week period. Goals #1 and 2 were addressed from the start and were emphasized during the first three treatments. Goal #3 was addressed at the fourth visit. Stability exercises were reviewed and progressed throughout all the treatment sessions.

Goal #1. Correct posture and recruit local muscles of the trunk and posterior hip muscles: to improve dynamic control and thus decrease strain on the R SIJ.

It was felt that this patient, whose symptoms are all aggravated by weight bearing, first needed to change her sway-back posture in standing to adopt a more active posture and to recruit her local muscles in order to help her maintain that good posture. She was first shown how to recruit her TA in supine and how to maintain her contraction while adding movements with her right leg (hip flexion, leg slide on the bed, knee opening) without moving her Lx spine or pelvis. Recruitment of her R gluteus medius and lateral rotators of her hip was also taught in sidelying with first contracting her TA to avoid any back or pelvic movement. Once this was mastered, the patient was shown how to recruit her R sacral multifidi, also in sidelying, so that it could be incorporated into her exercise routine. In standing, exercises were done to actively correct her sway-back by aligning her upper sternum and symphysis pubis while recruiting her local muscles. Sitting to standing exercises from a

Continued

Case study 7.1—cont'd

chair were practised in front of a mirror, consciously recruiting the external rotators of the hip to ensure good tracking of the knee and avoiding any pain. This exercise was progressed by transferring weight on the R leg without losing good alignment of the trunk and of the R lower extremity. Proper bending techniques using her hips and knees and keeping her lumbar spine neutral were reviewed. The patient was also made aware of the hypertonicity of her global muscles in the thoracolumbar area and was given stretching exercises (including costolateral breathing) and cues to learn to release them.

After the first two treatments, the patient was partially able to correct her sway and could control her femur about 50% on OLS. It took three treatments for her to learn to fully control her femur in OLS and in the ½ squat position. Both (P1) and (P4) started to improve after the first treatment and she had no more (P4) after three visits. Decreased unlocking of the R SIJ was seen on OLS when she recruited her local muscles prior to standing on the right leg.

Goal #2. Increase mobility of the lumbar spine and R SIJ: to take the stress off the R SIJ; decrease global muscle recruitment; improve lumbar ROM; improve posture.

Mobilizations of the lumbar spine were started on the first treatment and were used throughout the course of treatment. Unilateral P/A movements, grade IV to IV+ were used on S1 to T10 on the left and on T10 to L1 on the right. Specific right extension mobilizations were also used in sidelying from T12/L1 to L2/3 and at L5/S1, grade IV. Following these techniques, the tone in the global muscles started to release and the lumbar movements in extension and both SF improved. Less discomfort was felt in the right low lumbar area on active movements and (P3) was no longer produced on extension. Posture correction in standing was easier. Exercises were taught to maintain the lumbar mobility gained.

Mobilization of the R innominate in posterior rotation was added from the 3rd to the 6th treatment. The mobilizations were done in both supine and side-lying positions using contract–relax techniques + passive mobilizations with a grade III to III+. On re-assessment, there was a gradual increase in give on passive mobility testing of the SIJ in the A/P plane and an increase in range of posterior rotation of the innominate. Less (P1) and (P3) were felt on weight bearing, there was less unlocking of the R SIJ on OLS on the right and the SIJ provocation tests were much less painful. An exercise was taught to maintain posterior rotation of the right innominate.

Goal #3. Regain R hip mobility: improve the flexibility of the anterior hip muscles; learn to center the femoral head; increase hip extension; decrease the pull on R innominate into anterior rotation.

Active stretching exercises were given to improve the flexibility of the rectus femoris, tensor fascia lata muscles and iliotibial band. Mobilizations using A/P movements on the femoral head was used in neutral hip position, grade III to III+. Recruitment of the deep psoas muscle was taught to centralize the femoral head prior to doing any hip movement and the patient was taught how to actively release the tension in the groin muscles. Passive mobilizations to increase hip extension, grade IV to IV+ were added to further gain hip extension.

By the end of the eight treatment sessions, pain had resolved in all areas, the patient's standing posture and her mobility had much improved, she was able to function well without discomfort and she had learned proper body mechanics for lifting her baby. The recruitment of her local muscles had much improved but she needed to continue to consciously think of recruiting her muscles during any task that required bending and lifting. Her pelvic floor muscles were still weak and she still suffered from stress incontinence. She was then referred to a pelvic floor therapist.

References

Australian Acute Musculoskeletal Pain Guidelines Group (AAMPGG): *Evidence-based management of acute musculoskeletal pain*. Bowen Hills, Australia, 2003, Australian Academic Press.

Albert H, Godskesen M, Westergaard J: Evaluation of clinical tests used in classification procedures in pregnancy-related pelvic joint pain, *Eur Spine J* 9:161–166, 2000.

Apkarian AV, Robinson JP: Low back pain, *IASP Pain Clin Updat* VXIII(Issue 6), 2010.

Banks K, Hengeveld E: *Maitland's Clinical companion: an essential guide for students*, Elsevier, 2010, Churchill Livingstone.

Barker PJ, Briggs CA, Bogeski G: Tensile transmission across the lumbar fasciae in unembalmed cadavers: effects of tension to various muscular attachments, *Spine* 29(2):129–138, 2004.

Barker PJ: *Applied anatomy and biomechanics of the lumbar fascia: implications for segmental control.*

PhD thesis, Australia, 2005, University of Melbourne.

Beales DJ, O'Sullivan PB, Briffa NK: Motor control patterns during an active straight leg raise in chronic pelvic girdle pain subjects, *Spine* 34(9):861–887, 2009.

Bergmark A: Stability of the lumbar spine. A study in mechanical engineering, *Acta Orthop Scand* 230:1–54, Review, 1989.

Boissonault W: *Primary care for the physical therapist. examination and triage*, ed 2, Amsterdam, 2011, Elsevier-Saunders.

Buyruk HM, Stam HJ, Snijders CJ, et al: The use of colour Doppler imaging for the assessment of sacroiliac joint stiffness: a study on embalmed human pelvises, *Eur J Radiol* 21:112–116, 1995a.

Buyruk HM, Snijders CJ, Vleeming A, et al: The measurements of sacroiliac joint stiffness with colour Doppler imaging: a study on healthy subjects, *Eur J Radiol* 21:117–121, 1995b.

Cusi M, Saunders J, Hungerford B: The use of prolotherapy in the sacroiliac joint, *British Journal of Sports Medicine* 44(2):100–104, 2010.

Cyriax J: *Textbook of Orthopaedic Medicine*, ed 7, London, 1975, Ballière Tindall.

Damen L, Spoor CW, Snijders CJ: Does a pelvic belt influence sacroiliac joint laxity? *Clin Biomech (Bristol, Avon)* 17(7):495–498, 2002.

Dorman T: Pelvic mechanics and prolotherapy. In Vleeming A, Mooney V, Dorman T, Snijders C, Stoeckart R, editors: *Movement stability and low back pain*, Edinburgh, 1997, Churchill Livingstone.

Edwards I: *Clinical reasoning in three different field of physiotherapy. a qualitative case study*. PhD Thesis, Adelaide, 2000, School of Physiotherapy. Division of Health Sciences. University of South Australia.

Edwards I, Jones M, Carr J, et al: Clinical reasoning strategies in physical therapy, *Phys Ther* 84:312–330, 2004.

Fortin JD, Dwyer AP, West S, et al: Sacroiliac joint: pain referral maps upon applying a new injection/arthography technique. Part 1: Asymptomatic volunteers, *Spine* 19(13):1475–1482, 1994.

Gibbons S: Clinical anatomy and function of psoas major and deep sacral gluteus maximus. In Vleeming A, Mooney V, Stoeckart R, editors: *Movement , stability and lumbopelvic pain*, ed 2, Edinburgh, 2007, Elsevier.

Goodman CC, Snyder TEK: *Differential diagnosis for physical therapists: screening for referral*, ed 4, Amsterdam, 2007, Elsevier-Saunders.

Hansen HC, Helm S: Sacroiliac joint pain and dysfunction, *Pain Physician* 6:173–189, 2003.

Hengeveld E: *Psychosocial issues in physiotherapy: manual therapists' perspectives and observations*. MSc Thesis, London, 2000, Dept. of Health Science. University of East London.

Hengeveld E, Banks K: *Maitland's Peripheral manipulation*, ed 4, Edinburgh, 2005, Elsevier Butterworth-Heinemann.

Hengeveld E, Banks K: *Maitland's Peripheral manipulation*, ed 5, Edinburgh, 2014, Elsevier Butterworth Heinemann.

Hodges PW: Lumbopelvic stability: a functional model of the biomechanics and motor control. In Richardson C, Hodges PW, Hides J, editors: *Therapeutic exercise for lumbopelvic stabilisation. A Motor Control Approach for the Treatment and Prevention of Low Back Pain*, ed 3, Edinburgh, 2004, Churchill Livingstone.

Hodges PW, Cholewicki J: Functional control of the spine. In Vleeming A, Mooney V, Stoeckart R, editors: *Movement , stability and lumbopelvic pain*, ed 2, Edinburgh, 2007, Elsevier.

Hodges PW, Richardson CA: Delayed postural contraction of transversus abdominis in low back pain associated with movement of the lower limbs, *J Spinal Disord* 11(1):46–56, 1998.

Hodges PW, Kaigle Holm A, Holm S, et al: Intervertebral stiffness of the spine is increased by evoked contraction of transversus abdominis and the diaphragm: in vivo porcine studies, *Spine* 28(23):2594–2601, 2003.

Huijbregts P: Sacroiliac joint dysfunction: Evidence based diagnosis. Orthopaedic division review. May/June 2004, www.orthodiv.org, 2004.

Hungerford B, Gilleard W, Hodges P: Evidence of Altered Lumbopelvic Muscle Recruitment in the Presence of Sacroiliac Joint Pain, *Spine* 28(14):1583–1600, 2003.

Hungerford B, Gilleard W, Lee D: Altered patterns of pelvic bone motion determined in subjects with posterior pelvic pain using skin markers, *Clin Biomechanics* 19:456–464, 2004.

Hungerford B, Gilleard W, Moran M, et al: Evaluation of the Ability of Physical Therapists to Palpate Intrapelvic Motion with the Stork test on the Support Side, *Phys Ther* 87(7):879–887, 2007.

Jones M: Clinical reasoning and pain, *Man Ther* 1:17–24, 1995.

Jones M, Rivett D, editors: *Clinical Reasoning for Manual Therapists*, Edinburgh, 2004, Butterworth-Heinemann, Elsevier.

Kapandji AI: *Physiology of the joints, Volume 3, the spinal column, pelvic girdle and head*, Edinburgh, 2008, Churchill Livingstone, Elsevier.

Kissling RO, Jacob HAC: The mobility of sacroiliac joints in healthy subjects. In Vleeming A, Mooney V, Dorman T, Snijders C, Stoeckart R, editors: *Movement, stability & low back pain: the essential role of the pelvis*, New York, 1997, Churchill Livingstone-Elsevier.

Koes BW, Assendelft WJ, van der Heijden GJ, et al: Spinal manipulation for low back pain. An updated systematic review of randomized clinical trials, *Spine* 21(24):2860–2871, 1996.

Laslett M: Evidence-based clinical testing of the lumbar spine and pelvis. In Vleeming A, Mooney V, Stoeckart R, editors: *Movement , stability and lumbopelvic pain*, ed 2, Edinburgh, 2007, Elsevier.

Laslett M: Evidence-based diagnosis and treatment of the painful sacroiliac joint, *J Man Manipulative Ther* 16(3):142–152, 2008.

Laslett M, Williams W: The reliability of selected pain provocation tests for sacroiliac joint pathology, *Spine* 19(11):1243–1249, 1994.

Laslett M, Young SB, April CN, et al: Diagnosing painful sacroiliac joints: A validity study of a McKenzie evaluation and sacroiliac provocation tests, *Aust J Physiother* 49(2):89–97, 2003.

Laslett M, Aprill CN, McDonald B, et al: Diagnosis of Sacroiliac Joint Pain: Validity of individual provocation tests and composites of tests, *Man Ther* 10:207–218, 2005.

Lee D: *The pelvic girdle: an approach to the examination and treatment of the lumbopelvic-hip region*, Edinburgh, 2004, Churchill Livingstone. Elsevier.

Lee DG, Vleeming A: An integrated therapeutic approach to the treatment of pelvic girdle pain. In Vleeming A, Mooney V, Stoeckart R, editors: *Movement , stability and lumbopelvic pain*, ed 2, Edinburgh, 2007, Elsevier.

Lee D, Lee LJ: *The pelvic girdle, an integration of clinical expertise and research*, ed 4, Edinburgh, 2010, Churchill Livingstone. Elsevier.

Maigne JY, Aivalikidis A, Pfefer F: Results of sacroiliac joint double blocks and value of pain provocations tests in 54 patients with low back pain, *Spine* 21:1889–1892, 1996.

Maitland GD: *Vertebral manipulation*, ed 5, Oxford, 1986, Butterworth Heinemann.

Maitland GD, Hengeveld E, English K, et al: *Maitland's Vertebral Manipulation*, ed 7, Edinburgh, 2005, Elsevier – Butterworth-Heinemann.

Mens J, Vleeming A, Stoeckart R, et al: Understanding Peripartum Pelvic Pain: Implications of a Patient Survey, *Spine* 21(11):1363–1369, 1996.

Mens JMA, Vleeming A, Snijders C, et al: The active straight leg raising test and mobility of the pelvic joints, *Eur Spine J* 8(6):468–473, 1999.

Mens JMA, Vleeming A, Snijders CJ, et al: Reliability and validity of the active straight leg raise test in posterior pelvic pain since pregancy, *Spine* 26(10). 1167–1171, 2001.

Mens JMA, Vleeming A, Snijders CJ, et al: Validity of the active straight leg raise test for measuring disease severity in patients with posterior pelvic pain after preganancy, *Spine* 27(2):196–200, 2002.

Orthopaedic Divison of the Canadian Physiotherapy Association: *Level IV/V manual therapy course notes*, 2006,

Ostgaard HC: What is pelvic girdle pain? In Vleeming A, Mooney V, Stoeckart R, editors: *Movement , stability and lumbopelvic pain*, ed 2, Edinburgh, 2007, Elsevier.

O'Sullivan P, Beales DJ: Diagnosis and classification of pelvic girdle pain disorders – Part 1: A mechanism based approach within a biopsychosocial framework, *Man Ther* 12:86–97, 2007a.

O'Sullivan P, Beales DJ: Diagnosis and classification of pelvic girdle pain disorders – Part 2: Illustration of the utility of a classification system via case studies, *Man Ther* 12:e1–e12, 2007b.

O'Sullivan P, Twomey L, Allison G: Evaluation of specific stabilizing exercise in the treatment of chronic low back pain with radiologic diagnosis of sondylolysis or spondylolisthesis, *Spine* 22(24):2959–2967, 1997.

O'Sullivan P, Beales D, Beetham J, et al: Altered motor control

strategies in subjects with sacroiliac joint pain during the active straight leg raise test, *Spine* 27(1):E1, 2002.

Palastanga N, Field D, Soames R: *Anatomy and Human Movement. Structure and Function*, Oxford, 1994, Butterworth-Heinemann.

Panjabi MM: The stabilizing system of the spine. Part 1: function, dysfunction, adaptation and enhancement, *J Spinal Disord* 5(4):383–389, 1992.

Payton O: Clinical reasoning processes in physical therapy, *Phys Ther* 65:924–928, 1987.

Pel JJM, Spoor CW, Pool-Goudzwaard AL, et al: Biomechanical analysis of reducing sacroiliac joint shear load by optimization of pelvic muscle and ligament forces, *Ann Biomed Eng* 36(3):415–424, 2008.

Pool-Goudzwaard A, Hoek van Dijke G, van Gurp M, et al: Contribution of pelvic floor muscles to stiffness of the pelvic ring, *Clin Biomech* 19:564–571, 2004.

Richardson CA, Jull GA, Hodges PW, et al: *Therapeutic exercise for spinal segmental stabilization in low back pain – scientific basis and clinical approach*, Edinburgh, 1999, Churchill Livingstone.

Richardson CA, Snijders CJ, Hides JA, et al: The relationship between the transversely oriented abdominal muscles, sacroiliac joint mechanics and low back pain, *Spine* 27(4): 399–405, 2002.

Richardson C, Hodges PW, Hides J: *Therapeutic exercise for lumbopelvic stabilisation. a motor control approach for the treatment and prevention of low back pain*, ed 3, Edinburgh, 2004, Churchill Livingstone.

Robinson HS, Brox JI, Robinson R, et al: The reliability of selected motion and pain provocation tests for the sacroiliac joint, *Man Ther* 12:72–79, 2007.

Sackett DL, Richardson WS, Rosenberg W, et al: *Evidence-Based Medicine – How to practice and teach EB*, Edinburgh, 1998, Churchill-Livingstone.

Sapsford R: The pelvic floor – A clinical model for function and rehabilitation, *Physiotherapy* 87(12):620–630, 2001.

Sapsford R: Rehabilitation for pelvic floor muscles utilizing trunk stabilisation, *Man Ther* 9:3–12, 2004.

Sapsford R, Hodges PW: Contraction of Pelvic Floor Muscles During Abdominal Maneuvers, *Arch Physical Medicine & Rehabilitation* 82:1081–1088, 2001.

Schwartzer AC, Aprill CN, Bogduk N: The sacroiliac joint in chronic low back pain, *Spine* 20(1):31–37, 1995.

Smith MD, Russell A, Hodges PW: Disorders of breathing and continence have s stronger association with back pain than obesity and physical activity, *Aust J Physiother* 52:11–16, 2006.

Snijders CJ, Vleeming A, Stoeckart R: Transfer of lumbosacral load to iliac bones and legs. Part 1: Biomechanics of selfbracing of the sacroiliac joints and its significance for treatment and exercise. *Clin Biomech* 8:285–294. 1993.

Stuge B, Vøllestad NK: Important aspects for efficacy of treatment with specific stabilizing exercises for postpartum pelvic girdle pain. In Vleeming A, Mooney V, Stoeckart R, editors: *Movement , stability and lumbopelvic pain*, ed 2, Edinburgh, 2007, Elsevier.

Stuge B, Laerum E, Kirkesola G, et al: The efficacy of a treatment program focusing on specific stabilizing exercises for pelvic girdle pain after pregnancy, *Spine* 29(4):351–359, 2004.

Sturesson B, Uden A, Vleeming A: A Radiostereometric Analysis of Movements of the Sacroiliac Joints During the Standing Hip Flexion Test, *Spine* 25(3):364–368, 2000a.

Sturesson B, Uden A, Vleeming A: A Radiostereometric Analysis of Movements of the Sacroiliac Joints in the Reciprocal Straddle Position, *Spine* 25(3):214–217, 2000b.

Szadek KM, van der Wurff P, van Tulder MW, et al: Diagnostic validity of criteria for sacroiliac joint pain: A systematic review, *J Pain* 10(4):354–368, 2009.

Thomas-Edding D: Clinical Problem solving in physical therapy and its implications for curriculum development. Proc. 10th Int'l Congress of the World Confederation of Physical Therapy, Sydney, 1987.

van Deursen LL, Patijn J, Ockhuysen AC: The value of some clinical tests of the sacroiliac joint, *Man Med* 5:96–99, 1990.

van der Wurff P, Magmeijer RHM, Meyne W: Clinical Tests of the sacroiliac joint: a systematic methodological review: Part 1: Reliability, *Man Ther* 5(1):30–36, 2000.

van Tulder M, Koes B: Evidence based medicine for chronic low back pain. In: *Proceedings from the 7th Interdisciplinary World Congress on low back and pelvic pain*, Los Angeles, 2010.

van Wingerden JP, Vleeming A, Buyruk HM, et al: Stabilization of the sacroiliac joint in vivo: verification of muscular contribution to force closure of the pelvis, *Eur Spine J* 13(3):199–205, 2004.

Vleeming A, Stoeckart R, Snijders CJ: Relation between form and function in the sacroiliac joint. 1: Clinical anatomical aspects, *Spine* 15(2):130–136, 1990.

Vleeming A, Buyruk H, Stoeckart R, et al: An integrated therapy for peripartum pelvic instability: a study of the biomechanical

effects of pelvic belts, *Am J Obstet Gynecol* 166(4):1243–1247, 1992.

Vleeming A, Pool-Goudzwaard A, Stoeckart R, et al: The posterior layer of the thoracolumbar fascia: its function in load transfer from spine to legs, *Spine* 20:753–758, 1995.

Vleeming A, Pool-Goudzwaard AL, Hammudoghlu D, et al: The function of the long dorsal sacroiliac ligament: its implication for understanding low back pain, *Spine* 21(5):556–562, 1996.

Vleeming A, Snijders CJ, Stoeckart R, et al: The role of the sacroiliac joints in coupling between spine, pelvis, legs and arms. In Vleeming A, Mooney V, Dorman T, et al, editors: *Movement, Stability & Low Back Pain – The essential role of the pelvis*, New York, 1997, Churchill Livingstone-Elsevier.

Vleeming A, de Vries HJ, Mens JM, et al: Possible role of the long dorsal sacroiliac ligament in women with peripartum pelvic pain, *Acta Obstet Gynecol Scand* 81(5):430–436, 2002.

Vleeming A, Stoeckart R: The role of the pelvic girdle in coupling the spine and the legs: a clinical-anatomical perspective on pelvic stability. In Vleeming A, Mooney V, Stoeckart R, editors: *Movement , stability and lumbopelvic pain*, ed 2, Edinburgh, 2007, Elsevier.

Vleeming A, Albert HB, Östgaard HC, et al: European Guidelines for the diagnosis and treatment of pelvic girdle pain, *Europ Spine J* 17:794–819, 2008.

World Health Organization (WHO) : *The International Classification of Functioning, Disability and Health (ICF)*, Geneva, 2001, World Health Organization.

Sustaining functional capacity and performance

8

Elly Hengeveld

CHAPTER CONTENTS

Role of passive movement in promotion of
active movement and physical activity 381

Underlying mechanisms of passive
movement. 384

Functional restoration programmes and
self management 386

Cognitive behavioural principles. 390

Recognition of potential barriers to full
functional recovery. .390

Collaborative goal setting 395

Phases of behavioural change 396

Compliance enhancement. 398

Patient education. 400

Key words

Movement continuum theory, compliance, patient-
education, phases of change, collaborative goal-
setting, yellow flags

Introduction

Physiotherapists play a central role in the maintenance and improvement of the movement capacity
of individuals in a society. The overall objective of
physiotherapeutic treatment may be summarized as
follows: to enhance movement functions, overall
wellbeing and purposeful actions in daily life, in order
to allow a patient to participate in their chosen activities of life (in their roles as spouse, family member,
friend; in sports, leisure activities and work).

Within the description of physiotherapy by the
World Confederation of Physical Therapy (WCPT
1999) the core of the profession is described as
follows:

- Human movement is central to the skills and
  knowledge of the physiotherapist
- These skills are particularly important in
  circumstances where movement and function
  are threatened by the process of ageing, or that
  of injury and disease
- Physiotherapy places full and functional
  movement at the heart of what it means to be
  healthy.
- Physiotherapists are concerned with identifying
  and maximizing movement potential, within the
  spheres of promotion, prevention, treatment
  and rehabilitation
- Intervention is implemented and modified in
  order to reach agreed goals and may include:
  manual handling; movement enhancement;
  physical, electrotherapeutic and mechanical
  agents; functional training; provisions of aids
  and appliances; patient-related instruction;
  documentation, coordination and
  communication
- Intervention may also be aimed at prevention of
  impairments, functional limitations, disability
  and injury including the promotion and
  maintenance of health, quality of life, and
  fitness for all ages and populations.

Within physiotherapy many treatment methods
exist to achieve the above-mentioned aims. It has
been discussed that many physiotherapists appear to

identify with various treatment methods (KNGF 1992), without identifying with a central core of movement rehabilitation. This notion was formed a few decades ago; however, it still seems valid now, as other 'new' treatment methods appear to have become dominant and often exclusively applied. In spite of specializations within the field of physiotherapy, it is necessary for physiotherapists to develop skills in a wide range of treatment methods, including communication and patient education.

The following quote may demonstrate this principle:

> Many of these approaches are practised to the exclusion of others. A manipulative physiotherapist may not take account of functional restoration. A Feldenkrais practitioner may not be concerned about fitness and functional restoration programmes may emphasize strength and stability at the expense of moving with ease. Self-management as the total solution can ignore the benefits of 'hands-on' therapy such as massage. Strength, mobility, fitness and relaxation all contribute to full functioning. Can practitioners afford to practise one method to the exclusion of others, or even worse, actively discourage others?
>
> (McIndoe 1995, p. 156)

In the decades since the first development of the Maitland Concept of neuromusculoskeletal (manipulative) physiotherapy, many societal changes have occurred including immense changes in the lifestyles of many people. Furthermore, the viewpoints within medical and physiotherapeutic practice and science have changed from dualistic, biomedical to more holistic, bio-psychosocial paradigms.

Naturally these changes are also reflected in the workings of this concept; however, its core principles for the clinical work of physiotherapists are as valid as in its initial stages.

Lifestyle and physical activity

Lifestyles in the industrialized world have become more sedentary with different diets over the decennia since the Second World War. The impact of inactivity and diet on health issues is increasingly acknowledged and it has been recognized that regular physical activity is effective in the primary and secondary prevention of several diseases, for example cardiovascular disease, diabetes, some forms of cancer, hypertension, obesity, depression, osteoarthritis and osteoporosis. Furthermore, there

is indication that musculoskeletal fitness is of particular importance in the elderly to maintain their independence (Warburton et al. 2006). It is estimated that each year 1.9 million people die as a result of physical inactivity, and that at least 30 minutes of moderate intensity physical activity 5 days per week reduces the risk of several of these common non-communicable diseases (WHO 2004). Global programmes to promote healthier lifestyles have been developed (WHO 2008) and it is acknowledged that the unique role of physiotherapists with their specific knowledge in sustaining movement capacity and health promotion will increase in these programmes in the near future (WCPT 2012).

Role of passive movement in promotion of active movement and physical activity

With the changing role of physiotherapists towards health promotion and prevention, as well as the focus on secondary prevention of ongoing disability due to pain, it may seem that passive movement as an element of treatment would become less relevant, or even obsolete. One of the listed psychosocial factors hindering full restoration of function is 'overly depending on passive modalities' and 'excessive downtime because of the pain' (Kendall et al. 1997). This has led to a somewhat polarized discussion of 'hand-on' versus 'hands-off' therapy by manipulative physiotherapists. In this debate it was assumed that passive modalities would make a patient dependent upon the treatment, and active movement would enhance active coping strategies. It seems that within this discussion no cognitive-behavioural perspectives on passive and active treatment modalities have been taken into consideration. Currently it appears sometimes that manipulative physiotherapists have to justify the selection of passive mobilization and manipulation in the treatment of their patients with painful movement disorders.

However, over the years an extensive body of randomized controlled trials (RCTs), reviews and practice guidelines report that in acute and sub-acute phases passive mobilizations and manipulations in combination with self-management strategies appear to lead to better treatment outcomes than single active or passive treatment-modalities (e.g. Gross et al. 2002, Jull et al. 2002, Vicenzino 2003,

AAMPGG 2003, Van Tulder et al. 2006, Walker et al. 2008). In a recent editorial in the journal manual therapy it was commented that:

> ... Hands on, hands off? There is ample evidence of changes in motor control in association with neck and back pain. Thus there is no argument that exercise and activity are important components of any rehabilitation program to address these deficits. There is also ample evidence that zygapophysial joints and discs are common sources of pain. Manipulative/manual therapy is directed towards the painful joint dysfunction and there is a considerable body of research into the mechanisms of effect and effectiveness of manipulative therapy. Manipulative/manual therapy has proven pain relieving effects. [...] the evidence suggests that the use of manipulative/manual therapy should not be forgotten. Painful joint dysfunction is present in the vast majority of neck and low back pain patients ...
>
> (Jull & Moore, 2012; p. 200)

Hence, also in contemporary perspectives, the art of passive mobilization and manipulation still plays a central role in the treatment of many movement disorders. Particularly in acute and sub-acute phases of nociceptive and peripheral neurogenic disorders to influence pain, passive mobilization and manipulation may give short-term effects on pain reduction. Furthermore passive mobilization techniques can be employed to optimize mobility of joints, neurodynamic structures, soft tissues and muscles. The discussion should revolve around the question of how active and passive treatment modalities can complement each other to achieve optimum treatment results, rather than a somewhat polarized selection of either one or the other treatment form. If passive mobilizations, and possibly also manipulations, are being applied within a cognitive behavioural approach to treatment, it is possible that better results are being achieved (Bunzli et al. 2011), both in the treatment of acute and sub-acute pain as well as in the treatment on ongoing pain and disability.

To summarize, with the application of passive mobilizations and/or manipulations within the overall physiotherapeutic management, the following aspects may need to be taken into consideration:

- Passive mobilizations serve as a kick-start to active movement.
- Passive movements also may play a role in the diagnostics of movement disorders, particularly within a framework of dominant peripheral nociceptive and neurogenic pain mechanisms. The abnormalities detected as for example pain-reproduction and restricted range of

motion as well as the outcome in reassessment procedures after the application of the passive techniques, may be indicative of the source of the patient's symptoms.

However, in cases on central nervous system modulation with peripheral sensitization of tissue-reactions and more generalized tenderness false-positive results may occur. Nonetheless, in these circumstances hypotheses may be developed regarding reactivity and possible pathophysiological, cognitive, emotional and behavioural contributing factors to the pain experience. The reactivity to passive movement and touch, as well as generalized tenderness, may serve as a parameter in reassessment procedures.

Hence, touch and palpation also need to be seen as an important part of communication with the tissues and the understanding of responses of these tissues to touch and passive movement. On the one hand, touch and palpation allow the therapist to compare the state of the tissues encountered and, on the other hand, to be able to identify with the patient and gain an understanding of why and how protective responses have developed.

- In principle passive movement may find a place on the level of 'body parts' on Cott et al.'s (1995) movement continuum (see Chapter 1 (and 2) of Volume 2). It is postulated that all levels on the movement continuum are interdependent. For example, painfully restricted hip movements may limit activities such as getting up from a chair, bending down or walking, adding to a lack of confidence in everyday activities and may become a contributing factor for loss of independence in elderly people. Therefore the optimization of the movement potential on this level of 'body parts' may be a central condition towards the restoration of full movement capacity. Based on information from subjective examination, the goals of rehabilitation of the movement levels of the person in the environment and society may be defined. However, the manipulative physiotherapist's specific physical examination procedures, including passive motion tests, will reveal if the conditions on the movement level of 'body parts' are being fulfilled and need to be defined in the treatment objectives.

- Passive mobilization may be necessary to optimize joint function in the so-called 'functional corners', e.g. shoulder-quadrant, extension abduction and extension adduction of the elbow or knee, or flexion/adduction (F/AD) of the hip (Maitland 1991). This will ensure that the joints have a functional reserve capacity when the movement system is asked to do a little more than it does normally. This functional reserve capacity may be a contributing factor in the reduction of the incidence of recurrent episodes.

- Frequently, treatment with passive mobilization and/or manipulation may be considered to achieve pain reduction on a short-term basis; however, in order to maintain long-term treatment effects, active movement to control pain and movement impairments, such as mobility and motor control, need to be integrated in an early phase of treatment.

- It appears that the integration of a cognitive behavioural approach to manipulative physiotherapy may enhance treatment outcomes (Bunzli et al. 2011). This includes addressing a patient's worries, assessing the patient's cognitions about causes of and treatment options for their problem, collaborative goal-setting, following a motivational phase of change model and compliance enhancement strategies, including education. Furthermore, being alert towards patients' key gestures or remarks during the various examination and treatment procedures and responding to them is important. For example, during palpation and the examination of accessory movements, a patient may say 'that spot you're pressing on is hurting me!' Your explanation may need to be: 'This spot especially needs treatment, not the ones that are fully painfree; however, I'm going to gently move this spot in such a way that it remains below the threshold of pain'. Or during reassessment procedures: 'Why do you always make me perform movements which hurt me?' In the latter case it may be useful to take a moment to explain the purpose of the reassessment procedures and the patient's observational role in them to compare the pain sensation and movement-ability.

- A multidimensional attitude towards touch as well as passive and active movement is needed.

The following quotes demonstrate dimensions of therapeutic touch beyond joint mechanics and anatomy:

Through the skin every human being is subject to a multitude of impressions by which he perceives the objects with which he is in contact. Further he may have bodily sensations. Through these manifestations each individual assumes his corporeal identity and without this he could not define his immediate 'life-world'.

(Rey 1995, p. 5)

Although manipulation starts at a local anatomical site, its remote influence on the human experience can be as far as the infinite expansion of the psyche. Manipulation is not limited by anatomical boundaries but involves the abstract world of the imagination, emotions, thoughts and full-life experience of the individual. The body is the centre of orientation in our perception of our environment, focus of subjective experience, field of reference, organ of expression and articulatory node between the self and the environment. When we touch the patient, we touch the whole of this experience

(Ledermann 1996, p. 158)

- It is postulated that active movement can occur without active (cognitive and emotional) participation of the patient, while passive movement, in combination with in-depth communication skills, can require strong participation of the patient, thus enhancing bodily awareness (Banks & Hengeveld 2010). During touching, passive movement and communication, the physiotherapist may mirror certain bodily reactions and guide the patient towards increased awareness of use of the body. This may be essential for many (chronic) pain patients, as they do not seem to have a sense of how they use (and tense) their body in many life situations. In fact touch (and passive movement) may be essential in many bodily-perception trainings. Furthermore, touch deprivation may be one essential aspect of chronic pain and suffering.

- Gentle passive movements, especially passive physiological movements, may guide patients to assist in active moving, followed by active movements (Zusman 1991). This approach may be particularly beneficial in those cases in which active movement does not seem to be possible.

- In those cases where touch and passive movement do not seem to be possible, active movement frequently is also difficult. A salutogenic approach towards active testing and passive movement may enhance selection of treatment interventions, including passive movement and touch (see Chapter 2).

- As manipulative physiotherapists frequently will select and apply other interventions beyond passive mobilizations to optimize the movement potential of the patient, it is essential to monitor the treatment outcomes of each intervention by regular re-assessment procedures.
- Summarizing the treatment effects in the reassessment phase after a passive mobilization technique is an essential feature of a cognitive behavioural attitude towards treatment, 'since we moved your neck, it seems now that you move more freely, like you said. Now we should seek similar movements, which you can perform by yourself, so that you can keep control over the pain by yourself.'

If passive movements are used judiciously in combination with self-management strategies, patient education and communication, musculoskeletal (manipulative) physiotherapists have a lot to offer in the treatment of painful movement disorders and the secondary prevention of chronic disability due to pain.

Figure 8.1 delineates the possible role of passive mobilization and/or manipulation within the overall physiotherapeutic process.

Underlying mechanisms of passive movements

The underlying mechanisms of passive manipulative treatment have been described from different perspectives as biomechanics, tissue biology, neurophysiology and, partially, biochemistry. Early explanations included adjusting joint subluxations, restoring bony alignment and reducing nuclear protrusions. However it has been demonstrated that these theories have not found an acceptable scientific basis (Twomey 1992). Based on a literature review, it is postulated that the biological effects may be found in improvement of nutrition of spinal discs and vertebral joints, metabolic effects in synovia, subchondral bone and ligamentous and capsular structure, as well as fluid exchange between tissues (Twomey 1992). Neurophysiological effects, in particular, have received much attention in many publications (Wright 1995). In a study with 38

subjects with mild or moderate knee pain, passive accessory movements were compared with manual contact and no contact interventions. Pain pressure thresholds were described as increasing significantly in the mobilization group, locally in the knee, but also more distal from the affected joints (Moss et al. 2007). Similar results have been achieved in other studies on the spine (Vicenzino et al. 1998b, Sterling et al. 2001), elbow (Paungmali et al. 2003) and ankle (Yeo & Wright 2011). The authors postulated that local physiological, cellular mechanisms, such as alteration in concentration of inflammatory agents e.g. prostaglandin PGE_2, as well as central nervous system mechanisms, could be involved in this phenomenon. The central mechanisms could include activation of local segmental inhibitory pathways in the spinal cord as well as descending inhibitory pathways from the brainstem (Moss et al. 2007). Sympathoexcitory effects have been described by various authors (Chiu & Wright 1996, Sterling et al. 2001), with effects on cardiorespiratory systems, as well as sudomotor and peripheral vasomotor changes (Vicenzino et al. 1998a). Based on a literature-review, Schmid et al. (2008) conclude that descending pathways may play a key role in manipulative physiotherapeutic induced hypoalgesia, with consistency for concurrent hypoalgesia, sympathetic nervous system excitation and changes in motor function. These notions are confirmed by Bialosky et al. (2008), who suggest a model in which a cascade of neurophysiological responses from the peripheral and central nervous system may be responsible for the therapeutic effects. Zusman (2004) proposes three neurological mechanisms as an explanation for the effects of manipulative physiotherapy:

1. Input by repeated stimuli, for example oscillatory passive movement and its progression, would lead to a desensitization of the nervous system with restoration of normal system sensory processing

2. Based on central learning theory and neuroplasticity, habituation of sensomotor processes, in which synaptic learning would lead to decreased behavioural responses to repeated stimulation; and

3. (Averse memory) extinction of protective, unfavourable sensomotoric patterns, by offering the nervous system different, normal sensomotor stimuli with passive and active movements.

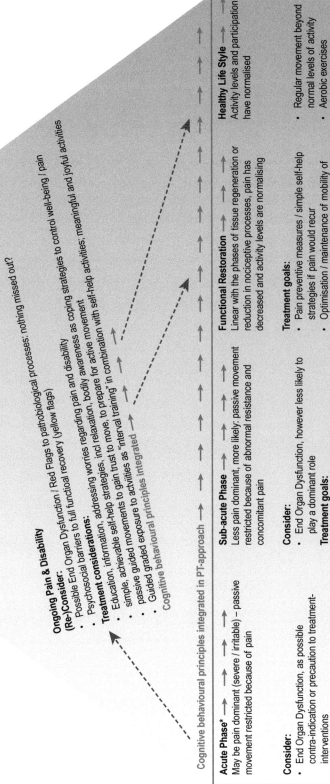

Cognitive behavioural principles integrated in PT-approach →

Ongoing Pain & Disability
(Re-)Consider:
· Possible End Organ Dysfunction / Red Flags to pathobiological processes: nothing missed out?
· Psychosocial barriers to full functioal recovery (yellow flags)

Treatment considerations:
· Education, information, addressing worries regarding pain and disability
· simple, achievable self-help strategies, incl relaxation, bodily awareness as coping strategies to control well-being / pain
· passive guided movements to gain trust to move, to prepare for active movement
· Guided graded exposure to activities as "interval training" in combination with self-help activities; meaningful and joyful activities
· Cognitive behavioural principles integrated

Healthy Life Style
Activity levels and participation have normalised

· Regular movement beyond normal levels of activity
· Aerobic exercises
· Flexibility exercises
· Agility exercises
· Resistance exercises

Functional Restoration
Linear with the phases of tissue regeneration or reduction in nociceptive processes, pain has decreased and activity levels are normalising

Treatment goals:
· Pain preventive measures / simple self-help strategies if pain would recur
· Optimisation / maintenance of mobility of movement-components as joints ("functional corners"), neurodynamic structures, muscles, soft tissues (e.g. scar tissue)
· Optimisation / maintenance muscular control (local, global stabilisers) during functional activities
· Confidence to use the body
· Optimisation / maintenance of general fitness (aerobic, flexibility, agility, resistance exercises)

Treatment interventions:
· Elements of active movement therapies

Sub-acute Phase
Less pain dominant, more likely: passive movement restricted because of abnormal resistance and concomitant pain

Consider:
· End Organ Dysfunction, however less likely to play a dominant role

Treatment goals:
· Pain reduction / pain control
· secondary prevention: maintain activity levels as much as possible
· Normalisation of mobility of joints, neurodynamics (soft tissues, muscles)
· Optimisation of contributing factors as muscular control, posture, unhelpful thoughts, confidence to move

Treatment interventions:
· as in acute phase
· progression of treatment with passive mobilisation towards resistance / optimising mobility
· Self-management as in acute phase, may follow progression of treatment; include auto-mobilisations, muscular control, relaxation where necessary

Acute Phase*
May be pain dominant (severe / irritable) – passive movement restricted because of pain

Consider:
· End Organ Dysfunction, as possible contra-indication or precaution to treatment-interventions
· Neurophysiological pain mechanisms: likely peripheral nociceptive and/or peripheral neurogenic

Treatment goals:
· Pain reduction / pain control
· secondary prevention of ongoing pain and disability: maintain activity levels as much as possible and self-management strategies

Treatment interventions:
· address worries, information and education;
· check possible DLA inspite of pain – relate self-help strategies to pain control where necessary
· passive mobilisation / manipulation to control pain
· self-management strategies to control pain
· other modalities to control pain

*Overlap between all phases is possible

Figure 8.1 • Therapeutic process: phases of functional restoration towards full movement capacity and the role of passive mobilization within this process. Some patients develop on-going pain and disability, which needs to be recognised in a phase as early as possible, in order to adapt the treatment to the specific needs of the patient.

Functional restoration programmes and self-management

With the development of functional restoration programmes to sustain optimum movement capacity of an individual, it is essential to consider the person's context, lifestyle, needs and preferences. Some like the challenges of medical training and fitness machines, whilst others prefer to run and do exercises in a forest rather than in a gymnasium. Others may favour exercising to gentle music and following movement programmes that enhance a sense of inner contemplation, rather than intense training accompanied by loud music. Furthermore, with regard to contextual aspects: a mother who has three young children, and who takes care of a sick father-in-law, may need simple relaxation techniques and exercises which can be adapted to her daily life, rather than a pre-set exercise programme which demands that she reserves extra time in her schedule.

In a more traditional multidimensional approach to management, manipulative physiotherapists set the priorities of treatment firstly in reduction and control of the pain, in parallel with improvement of the movement-impairments. Often it is assumed that the patients themselves take the responsibility of rehabilitation on activity and participation levels: *'Now that my shoulder is better, I have resumed training in volleyball. Also I spoke with the boss and I'll start working again next week'.* Furthermore, it is assumed that the patient immediately understands and applies preventive and self-management measures at appropriate moments, and regains confidence to move and use the body again (Fig. 8.2). If these situations indeed do occur, the manipulative physiotherapist does not need to consider many treatment objectives of functional restoration or motivation to change lifestyle. However, probably more often than not, therapists needs to ask themselves why patients do not resume their activities, or do not seem to apply the suggestions/exercises of the therapist, or why they do not appear to have confidence to use the body in daily life.

Usually the hypotheses regarding the movement dysfunctions and concomitant neurophysiological pain mechanisms, precautions to treatment and the individual illness experience with assessment and probationary treatments will have been established after the first two–three therapy sessions. In order to plan a comprehensive treatment 'thinking from the end' can be a useful tool to help plan further treatment in this phase (Fig. 8.3), by asking the following questions:

- Which movement-impairments should be improved, if an ideal state could be achieved?
- Which activities must improve? Do any activities regarding participation need to be followed up?
- Is the general level of activity in daily life optimal, too low, or relatively high? If too low: how does one motivate the patient to increase levels of fitness and apply a fitness programme? If relatively high: are there any relaxation strategies that the patient may employ during daily life? Is there any disuse of structures by habituated movement patterns in daily life, which need to be addressed?
- Does the patient seem to trust the movement of his or her body in daily life? (If not: how can the manipulative physiotherapist guide the patient to the *experience*?)
- Does the patient move with an overly increased bodily awareness (and guarding) or seem to 'forget' the body during meaningful activities?

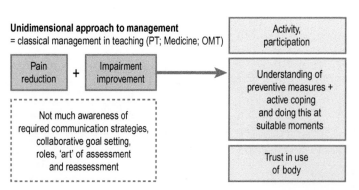

Unidimensional approach to management
= classical management in teaching (PT; Medicine; OMT)

Pain reduction + Impairment improvement →

Not much awareness of required communication strategies, collaborative goal setting, roles, 'art' of assessment and reassessment

Activity, participation

Understanding of preventive measures + active coping and doing this at suitable moments

Trust in use of body

Figure 8.2 • One-dimensional approach to treatment. Reproduced from Hengeveld (2000) with permission from Elsevier and Elly Hengeveld.

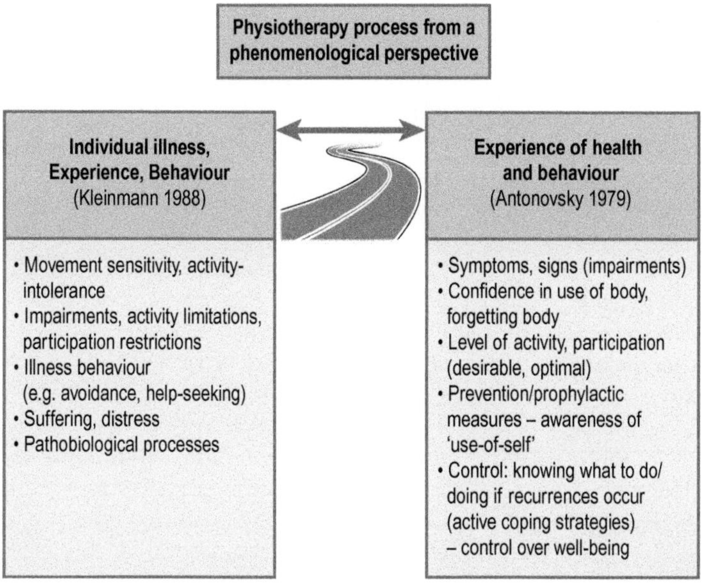

Physiotherapy process from a phenomenological perspective

Individual illness, Experience, Behaviour (Kleinmann 1988)	Experience of health and behaviour (Antonovsky 1979)
• Movement sensitivity, activity-intolerance • Impairments, activity limitations, participation restrictions • Illness behaviour (e.g. avoidance, help-seeking) • Suffering, distress • Pathobiological processes	• Symptoms, signs (impairments) • Confidence in use of body, forgetting body • Level of activity, participation (desirable, optimal) • Prevention/prophylactic measures – awareness of 'use-of-self' • Control: knowing what to do/doing if recurrences occur (active coping strategies) – control over well-being

Figure 8.3 • Manipulative physiotherapists guide patients on a disease-health continuum, towards a sense of health and well-being in movement functions. This approach guides physiotherapists in planning comprehensive treatment objectives. Reproduced from Hengeveld & Banks (2005) with permission from Elsevier.

- Is the patient aware of any preventive measures and how to use his or her body in everyday situations?
- Does the patient seem to have an adequate sense of control of the pain or well-being? If not, which measures or specific coping strategies should be undertaken?

Purposes of functional restoration programmes

Functional restoration programmes may fulfil different purposes:

- Self-help strategies to control pain and to promote a sense of well-being
- Rehabilitation of movement impairments
- Prevention of new episodes of symptoms
- Increase bodily awareness and relaxation, including the change in habitual movement patterns
- Enhancing trust to move and to participate with confidence in daily life activities
- Increase general fitness and optimization of activity levels.

1. Self-help strategies to control pain and to promote a sense of well-being. These may include:
   a. Repeated movements
   b. Automobilizations
   c. Relaxation strategies, including pendular exercises, visualization techniques, distraction
   d. Body and proprioceptive awareness
   e. Muscle control exercises
   f. Other pain management strategies, e.g. hot packs, cold packs.

   The therapist first needs to establish the sources of nociception and movement dysfunction with the specific examination procedures of manipulative physiotherapy. Then the way in which the movement dysfunction should be treated needs to be determined collaboratively with the patient 1) by means of the therapist with passive movement and touch and 2) by self-management strategies of the patient, to maintain the gains from treatment. Exercises and other self-management strategies primarily need to be based on information of the subjective examination (24-hour behaviour of symptoms; history; contributing factors) rather than information from inspection and active testing alone. For example, a woman with a flat thoracic spine, who usually works in flexed positions may control her pain best by repeated movements in extension and/or rotation, in spite of the flattened thoracic spine.

2. Rehabilitation of movement impairments such as joint mobility, neurodynamics and

muscle function, including automobilization exercises, neurodynamic 'slider and tensioner' techniques, muscle stretching/inhibition and muscular recruitment. The following aspects need to be taken into account:

a. Most of the exercises should maintain the gains from treatment with passive mobilization

b. The exercises need to reflect the current clinical stages of the patient's disorder, similarly to the selection and progression of treatment with passive movement

c. Particularly in peripheral joints, automobilizations can be similar to the passive mobilizations as performed by the therapist.

3. Prevention of new episodes of symptoms.

a. This may include recommendations from back-schools, muscular recruitment in everyday activities such as lifting things, increased awareness of body use (see above) and regular repetitive movements to compensate habitual patterns (e.g. repeated extension movements of the spine after sitting or pendular movements of the shoulder or knee after having been in an end-of-range position for a while).

b. Passive mobilization may be necessary to optimize joint function in the so-called 'functional corners', as for example shoulder-quadrant, extension abduction and extension adduction of the elbow or knee, or F/AD of the hip. This will ensure that the joints have a functional reserve capacity, when the movement system is asked to do a little more than it does normally. This functional reserve capacity will be a contributing factor to reduce the incidence of recurrent episodes, which is based on the following principle: 'the more limited a movement is, the more vulnerable the structures will be if moved beyond their currents limits'.

4. Increase bodily awareness and relaxation, including the change in habitual movement patterns.

a. Within the change of habits in work movements and postures, training of awareness of the use of the body may be necessary. Many patients may not be aware of how they use their bodies with tension and guarded movements, which in itself may be a contributing factor to ongoing pain and hypersensitivity of structures.

b. Often, patients need to learn the pacing of daily life activities. They may perform certain activities for too long in the same manner. However, the education of pacing strategies needs to be considered from a cognitive behavioural perspective, as the physiotherapist enters the patient's world of personal values and meanings. It may not always be easy to change habits that have evolved over many years of a lifetime.

c. The therapist may guide the patient by gentle communication techniques and touch towards a different perception of the use of the body, e.g. a woman who habitually sits with her shoulder pulled into elevation and protraction and flexion of her thoracic spine (Table 8.1).

5. Enhancing trust to move and to participate with confidence in daily life activities.

a. Frequently it is necessary for the manipulative physiotherapist to monitor whether the patient has regained trust to move in daily life situations. For example, is the patient confident to cross a street after a period of acute neck pain (requiring quick rotational movements)? Can the patient perform long periods of work that requires a lot of concentration (after an acceleration injury of the neck), or run to catch a bus after an episode of acute back pain? Frequently these automatic motor patterns have to be retrained, but it needs to be done in circumstances, which mirror the daily life situations as much as possible.

b. Another important element of moving with confidence is that a person normally is not aware of the body during meaningful activities. This 'forgetting of the body' is in a sense an aspect of a healthy experience. However, if symptoms should recur after a while, the patient ideally should integrate some of the recommended self-management strategies automatically.

c. Passive mobilizations may be a means to let patients experience movements again, which they did not dare to perform before. Again, passive mobilization may kickstart active movement.

Table 8.1 Various communication styles leading to different responses and awareness

Directive communication style	Mirroring, guiding by asking questions as a communication technique
PT: You should not sit like this. That will certainly provoke pain. I think it is better to observe in your daily life that you do not sit in so much tension. I will show it to you once again and I suggest you do this exercise three times a day and, of course, when it hurts as well *(shows the patient once again how to relax the shoulders more towards a neutral position)* Pat: Okay PT: I'll see you then, next time	PT: How are you now? Pat: It hurts me at my shoulder PT: Do you notice anything different about your posture? Pat: No PT: I observe that you have pulled you shoulder forwards and upwards (mirrors the positions) Pat: *(Observes herself now)* – Oh yes, that's right (but does not change anything immediately) PT: Would you be able to change something? Pat: *(Pulls shoulders very far down and in retraction)* Like this? PT: Maybe a bit less *(guides the movement)* How does it feel now? Pat: That feels fine PT: Does anything hurt you right now? Pat: No PT: You mean there is none of that shoulder pain you had just now? Pat: No PT: Could you please pull your shoulder upwards and forwards, like you did before? Pat (Performs the movement) PT: How does it feel right now? Pat: That hurts at my shoulder (but does not change automatically) PT: How about trying to relax your shoulder again? *(Guides the movement with contact)* Pat: Now it's gone indeed PT: Could you please do this again? Pat: *(Pulls the shoulder up again)* That hurts again
Next session	PT: And if you change the position again?
PT: How have you been since last time? Pat: I still have pain PT: Have you been able to do that exercise which I showed you last time? Pat: Yes PT: Could you show me once again? Pat: Hmm, I don't know if I have done it right, could you show me once again? In such cases the physiotherapist (PT) may be disappointed that the patient (Pat) seems to have forgotten the exercise. However, this may be due to that particular moment during the session (in the last few minutes) and the quality of communication.	Pat: *(Performs the movements without the aid of the physiotherapist)* Now it is much better again In this case the reassessment is not only the evaluation of the symptom responses, but also if the patient automatically changes her movement behaviour, as happened in the third repetition. To follow the sequence with cognitive reinforcement and explanation will often be useful. PT: I suggest you observe yourself now and again during the day, this afternoon and tomorrow. Maybe you'll notice that you pull up your shoulders more often. We all move often automatically, without thinking. I notice that with myself as well. Shall I explain what may happen in your body when you perform such movements? Pat: Yes, please PT: *Explains the principle of the bent finger* (McKenzie 1981) Pat: Ahah! PT: Could you imagine that similar things happen in your shoulder? Pat: Oh well, yes PT: I have explained a lot to you – however, I am not sure if I've done a good job. Would you mind telling me in your own words what you've understood? Pat: If I am sitting in such a tensed position, the blood circulation is in trouble. If I move differently it is better This has been a reassessment on a cognitive level. If the patient is invited to explain in her own words, the physiotherapist immediately understands whether the explanation 'touched ground', and in patients themselves deeper understanding may be enhanced. PT: Then I would like to suggest that you pay attention a few times during the day, if you happen to pull your shoulders upwards. Especially when you feel that it is hurting again. Maybe you could just try this simple exercise then. If it helps you enough, then we come closer to the understanding of your problem. If it does not help you enough, then we have to look for alternatives. So, please, if you could try it, and feel free to tell me if you feel it is not successful enough …

Reproduced from Banks and Hengeveld (2010) with permission from Elsevier.

6. Increase general fitness, optimization of activity levels and changes in lifestyle.

   a. Many patients may need to increase their general physical fitness levels with physiological stimuli to improve cardiovascular condition, overall strength and agility.

   b. Persons who have been avoiding activities may be physically deconditioned and may need reconditioning programmes with graded exposure to activity.

   c. However, passive movement may be considered as a graded loading of structures and may become, in combination with well-guided reassessment procedures, a first step in the graded exposure to activities. In fact passive movement may be of support in the restoration of movement tolerance and acceptance, particularly in those cases where the patient has lost confidence in any active movement.

   d. Furthermore, passive movement may ensure reserve capacity in mobility to maximize performance. This follows the same principle as stated above under the heading of prevention (optimizing mobility in 'functional corners' of, for example, the shoulder, hip, elbow, knee).

In planning functional restoration programmes, cognitive behavioural principles should be considered to enhance treatment outcomes.

Cognitive behavioural principles

As stated in Chapter 2 physiotherapists play an important role in changing patients' behaviour, particularly in relation to movement and functional capacity. It has been postulated that the integration of cognitive behavioural principles may enhance therapeutic outcome (Bunzli et al. 2011). It is essential to see these principles as an integral part of physiotherapy practice and not as a substitute.

It is recognized that behaviour and habits will not change overnight after a single instruction of an exercise. Part of the work of physiotherapists involves change management, in which motivation, increasing awareness and careful planning of all steps in the therapeutic process are essential. It is necessary to recognize that patients may go through different motivational phases, in which the recognition

and guidance by the therapist may be crucial to final therapeutic outcomes.

The role of cognitive behavioural practice will apply in both the application of mobilization and manipulation, and more particularly in achieving the desired effect of maximizing functional capacity. This may encompass:

- Changes in movement behaviour in daily life – if pain or discomfort occurs, individuals learn to perform certain movements
- Changes in habitual patterns of movement in daily life, which may be a causative factor of pain
- Motivation to change behaviour with regard to training and maintaining fitness
- By means of information and educational strategies patients may develop a different perspective on their problem, for example, the meaning of pain as a threat may change; therefore, the patient is empowered to develop different coping strategies.

Next to skilled communication, the key cognitive behavioural aspects that may need to be integrated into physiotherapeutic approaches include:

- Recognition of potential barriers to full functional recovery
- The process of collaborative goal-setting
- Phases of change
- Compliance enhancement
- Patient education.

Recognition of potential barriers to full functional recovery

If individuals may not recuperate to full functional activities, it is recommended to take a biopsychosocial perspective. On the one hand, it is essential to consider possible pathobiological processes ('red flags'), which may have been missed out in the initial diagnostic process or psychosocial aspects, contributing to the pain and disability. It is important not to neglect the 'bio' viewpoint on patients' problems, even in the presence of psychosocial aspects (Box 8.1; Hancock et al. 2011).

On the other hand several potential psychosocial barriers to full functional recovery have been described and summarized in the term 'yellow flags' (Kendall et al. 1997, Watson & Kendall 2000, Waddell 2004). They have been described in a

Box 8.1

Screening of bodily systems

When indicated, various body systems should be screened in the first physiotherapy consultation or if patients do not seem to recuperate to full functional activities, in order to identify pathological processes which require the attention and diagnosis of another specialist. Screening of the following bodily systems is suggested:

- Cardiovascular system
- Pulmonary system
- Gastrointestinal system
- Urogenital system
- Endocrine system
- Nervous system
- Pathological origins of head and facial pain
- Musculoskeletal system disease
- Rheumatic disease
- Psychiatric disorders
- Skin disorders.

For detailed reading, consult Boissonnault (2010) and Goodman & Snyder (2012).

In general, information from the basic examination procedures of the manipulative physiotherapist may highlight situations in which patients need referral to an appropriate medical practitioner (Refshauge & Gass 1995):

- Any severe unremitting pain
- Any severe unremitting pain that stays the same or worsens despite rest, analgesia or appropriate intervention
- Severe pain with little disturbance of movement
- Severe night pain
- Worsening neurological deficit despite appropriate intervention
- Non-mechanical behaviour (e.g. excellent response to anti-inflammatory medication, little movement disturbance, lack of response to analgesia, unusual pain patterns, inability to ease symptoms by positioning or postures or movement, heat or other modalities, long-lasting morning stiffness)
- Severe pain without major trauma (or severe undiagnosed pain following major trauma) or a relatively minor incident in history leading to severe pain and disability
- Severe muscle reactions ('spasm')
- Marked trauma prior to the current symptoms.

---

mnemonic 'ABCDEFW', which does *not* indicate a ranking in relative importance (Kendall et al. 1997). The yellow flags as they are related to physiotherapy practice are outlined in Box 8.2.

It is critical to avoiding pejorative labelling of patients with yellow flags as this will have a negative effect on the attitudes of clinicians and management of the patient's problem (Kendall et al. 1997). Predicting poor outcomes in acute nociceptive pain states with the presence of relevant yellow flags should lead to different approaches to treatment rather than denying therapy or shifting patients over to psychiatrists.

Within the physiotherapeutic process the most relevant yellow flags may be summarized as below (Hengeveld 2003). They need to be considered in clinical reasoning processes with the hypotheses categories 'individual illness experience' or 'contributing factors'.

'Perceived disability'

The perceived disability is an important element of the individual illness-experience. If this perception does not seem related to the phases of tissue regeneration or normalization of nociceptive processes, it needs to be specifically addressed in treatment, whether with educational strategies or direct experiences with activities which the patient feels may not be possible. However, this may need patience and careful planning by the therapist. A first impression of the perceived disability may be gained when at initial assessment the therapist asks about the patient's main problem and then completes the question with a more general question: 'how does this problem interfere with your daily life: none at all, moderate or strong?'

'Beliefs and expectations'

'Beliefs and expectations' can refer to the causes of the problem, as well to as the possible treatment options.

- Regarding causes and treatment option, the therapist needs to be aware that the patient may follow different paradigms from the therapist. If the patient has a more biomedical, structural oriented paradigm, while the

Box 8.2

Psychosocial risk factors to long-term disability with relevance to physiotherapy practice

Attitudes and beliefs about pain

- Belief that pain is harmful or disabling resulting in fear avoidance behaviour (e.g. the development of guarding movements and fear of movement)
- Belief that all pain must be abolished before attempting to return to work or normal activity
- Expectation of increased pain with activity or work, lack of ability to predict capability
- Catastrophizing, thinking the worst, misinterpreting bodily symptoms
- Belief that pain is uncontrollable
- Passive attitude to rehabilitation.

Behaviours

- Use of extended rest, disproportionate 'downtime'
- Reduced activity levels with significant withdrawal from daily activities, avoidance of normal activities and progressive substitution of lifestyle away from productive activity
- Irregular participation or poor compliance with physical exercise
- Excessive reliance on use of aids or appliances
- Increased intake of alcohol or other substances since onset of pain.

Compensation issues

- Lack of financial incentive to return to work
- History of claim(s) due to other pain problems
- Previous experience of ineffective case management (e.g. absence of interest, perception of being treated punitively).

Diagnosis and treatment

- Health professionals sanctioning disability, not providing interventions that will improve function
- Experience of conflicting diagnoses and explanations, resulting in confusion

- Diagnostic language leading to catastrophizing and fear
- Dramatization of back pain by health professional producing dependency on treatments, and continuation of passive treatment
- Advice to withdraw from job and other relevant activities.

Emotions

- Fear of increased pain with activity or work
- Long-term low mood, loss of sense of enjoyment
- Anxiety about and heightened awareness of bodily sensations
- Feeling under stress and unable to maintain a sense of control
- Feeling useless and not needed.

Family

- Overprotective partner/spouse; solicitous behaviour of spouse (e.g. taking over tasks)
- Extent to which family members support any attempt to return to work or other relevant activities
- Lack of support person to talk with about problems.

Work

- Job involving high biomechanical demands with maintenance of constrained or sustained postures; inflexible work schedule preventing appropriate breaks
- Belief that work is harmful, that it will cause damage or be dangerous
- Minimal availability of selected duties and graduated return to work pathways, with unsatisfactory implementation of these
- Absence of interest of employer

Adapted from Kendall et al. 1997.

---

physiotherapist follows a movement paradigm, confusion and insecurity may result if this is not clarified in the early phases of a treatment series. Therefore, time should be allocated in the 'welcoming phase' of treatment, to address the various approaches which may be possible and to emphasize the paradigms of the physiotherapist as a specialist for the diagnosis and treatment of movement dysfunctions. Some communication examples are given in

Chapter 3, Communication and the therapeutic relationship.

- Over the course of treatment, if patients seem to relate their pain and disability strongly to an incident which lies many years back, it may be useful to invest time on educational strategies, in which it is gently clarified that the things which caused that start of the nociceptive processes may not be those aspects which maintain them. It is discussed that a pain experience often changes over time, due to interactions between the individual, his or her environment and medical professionals (Delvecchio Good et al. 1992), and due to an increasing influence of cognitive, emotional and behavioural factors (Vlaeyen & Crombez 1999).

- In addressing the coping strategies that the patient performs when the pain occurs, it is possible that patients perceive a sense of helplessness, by stating that 'they cannot do anything to influence the pain'. In these cases it is essential to look for any instinctive postures or intuitive movements made by the patients. Very often these particular postures and movements may be integrated into therapy; for example, patients may state that they cannot do anything to help their pain while simultaneously placing their hands on their back and bending slightly away from the painful side. By making the patient aware that they already do something instinctively to help their pain, the therapist could suggest that this might even be a useful strategy if done deliberately, repeated and in a more relaxed way – and so, from the perspective of passive movements, the therapist may start treatment in combined flexion/sideflexion directions away from the painful side. Often patients may not be aware that they instinctively perform very useful strategies; the therapists' role may be to make the patient aware and to reinforce this behaviour by encouragement and subtle guidance.

Confidence in own capabilities

The topic of patients' confidence in their own capabilities to control pain and/or well-being is linked to beliefs and expectations, as discussed above.

If a patient shows little confidence and demonstrates strong protective movement behaviour or even a fear to move the performance of physical examination may be challenging, particularly if the physiotherapist emphasizes pain reproduction as the sole parameter to assessment. It has been acknowledged that a clinician's behaviour may reinforce the illness behaviour and experience of the patient (Hadler 1996, Pilowsky 1997). In such a situation it may be possible that careful guiding only until the onset of pain ('P$_1$') and *immediately* away from the point of pain, in fact may *reinforce* the maladaptive or unhelpful behaviour. Test movements may be taken '*slightly beyond* the onset of pain', rather than

'until the onset of pain'. A point in the movement may occur where the patient indicates that the pain increases. The therapist then gently moves back in the movement to check if the pain subsides quickly enough, then progresses to the onset of pain again, at the same time enquiring if the patient has the trust to move a bit further. For example, if the patient is able to move until 90° of arm flexion before the pain starts, but stills trusts to move until 110°, the therapist has found two important variables in the test movement:

- P$_1$ at 90° of flexion
- 'Trust 1' at 110° of flexion, indicating the point in the movement at which the patient trusted to move to, in spite of the pain.

In fact, this approach to physical examination in cases of strong fear-avoidance behaviour may be considered as a first step toward *guided graded-exposure-to-activity*.

The communication example in Box 8.3 may explain some of the subtleties of the examination process in these circumstances.

Sense-of-control over well-being and movement behaviour when pain occurs

A patient's sense of control over their own well-being and movement behaviour when the pain occurs are both partially linked to beliefs and expectation, but also to direct behaviour.

The subjective examination phase, in which it is assessed when symptoms would increase, is particularly important for obtaining information about the sense of control and the behaviour leading to the increase in pain, as well as the behaviour used in controlling the pain or well-being. This phase of the examination may be an important learning stage for the patient, to link the activities to the onset of pain, as well as to the reduction of pain. Therefore, the potential of 'patient-empowerment' (Klaber Moffet & Richardson 1997) is very high at this initial stage of examination.

Opinions of other clinicians

If a patient has seen various clinicians, e.g. different medical specialists but also more than one physiotherapist, they may be left feeling insecure and confused from all the different opinions they may have received. In particular this may be the case if the patient's implicit expectation is that there is only one cure to the problem, and that the problem will

Box 8.3

Verbatim example of a possible approach to examination procedures in case of extreme guarding of movements

(ET, Examiner's thoughts; Q, question; A, answer)

Q 'I would like to examine the movements of your arm – how far you may be able to move the arm, and if some movements are okay but others provoke discomfort. However, I would not like to push you into any movements that you are not confident of doing yourself. Will you give me a sign if that happens?'

A 'Oh yes.'

Q 'Could you lift your arm up, as far as you trust yourself to do?'

A (*moves until c. 90° flexion*) 'Oh no, not further than this.'

Q (*takes off the weight of the arm and slightly back to c. 80° of flexion*) 'And if I move it like this?'

A 'Now it is alright again.'

Q (*moves arm gently back to 90° of flexion*) 'And now here again?'

A (*grimaces*) 'Oh, there it hurts again.'

Q (*back to 80° of flexion*) 'Now, okay again?'

A 'Yes.'

Q 'Was the pain the second time the same as the first time? Or did it get worse the second time?'

A 'No, it was the same.'

ET If the pain had increased the second time I would stop the testing now. However, it seems to have more of an 'on–off' character than I initially thought. I want him to move the arm gently 'beyond P$_1$'.

Q 'Okay, could I gently take you back to that point of pain?'

A 'Okay.'

Q 'Now it hurts again?'

A 'Yes.'

Q 'Would you trust yourself to move a bit further in spite of the pain? Only as far as what you trust to move!'

A (*grimaces and moves until c. 110°*) 'Until here.'

Q 'Okay, and back again. How are you now?'

A 'It's alright again.'

Q 'I would like you to remember this movement, as we will check it later in therapy again – maybe your pain has changed after the treatment or maybe you will trust to lift your arm a bit higher.'

Performance of an examination in such a manner requires an awareness of the subtleties of communication and the effects of touch during the examination process. In fact the patient may learn various aspects from the examination procedures, for example:

- The pain may be more movement dependent than initially believed
- There may be movements which provoke more discomfort and there may be movements which are less uncomfortable instead of believing that everything hurts all the time in the same manner
- It is not dangerous to move carefully beyond the point where a pain has commenced
- The patient may learn to trust the physiotherapist, as the questioning and testing indicated to the patient that they would not be forced to move in ways in which they themselves did not trust.

A procedure performed in such a manner may be seen as an expression of a bio-psychosocial approach to initial treatment of fear avoidance behaviour with regard to movements and activities. Hence, the gradual exposure to activities may start with the first physical examination procedures.

---

be just normalized or removed. A possible remark indicating this could be, for example: 'everybody says something different, why don't they find it and fix it?' It may be essential to take time and discuss with the patient the challenges and possibilities which may lie in all the different paradigms and viewpoints they may have encountered during their quest to relieve their pain. In fact, it may be necessary to address the issue of the numerous encounters explicitly, in order to gain the patient's trust:

> Team members must, therefore, take great care with not only what they say, but also how they speak and behave. They should have the ability to put patients at

their ease. Patients will disclose more information if they have confidence that clinicians are being honest and non-judgemental. Patients will have been seen by a number of other specialists. Usually these consultations have been very short, often not with a consultant, but with a trainee, whose communication skills may not be well developed. It may have been implied, that the pain is 'all in the head' or that patients are exaggerating their pain. The patient may even have been invited to see a psychiatrist.

> The team member, therefore, generally has a considerable amount of repair work to do in order to gain the patient's confidence and impress upon the patient that this consultation will be different.

(Main & Spanswick, 2000; pp. 120 &121)

Level of activities and participation

The level of activities may be low and the patient may have been labelled as 'physically deconditioned' and suffering from 'kinesiophobia'. Although reconditioning programmes towards a better physical condition will be necessary in many cases, it is important to realize that a term such as 'kinesiophobia' is somewhat awkward, as the behaviour leading to the avoidance of activities is in principle healthy, protective behaviour, which has become maladaptive over the course of time. A phobia is a psychiatric term described in DSM-IV (Diagnostic and Statistical Manual of Mental Disorders, 4e; American Psychiatric Association 2000) and should stay in the realm of psychopathology. In fact, avoidance behaviour may be linked to aspects other than an avoidance to move, e.g. avoiding meaningful social activities such as accepting dinner invitations or going to the theatre (Philips & Jahanshani 1986, Philips 1987). Therefore this kind of behaviour may be considered to be a social avoidance of meaningful and joyful stimuli.

Reactions of social environment

It has been recognized for a long time that the social environment (e.g. spouse, boss, colleagues, friends) may have a direct influence on the behaviour and perception of a person with pain (Kleinmann 1988, Pilowsky 1997, Delvecchio Good et al. 1992, Kendall et al. 1997). Illness behaviour, with stress reactions or a sense of threat, may be reinforced by certain rewards, but also by punishing behaviour of the social environment. Constructs of 'gain' are likely placed under the umbrella of 'reactions of the environment'. Secondary gain, which is claimed to play a role in the generation and maintenance of illness behaviour, may too readily lead to stigmatizing towards malingering (Fishbain 1994). Secondary gain is described as a social advantage attained by a person as a consequence of an illness; however, tertiary gains may also exist, in which others in the direct environment benefit from the illness of the person. It is warned not to focus solely on the secondary gain of a person with pain without asking what may be the secondary losses to the person as well (Fishbain 1994).

The process of collaborative goal-setting

The development of a therapeutic relationship is an essential element of a cognitive behavioural approach to treatment. It has been postulated that a constructive therapeutic relationship supports patients' satisfaction of treatment and aids in the development of trust (May 2001). It appears to enhance treatment outcomes (Foster et al. 2008, Bunzli et al. 2011). It is recommended that within a therapeutic relationship patients need to be treated as equals and experts in their own right. Within this practice following a process of collaborative goal-setting is recommended (Main & Spanswick 2000).

There are indications that compliance with the recommendations, instructions and exercises may increase if treatment objectives are defined in a collaborative rather than a directive way (Riolo 1995, Sluys et al. 1993, Bassett & Petrie 1997, Middleton 2004, McLean et al. 2010).

It is essential to consider collaborative goal-setting as a process throughout all treatment sessions rather than only at the beginning of the treatment series. In fact, ongoing information and goal-setting may be considered essential elements of the process of informed consent.

Various agreements between the physiotherapist and patient may be made in the process of collaborative goal-setting:

- Initially the physiotherapist and patient need to define treatment objectives collaboratively
- Additionally, the parameters to monitor treatment results may be defined in a collaborative way
- The physiotherapist and patient need to collaborate on the selection of interventions to achieve the desired outcomes
- In situations where 'sensitive practice' seems especially relevant, some patients may need to be given the choice of a male or a female physiotherapist or may express their preference regarding a more open or an enclosed treatment room (Schachter et al. 1999).

Frequently, physiotherapists may ask a patient at the end of the subjective examination what would be the goal of treatment. Often the response will be that the patient would like to have less pain and no further clarification of this objective takes place. In some cases this approach may be too superficial, especially if the prognosis is that diminution of pain intensity and frequency may not be easily achieved. This may be the case in certain chronic pain states or where secondary prevention of chronic disability seems necessary. Patients commonly state that their goal of treatment is 'having less pain'; however, after being asked some clarifying questions it often transpires that they wish to find more control over their well-being with regard to pain, in order to be able to resume certain activities.

In the initial session during subjective examination, various stages occur in which collaborative goal-setting may take place by the communication technique of summarizing:

- After establishment of the main problem and the areas in which the patient may feel the symptoms
- After the establishment of the 24-hour behaviour of symptoms, activity levels and coping strategies
- After establishment of the history
- After completion of the physical examination (at this stage it is essential to establish treatment objectives collaboratively, not only in the reduction of pain, but also to define clear goals on the levels of activity which need to be improved and in which circumstances the patient may need self-management strategies to increase control over wellbeing and pain).

The relatively detailed process of collaborative goal-setting needs to be continued during the initial phase of each session. It is essential to clarify if the earlier agreed goals are still to be followed up. If possible, it is useful to explain to the patient the diverse treatment options on how the goals may be achieved and then let the patient make the choice of the interventions.

Another phase of collaborative goal-setting takes place in later stages during retrospective assessment procedures. In this phase a reconsideration of treatment objectives is often necessary. Initially the physiotherapist and patient may have agreed to work on improvement of pain, pain control with self-management strategies, educational strategies with regard to pain and movement, and to treat impairments of local functions, such as pain-free joint movement and muscular recruitment. In later stages it is essential to establish goals with regard to activities that are meaningful for the patient. If a patient is able to return to work after a certain period of sick leave, it is important to know about those activities which the patient seems most concerned about and where the patient expects to develop symptoms again. For example, an electrician who needs to kneel down in order to perform a task close to the floor may be afraid that in this case his back will start to hurt again. It may be necessary to include this activity in the training programme in combination with simple self-management strategies, which can be employed immediately in the work place.

This phase of retrospective assessment, including a prospective assessment with redefinition of treatment objectives on activity and participation levels, is considered to be one of the most important phases of the rehabilitation of patients with movement disorders (Maitland 1986).

To summarize, the process of collaborative goal-setting should include the following aspects (Brioschi 1998):

- The reason for referral to physiotherapy
- The patient's definition of the problem, including goals and expectations
- Clarification of questions with regard to setting, frequency and duration of treatment
- Hypotheses and summary of findings of the physiotherapist, and clarification of the possibilities and limitations of the physiotherapist, resulting in agreements, collaborative goal definitions, and a verbal, or sometimes written, treatment contract.

Phases of change

It has been suggested that individuals may go through various phases of motivation before they start to change behaviour (Box 8.4; Prochaska & DiClemente 1994, van der Burght & Verhulst 1997, Dijkstra 2002). Habits rarely change overnight and people will go through phases in which the intention may exist to change behaviour, but distractions and tasks in daily life, as well as other habits, may hinder the patient from automatically and consequently incorporating the suggested behaviour immediately. Physiotherapists have to be aware of these phases and adapt their instructions, recommendations and treatment accordingly.

It appears that explicitly recognizing and working with the phases of change may enhance compliance or adherence to suggestions and exercises more than other interventions, for example supporting materials. Based on a literature-review, McLean et al. (2010) concluded that there was moderate evidence that a motivational cognitive behavioural (CB) programme can improve attendance at exercise-based clinic sessions.

Box 8.4

Phases of change model

1. Pre-contemplation: in this phase it is not considered to change behaviour
2. Contemplation: change of behaviour is considered; however, no concrete plan exists
3. Preparation: plans are developed actively to change behaviour in the short term
4. Action: phase in which the desired behaviour is performed
5. Consolidation: the desired behaviour is maintained, also without contact with the clinician, and fall-backs in behaviour are being prevented.

1. Pre-contemplation

- Investigation of beliefs and expectations of the patient
- Process of collaborative goal-setting is essential
- Information and education with regard to pain mechanisms; usefulness of movements to enhance well-being, to influence pain and to support healing processes (e.g. with discal problems or osteoarthritis)
- Patient needs to experience directly that the exercises contribute to well-being (by skilled reassessment procedures)
- Attention to the quality of the educational processes is essential – did the education contribute to more understanding and motivation?

2. Contemplation

- Frequently neglected in educational sessions: has the patient understood the educational message?
- Does the patient consider the given information useful?
- Allow time to ask questions concerning the information given
- Furthermore, over a period of several sessions it is essential to give the patient sufficient time to ask questions and seek clarifications
- Enhance positive feedback by performing a reassessment after an exercise has been instructed (sometimes only seeking information of the sense of pain or well-being respectively – 'present pain')
- What kind of plans or possibilities would the patients see themselves to change the behaviour? Where would they perceive barriers? In which way would they be able to overcome the barriers and implement the plan to change behaviour?

Adapted from Prochaska & DiClemente 1994.

3. Preparation

- It is often useful to suggest one or two exercises to perform in daily life
- In this phase it is essential that the patient can experience that movement and relaxation may contribute to well-being. Perceived success, including a sense of achievement, appears to be a relevant factor in compliance to exercises (Courneya et al. 2004). Hence, reassessment of subjective findings and physical examination tests will contribute to a sense of success.
- Check regularly in reassessment procedures at the beginning of follow up sessions, if the patient has been capable of performing the exercises at the moment that pain occurred.
- Clear information is needed: when to do the exercises in daily life, in which frequency, what the patient should observe during and after the exercise.
- Confirm with the patient when it was possible to do the exercises and when difficulties existed. What did the patient experience during and after the exercise?
- Control whether the suggested interventions brought the desired results.

4. Action

- The exercises and other recommendations should be simple, manageable and achievable as well as integrated into daily life situations and provide a sense of success
- If an exercise/instruction appears to be useful during the treatment session, the therapist needs to find out if the exercises can be performed in the same manner during daily life situations – if not, variations of the same movement need to be sought in a collaborative problem-solving process with the patient
- It is essential that the physiotherapist keeps checking in reassessment procedures if the patient is able to apply the suggested (movement) behaviour, or if adaptations are necessary

5. Consolidation

- Anticipation on likely future difficulties and possible strategies, which could be employed if the given difficulty would (re)occur.

Compliance

Compliance is described as the degree to which the behaviour of a client coincides with the recommendations of the clinician (Schneiders et al. 1998). At times the word 'adherence' is used as well. However, both terms are somewhat awkward, as they indicate too strongly an authoritarian one-dimensional patient–clinician relationship in which the patient has to follow the orders of the clinician in a passive role (Kleinman 1997). Within this context a focus on the change of unfavourable (movement) behaviours in daily life is recommended, hence taking a cognitive–behavioural perspective in which the term 'compliance' is associated with a more active role for the patient.

Barriers to compliance

It seems that compliance to medical or physiotherapy interventions ranges from 15 to 94%, depending on the way the studies were performed (Sluys & Hermans 1990, Ferri et al. 1998). There appear to be different opinions as to why patients do not follow the advice, recommendations or exercises given by a physiotherapist. It appears that many physiotherapists contribute this to patients' lack of motivation or discipline (Kok & Bouter 1990).

However, a profound study indicates several categories of barriers perceived by patients to the suggested behaviours (Sluys 1991):

- Barriers to incorporating the suggestions and exercises into daily life (e.g. exercises in supine cannot be performed in a work setting; not enough time to exercise every day for 30 minutes; directive goal-setting such as 'you should take more time off for yourself'; too many instructions and suggestions in one treatment session)
- Lack of positive feedback (insecurity as to whether the exercises are performed in the correct manner; no experience if the exercises truly are helpful)
- Sense of helplessness (the patient does not experience an ability to influence the situation positively).

Compliance enhancement

Various strategies may need to be employed to enhance the patient compliance to the physiotherapist's suggestions, recommendations and instructions. This may include motivational phases, short-term and long-term compliance:

- *Motivational phase:*
  - Consider the various phases of changes through which a patient may go and adapt the treatment accordingly (see above).
  - Include patient education sessions on pain, neurophysiological pain mechanisms and the role of movement in tissue regeneration or modulation/neuroplastic changes of nociceptive processes.
- *Short-term compliance:*
  - The phase of short-term compliance starts once the patient begins to experiment with a few simple exercises in daily life.
  - The desired effect should not be expected immediately, nor should the patient be expected to perform the exercises at all the appropriate moments in his/her daily life.
  - Often it is better to start off with one or two exercises and to check whether they are helpful, before integrating others into the self-management pain control programme.
  - Regular contact between the physiotherapist and patient is essential, in which the patient can ask questions and the physiotherapist can give corrections or suggestions.
  - The physiotherapist may need to motivate the patient to 'hang on' to the exercises, even if no immediate results are experienced yet.
  - During the subjective reassessment in follow-up sessions, the physiotherapist should find out whether the patient has been able to perform the exercises and if they have done them at appropriate times of the day. Patients may do the exercises at fixed times of the day; however, when pain increases they often stay in the habituated behaviour of resting or taking medication, rather than trying out the suggested interventions. It is essential that the physiotherapist does not consider this as a lack of motivation, but as a new help-seeking behaviour which has not been habituated yet. The style of communication may substantially influence this process of learning and experimenting with exercises in various daily life situations.

* *Long-term compliance:*
  ○ The patient maintains the behaviour after completion of the therapy (long-term compliance).
  ○ This phase needs to be well prepared.
  ○ It usually takes place towards the end of the treatment series and is completed with the final analytical assessment.
  ○ Collaboratively with the physiotherapist, the patient needs to anticipate future situations in which pain recurrences are likely to occur.
  ○ The physiotherapist and patient discuss and repeat the behaviours which may be useful to influence the discomfort if the situation should occur.
  ○ Repetition of prophylactic measures is frequently helpful in this phase as well.

Selection of meaningful exercises to enhance compliance: algorithm of actions and decisions

In order to find simple exercises which are meaningful to the patient, several decisions and actions may need to be taken:

* Find the sources of the movement dysfunction by examination and reassessment procedures.
* Make a decision collaboratively with, rather than for, the patient with regard to treatment goals and interventions.
* In the planning phase of treatment and the selection of interventions decide which physiotherapist-directed interventions (e.g. passive mobilizations) and which self-management strategies are to be employed.
* Consider the objectives of the strategies: does the patient need to perform the exercises for a limited period (e.g. postoperative treatment), or does the patient have to do the exercises for an indefinite period?
* For those patients whose main complaint is pain, it is essential to teach coping strategies that have an influence on the pain prior to the employment of interventions, which should influence contributing factors like posture and general fitness. With these coping strategies, patients may perceive a sense of success and control over their well-being; hence, they may develop the trust to perform exercises that they initially believed to be harmful.

Guidance towards a healthy lifestyle with increased activities needs education and the direct experience of a sense of control over the pain. Without effective coping strategies addressing pain and well-being, it may become an almost insurmountable task to develop an active lifestyle for persons suffering from pain and lack of confidence to move.

Compliance enhancement: general remarks

* One of the most essential goals of a self-management strategy is guiding patients to a sense-of-control over their wellbeing (Harding et al. 1998).
* Coping strategies for pain control should mainly be based on difficulties in daily life. In these cases, information from the subjective examination is frequently more important in decision-making than data from inspection or active movement testing (especially data from '24-hour behaviour' and precipitating factors in history). For example, a woman who works at a sewing machine in a factory develops pain in the thoracic area after 6 hours of work. Although physical examination shows that she has a flattened thoracic kyphosis, her self-management strategies to alleviate the pain are variations of repeated extension and rotation movements.
* Exercises that need to be employed long-term should be integrated into normal routines (e.g. no exercises in supine lying). Provide simple, achievable exercises that can be easily incorporated into the daily life.
* Exercises need to contribute to a sense of success.
* It is essential not to teach a single intervention, but to work collaboratively with the patient on modifications of the exercise/instruction according to the demands of the various daily life situations. The patient needs to know that the adaptations are not different exercises, but 'variations on the same theme'.
* Follow an instruction and education plan in which an awareness of all the instructions given during one session is necessary. Repeat the given information over various sessions; give pieces of information, rather than everything at once.
* Take time to teach the exercises, rather than telling the patient what to do in the last few

minutes of a session. Allocate time for the patient to ask questions.

- If a patient believes that moving may be harmful when activities and work-situations provoke pain, the physiotherapist can guide the patient with educational strategies that are complementary to passive mobilizations and other self-management interventions. At times the physiotherapist may use the following axioms in the educational process:

It's not what you move, but how you move.

(Sahrmann 1999)

It's not necessarily the work-task, but the working-style which provokes symptoms.

(Watson 1999)

- Written information as a mnemonic may enhance understanding. At times, patients may do this by themselves. A 'pain, activities and exercise-diary' may be incorporated.
- Ensure that the exercises can be implemented in daily life situations – therefore the patient frequently needs to be provided with variations of the same exercise (especially in those situations where the patient needs to develop a new behaviour, which needs to last for a long time, maybe even a lifetime).
- Anticipate difficulties: after the selection and instruction of an exercise, the physiotherapist needs to discuss with the patient whether and where he or she anticipates difficulties; certain exercises may be very useful but perhaps not during a given work situation. Collaborative problem-solving for such a situation is essential and modifications of the exercise need to be worked out.
- At the completion of a treatment series, in order to enhance long-term compliance, further anticipation of possible future recurrences and their solutions needs to take place.

Conclusion: compliance enhancement

Before instructing an exercise the physiotherapist may go through the following steps and questions:

- What are the goals of the exercise?
- When should the exercises be employed in daily life?
- Have I explained the objectives of the exercises to the patient?

- Have I checked if the patient has understood?
- Were the exercises reassessed immediately after the exercise? Did they contribute to a sense-of-success?
- Did I anticipate collaboratively with the patient whether and when difficulties may occur in performing the exercises?
- Which solutions have I worked out collaboratively with the patient?

Patient education

In order to promote motivation and enhance motivation of the patient, education has found an important place in physiotherapy practice (Sluys 2000, Butler & Moseley 2003). Patient education is considered a core task in physiotherapy practice, as the definition of physiotherapy by the World Confederation of Physical Therapy (WCPT 1999) states:

> **Intervention/treatment** is implemented and modified in order to reach agreed goals and may include manual handling; movement enhancement; physical, electro-therapeutic and mechanical agents; functional training; provision of assistive technologies; patient related instruction and counselling; documentation and co-ordination, and communication.
>
> (p. VII)

Some educational principles

It has been recognized that in physiotherapy much information is given; however, it does not seem to follow explicit principles of cognitive-behavioural therapy, information technology or education (Sluys & Hermans 1990). It seems that many therapists do employ the principles, but in a more implicit, intuitive sense (Hengeveld 2000, Green et al. 2008, Sandborgh et al. 2010). Before embarking on an educational session, it is important to consider several educational principles (Brioschi 2005):

- What is the objective of the educational session(s)? For example, explain pain and the role of movement/activity in the management of pain; the role of movement and relaxation in the maintenance of health; the role of active movement in the regeneration of disc or cartilage tissue.
- Establish the cognitive level of the patient – at what complexity the education should be delivered?

- Develop an educational strategy – the information may be given (and reassessed) piecemeal over further sessions; a progression of information may enhance the educational process.
- Develop simple metaphors to explain aspects of pain and its treatment from the physiotherapist's perspective.
- Prepare educational material to support the educational process.
- Consider ways to reassess the process, e.g. by asking patients to repeat in their own words what they remember from the session.
- Ask yourself: does the given information contribute to more understanding or to more confusion in the patient?
- Give the patient time to ask questions; also in follow-up sessions.

In addition, the choice of words should be selected in such a way that the patient is directly integrated in the discussion, i.e. talking *with* rather than to the patient. It is pertinent to note that patients may be motivated faster, and on a long-term basis, if they hear themselves making statements about their options and possibilities.

A language that enhances change should revolve around five aspects:

1. Wishes ('I would like to be able to play with my kids again')
2. Reasons ('I come to the physiotherapy because I want to learn what I could do myself')
3. Possibilities ('I could go swimming more regularly')
4. Confidence ('Going on my bike to work is something I could try, as I have done that before')
5. Necessity ('If I don't do anything, I think my back will only get worse')

If a person is changing in motivation, they may use language indicating commitment to the change. Clinicians should develop sensitivity towards these subtleties of language. Patients may state, for example (van Merendonk et al. 2012):

- I will think about it
- I will do it when I have time
- I'll do my best to plan it into my schedule
- I expect that I can start with it by tomorrow
- Yes I certainly will do that.

It is stated that patient education is of particular relevance when the clinical presentation is characterized and dominated by central nervous system modulation of a pain experience and/or where maladaptive illness perceptions and behaviour is present (Nijs et al. 2011). However, it may be argued that each person, regardless of the clinical problem, needs adequate information in order to understand the physiotherapist's reasoning in the determination of a meaningful, individualized therapy.

Conclusion

Musculoskeletal (manipulative) physiotherapists have a core task in the treatment of patients with movement disorders and the guidance towards functional restoration and a healthy lifestyle. At certain times in the process the art of passive movement should not be neglected, and the incorporation of cognitive behavioural principles should be considered throughout all phases of the process. In order to provide optimum patient care, these elements deserve their justified place in contemporary practice as much as any other information gained from contemporary evidence-based practice.

References

AAMPGG (Australian Acute Musculoskeletal Pain Guidelines Group): *Evidence-based management of acute musculoskeletal pain*, Bowen Hills, 2003, Australian Academic Press.

American Psychiatric Association: *Diagnostic and Statistical Manual of Mental Disorders*, ed 4, Arlington, VA, 2000, American Psychiatric Association.

Banks K, Hengeveld E: *Maitland's Clinical Companion: an essential guide for students*, Edinburgh, 2010, Churchill Livingstone Elsevier.

Bassett SF, Petrie KJ: The effect of treatment goals on patient compliance with physiotherapy exercise programmes, *Physiother Can* 85:130–137, 1997.

Bialosky JE, Bishop MD, Price DD, et al: The mechanisms of manual therapy in the treatment of musculoskeletal pain. A comprehensive model, *Man Ther* 13(1):1–8, 2008.

Boissonnault W: *Primary care for the physical therapist. Examination and triage*, ed 2, St. Louis, 2010, Elsevier – Saunders.

Brioschi R: Kurs: die therapeutische Beziehung. Leitung: Brioschi R & Hengeveld E. Fortbildungszentrum Zurzach, Mai 1998.

Brioschi R: *Course on interdisciplinary pain management – ZST*, Switzerland, 2005, Zurzach.

Bunzli S, Gillham D, Esterman A: Physiotherapy-provided operant conditioning in the management of low back pain disability: a systematic review, *Physiother Res Int* 16(2011): 4–19, 2011.

Butler DS, Moseley GL: *Explain pain*, Adelaide, Australia, 2003, Noigroup Publications.

Chiu TW, Wright A: To compare the effects of different rates of application of a cervical mobilisation technique on the sympathetic outflow to the upper limb in normal subjects, *Man Ther* 1(4):198–203, 1996.

Cott CA, Finch E, Gasner D, et al: The movement continuum theory for physiotherapy, *Physiother Can* 47:87–95, 1995.

Courneya KS, Friedenreich CM, Sela RA, et al: Exercise motivation and adherence in cancer survivors after participation in a randomized controlled trial: an attribution theory perspective, *Int J Behav Med* 11(1):8–17, 2004.

Delvecchio Good MJ, Brodwin PE, Good B, et al: *Pain as human experience. An anthropological perspective*, Berkeley, 1992, University of California Press.

Dijkstra A: Het veranderingsfasenmodel als leidraad bij het motiveren tot en begeleiding van gedragsverandering bij patienten, *Ned Tijdschr Fysio* 112:62–68, 2002.

Ferri M, Brooks D, Goldstein RS: Compliance with treatment – an ongoing concern, *Physiother Can* 50:286–290, 1998.

Fishbain DA: Secondary gain concept. Definition of problems and its abuse in medical practice, *Am Pain Soc J* 3:264–273, 1994.

Foster NA, Bishop A, Thomas E, et al: Illness perceptions of low back pain patients in primary care: what are they, do they change and are they associated with outcome? *Pain* 136:177–187, 2008.

Goodman CBC, Snyder TEK: *Differential diagnosis for physical therapist: screening for referral*, ed 5, St. Louis, 2012, Elsevier-Saunders.

Green A, Jackson DA, Klaber Moffet JA: An observational study of physiotherapists' use of cognitive behavioural principles in the management of patients with back pain and neck pain, *Physiotherapy* 94:306–313, 2008.

Gross AM, Kay TM, Kennedy C, et al: Clinical practice guideline on the use of manipulation or mobilization in the treatment of adults with mechanical neck disorders, *Man Ther* 7(4):193–205, 2002.

Hadler NM: If you have to prove you are ill, you can't get well, *Spine* 20:2397–2400, 1996.

Hancock MJ, Maher CG, Laslett M, et al: Discussion paper: what happened to the 'bio' in the bio-psycho-social model of low back pain? *Eur Spine J* 20:2105–2110, 2011.

Harding VR, Simmonds MJ, Watson PJ: Physical therapy for chronic pain, *Pain, Clin Updates (IASP)* VI:1–4, 1998.

Hengeveld E: Psychosocial issues in physiotherapy: manual therapists' perspectives and observations. MSc Thesis. London, 2000, Department of Health Sciences, University of East London.

Hengeveld E: Das biopsychosoziale Modell. In van den Berg F, editor: *Angewandte Physiologie, Band 4: Schmerzen verstehen und beeinflussen*, Stuttgart, 2003, Thieme Verlag, Kap 1.4.

Hengeveld E, Banks K: *Maitland's Peripheral manipulation: management of neuromusculoskeletal disorders* (vol 2), ed 4, Edinburgh, 2005, Butterworth Heinemann Elsevier.

Jull G, Trott P, Potter H, et al: A randomized controlled trial of exercise and manipulative therapy for cervicogenic headache, *Spine* 27(17):1835–1843, 2002.

Jull G, Moore A: Editorial: Hands on, hands off? The swings in musculoskeletal physiotherapy practice, *Man Ther* 17:199–200, 2012.

Kendall NAS, Linton SJ, Main CJ, et al: *Guide to assessing psychosocial yellow flags in acute low back pain: risk factors for long-term disability and work loss*, Wellington, New Zealand, 1997, Accident Rehabilitation and Compensation Insurance Corporation of New Zealand and the National Health Committee.

Klaber Moffet J, Richardson PH: The influence of the physiotherapist-patient relationship on pain and disability, *Physiother Theory and Pract* 13:89–96, 1997.

Kleinmann A: *The illness narratives: suffering, healing and the human condition*, New York, 1988, Basic Books Harpers.

Kleinman A: In Fadiman A, editor: *The spirit catches you and you fall down: a Hmong child, her American doctors and the collision of two cultures*, New York, 1997, Farrar, Strauss and Giroux.

KNGF: *Visie op Fysiotherapie*, Amersfoort, 1992, Koninklijk Nederlands Genootschap voor Fysiotherapie [Royal Dutch Society for Physiotherapy; in Dutch].

Kok J, Bouter L: Patientenvoorlichting door fysiotherapeuten in de eerste lijn, *Ned Tijdschr Fysio* 100:59–63, 1990.

Ledermann E: *Fundamentals of manual therapy: physiology, neurology and psychology*, New York, 1996, Churchill-Livingstone.

Main CJ, Spanswick CS: *Pain management: an interdisciplinary approach*, Edinburgh, 2000, Churchill Livingstone.

Maitland GD: *Vertebral manipulation*, ed 5, Oxford, 1986, Butterworth Heinemann Elsevier.

Maitland GD: *Peripheral manipulation*, ed 3, Oxford, 1991, Butterworth Heinemann.

May S: Patient satisfaction with management of back pain. Part 1: What is satisfaction? Review of satisfaction with medical management; Part 2: An explorative, qualitative study into patients' satisfaction with physiotherapy, *Physiotherapy* 87:4–20, 2001.

McIndoe R: Moving out of pain: hands-on or hands-off. In: Shacklock M, editor: *Moving in on pain*, Melbourne, 1995, Butterworth Heinemann.

McKenzie RA: *The lumbar spine: mechanical diagnosis and therapy*, Waikanae, New Zealand, 1981, Spinal Publications.

McLean SM, Burton L, Littlewood C: Interventions for enhancing adherence with physiotherapy, *Man Ther* 15:514–521, 2010.

Middleton A: Chronic low back pain: patient compliance with physiotherapy advice and exercise, perceived barriers and motivation, *Phys Ther Rev* 9:153–160, 2004.

Moss P, Sluka K, Wright A: The initial effects of knee joint mobilisation on oateoarthritic hyperalgesia, *Man Ther* 12:109–118, 2007.

Nijs J, van Wilgen CP, van Oosterwijck J, et al: How to explain central sensitization to patients with 'unexplained' chronic musculoskeletal pain: practice guidelines, *Man Ther* 16:413–418, 2011.

Paungmali A, O'Leary S, Souvlis T, et al: Hypoalgesic and sympathoexcitatory effects of mobilisation with movement for lateral epicondylalgia, *Phys Ther* 83:374–383, 2003.

Philips HC: Avoidance-behaviour and its role in sustaining chronic pain, *Behav Res Ther* 25:273–279, 1987.

Philips HC, Jahanshani M: The components of pain behaviour Report, *Behav Res Ther* 24:117–124, 1986.

Pilowsky I: *Abnormal illness behaviour*, Chichester, 1997, John Wiley.

Prochaska J, DiClemente C: Stages of change and decisional balance for twelve problem behaviours, *Health Psychol* 13:39–46, 1994.

Refshauge K, Gass E: *Musculoskeletal physiotherapy*, Oxford, 1995, Butterworth Heinemann.

Rey R: *The history of pain*, Cambridge, MA, 1995, Harvard University Press.

Riolo L: Commentary, *Phys Ther* 73:784–786, 1995.

Sahrmann S: *Course on the assessment and treatment of movement impairments*. Zurzach, Switzerland, 1999.

Sandborgh M, Asenlof P, Lindberg P, et al: Implementing behavioural medicine in physiotherapy treatment. Part II: Adherence to treatment protocol, *Adv Physiother* 12:13–23, 2010.

Schachter CL, Stalker CA, Teram E: Towards sensitive practice: issues for physical therapists working with survivors of childhood abuse, *Phys Ther* 79:248–261, 1999.

Schmid A, Brunner F, Wright A, et al: Paradigm shift in manual therapy? Evidence for a central nervous system component in the response to passive cervical joint mobilisation, *Man Ther* 13:387–396, 2008.

Schneiders A, Zusman M, Singer KP: Exercise therapy compliance in acute low back pain patients, *Man Ther* 3:147–152, 1998.

Sluys E, Hermans J: Problemen die patienten ervaren bij het doen van huiswerkoefeningen en bij het opvolgen van adviezen, *Ned Tijdschr Fysio* 100:175–179, 1990.

Sluys E: Patient education in physiotherapy: towards a planned approach, *Physiotherapy* 77:503–508, 1991.

Sluys EM, Kok GJ, van der Zee J, et al: Correlates of exercise compliance in physical therapy, *Phys Ther* 73:771–786, 1993.

Sluys EM: *Therapietrouw door voorlichting*, Amsterdam, 2000, SWP.

Sterling M, Jull G, Wright A: Cervical mobilisation: concurrent effects on pain, sympathetic nervous system activity and motor activity, *Man Ther* 6:72–81, 2001.

Twomey L: A rationale for the treatment of back pain and joint pain by manual therapy, *Phys Ther* 72(12):885–892, 1992.

Van der Burght M, Verhulst H: Van therapietrouw naar zelf-management: voorlichting op maat, *Fysiopraxis* 12:4–7, 1997.

Van Merendonk S, Hulseboom M, Poelgeest A: Verandertaal en commitmenttaal, *FysioPraxis* 21(4):26–28, 2012.

Van Tulder M, Becker A, Bekkering T, et al: European Guidelines for the Management of Acute Low Back Pain, *Eur Spine J* 15:(Suppl. 2): 131–300, 2006.

Vicenzino B, Cartwright T, Collins D, et al: Cardiovascular and respiratory changes produced by lateral glide mobilization of the cervical spine, *Man Ther* 3(2):67–71, 1998a.

Vicenzino B, Collins D, Benson H, et al: An investigation of the interrelationship between manipulative therapy induced hypoalgesia and sympathoexcitory effects, *J Manipulative Physiol Ther* 21(7):448–453, 1998b.

Vicenzino B: Lateral epicondylalgia: a musculoskeletal physiotherapy perspective, *Man Ther* 8(2):66–79, 2003.

Vlaeyen JWS, Crombez G: Fear of movement/(re)injury, avoidance and

pain disability in chronic low back pain patients, *Man Ther* 4:187–195, 1999.

Waddell G: *The Back Pain Revolution*, ed 2, Edinburgh, 2004, Elsevier-Churchill Livingstone.

Walker MJ, Boyles RE, Young BA, et al: The effectiveness of manual physical therapy and exercise for mechanical neck pain. A randomized clinical trial, *Spine* 33(22):2371–2378, 2008.

Warburton DER, Nicol CW, Bredin SSD: Health benefits of physical activity: the evidence, *CAMJ* 174(6):801–809, 2006.

Watson P: *Psychosocial assessment*, Zurzach, Switzerland, 1999, IMTA Educational Days.

Watson PJ, Kendall N: Assessing psychosocial yellow flags. In Gifford L, editor: *Topical Issues in Pain 2. Bio-psychosocial assessment and management. Relationships and pain*, Falmouth, 2000, CNS Press.

WCPT: *Description of physical therapy*, London, 1999, World Confederation of Physical Therapy.

WCPT: Physical therapy, physical activity and health. World Confederation of Physical Therapy: 2012. Online. Available, http://www.wcpt.org/node/33329.

WHO: *Global strategy on diet, physical activity and health*, Geneva, 2004, World Health Organization.

WHO: *WHO global strategy on diet, physical activity and health – a framework to monitor and evaluate implementation*, Geneva, 2008, World Health Organization.

Wright A: Hypoalgesia post-manipulative therapy: a review of a potential neurophysiological mechanism, *Man Ther* 1(1):11–16, 1995.

Yeo H, Wright A: Effects of performing a passive accessory mobilization technique in patients with lateral ankle pain, *Man Ther* 16:373–377, 2011.

Zusman M: Central nervous system contribution to mechanically produced motor and sensory responses, *Aust J Physiother* 38:245–255, 1991.

Zusman M: Mechanisms of Musculoskeletal Physiotherapy, *Physiother Rev* 9(1):39–49, 2004.

Movement diagram theory and compiling a movement diagram

Appendix 1 remains as it was presented by Geoff Maitland in the 3rd edition of this book (1991). However, in view of contemporary developments arising from research and peer review of this subject, it was felt necessary by the current authors to add a contemporary perspective. What is clear is that movement diagrams remain a valuable tool for both current and developing clinical practice (Chesworth et al. 1998).

A contemporary perspective on defining resistance, grades of mobilization and depicting movement diagrams

Petty et al. (2002) in their peer review article *'Manual examination of accessory movement-seeking R_1'* have rightly challenged the long-held belief that for an asymptomatic joint, the resistance first felt by the therapist (R_1) when the joint is moved passively occurs towards the end of the range. R_1 is considered to be at the transitional point between the toe and linear regions of a load displacement curve (Lee & Evans 1994) (Fig. A1.1).

Petty et al. (2002) used a spinal assessment machine which applied a posteroanterior force to the L3 spinous process whereby resistance was found to commence at the beginning of the range, the curve ascending as soon as the force was applied (Fig. A1.2).

The suggestions, therefore, are that there is no clear transition point between the toe and linear regions, this having previously been to the point of definition of R_1. The lack of definite transition may explain the poor reliability of therapists in judging the onset of resistance to passive movement (R_1) (Latimer et al. 1996).

Petty et al. (2002) suggest that R_1 should be depicted as early as A on the movement diagram, A being the starting point of the range of movement. The consequence of this would be to call into question the accuracy of the resistance-based defined treatment grades of mobilization/manipulation (grades I–V) resulting in the loss of grades I and II and limiting the definitions to grades III and IV.

After due consideration of the case presented by Petty et al. (2002), the authors of this edition of *Maitland's Peripheral Manipulation* have proposed a reappraisal of the following:

1. The retention of grades I and II in the context of the redefinition of R_1
2. The redefining of resistance
3. The depiction of movement diagrams.

The authors, therefore, are minded that such a reappraisal may affect the future direction of qualitative or quantitative research into movement diagrams, particularly in relation to the reliability of therapists' definition of R_1 and the accurate calibration of treatment grades of mobilization and manipulation.

Redefining grades of mobilization

When a joint is moved passively (accessory or physiological, vertebral or peripheral) a variety of resistances are encountered, for example:

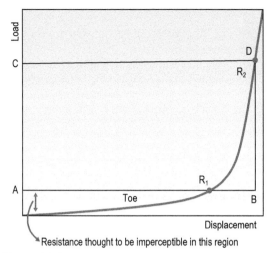

Figure A1.1 • Relationship of movement diagram (ABCD) to load-displacement curve. Reproduced by kind permission from Petty et al. (2002).

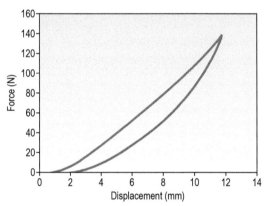

Figure A1.2 • Typical force-displacement curve of a central PA applied to L3 obtained using the spinal assessment machine. The left-hand curve is loading and the right hand curve is unloading curve. Reproduced by kind permission from Petty et al. (2002).

- The *soft*, immediate resistance to movement which fits to the laws of physics
- A *firmer* resistance to movement when the joint is nearing its end of range or its impaired limit (a stiff joint)
- The through-range resistance encountered when arthritic joints are moved with their joint surfaces squeezed together
- The resistance of involuntary protective muscle spasm
- The resistance of voluntary holding.

The original resistance-defined grades of mobilization/manipulation (Maitland 1991) relate to resistance (R) being defined in terms of spasm-free

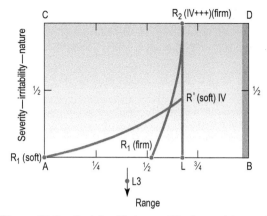

Figure A1.3 • R_1 defined in terms of the firm resistance of a stiff, hard end-feel.

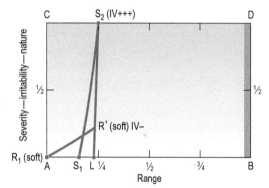

Figure A1.4 • Protective involuntary muscle spasm as a resistance.

resistance (stiffness) or hard and soft end-feel in the ideal or *normal* joint (Maitland 1992).

From the authors' viewpoint, therefore, the reference to resistance refers to the *firmer* resistance felt when a joint is nearing its end range or impaired limit (Fig. A1.3), rather than the *soft* resistance to movement which is felt immediately the joint is moved. It is clear that this definition of resistance can also be related to the resistance encountered due to protective involuntary muscle spasm (Fig. A1.4).

If such an argument is valid – and it may not be – then the grading system I, II, III, IV and V can still be retained but redefined as follows:

- *Grade I* – a small amplitude movement at the beginning of the available range where there is soft resistance but no firm resistance (a note should also be made that A is the starting point of the movement and can be varied according to where the start of the movement needs to be for best effects).

- *Grade II* – a large amplitude movement performed within the available range where there is soft resistance but no firm resistance.
- *Grade III* – a large amplitude movement performed into firm resistance or up to the limit of the available range.
- *Grade IV* – a small amplitude movement performed into firm resistance or up to the limit of the available range.
- *Grade V* – a small amplitude high velocity thrust performed usually, but not always, at the end of the available range.

Redefining resistance

Resistance (R_1), in this context, would be redefined as follows:

- R_1 (soft) – the onset of resistance encountered at the immediate moment that movement commences. Minimal; may even be imperceptible.
- R_1 (firm) – the onset of resistance encountered due to: stiffness, the joint surfaces being squeezed together and moved, the hard and soft end-feel of a normal joint, protective involuntary muscle spasm (S_1 would be the qualifying term in this case) or voluntary holding.

Movement diagram: parameters of reliability

In view of the low intertherapist reliability in detecting the relevant reference points and measurable parameters of a movement diagram, the authors suggest a redefining of some of these parameters. Maitland (1991) depicts B as a thickened point to account for the variation in the therapist's judgement of the end of the normal average range of passive movement. This should be extended to other reference points and parameters of measurement so that margins of error can be accounted for and clinical variations between individual therapist's perceptions can be recognized. Therefore:

- A still remains a fixed starting point but can be varied (all movements have a definite starting point)
- B has already been recognized as a thickened line

- R_1 (soft) is easy to represent because it can be assumed its onset corresponds to the start of the movement at A
- R_1 (firm) should be represented as a thickened line as is B in order to account for the margins of error in the individual perceptions of the onset of firm resistance
- L being the limit of impaired range should also be a thickened line to take account of the margins of error encountered in determining the limit of the impaired movement by P_2, R_2 or S_2
- **The lines P_1 to P_2 (P′), R_1 to R_2 (R′) (soft or firm) and S_1 to S_2 (S′) should all be depicted with margins of error to account for individual variations in their perception.**

Figures A1.5 and A1.6 show the representation of such natural variations on movement diagrams.

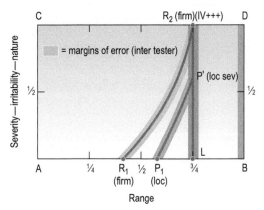

Figure A1.5 • Movement diagram depicting margins of error.

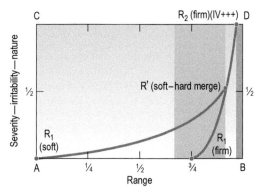

Figure A1.6 • Pictorial relationship between soft and firm resistance (soft end-feel). The transitional shaded area between the toe and linear phases of the compliance curve is the area which is probably least reliable (intertherapist) during passive movement testing.

The movement diagram: a teaching aid, a means of communication and self-learning

> Geography would be incomprehensible without maps. They've reduced a tremendous muddle of facts into something you can read at a glance. Now I suspect … economics [read passive movement] is fundamentally no more difficult than geography except it's about things in motion. If only somebody would invent a dynamic map.
>
> SNOW (1965).

The movement diagram is intended solely as a teaching aid and a means of communication. When examining, say, a posteroanterior movement of the acromio-clavicular joint produced by pressure on the clavicle, newcomers to this method of examining will find it difficult to know what they are feeling. However, the movement diagram makes them analyse the movement in terms of range, pain, resistance and muscle spasm. Also, it makes them analyse the manner in which these factors interact to affect the movement.

Movement diagrams (and also the grades of movement) are not necessarily essential to using passive movement as a form of treatment. However, they are essential to understanding the relationship that the various grades of movement have to a patient's abnormal joint signs. Therefore, although they are not essential for a person to be a good manipulator, they are essential if the teaching of the whole concept of manipulative treatment is to be done at the highest level.

Movement diagrams are essential when trying to separate the different components that can be felt when a movement is examined. They therefore become essential for either teaching other people, or for teaching one's self and thereby progressing one's own analysis and understanding of treatment techniques and their effect on symptoms and signs.

The components considered in the diagram are *pain, spasm-free resistance* (i.e. stiffness) and *muscle spasm* found on joint examination, their relative strength and behaviour in all parts of the available range and in relation to each other. Thus the response of the joint to movement is shown in a very detailed way. The theory of the movement diagram is described in this appendix by discussing each component separately at first (for the practical compilation of a diagram for one direction of movement of one joint in a particular patient, see 'Compiling a movement diagram' below).

Each of the above components is an extensive subject in itself and it should be realized that discussion in this appendix is deliberately limited in the following ways:

- The spasm referred to is protective muscle spasm secondary to joint disorder
- Spasticity caused by upper motor neurone disease and the voluntary contraction of muscles is excluded.

Frequently this voluntary contraction is out of all proportion to the pain experienced yet in very direct proportion to the patient's apprehension about the examiner's handling of the joint. Careless handling will provoke such a reaction and thereby obscure the real clinical findings. Resistance (stiffness) free of muscle spasm is discussed only from the clinical point of view, i.e. discussion about the pathology causing the stiffness is excluded.

A movement diagram is compiled by drawing graphs for the behaviour of pain, physical resistance and muscle spasm, depicting the position in the range at which each is felt (this is shown on the horizontal line AB) and the intensity, nature or quality of each (which is shown on the vertical line AC) (Fig. A1.7).

The baseline AB represents any range of movement from a starting position at A to the limit of the average normal passive range at B, remembering that when examining a patient's movement of any joint, it is only considered normal if firm proportionate overpressure may be applied without pain. It makes no difference whether the movement

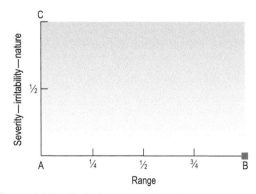

Figure A1.7 • Beginning a movement diagram.

depicted is large or small, whether it involves one joint or a group of joints working together, or whether it represents 2 mm of posteroanterior movement or 180° of shoulder flexion.

Because of soft-tissue compliance, the end of range of any joint (even 'bone to bone') will have some soft tissue component, physiological or pathological. Thus the range of the 'end of range' (B) will be a moveable point, or have a depth of position on the range line. To locate halfway through the range of the 'end of range' as a grade IV and to fit in either side of it a plus sign (1) and a minus sign (2) allows the depiction of the force with which this 'end of range' point is approached (Edwards, A., unpublished observations).

Point A, the starting point of the movement, is also variable: its position may be the extreme of range opposite B or somewhere in mid-range, whichever is more suitable for the diagram. For example, if shoulder flexion is the movement being represented and the pain or limitation occurs only in the last 10° of the range, the diagram will more clearly demonstrate the behaviour of the three factors if the baseline represents the last 20° rather than 90° of flexion. For the purpose of clarity, position A is defined by stating the range represented by the baseline AB. In the above example, if the baseline represents 90°, A must be at about 90°; similarly, if the baseline represents 20°, position A is with the arm 20° short of full flexion (assuming of course that the range of flexion is 180°).

As the movement diagram is used to depict what can be felt when examining passive movement, it must be clearly understood that point B represents the extreme of *passive movement*, and that this lies variably, but very importantly, beyond the extreme of active movement.

The vertical axis AC represents the quality, nature or intensity of the factors being plotted; point A represents complete absence of the factor and point C represents the maximum quality, nature or intensity of the factor to which the examiner is prepared to subject the person. The word 'maximum' in relation to 'intensity' is obvious: it means point C is the maximum intensity of pain the examiner is prepared to provoke. 'Maximum' in relation to 'quality' and 'nature' refers to two other essential parts. They are:

1. *Irritability* – when the examiner would stop the testing movement when the pain was not necessarily intense but when it was assessed

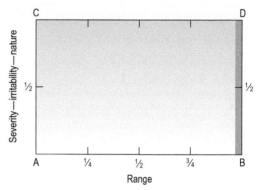

Figure A1.8 • A frame of a basic movement diagram.

that if the movement was continued into greater pain there would be an exacerbation or latent reaction.

2. *Nature* – when P_1 represents the onset of, say, scapular pain, but as the movement is continued the pain spreads down the arm. The examiner may decide to stop when the provoked pain reaches the forearm.

Thus meaning of 'maximum' in relation to each component is discussed again later.

The basic diagram is completed by vertical and horizontal lines drawn from B and C to meet at D (Fig. A1.8).

Pain

P_1

The initial fact to be established is whether the patient has any pain at all and, if so, whether it is present at rest or only on movement. To begin the exercise it is assumed that the patient only has pain on movement.

The first step is to move the joint slowly and carefully in the range being tested, asking the patient to report immediately when any discomfort is felt. The position at which this is first felt is noted.

The second step consists of several small oscillatory movements in different parts of the pain-free range, gradually moving further into the range up to the point where pain is first felt, thus establishing the exact position of the onset of the pain. There is no danger of exacerbation if:

• Sufficient care is used
• The examiner bears in mind that it is the very first provocation of pain that is being sought.

The point at which this occurs is called P_1 and is marked on the baseline of the diagram (Fig. A1.9).

Thus there are two steps establishing P_1:

1. A single slow movement first.

2. Small oscillatory movements.

If the pain is reasonably severe then the point found with the first single slow movement will be deeper in the range than that found with oscillatory movements. Having thus found where the pain is first felt with a slow movement, the oscillatory test movements will be carried out in a part of the range that will not provoke exacerbation.

L (1 of 3) where (L 5 limit of range)

The next step is to determine the available range of movement. This is done by slowly moving the joint beyond P_1 until the limit of the range is reached. This point is marked on the baseline as **L** (Fig. A1.10).

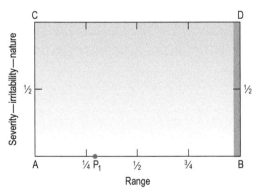

Figure A1.9 • Onset of pain.

L (2 of 3) what

The next step is to determine what component it is that prevents or inhibits further movement. As we are only discussing pain at this stage, P_2 is then marked vertically above L at maximum quality, nature or intensity (Fig. A1.11). The intensity or quality of pain in any one position is assessed as lying somewhere on the vertical axis of the graph (i.e. between A and C) between no pain at all (i.e. A) and the limit (i.e. C).

It is important to realize that maximum intensity or quality of pain in the diagram represents the maximum the physiotherapist is prepared to provoke. This point is well within, and quite different from, a level representing intolerable pain for the patient. Estimation of 'maximum' in this way is, of course, entirely subjective, and varies from person to person. Though this may seem to some readers a grave weakness of the movement diagram, *yet it is in fact its strength*. When a student's 'L', 'P_2' is compared with the instructor's, the differences that may exist will demonstrate whether the student has been too heavy handed or too 'kind-and-gentle'.

L (3 of 3) qualify

Having decided to stop the movement at L because of the pain's 'maximum "quality or intensity"' and therefore drawn in point P_2 on the line CD, it becomes necessary to qualify what P_2 represents: if it is the intensity of the pain that is the reason for stopping at L, then P_2 should be qualified thus: 'P_2 (intensity)'.

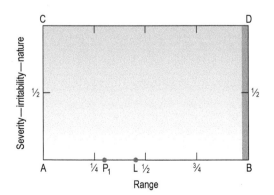

Figure A1.10 • Limit of the range.

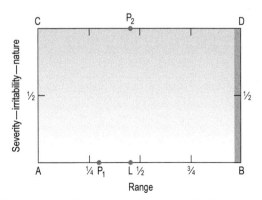

Figure A1.11 • Maximum quality or intensity of pain.

If, however, the examiner believes that there may be some latent reaction if the joint is moved further even though the pain is not severe, then P_2 should be qualified thus: 'P_2 (latent)' (Fig. A1.12).

P_1P_2

The next step is to depict the behaviour of the pain during the movement between P_1 and P_2. If pain increases evenly with movement into the painful range, the line joining P_1 and P_2 is a straight line (Fig. A1.13). However, pain may not increase evenly in this way. Its build-up may be irregular, calling for a graph that is curved or angular. Pain may be first felt at about quarter range and may initially change quickly, and then the movement can be taken further until a limit at three-quarter range is reached (Fig. A1.14).

In another example, pain may be first felt at quarter range and remain at a low level until it

suddenly changes, reaching P_2 at three-quarter range (Fig. A1.15).

The examples given demonstrate pain that prevents a full range of movement of the joint, but there are instances where pain may never reach a limiting intensity. Figure A1.15 is an example where a little pain may be felt at half range but the pain scarcely changes beyond this point in the range and the end of normal range may be reached without provoking anything approaching a limit to full range of movement. There is thus no point L, and P' (P' means P prime) appears on the vertical line BD to indicate the relative significance of the pain at that point (Fig. A1.16). The mathematical use of 'prime' in this context is that it represents 'a numerical value which has itself and unity as its only factors' (*Concise Oxford Dictionary*).

If we now return to an example where the joint is painful at rest, mentioned above, an estimate must be made of the amount or quality of pain present at rest, and this appears as P on the vertical axis AC (Fig. A1.17). Movement is then begun slowly and

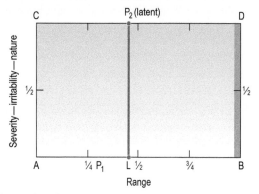

Figure A1.12 • Latent reaction of maximum quality or intensity of pain.

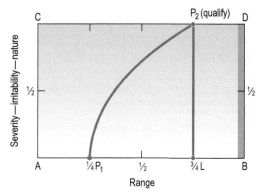

Figure A1.14 • Early increase of pain.

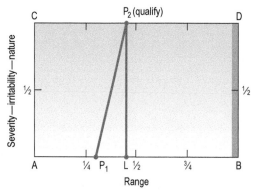

Figure A1.13 • Pain increasing evenly with movement.

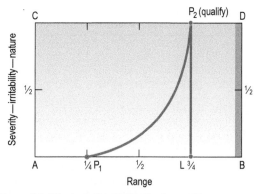

Figure A1.15 • Later increase of pain reaching a maximum at three-quarter range.

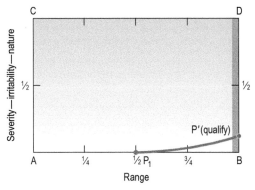

Figure A1.16 • Pain with no limiting intensity.

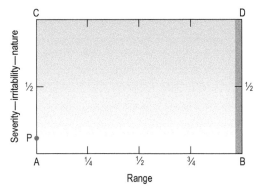

Figure A1.17 • Pain at rest.

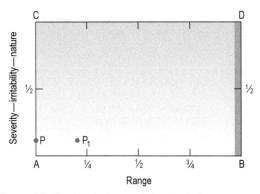

Figure A1.18 • Level where pain begins to increase.

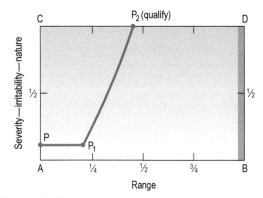

Figure A1.19 • Pain due to subsequent movement.

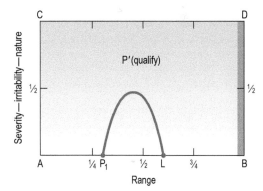

Figure A1.20 • Arc of pain.

Again it must be emphasized that this evaluation of pain is purely subjective. Nevertheless, it presents an invaluable method whereby students can learn to perceive different behaviours of pain, and their appreciation of these variations of pain patterns will mature as this type of assessment is practised from patient to patient and checked against the judgment of a more experienced physiotherapist.

An arc of pain provoked on passive movement might be depicted as shown in Figure A1.20.

Resistance (free of muscle spasm/motor responses)

These resistances may be due to adaptive shortening of muscles or capsules, scar tissue, arthritic joint changes and many other non-muscle-spasm situations.

A normal joint, when completely relaxed and moved passively, has the feel of being well oiled and friction free (Maitland 1980). It can be likened to wet soap sliding on wet glass. It is important for the

carefully until the original level of pain begins to increase (P_1 in Fig. A1.18). The behaviour of pain beyond this point is plotted in the manner already described, and an example of such a graph is given in Figure A1.19. When the joint is painful at rest the symptoms are easily exacerbated by poor handling. However, if examination is carried out with care and skill, no difficulty is encountered.

physiotherapist using passive movement as a form of treatment to appreciate the difference between a free-running, friction-free movement and one that, although being full range, has minor resistance within the range of movement. A strong recommendation is made for therapists to feel the movements suggested in the article.

When depicting a compliance diagram of the forces applied to stretching a ligament from start to breaking point, the graph includes a 'toe region', a 'linear region' and a 'plastic region'; the plastic region ends at the 'break point' (Fig. A1.21).

When a physiotherapist assesses abnormal resistance present in a joint movement, physical laws state that there must be a degree of resistance at the immediate moment that movement commences. The resistance is in the opposite direction to the direction of movement being assessed, and it may be so minimal as to be imperceptible to the physiotherapist. This is the 'toe region' of the compliance diagram, and it is omitted from the movement diagram as used by the manipulative physiotherapist.

The section of the compliance graph that forms the movement diagram represents the clinical findings of the behaviour of resistance when examining a patient's movement in the linear region only (Fig. A1.22).

R₁

When assessing for resistance, the best way to appreciate the free running of a joint is to support and hold around the joint with one hand while the other hand produces an oscillatory movement back and forth through a chosen path of range. If this movement is felt to be friction free then the oscillatory movement can be moved more deeply into the range. In this way the total available range can be assessed. With experience, by comparing two patients, and also comparing a patient's right side with the left side, the physiotherapist will quickly learn to appreciate minor resistance to movement. Point R_1 is then established and marked on the baseline AB (Fig. A1.23).

L – where, L – what

The joint movement is then taken to the limit of the range. If resistance limits movement, the range is assessed and marked by L on the baseline. Vertically above L, R_2 is drawn on CD to indicate that it is resistance that limited the range. R_2 does not necessarily mean that the physiotherapist is too weak to push any harder; it represents the strength of the resistance beyond which the physiotherapist is not prepared to push. There may be factors such as rheumatoid arthritis which will limit the strength

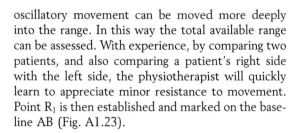

Figure A1.22 • Movement diagram (ABCD) within compliance diagram. The dotted rectangular area (ABCD) is that part of the compliance diagram that is the basis of the movement diagram used for representing abnormal resistance (R_1R_2 or R_1R').

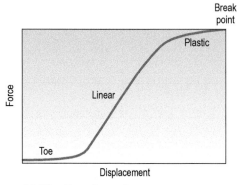

Figure A1.21 • Compliance diagram.

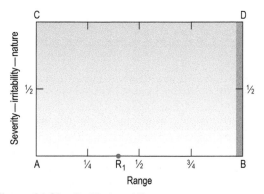

Figure A1.23 • Positioning of R_1.

represented by R_2 to being moderately gentle. Therefore as with P_2, R_2 needs to be qualified. The qualification needs to be of two kinds if it is gentle (e.g. R_2 (IV−, RA)), the first indicating its strength and the second indicating the reason why the movement is stopped even though the strength is weak (Fig. A1.24). When R_2 is a strong resistance (e.g. R_2 (IV++)), its strength only needs to be indicated (Fig. A1.24).

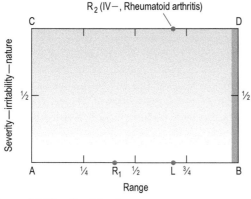

Figure A1.24 • Qualifying R_2.

R_1R_2

The next step is to determine the behaviour of the resistance between R_1 and L, i.e. between R_1 and R_2. The behaviour of resistance between R_1 and R_2 is assessed by movements back and forth in the range between R_1 and L, and the line depicting the behaviour of the resistance is drawn on the diagram (Fig. A1.25). As with pain, resistance can vary in its behaviour, and examples are shown in Figure A1.25.

The foregoing resistances have been related to extra-articular structures. However, if the joint is held in such a way as to compress the surfaces, intra-articular resistance might be depicted as in Figure A1.26.

Muscle spasm/motor responses

There are only two kinds of muscle spasm/motor responses that will be considered here: one that always limits range and occupies a small part of it,

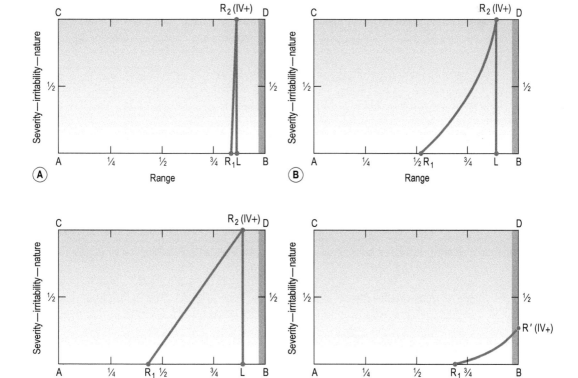

Figure A1.25 • Spasm-free resistance.

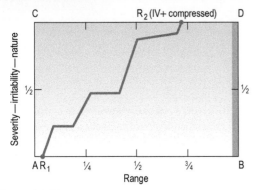

Figure A1.26 • Crepitus.

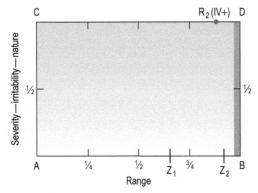

Figure A1.27 • Resistance to passive movement felt between Z_1 and Z_2.

and the other that occurs as a quick contraction to prevent a painful movement.

Whether it is a spasm or stiffness that is the limiting factor, the range can frequently only be accurately assessed by:

1. repeated movement taken somewhat beyond the point at which resistance is first encountered

2. being performed at different speeds.

Muscle spasm shows a power of active recoil. In contrast, resistance that is free of muscle activity does not have this quality; rather it is constant in strength at any given point in the range.

The following examples may help to clarify the point. If a resistance to passive movement is felt between Z_1 and Z_2 on the baseline AB of the movement diagram (Fig. A1.27), and if this resistance is 'resistance free of muscle spasm', then at point 'O', between Z_1 and Z_2 (Fig. A1.28), the strength of resistance will be exactly the same irrespective of how quickly or slowly a movement is oscillated up to it. Furthermore, any increase in strength will be

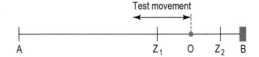

Figure A1.28 • Differentiating resistance from spasm.

directly proportional to the depth in range, regardless of the speed with which the movement is carried out, i.e. the resistance felt at one point in the movement will always be less than that felt at a point deeper in the range. However, if the block is a muscle spasm and test movements are taken up to a point 'O' at different speeds, the strength of the resistance will be greater, with increases in speed.

The first of the two kinds of muscle spasm will feel like spring steel and will push back against the testing movement, particularly if the test movement is varied in speed and in position in the range.

S_1

Testing this kind of spasm is done by moving the joint slowly to the point at which the spasm is first elicited, and at this point it is noted on the baseline as S. Further movement is then attempted. If maximum intensity is reached before the end of range, spasm thus becomes a limiting factor.

L – where, L – what

This limit is noted by L on the baseline and S_2 is marked vertically above on the line CD. As with P_2 and R_2, S_2 needs to be qualified in terms of strength and quality, for example S_2 (IV–, very sharp).

S_1S_2

The graph for the behaviour of spasm is plotted between S_1 and S_2 (Fig. A1.29). When muscle spasm limits range it always reaches its maximum quickly, and thus occupies only a small part of the range. Therefore, it will always be depicted as a near-vertical line (Fig. A1.29A,B). In some cases when the joint disorder is less severe, a little spasm that increases slightly but never prohibits full movement may be felt just before the end of the range (Fig. A1.29C).

The second kind of muscle spasm is directly proportional to the severity of the patient's pain: movement of the joint in varying parts of the range causes

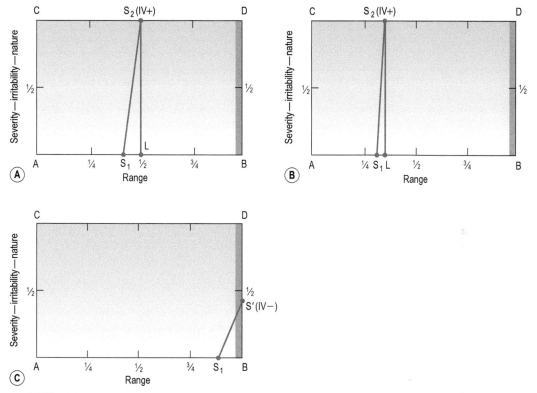

Figure A1.29 • Muscle spasm.

sharply limiting muscular contractions. This usually occurs when a very painful joint is moved without adequate care and can be completely avoided if the joint is well supported and moved gently. This spasm is reflex in type, coming into action very rapidly during test movement. A very similar kind of muscle contraction can occur as a voluntary action by the patient, indicating a sharp increase in pain. If the physiotherapist varies the speed of the test movements it should be possible to distinguish quickly between the reflex spasm and the voluntary spasm by the speed with which the spasm occurs – reflex spasm occurs more quickly in response to a provoking movement than voluntary spasm. This second kind of spasm, which does not limit a range of movement, can usually be avoided by careful handling during the test.

To represent this kind of spasm, a near-vertical line is drawn from above the baseline; its height and position on the baseline will signify whether the spasm is easy to provoke and will also give some indication of its strength. Two examples are drawn of the extremes that may be found (Fig. A1.30A, B).

Modification

There is a modification of the baseline AB which can be used when the significant range to be depicted occupies only, say, 10° yet it is 50° short of B. The movement diagram would be as shown in Figure A1.31 and, when used to depict a movement, the range between 'L' and 'B' must be stated.

The baseline AB for the hypermobile joint movement to be depicted would be the same as that shown earlier where grades of movement are discussed, and the frame of the movement diagram would be as in Figure A1.32.

Having discussed at length the graphing of the separate elements of a movement diagram, it is now necessary to put them together as a whole.

Compiling a movement diagram

This book places great emphasis on the kinds and behaviours of pain as they present with the different movements of disordered joints. Pain is of major

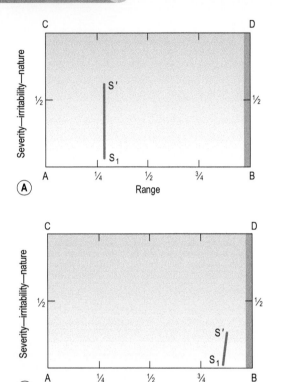

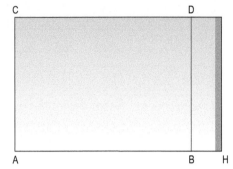

Figure A1.32 • Frame of movement diagram for hypermobile joint.

Figure A1.30 • Spasm that does not limit range of movement.

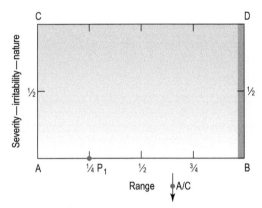

Figure A1.33 • Point at which pain is first felt.

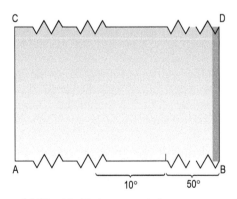

Figure A1.31 • Modified movement diagram.

importance to the patient and therefore takes priority in the examination of joint movement. The following demonstrates how the diagram is formulated. When testing the acromioclavicular (A/C) joint by posteroanterior pressure on the clavicle (for example) the routine is as follows.

Step 1. P_1

Gentle, increasing pressure is applied very slowly to the clavicle in a posteroanterior direction and the patient is asked to report when pain is first felt. This point in the range is noted and the physiotherapist then releases some of the pressure from the clavicle and performs some oscillatory movements, again asking if the patient feels any pain. If pain is not felt, the oscillation should then be carried out slightly deeper into the range. Conversely, if pain is felt, the oscillatory movement should be withdrawn in the range. By these oscillatory movements in different parts of the range, the point at which pain is first felt with movements can be identified and is then recorded on the baseline of the movement diagram as P_1 (Fig. A1.33). The estimation of the position in the range of P_1 is best achieved by performing the oscillations at what the physiotherapist feels is one-quarter range, then at one-third range and then at half range. By this means, P_1 can be very accurately

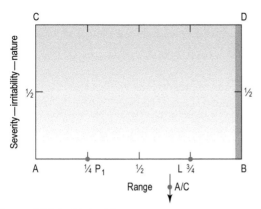

Figure A1.34 • Limit of the range.

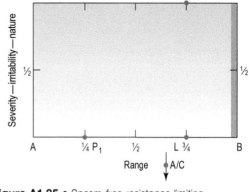

Figure A1.35 • Spasm-free resistance limiting movement.

assessed. Therefore the two steps to establishing P_1 are:

1. A single slow movement.

2. Small oscillatory movements.

Step 2. L – where

Having found P_1 the physiotherapist should continue further into the range with the posteroanterior movements until the limit of the range is reached. The therapist identifies where that position is in relation to the normal range and records it on the baseline as point L (Fig. A1.34).

Step 3. L – what

For the hypomobile joint the next step is to decide why the movement was stopped at point L. This means that the joint has been moved as far as the examiner is willing to go but has not made it reach 'B'. Having decided *where* 'L' is, the examiner has to determine the reason for stopping at L; *what* it was that prevented the examiner reaching 'B'. Assume, for the purpose of this example, that it was physical resistance, free of muscle spasm that prevented movement beyond L. Where the vertical line above L meets the horizontal projection CD, it is marked as R_2 (Fig. A1.35). The R_2 needs to be qualified using words or symbols to indicate what it was about the resistance that prevented the examiner stretching it further; for example the patient may have rheumatoid arthritis and the examiner may not be prepared to go further (see Fig. A1.24) or to push harder than grade IV (Fig. A1.35).

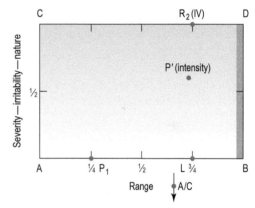

Figure A1.36 • Quality of intensity of pain at L.

Step 4. P′ and defined

The physiotherapist then decides the quality, nature or the intensity of the pain at the limit of the range. This can be estimated in relation to two values:

1. what maximum would feel like

2. what halfway (50%) between no pain and maximum would feel like.

By this means the intensity of the pain is fairly easily decided, thus enabling the physiotherapist to put P′ on the vertical above L in its accurately estimated position (Fig. A1.36).

If the limiting factor at L were P_2, then Step 4 would be estimating the quality or intensity of R′ and defining it (Fig. A1.37).

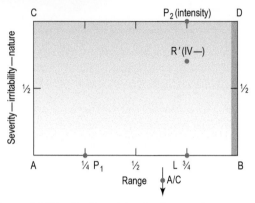

Figure A1.37 • Quality or intensity of spasm-free resistance.

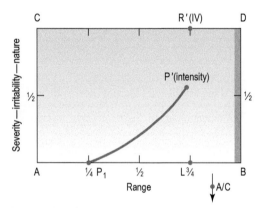

Figure A1.38 • Behaviour of the pain.

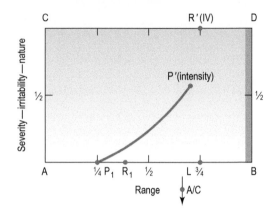

Figure A1.39 • Commencement of resistance.

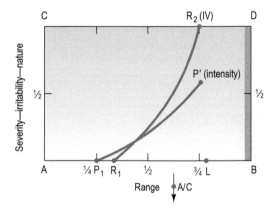

Figure A1.40 • Behaviour of resistance.

Step 5. Behaviour of pain P_1P_2 or P_1P'

The A/C joint is then moved in a posteroanterior direction between P_1 and L to determine – by watching the patient's hands and face and also by asking the patient – how the pain behaves between P_1 and P_2 or between P_2 and P': in fact it is better to think of the pain between P_1 and L because at L, pain is going to be represented as P_2 or P'. The line representing the behaviour of pain is then drawn on the movement diagram, i.e. the line P_1P_2 or between P_1 and P' is completed (Fig. A1.38).

Step 6. R_1

Having completed the representation of pain, resistance must be considered. This is achieved by receding further back in the range than P_1, where, with carefully applied and carefully felt oscillatory movements, the presence or not of any resistance is ascertained. Where it commences is noted and marked on the baseline AB as R_1 (Fig. A1.39).

Step 7. Behaviour of resistance R_1R_2

By moving the joint between R_1 and L the behaviour of the resistance can be determined and plotted on the graph between points R_1 and R_2 (Fig. A1.40).

Step 8. S_1S'

If no muscle spasm has been felt during this examination and if the patient's pain is not excessive, the physiotherapist should continue the oscillatory posteroanterior movements, but perform them more sharply and quicker to determine whether any spasm can be provoked. If no spasm can be provoked, then there is nothing to record on the

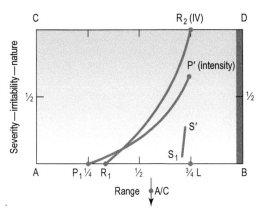

Figure A1.41 • Strength of spasm.

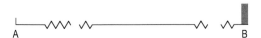

Figure A1.42 • Modified diagram baseline.

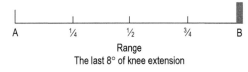

Range
The last 8° of knee extension

Figure A1.43 • Diagram showing restricted range.

Table A1.1 Steps taken in compiling a movement diagram

Where resistance limits movement	Where pain limits movement

1. P_1 (a) slow
    (b) oscillatory
	1. P_1 (a) slow
	    (b) oscillatory

2. L – where	2. L – where
3. L – what (and define) R_2	3. L – what (and define) P_2
4. P' (define)	4. P_1 P_2 (behaviour)
5. P_1 P' (behaviour)	5. R_1
6. R_1	6. R' (define)
7. R_1 R_2 (behaviour)	7. R_1 R' (behaviour)
8. S (defined)	8. S (defined)

movement diagram. However, if with quick, sharper movements a reflex type of muscle spasm is elicited to protect the movement, this should be drawn on the movement diagram in a manner that will indicate how easy or difficult it is to provoke (i.e. by placing the spasm line towards A if it is easy to provoke, and towards B if it is difficult to provoke). The strength of the spasm provoked is indicated by the height of the spasm line, S_1S' (Fig. A1.41).

Thus the diagram for that movement is compiled showing the behaviour of all elements. It is then possible to access any relationship between the factors found on the examination. The relationships give a distinct guide as to the treatment that should be given, particularly in relation to the 'grade' of the treatment movements, i.e. whether 'pain' is going to be treated or whether the treatment will be directed at the resistance.

Summary of steps

Compiling a movement diagram may seem complicated, but it is not. It is a very important part of training in manipulative physiotherapy because it forces the physiotherapist to understand clearly what is felt when moving the joint passively. Committing those thoughts to paper thwarts any guesswork, or any 'hit-and-miss' approach to treatment. Table A1.1 summarizes the steps taken in compiling a movement diagram where resistance limits movement, and the steps taken where pain limits movement.

Modified diagram baseline

When either the limit of available range is very restricted (i.e. L is a long way from B), or when the elements of the movement diagram occupy only a very small percentage of the full range, the basis of the movement diagram needs modification. This is achieved by breaking the baseline as in Figure A1.42. The centre section can then be identified to represent any length, in any part of the minimal full range. When the examination findings are only to be elicited in the last, say, 8° of a full range, point A in the range is changed and the line AB is suitably identified as in Figure A1.43. This example demonstrates that from A to B is 8°, and A to one-quarter is 2°, and so on.

Example – range limited by 50%

Marked stiffness, with 'L' a large distance before 'B', necessitates a modified format of the movement

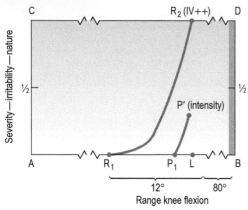

Figure A1.44 • Using a modified diagram.

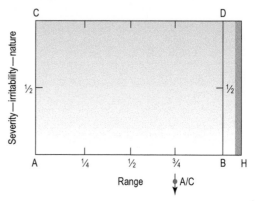

Figure A1.46 • Movement diagram for hypermobile range.

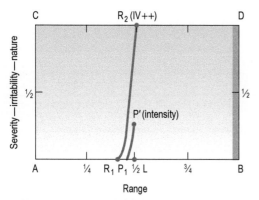

Figure A1.45 • Range limited by 50%, shown on an unmodified diagram (160° knee flexion).

diagram. The example will be restricted knee flexion, a longstanding condition following a fracture.

The first element is R_1 and the distance between R_1 and L is only 12°. Pain is provoked only by stretching (Fig. A1.44). If the movement diagram were drawn on an unmodified format it would be as in Figure A1.45. Figure A1.45 clearly wastes considerable diagram space and is difficult to interpret. With the same joint movement findings represented on the modified format of the movement diagram it becomes clearer and much more useful. The modified format of the baseline of the diagram (Fig. A1.44) requires only two extra measurements to be stated:

1. The measurement between L and B.

2. The measurement between R_1 and L.

Knowing that R_1 to L equals 12° makes it easy to see that R_1 is approximately 7° before P_1. Because of the increased space allowed to represent the

elements of the movement, the behaviour is also far easier to demonstrate.

Clinical example – hypermobility

This example is included for the express purpose of clarifying the misconceptions that exist about hypermobility and the direct influence that some authors and practitioners afford it in restricting passive movement treatment.

If the movement (using the same acromioclavicular joint being tested with posteroanterior movements), before having become painful, were hypermobile, the basic format of the movement diagram would be shown as in Figure A1.46.

If it becomes painful and requires treatment the movement diagram could be as follows.

Step 1. P_1

The method is the same as in Example 1; see also Figure A1.47.

Step 2. L – where

The method is the same as in Example 1; see also Figure A1.48.

Step 3. L – what (and define)

The method is the same as in Example 1; see also Figure A1.49.

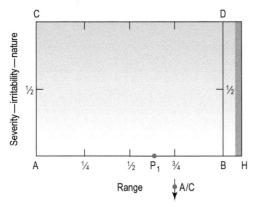

Figure A1.47 • P₁ hypermobile joint.

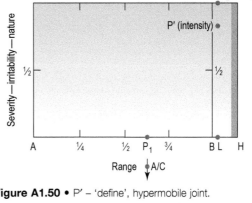

Figure A1.50 • P′ – 'define', hypermobile joint.

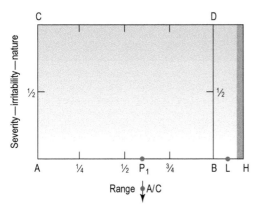

Figure A1.48 • L – 'where,' hypermobile joint.

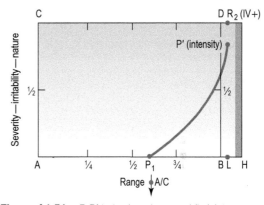

Figure A1.51 • P₁P′ behaviour, hypermobile joint.

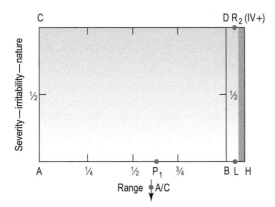

Figure A1.49 • L – 'what' (and define), hypermobile joint.

Step 4. P′ define (Fig. A1.50)
Step 5. P₁P′ behaviour (Fig. A1.51)
Step 6. R₁ (Fig. A1.52)
Step 7. R₁R₂ behaviour (Fig. A1.53)

Treatment

Hypermobility is not a contraindication to manipulation. Most patients with hypermobile joints, one of which becomes painful, have a hypomobile situation at that joint. They are therefore treated on the same basis as is used for hypomobility. It makes no difference whether the limit (L) of the range, on examination, is found to be beyond the end of the average-normal range (as in the example above, L being beyond B) or before it (L being on the side of B). Proof of hypomobility is validated by assessment at the end of successful treatment.

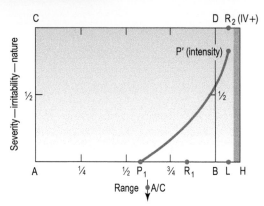
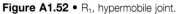

Figure A1.52 • R_1, hypermobile joint.

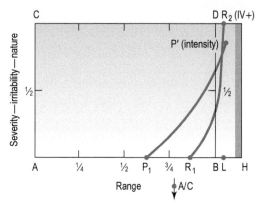

Figure A1.53 • R_1R_2 behaviour, hypermobile joint.

References

Chesworth BM, MacDermid JC, Roth JH, et al: Movement diagram and 'end-feel' reliability when measuring passive lateral rotation of the shoulder in patients with shoulder pathology, *Phys Ther* 78:593–601, 1998.

Latimer J, Lee M, Adams R: The effects of training with feedback on physiotherapy students' ability to judge lumbar stiffness, *Man Ther* 1, 266–270, 1996.

Lee R, Evans J: Towards a better understanding of spinal posteroanterior mobilization, *Physiotherapy* 80:68–73, 1994.

Maitland GD, The hypothesis of adding compression when examining and treating synovial joints, *J Orthop Sports Phys Ther* 2:7–14, 1980.

Maitland GD: *Peripheral Manipulation*, ed 3, Oxford, 1991, Butterworth-Heinemann.

Maitland GD: *Neuro/musculoskeletal Examination and Recording Guide*, ed 5, Adelaide, 1992, Lauderdale Press.

Petty N, Maher C, Latimer J, et al: Manual examination of accessory movements-seeking R_1, *Man Ther* 7:39–43, 2002.

Snow CP: Strangers and Brothers, London, 1965, Penguin Books, p 67.

Clinical examples of movement diagrams

CHAPTER CONTENTS

Hypermobility 423
   Step 1. P_1 423
   Step 2. L – where. 423
   Step 3. L – what (and define) 423
   Step 4. P' define 423
   Step 5. P_1P' behaviour 423
   Step 6. R_1 423
   Step 7. R_1R_2 behaviour 423
Scheuermann's disease. 424
   The spondylitic cervical spine. 425

Hypermobility

This example is included for the express purpose of clarifying the misconceptions that exist about hypermobility, and the direct influence that some authors and practitioners afford it in restricting treatment.

If the movement (using the same C3/4 joint being tested with PAs on C3, pages 421–424), before having become painful, were hypermobile, the basic format of the movement diagram would be as shown in Figure A2.1.

Step 1. P_1

The method is the same as in Example 1 (*see* Figure A2.2).

Step 2. L – where

The method is the same as in Example 1 (*see* Figure A2.3).

Step 3. L – what (and define)

The method is the same as in Example 1 (*see* Figure A2.4).

Step 4. P' define

(Figure A2.5)

Step 5. P_1P' behaviour

(Figure A2.6)

Step 6. R1

(Figure A2.7)

Step 7. R_1R_2 behaviour (Figure A2.8)

Treatment

Hypermobility is not a contraindication to manipulation. Most patients with hypermobile joints, one of which becomes painful, have a hypomobile situation at that joint. They are therefore treated on the

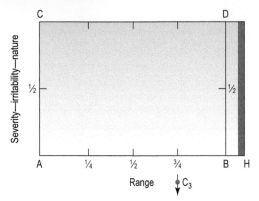

Figure A2.1 • Movement diagram for hypermobile range

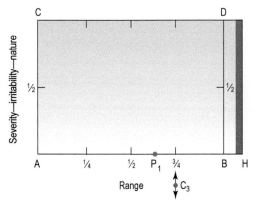

Figure A2.2 • P₁, hypermobile joint

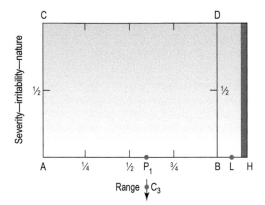

Figure A2.3 • L – where, hypermobile joint

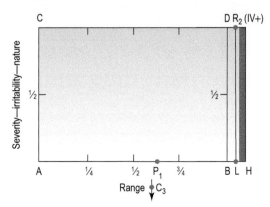

Figure A2.4 • L – what (and define), hypermobile joint

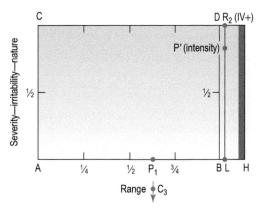

Figure A2.5 • P' – define, hypermobile joint

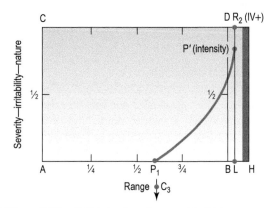

Figure A2.6 • P₁P' behaviour, hypermobile joint

same basis as is used for hypomobility. It makes no difference whether the limit (L) of the range, on examination, is found to be beyond the end of the average–normal range (as in the example above, L being beyond B) or before it (L being on the side of B).

Scheuermann's disease

Manipulative physiotherapists are frequently asked to treat patients who have back pain related to the stiffness resulting from old, inactive Scheuermann's

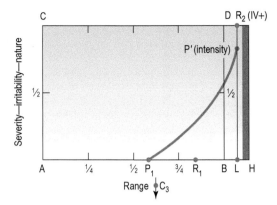

Figure A2.7 • R_1, hypermobile joint

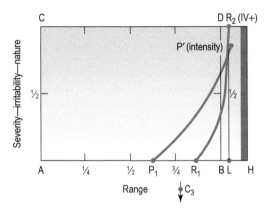

Figure A2.8 • R_1R_2 behaviour, hypermobile joint

disease. The purpose of presenting this series of movement diagrams is to emphasize the 'end-feel' characteristic of posteroanterior central vertebral pressures on a Scheuermann's spine.

These movement diagrams only represent the resistance (free of muscle spasm) element. It is assumed that the peak of the characteristic kyphosis is at L1, and that the patient is lying prone, which puts the main vertebra(e) involved at the limit of their range of extension and posteroanterior movement (point A on the base line of the diagram) (Figure A2.9).

It may be of interest to comment that in the young adolescent it is possible to know, by the feel of resistance to posteroanterior pressures over five adjacent vertebrae, that osteochondritis ('Scheuermann's disease') is present even before the radiological evidence is obvious. Of the five vertebrae referred to, the top and bottom ones will have a normal range, and the middle one of the five will have a

slightly prominent spinous process and will be resistant to the posteroanterior pressures. The adjacent vertebrae to the central prominent and stiff one will have a degree of resistance to the pressures that is equal at the two vertebrae, and a degree of stiffness that is halfway between that of the two normal vertebrae.

The spondylitic cervical spine

Many or most of the elderly patients referred for treatment of local cervical symptoms have underlying wear-and-tear degenerative changes. These changes of themselves are not necessarily responsible for the present problem, although they may account for some restriction of movement and a degree of discomfort which the patient considers to be normal. This being so, the manipulative physiotherapist does not have as her goal the restoration of a FULL pain-free range of movement. The goal is a 'compromise goal', which infers that the range of movement will be restored to what it was before it became symptomatic, and the symptoms will have either been cleared or restored to what the patient had considered to be his normal.

Such circumstances occur so often that they are worthy of description in terms of the movement diagram.

The example will be of an elderly man who has sought treatment because he is having increasing discomfort in the right mid-cervical area, which he notices with turning his head to the right, particularly when trying to reverse his car.

Prior to seeking treatment he believed he could turn his head equally to left and right, and the movements were painless. As is so often the case, his normal range of cervical rotation was only approximately 35–40°. Representing this on a movement diagram (that is, as rotation for the whole cervical spine rather than for one particular intervertebral level) at a time when he considered that he was normal, the diagram would be something like that shown in Figure A2.10.

At the time when he had had his right-sided cervical pain, the movement diagram of his cervical rotation to the right differed in small but significant ways from the above (Figure A2.11). The differences are:

1. P_1P' (a significant change in the pain sensation).

2. R_1R_2 (the altered behaviour of the resistance).

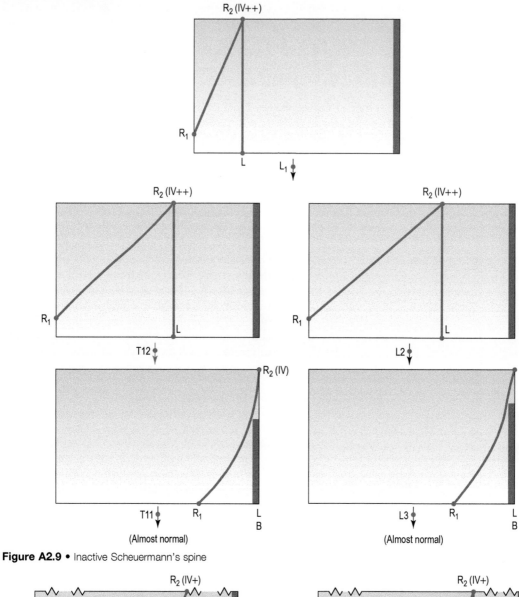

Figure A2.9 • Inactive Scheuermann's spine

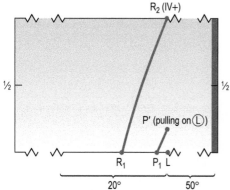

Figure A2.10 • Cervical rotation right, normal movement diagram (spondylitic spine)

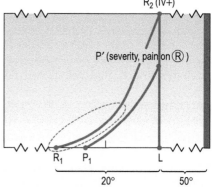

Figure A2.11 • Cervical rotation right, symptomatic movement diagram (spondylitic spine)

The P_1 of *Figure A2.11* will only return to his 'normal' if the new curved first part (encircled) of the R_1R_2 behaviour of the resistance is cleared. If treatment is successful, the R_1R_2 line will change so that the behaviour of resistance will return to its original straight line (R_1R_2 in *Figure A2.10*). P_1P' of *Figure A2.11* will also resume to being the P_1P' of *Figure A2.10*.

Readers may believe that it is impossible to assess such small changes in resistance (encircled part in Figure A2.11). However, if they apply themselves to the discipline required for compiling movement diagrams – that is, doing passive movements critically and analysing what they feel, rather than doing passive movements by instinct – they will be surprised at just how precise their judgements can become (Evans 1982).

Tip

It is surprising how precise a judgement of small changes in resistance can be.

Reference

Evans DH: *Accuracy of Palpation Skills*. Unpublished thesis, 1982, South Australian Institute of Technology.

Examination refinements and movement diagrams

CHAPTER CONTENTS

Varied inclinations and contact points 428

Sagittal posteroanterior movements in
combined positions 430

Diagrams of different movements on a
patient with one disorder 431

Varied inclinations and contact points

> **Tip**
>
> The aim of varying the angle of inclination and point of contact is to find the movement that provokes the symptoms which are comparable with those of the patient.

In Chapter 6 it was stated that palpation examination techniques need to be varied (1) in their angle of inclination by amounts even as small as 1–2°; and (2) in their contact points, which similarly may be as little as 1 mm or less apart. The aim of this examination technique is to find the movement that provokes symptoms comparable with the patient's symptoms. If posteroanterior central vertebral pressure is the movement being examined, the sagittal direction can be inclined:

1. Cephalad/caudad
2. Left/right
3. In various combinations of these.

The point of contact on each spinous process can be changed from the standard two bifid processes to:

1. One process
2. Higher/lower on the one process
3. Medially/laterally on the one process
4. Various combinations of these
5. The same variations (1)–(4) in contact with both processes (when (3) would read 'left/right').

As an example of this, a patient may have an area of general mid-cervical pain spreading across the top of the trapezius on the right and reaching to the top of the right shoulder. On examination by palpation, moving the spinous process of C5 in variations of inclinations and contact points, the movement diagrams may be as follows:

1. The exact sagittal posteroanterior movement with each thumb contacting each bifid spinous process of C5 (Figure A3.1).
2. When the sagittal posteroanterior movement is emphasized onto the right bifid process the diagram changes in its pain response and is closer to being 'comparable' than in (1) above (Figure A3.2).
3. When the contact point is changed to the lateral side of the left bifid process and directed 10° towards the right, a quite different response results (Figure A3.3). Obviously this test movement is insignificant compared with the preceding two tests.
4. If the examination has been carried out in the sequence represented here, the thought may

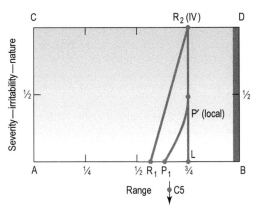

Figure A3.1 • Exact sagittal posteroanterior movement, thumbs contacting each of C5's bifid spinous processes

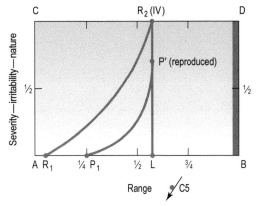

Figure A3.4

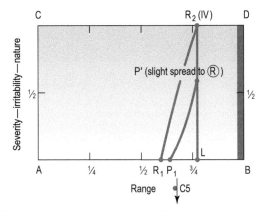

Figure A3.2 • Sagittal posteroanterior movement, emphasized on to right bifid spinous process of C5

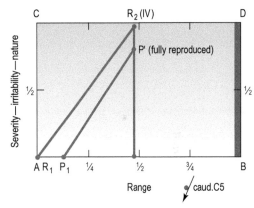

Figure A3.5

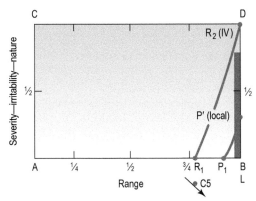

Figure A3.3 • Sagittal posteroanterior movement, contact point on lateral side of left bifid spinous process of C5 and directed 10° to the right

be: 'Well, pushing on the right bifid process is the most limited movement so far, and the pain response does produce some spread of pain to the supraspinous fossa. I wonder what the pain response will be if I move my contact point to the lateral side of the right bifid process and incline the PA say 20° towards the left? (Figure A3.4). This pain response is much more comparable with his symptoms, and the movement is both stiffer and has a more similar behaviour to that of the pain than have any of the preceding movements.

5. 'I wonder if this is sufficiently comparable to be used as the treatment technique? I think I'll just try adding a bit of caudad inclination through the same contact point.' (Figure A3.5).

This pain response, being such a clear 'reproduced pain', is very favourable. Another element indicating good comparability with the patient's symptoms is the similarity of the behaviour of the resistance element to the pain element.

This discussion can be carried one stage further, but in a somewhat different direction. If the manipulative physiotherapist chooses to use her thumb palpation movement as her treatment technique, she has to choose between the following:

1. Avoiding the patient's pain and therefore using *Figure A3.3* as the treatment technique.
2. Reproducing his symptoms and therefore using *Figure A3.5*.
3. Taking a reasonably safe pathway by using *Figure A3.4* but doing it as a grade IV movement, or even grade IV, so that a lesser degree of pain is provoked.

Sagittal posteroanterior movements in combined positions

> **Tip**
>
> Posteroanterior movements in combined positions are valuable as a means of finding the movement which provokes the patient's symptoms. This can then be used as a treatment technique or progression of treatment.

The value of combined movements in examination and treatment has been emphasized in this edition. Imagine a patient who has left suprascapular symptoms that are provoked by compressing type movements, such as extension, lateral flexion left, rotation left, and central posteroanterior movements on the left articular pillar of C5:

1. If the central posteroanterior movements are performed with the patient's head straight, the movement diagram may be as in Figure A3.6.
2. If the same sagittal posteroanterior movement is performed with the head rotated to the left, the diagram will be different, as shown in Figure A3.7.

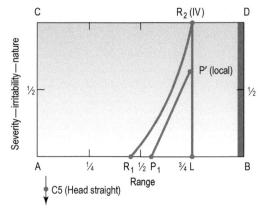

Figure A3.6 • Central posteroanterior movements, with patient's head straight

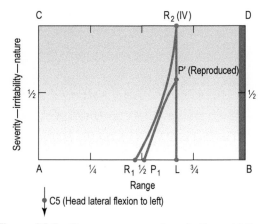

Figure A3.7 • The same movements as in *Figure A3.6*, with head in lateral flexion to the left and rotation to the left

3. Sagittal posteroanterior movements performed with the head in lateral flexion to the left may have the movement diagram shown in Figure A3.7.
4. If the patient's head is first laterally flexed to the left and then while in this position is rotated to the left, posteroanterior movements in this combination might be as shown in Figure A3.8.

Because the computations are endless, the manipulative physiotherapist should be aware of the possibilities available to her and be capable of exploiting them if progress is not up to the expectations.

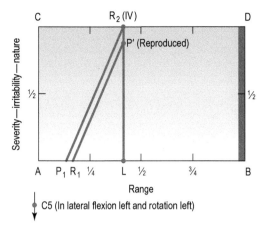

C5 (In lateral flexion left and rotation left)

Figure A3.8 • Sagittal posteroanterior movements, with patient's head first laterally flexed to the left and rotated to the left

Diagrams of different movements on a patient with one disorder

Tip

To draw diagrams for different movement directions in a patient with one disorder will help to determine which of these directions is likely to be more effective as a treatment technique. Furthermore, reassessment will determine the relationship between the patient's signs and symptoms and the movement diagram.

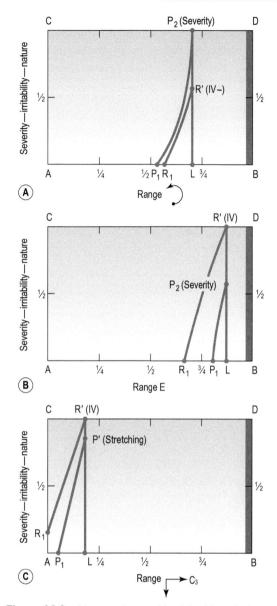

Figure A3.9 • Movements provoking left mid-cervical pain. (A) Cervical rotation to the left. (B) Extension. (C) Posteroanterior unilateral vertebral pressure on left side of C3 (4 mm)

When examining a patient's movements, there may be three main movements that provoke his (say) left mid-cervical pain. Assume that the movements are cervical rotation to the left, extension, and posteroanterior unilateral vertebral pressure on the left side of C3. The movement diagrams of each movement might be as in Figure A3.9.

The three movement diagrams are different from each other, and seeing that they are different helps in determining which will be used (if any of them are) as a treatment technique. Also, if one *is* chosen, and it is successful, it would be hoped that all three diagrams would show the same kind of improvement. If, however, two of them did improve and the third did not, and also if the patient did not feel he was getting better, then perhaps the unchanged movement diagram would then be used as the treatment technique.

There is one other important aspect to bear in mind. As well as the three diagrams depicted, cervical rotation to the right might prove a useful diagram, and be useful as a treatment technique (Figure A3.10).

Figures A3.9 and A3.10 are related to the standard physiological and accessory movements. It becomes more complicated when combined movements are introduced. However, when combined movements are used as part of the examination, diagrams can be used for them in the same way as described earlier in this appendix.

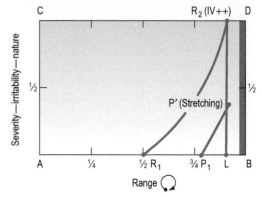

Figure A3.10 • Cervical rotation to the right in the same patient as in Figure A3.9

Recording

Elly Hengeveld

CHAPTER CONTENTS

Introduction 433

Asterisks 435

Conditions. 435

Some remarks with regards to recording. 435

Recording of subjective examination
findings 436

Recording of physical examination
findings 437

Active movements 440

Passive movements 440

Recording of treatment interventions 441

Information, instructions, exercises,
warning at the end of a session 441

Recording of follow-up sessions 442

Retrospective assessment 442

Written records by the patient 443

Conclusion 443

Key words

Recording, reassessment, SOAP notes

Introduction

Assessment and treatment require an in-depth written record of the findings and results at each session. Ideally, documentation which is systematic, consequent and easy to (re-)read in a short time provides the physiotherapist with a framework that should lead the therapist throughout the overall therapeutic process. Systematic records serve as a mnemonic and a means of communication to other professionals. They support the physiotherapist in various ways:

- To reflect upon the decisions made
- To control the actions taken
- If necessary, to quickly adapt the therapy to a changing situation.

Hence, written records are essential in the process of ongoing quality management.

It is argued that many physiotherapists consider documentation of sessions as a necessary evil. As a consequence many records frequently seem superficial and incomplete (Cohen 1997). Although probably recording will not be encountered with a lot of positive expectations in learning the 'art of physiotherapy', there are various reasons why physiotherapists should consider the recording of the sessions they shape:

- Records serve as a mnemonic for the physiotherapist of what has been done, thought and planned
- Systematic recording serves clinical reasoning and learning processes: committing thoughts to paper forces therapists to think more precisely and accurately and to become aware of their own reasoning processes. It enhances reflection and monitoring decisions made and actions taken

- Committing the essence of examination and treatment findings to paper is a valuable learning experience in itself. It forces one to identify the things that are essential, and record them, and leave out the less important information
- Committing thoughts to paper, with systematic recording, helps to clear the mind as the information and impressions gained throughout are organized
- Recording of patient information, actions and planning steps support the development of clinical patterns in memory. Therefore recording may be an essential process in the development of experiential knowledge (Higgs & Titchen 1995, Nonaka & Takeuchi 1995)
- Ideally, the records should document the trail along which assessment and treatment are moving
- Comprehensive, systematic patient records may serve as a basis for clinical case studies
- Records may be a mnemonic for the patient as well. In some cases, the patient may have forgotten how the disorder has been improved immediately following a treatment. If for other reasons a few days later the symptoms recur, the patient may easily interpret the condition as unchanged. Examination of the record made immediately following the treatment may guide the physiotherapist as well as the patient in the reassessment of the patient's condition over the whole period directly after the last session until the moment that symptoms increased again
- Records aid communication in team collaboration. If a colleague is absent from work, the physiotherapist may be able to continue with the initialized course of treatment, provided the records are such that they are understandable
- Recording for legal reasons – in many countries physiotherapists are enforced by law to store their patient records for a certain period of time. Furthermore, physiotherapy records may be used in litigation
- An increasing number of professional associations declare documentation as an integral part of the physiotherapy process (ÖPV 1998, WCPT 1999, Heerkens et al. 2003).

SOAP notes

Recording of therapy sessions must include detailed information, yet must be brief and provide a simple overview. Within this concept use has been made of the so-called 'SOAP' notes (Weed 1964, Kirk 1988). The acronym SOAP refers to the various parts of the assessment process:

1. Collection of subjective information
2. Collection of objective information
3. Performing an assessment
4. Develop and formulate a plan.

It is not mandatory to follow the guidelines and abbreviations as set out in this book; however, some method must be determined to suit the patient's comments and the therapist's pattern of thinking. The basic elements of the SOAP mnemonic may serve as a useful format to follow all the steps of the therapeutic process in a brief and comprehensive way.

It has been argued that the term 'objective' in the SOAP notes is somewhat awkward, due to the fact that the physiotherapist values the *subjective* experience of the patient while performing the test movements. Furthermore, it is argued that the physiotherapist as the 'measuring instrument' will give attention to those aspects of a test which seem most relevant at the time, and thus true objectivity in test procedures may not exist (Grieve 1988). It has therefore been decided to replace the term 'objective examination' with 'physical examination' (P/E).

There has been criticism that SOAP notes within problem oriented medical records (POMR) would confine the physiotherapist to focusing merely on biomedical data (French 1991); however, if the physiotherapist pays attention to key words and specific key phrases of the patient which are indicative of the individual illness experience, they may be recorded in parentheses and integrated in the documentation, thereby incorporating elements of the individual illness experience into the records.

At all times patient records should include the findings as well as the steps in planning –a trail is laid of what is done *and* what is thought. Recording encompasses ideally:

- Information on examination and assessment procedures
- Treatment interventions and results (reassessments)
- Planning steps and hypotheses formulated
- Important key words or phrases of the patient.

Asterisks

During the subjective examination the patient may state certain facts related to the disability which may prove to be valuable parameters for reassessment procedures. These should be highlighted in the records *immediately*, and an 'asterisk' sign may be used.

Although the use of asterisks is not mandatory, it may speed up the whole process. They are time savers, reminders and indicators of highly important facts for the particular person. Identifying these main assessment markers with a large, obvious asterisk not only enforces a commitment but also makes reassessment procedures quicker, easier, more complete and therefore more valuable.

Using asterisks is just as valuable for the physical examination parameters as it is for the subjective examination. Similarly, making use of the asterisks progressively *during* the physical examination rather than *after* is recommended. The same applies to each subsequent session.

At times it seems that the term 'asterisk' has become jargon; however, it is not meant in such a way. People teaching and working with this concept may frequently use the term 'subjective and physical examination asterisks'. Mostly this refers to information of subjective and physical examination parameters which will be reassessed at regular intervals over the whole therapeutic process in order to monitor progress in rehabilitation and the effects of treatment (Box A4.1).

Box A4.1

Use of asterisks

Asterisks are an invaluable aid in assessment procedures. The use of an asterisk in recording highlights the following aspects:
- Primary symptoms or activity limitations
- Signs that reproduce a patient's symptoms
- Other important comparable signs that will be followed up in reassessment procedures
- Other information that is important
- Key issues that need to be followed up
- 'Asterisk as you go along' indicates that it is important to immediately highlight relevant findings once they have been obtained rather than in retrospect. If the findings have been recorded straight away it will influence the physiotherapist in the further procedures of examination and assessment.

Conditions

Some people may prefer other ways of recording. However, regardless the method of recording, some conditions need to be fulfilled. Patient records need to be:
- Organized
- Clear
- Comprehensive
- Simple to (re)read
- Written concisely, in telegraphese
- Homogenous, consequent.

Some remarks with regards to recording

It is important to record related information even when the findings indicate normality. By their having been recorded, reference at a later date shows that the particular questions have been asked or physical examination tests have been carried out.

Recording normal findings on a 'record sheet' is a quick and simple procedure. For example, if a patient has pain in the shoulder area and the therapist has examined the acromioclavicular joint *comprehensively* and found it to have normal painless movements, all that might be recorded is:

$$AC ✓✓$$

The point is, *it must be recorded*.

There is much more to be recorded from an initial consultation than for subsequent sessions. However, the same detail is required and so the same details and abbreviations can be used. People have likes and dislikes about these symbols – this does not matter, provided the criteria for comprehensive recording are met.

Questionnaires as well as 'cheat sheets' as they are often termed, have advantages and disadvantages. The primary considerations are that they should not be regimented and they should not be detailed. A cheat sheet that has a list of questions requiring ticks and crosses, should not be used. They are inflexible and destroy independent thinking on the part of the examiner, and they completely obliterate any chance of following the patient's line of thought or the pursuit of hypotheses in greater detail.

Recording of subjective examination findings

With each patient there are many questions and answers that need to be entered in the recording, even if it is only to show that the question, which was important, has in fact been posed and answered.

It is a safe procedure to utilize the *patient's words* during the recording of subjective examination findings. For example, if a patient complains of a pulling in the arm while lifting the arm above the head, this needs to be recorded as the patient said it, rather than the physiotherapist's language of 'symptoms or pain with flexion', as this may immediately narrow down the physiotherapist's thinking.

Key words and phrases indicative of the personal illness experience may be put in quotation marks. It has been emphasized that such key words and phrases may be essential information to the shaping of the therapeutic process, hence they have to be recorded accordingly.

Organization of the information in the main categories of the subjective examination is essential to keep an overview over the process of subjective examination. While asking questions regarding the 'main problem', it is possible that the patient gives information on history mingled with, for example, bits of symptomatic behaviour. In such cases it is relevant to leave sufficient space on the paper to organize and record the information under sections 'history' or 'behaviour' rather than writing down every bit of information in a chronological manner. This will help the physiotherapist to keep an overview over the whole process of subjective examination, even if the communication technique of 'paralleling' has been chosen (Chapter 3).

Body chart

- Frequently, after establishment of the patient's main problem and receiving a more general statement about the perceived disability, the area, depth and nature, behaviour and chronology of the symptoms are clarified and recorded on a 'body chart' (Fig. A4.1).
- Reference to such a body chart provides a quick and clear reminder of the patient's symptoms and main problem.
- A well-drawn body chart helps to generate hypotheses on the sources of the movement

dysfunction or symptoms as well as on the neurophysiological pain mechanisms. Additionally, first hypotheses with regard to precautions and contraindications may be made.

- In principle, the body chart is drawn by the physiotherapist to facilitate recording and memory.
- Occasionally, in patients with chronic pain states, the body chart may be drawn by the patient. If different colours are used, as a metaphor for the pain experience they may become a guide in reassessment procedures.
- If the information on a body chart is recorded consistently at the same place all the time, self-monitoring mechanisms are more easily activated. If the physiotherapist forgets to ask certain questions, this may be noticed more easily when re-reading the information.
- The use of Arabic numerals in circles for the different symptom areas simplifies later recording: if there is a need to refer to the symptom areas, the numerals can be used rather than lengthy descriptions of the symptom areas.

Clinical tip

Always record the same information on the same spot of the body chart. This enhances self-monitoring – on re-reading the information it will be easier to discern if certain details are missing.

Behaviour of symptoms and activities

The information on the 'behaviour of symptoms' is essential to the expression of many hypotheses. Furthermore, the information usually serves in reassessment procedures of subsequent sessions. Therefore the information needs to be recorded in sufficient detail.

If activities or positions are found which aggravate the patient's symptoms, this has to be recorded meticulously. However, any easing factors also need to be written down straight away, on the same line as the activity which provokes the symptoms. This may sound pedantic to some; however, it will give the physiotherapist an immediate overview as to which activities and positions the patient has developed as useful coping strategies and with which ones the patient may need some help.

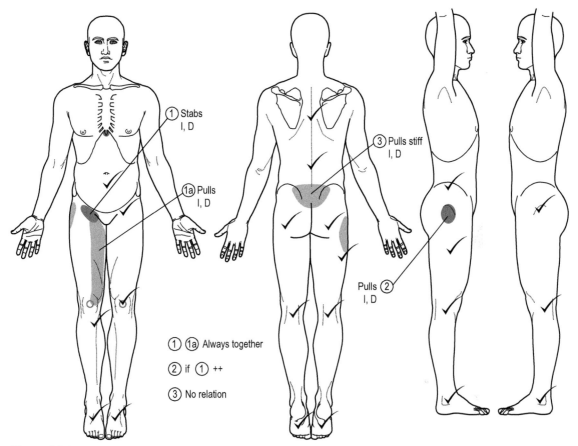

Figure A4.1 • Example of a body chart.

Some examples are:

- *① ↑ Gardening, pulling weeds, in squat position; after 10' P₁ ①, after 20' ①
  ↓ Gets up, walks around (few steps, shuttles leg):
  ①↓ 100% immed. May continue gardening.
- *① ↑ Putting on socks, in standing – activity possible as usual
  ↓①↓ 100% immed. as soon as leg is put down.
- *① ↑ Lying in bed – prone, right leg pulled up. Wakes up c. 03:00 ①
  ↓ Does not know how to ease. Gets up, walks c. 20' ① 'acceptable'

History

At times it may be difficult to keep an overview of all the information regarding the history of a patient's problem and to monitor if all the relevant data have been obtained. This may happen particularly in those circumstances where there have been more episodes and the problem has been recurrent for many years.A4.

Although not mandatory, the physiotherapist may draw a line indicative of the course of time to keep an overview of both the current and previous history (Figs A4.2, A4.3).

Recording of physical examination findings

Physical examination findings need to be recorded in sufficient detail and systematically in order to allow for quick referencing during subsequent reassessment procedures.

Making use of symbols helps speed up the process and enhances quick referencing (Table A4.1).

Current Hx

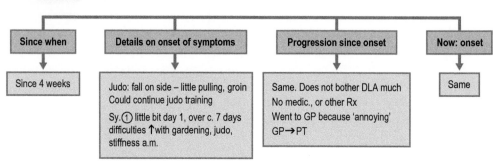

Figure A4.2 • Time line: current history.

Previous Hx

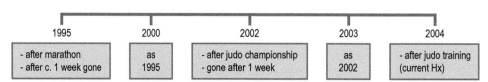

Between episodes: no symptoms, no disabilities
Current episode: does not disappear with little stretching exercises as in other episodes

Figure A4.3 • Time line: previous history.

Table A4.1 Recording symbols			
Peripheral joints		**Spine**	
F	Flexion	↕	Central posteroanterior pressure (PAs) ↙ with a Ⓛ inclination
E	Extension		
Ab	Abduction	↨	Central anteroposterior pressures (APs)
Ad	Adduction		
↺	Medial rotation	⌐•	Unilateral PAs on Ⓛ ◁ with a medial inclination
↻	Lateral rotation	⌐•	Unilateral APs on the Ⓛ
HF	Horizontal flexion	←•—	Transverse movement towards Ⓛ
HE	Horizontal extension		
HBB	Hand-behind-back	↻	Rotation towards Ⓛ
Inv	Inversion	↖	Lateral flexion towards Ⓛ
Ev	Eversion	←•→	Longitudinal movement (state cephalad or caudad)
DF	Dorsiflexion		
PF	Plantarflexion	⌐↓	Unilateral PAs at angle of Ⓡ 2nd rib
Sup	Supination	•—↓	Further laterally on Ⓡ on 2nd rib
Pron	Pronation		
El	Elevation	⌐↑	Unilateral APs on Ⓡ
De	Depression	CT ↗	Cervical traction in flexion
Protr	Protraction	CT ↑	Cervical traction in neutral (sitting)

Table A4.1 Recording symbols—cont'd

Peripheral joints		Spine	
Retr	Retraction	IVCT ↑	Sitting
Med	Medial	IVCT ↗	Lying
Lat	Lateral		
OP	Overpressure		
PPIVM	Passive physiological intervertebral movements	IVCT ↗ 10 3/0 15	Intermittent variable cervical traction in some degree of neck flexion, the strength of pull being 10 kg with a 3-second hold period, no rest period, for a treatment time lasting 15 minutes
PAIVM	Passive accessory intervertebral movements		
ULNT	Upper limb neural tests		
LLNT	Lower limb neural tests	LT	Lumbar traction
Q	Quadrant	LT 30/15	Lumbar traction, the strength of pull being 30 kg for a treatment time of 15 minutes
Lock	Locking position		
F/Ab	Flexion abduction	LT crk	Lumbar traction with hips and knees flexed: 15 kg
F/Ad	Flexion adduction	15/5	for 5 minutes
E/Ab	Extension abduction	IVLT 50 0/0 10	Intermittent variable lumbar traction, the strength of pull being 50 kg, with no hold period and no rest period, for a treatment time lasting 10 minutes
E/Ad	Extension adduction		
Distr	Distraction		
↕	Posteroranterior movement		
↥	Anteroposterior movement		
→→	Transverse movement in the direction indicated		
↕	Gliding adjacent joint surfaces		
>•<	Compression Longitudinal movement:		
Ceph	Cephalad		
Caud	Caudad		

Longitudinal movement is the direction of movement of a joint in line with the longitudinal axis of the body in its anatomical position. When that **same** movement is performed in any other position than the anatomical position, that movement of the joint is still called longitudinal movement even though it is not now in line with the longitudinal axis of the body

Spinal data reproduced by kind permission from Maitland, G. D., Hengeveld, E., Banks, K. & English, K. 2001. *Maitland's Vertebral Manipulation*, 6th edn. Oxford: Butterworth-Heinemann

Active movements

When recording the range and quality of movement and the symptomatic response to that movement, one should develop a pattern of recording and stick to it. By doing so, more facts can be remembered, while at the same time leaving the therapist's mental processes more time to take in other details. Active movement findings can be recorded as follows:

$$\text{Sup } \checkmark, \checkmark_{\text{IV++}}$$

This example means supination (sup) has a normal range and quality of movement (the first tick, $\checkmark$) and has no abnormal pain response when overpressure is applied (the second tick, $\checkmark$).

It is suggested relating the first tick ($\checkmark$) to movement responses such as range and quality of movement and the second tick ($\checkmark$) to symptom responses which occur during the test movement. It may be indicated with a grading of IV−, IV or IV+ how firm the overpressure has been. This is particularly relevant in those cases where the physiotherapist wants to test the movements with a certain amount of overpressure; however, factors in the 'nature of the disorder' may limit the physiotherapist in applying maximum overpressure.

A movement cannot be classed (or recorded) as normal unless the range is pain free both actively and passively. Further overpressure applied at the limit of the available range should not cause pain other than normal responses.

Abnormal findings may be recorded as follows:

$$\text{*Ab } 170°, \text{Dev. Ventr. } 120-170°, \text{①}_{\text{act. EOR}}$$
$$\text{Corr. Dev. } 130°, \text{①}11$$

This indicates that the range of abduction has been 170°, with a deviation of the movement between 120° and 170° of abduction; symptom reproduction occurred at the active end of range without application of overpressure. With correction of the deviation in the movement, the range decreased until 130° of abduction and the pain was clearly increased.

$$\text{*Hip F } 130°, \text{loc P groin}_{\text{IV}-}, \text{①}_{\text{IV}+}$$

This example shows that the overall range of hip flexion was 130°, without any deviations in the quality of the movement; local symptoms were produced with a light overpressure ('IV−'), symptom reproduction occurred with stronger overpressure ('IV+').

Passive movements

With passive movement the behaviour of pain, resistance and motor responses (spasm) is monitored. The physiotherapist is particularly interested in how these components behave and relate to each other. This is a very detailed examination procedure and may be considered as a part of the 'art of manipulative physiotherapy'. Most simply, but not mandatory, would be the drawing of a movement diagram, as delineated in Appendices 1–3. Otherwise abnormal findings regarding the behaviour of P_1 and P', R_1 and R_2, including their relationship, may be recorded verbally.

If certain passive movements are classed as normal, the same method ($\checkmark$), $\checkmark$)) as with active movements may be used. However, if relevant abnormal findings are present, this method is not sufficiently comprehensive.
Example:

$$\text{SLR}^®: R_1: 50°, \text{L 5 } R_2 \text{ } 70°; P_1 \text{ pulling hamstr. c. } 55°,$$
$$\text{P' only little } (3/10).$$

This example indicates that the physiotherapist first felt an increase in resistance with c. 50° of SLR, the movement was limited by resistance at c. 70° of SLR, only a little pulling sensation was provoked in the hamstrings area. Figure A4.4 illustrates the associated movement diagram.

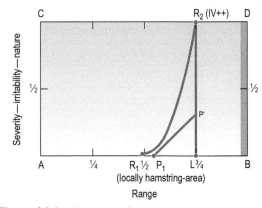

Figure A4.4 • Movement diagram.

Recording of treatment interventions

Before performing a treatment technique, the planning and the reasoning for its selection should be recorded. Next, the treatment and its effect should be written down. This needs to include sufficient details in order to be able to refer back at later stages when making retrospective assessments.

The treatment record for a passive mobilization technique should contain:

- the position of the patient
- the position of the joint
- selected treatment technique(s), including inclinations of the movements
- grade(s) of the technique
- rhythm in which the technique was performed
- duration (in number of repetitions or time units)
- symptomatic responses and the patient's reactions while the intervention is being performed ('assessment during treatment' – see Chapter 6)
- reassessment immediately following the technique (it is usually helpful to make comparisons or statements as to which parameters have improved and which ones have stayed unchanged).

It is essential not only to record the treatment by passive movement in detail but also active procedures, exercises or physical applications (e.g. ultrasound requires the same depth of recording).

Treatment is followed by a reassessment in which patients are asked to make a comparison of any changes of symptoms or in their sense of wellbeing resulting from the technique. This is then followed by a reassessment of the affected physical examination tests. Ideally, the records of the physical examination findings include a brief appraisal of the results in comparison with the assessment just before the application of the treatment technique.

Finally, at the end of a treatment session, the clinician should commit to paper thoughts on how treatment needs to be modified at the next session. Such an analysis not only forces the clinician to reflect on clinical reasoning processes, but also stimulates memory of the last treatment session.

Examples:

- **Passive movement:**

Rx G/H, Supine	C/O: 'same'
In: 150°F (before P₁)	P/E: F 160°, ① IV++
Do ✗: ↻, IV– to IV	☺
Smooth rhythm, rel. quick	('feels much freer, I can move higher')
Totally c. 6'	HBB: range & P ISQ
'Comfortable'; after 4' R₁ to L, especially with ✗	Plan: repeat same Rx; if HBB remains ISQ, do acc. mvt in EOR HBB
After c. 6' no further changes in P or R	

Other forms of treatment:

- **Exercises**

In sitting: do F/Ad hip R and L	C/O: 'lighter than before to stand'
5×, c. 10'', until slight pulling buttock	P/E: Lx F: <u>2 cm</u>, √, act EOR ☺
'Comfortable'	Hip F: 130°, ① IV+ ☺
	Plan: do ex. at/work; at least 3×/day A P buttock starts. 1–2 series; 5×/30'' each leg

- **Ultrasound**

Sitting, knee extended	C/O: 'not tender now'
Rx: US 3 MHz, large head; 1:2 int.	P/E: Squat: <u>full range</u>, √ ☺
1.0 W/cm²; 3'; on tender spot, medially knee	E/AB: √, ①, IV+ ☺
No pain	*(It is frequently useful to compare the results and to mark which elements may have improved following the intervention)*

Information, instructions, exercises, warning at the end of a session

Any information or instruction given during the treatment, any exercise that the patient should perform as a self-management strategy needs to be recorded as well.

At the beginning of a treatment series it is often important to warn the patient diplomatically for possible exacerbations. This also needs to be recorded.

Example

- Warned about possible increase; however, if spot gets smaller, may be a good sign.
- Should observe *and* compare:
  - mornings getting out of bed – changes in stiffness?
  - working in garden – anything different from before?
  - nights – anything changing in sleep pattern?
  - effect of exercise, if pain occurs?
- Instruction (e.g. remembers anything particular about fall during judo?).

Recording of follow-up sessions

When recording follow-up sessions, the first words must include a quotation of the patient's opinion of the effect of the previous treatment. This quotation must be worded in such a way that it is a 'comparison' rather than just a 'statement of fact'. The subjective reassessment is then completed in which the physiotherapist clarifies those activities that serve as parameters and have been highlighted with an asterisk in the records of previous sessions.

Following the subjective reassessment the record includes the physical examination tests which are being reassessed. These too are recorded as comparisons with the previous findings.

Changes in the physical examination findings will hopefully agree with the findings of the subjective assessment, so reinforcing each other. This will then make the total assessment more reliable.

Also during reassessment of physical examination tests it may be necessary to record key words and phrases; in the rehabilitation of, for example, shoulder problems it may be a good sign if the patient makes the spontaneous remark: *'the arm is mine again'*.

The following pattern may be used in recording follow-up sessions:

- Date, time of the day, Rx 3, D8 (indicating third session on eighth day since the initial consultation)
- C/O spontaneous information: 'better', 'felt lighter than before'
- C/O follow-up of subjective parameter: putting on socks today cf. yesterday: no pain (5 unusual! First time in 3 weeks!)
- PP
- P/E: reassessment of physical examination parameter (including statements of comparison with after/before the previous treatment)
- P/E: additional tests as planned
- Plan: e.g. stick to plan as stated after Rx 2
- Rx 3a (as above) …
- Rx 3b (as above)…
- Plan

Retrospective assessment

The record of retrospective assessment has to stand out from other parts of the treatment so that the information can be easily traced on reviewing progress in later sessions. This is particularly important when a patient has an extensive disorder and considerable treatment. To be practical, time must be a consideration, but not at the expense of detail and accuracy.

Especially within retrospective assessment, in the written record three requirements should be respected:

1. To stand out from other data (to be highlighted so that it is readily seen on checking back through the record).
2. To state with what time frame the comparison is made (e.g. Rx 5 cf. Rx 1).
3. To emphasize spontaneous information.

Retrospective assessments should include the following information and comparisons:

- General wellbeing compared with, for example, four sessions ago
- Symptoms compared with, for example, four sessions ago (know indicators of change – see Chapter 5)
- Level of activities compared
- Effect of interventions so far (P/E and passive movements)

- Effect of instructions, recommendations and exercises so far
- What has the patient learned so far – what was particularly relevant to the patient?
- Comparison of all the relevant physical examination parameters compared with, for example, four sessions ago
- Which interventions brought which results? (certain physical examination findings may improve more with some interventions than with others)
- Goals for the following phases of treatment (process of collaborative goal setting: redefinition or confirmation of agreed goals to treatment, interventions and the parameters to measure if the objectives are being achieved).

Written records by the patient

There are times when it is necessary for a patient to write a running commentary of the behaviour of the symptoms. For example, a patient may be a poor historian in which case he may be asked to write down how he feels immediately following treatment, how he feels that night and how he feels on first getting out of bed the next morning. Some people may feel this is encouraging a patient to become overly focussed on his symptoms. However, if the patient is asked not only to record how he feels, but also the level of activities, medication intake and possible self-management interventions, such a record may become a highly valuable teaching instrument which aids both the patient and the physiotherapist.

There are many different types of pre-printed form that can be used. However, it is essential that the forms leave space for information regarding:

- symptoms
- activities before and during the increase of symptoms
- activities throughout the day/week
- employment of self-management strategies to influence wellbeing, including the effects of the interventions.

When a written record by the patient is used, it should be handled by the manipulative physiotherapist in a particular sequence:

1. On receiving it from the patient, it should be laid down.
2. The patient should be asked to give a general impression of the effect of the last treatment.
3. The subjective assessment of the effect of the last treatment should be taken through to its conclusion.
4. The written record can then be assessed and any discrepancies clarified.

Conclusion

Although recording of examination findings, treatment interventions and results, and regular planning, may not be the most interesting part of learning, it is an essential element of the quality of the overall therapeutic process. It monitors the physiotherapist throughout the process and allows quick adaptation of interventions, if needed. When recording is accurate and succinct, and can be correctly interpreted by another person reading it, it is an invaluable self-teacher and may support physiotherapists on their path to expertise and maintaining this.

References

Cohen L: Documentation. In Wittink H, Hoskins Michel T, editors: *Chronic Pain Management for Physical Therapists*, Boston, 1997, Butterworth-Heinemann.

French S: Setting a record straight, *Therapy Weekly* 1:11, 1991.

Grieve GP: Critical examination and the SOAP mnemonic, *Physiotherapy* 74:97, 1988.

Heerkens YF, Lakerveld-Hey K, Verhoeven ALJ, et al: *KNGF – Richtlijn Fysiotherapeutische Verslaglegging*, Amersfoort, 2003, KNGF.

Higgs J, Titchen A: The nature, generation and verification of knowledge, *Physiotherapy* 81: 521–530, 1995.

Kirk D: *Problem Orientated Medical Records: Guidelines for Therapists*, London, 1988, Kings Fund Centre.

Nonaka I, Takeuchi, H: *The Knowledge-Creating Company*, New York, 1995, Oxford University Press.

ÖPV: *Broschüre Berufsbild Physiotherapeut*, Vienna, 1998, Österreichischer PhysiotherapieVerband.

WCPT: *Description of Physical Therapy*, London, 1999, World Confederation of Physical Therapy.

Weed L: Medical records, medical education and patient care, *Ir J Med Sci* 6:271–282, 1964.

Index

Page numbers followed by "f" indicate figures, "t" indicate tables, and "b" indicate boxes.

A

ABCDEFW mnemonic, 390–391
abdominal pain, 181f
Aβ fibres, 121, 122t
acceptance of patient, 2
accessory movements, 6
  lumbar spine, 265t–268t
    flexion, 299f
  PAIVMs see PAIVMs
  sacroiliac region, 358–362, 368–369
  testing, 7, 105
accuracy, clarification for, 30
ACTH, 129
active listening, 90
active movements, 381–384
  hip, 348–349
  lumbar spine, 273t–274t, 277–278
  promotion of, 381–384
  record-keeping, 440
  trunk, 345b, 347–348
active straight leg raising see straight leg raising
activities of daily living
  low back pain, 233
  pacing of, 388
  pelvic girdle pain, 344t
activity capabilities, 34, 93–94, 395
Aδ fibres, 121, 122t
adrenaline, 128
age of patient, 42
  cervical spine disorders, 116
  lumbar spine disorders, 254t, 265t–268t
alar ligament test, 151f
allodynia, 125, 179, 186
alternative questions, 90
analytical assessment, 8, 26, 98, 113

animals, response to noxious stimulation, 125
ankylosing spondylitis, 101, 254t
  excessive compression in, 367–368
  intra-articular injections for, 337t
antalgic posture, 123, 133, 140–141, 165, 168, 272, 346
anterior oblique sling of pelvic girdle, 330, 335–336
anterior superior iliac spine (ASIS), 352f, 353
anteroposterior vertebral pressure
  bilateral, cervical spine, 138f
  central, lumbar spine, 300f
  unilateral
    cervical spine, 138f, 218–220, 219f
    thoracic spine, 218–220, 219f
anxiety states, 21
appraisal, 47
arc of pain, 411, 411f
arm pain, thoracic spinal symptoms, 188f
arthrogenic impairment
  with myogenic impairment, 315f–318f
  with neurogenic impairment, 313f–315f, 318f
arthrogenic techniques, 305
assessment, 7–12
  analytical, 8, 98, 113
  asterisks in, 268, 277
  at initial examination, 41t, 96–97, 99–103
  cervical spine, 133
  diaphragm muscles, 364–365
  functional, 133
  listening see listening
  lumbar spine, 231–233, 308b–309b
  pain see pain
  pelvic floor muscles, 364
  pretreatment, 8–10
  progressive, 11

prospective, 308b–309b
resistance, behaviour of, 413, 413f–414f, 418f
retrospective, 11–12, 98, 112–113
  lumbar spine, 308b–309b
  record-keeping, 442–443
subjective, 8–9
treatment effects, 9–10
  at final examination, 12
  see also specific areas and conditions
assumptions, 47, 93
  causal, 48
  paradigmatic, 47–48
  prescriptive, 48
asterisks, 435
  in assessment, 268, 277
  use of, 435b
ATP, 122
auricular nerve, 137f
  neurodynamic testing, 143f
axoplasmic flow, 125, 125f

B

Babinski test, 134b
backache see low back pain
barriers to recovery, 390–395
  activity levels/participation, 395
  beliefs and expectations, 391–393
  confidence in own capabilities, 393
  perceived disability, 258, 391
  psychosocial risk factors, 392b
  second opinions, 393–394
  social environment, 395
bedside neurological examination, 134b
behaviour, 392b
  illness-related, 395
  pain-related, 87
  phases of change, 396
  of symptoms see symptoms, behaviour

beliefs and expectations, 391–393
bias, 15–16, 92–93
biceps femoris, 335
bilateral anteroposterior vertebral
    pressure
  cervical spine, 138f
  thoracic spine, 219f
biopsychosocial paradigm, 15, 18–19,
    174, 236
  cervical spine, 118–119, 118f, 119b
  facilitation of, 31–33
  low back pain, 242t
blocking of joint movements, 306b,
    414
blood flow, 124
bodily awareness, 111–112
bodily systems, screening of, 391b
body charts, 436, 437f
  lumbar spine, 259f–260f, 324f
body language, 87, 91
body-self neuromatrix, 36
bony changes in thoracic spine, 197
brachial plexus
  neurodynamic testing, 141
  palpation, 136–139
bradykinin, 122
brain
  changes in pain, 127, 127b
  pain-related areas, 126–127, 126b
'brainchild of ingenuity', technique as,
    6
breathing exercises, 129
'brick wall' model, 4t, 14–15
  thoracic spine, 190t
Brookfield, Steven, 16
Buteyko technique, 129

C

C fibres, 121, 122t
C1-2 (cervical spine) see cervical spine,
    C1-2 areas
C2-3 (cervical spine) see cervical spine,
    C2-3 areas
C2-7 (cervical spine) see cervical spine,
    C2-7 areas
C3-4 (cervical spine) see cervical spine,
    C3-4 areas
C7-T3 (thoracic spine) see thoracic
    spine, C7-T3 areas
C7-T4 (thoracic spine) see thoracic
    spine, C7-T4 areas
capability, definition of, 46
cardiac pain, 177f, 180f
case studies
  cervical spine, 164b–170b
  lumbar spine, 320
  sacroiliac region, 372b–376b
  thoracic spine, 178–182, 182f
catastrophizing, 21, 36, 156
causal assumptions, 48
central processing, 35–36
central sensitization
  cervical spine, 125–126, 130, 159
  headache, 126b

Centre for Epidemiologic Studies-
    Depression Scale, 24t
cerebral vascular accident, and cervical
    manipulation, 159
certainty matrix, 44, 44f
cervical anteroposterior unilateral
    vertebral pressure, 218–220,
    219f
cervical arterial dysfunction, 150, 150b
cervical lateral glide technique, 157,
    158f, 168f
cervical nerve roots
  lesions, 117–118, 121b
    context change, 128b, 153–155
    subjective examination, 131b
  palpation, 136–139
cervical spine, 116–163
  anteroposterior vertebral pressure
    bilateral, 138f
    unilateral, 138f, 218–220, 219f
  C1-2 areas, 185
  C2-3 areas, 185
  clinical reasoning applied to,
    118–119, 118f, 119b
  clinical syndromes
    cardiac pain, 177f, 180f
    headache, 117, 175f
    nerve root lesions, 117–118
    whiplash-associated disorder see
      whiplash-associated disorder
  extension, 150, 159f
  flexion, 142f–144f
    PPIVMs, 153–155
    rotatory test, 150
  ICFDH, 118
  manipulation (Grade V), 159–160
  mobilization, 123, 152–155
    anteroposterior bilateral vertebral
      pressure, 138f
    anteroposterior unilateral vertebral
      pressure, 218–220, 219f
    context change, 153–155, 159
    passive, 157, 158b, 158f
    posteroanterior unilateral vertebral
      pressure, 152b–153b, 152f
    treatment, 157–158
  pain epidemiology, 116–117
  PAIVMs, 152–153
  palpation, 135–139
    differentiation test, 164b–170b
  physical examination, 131–134,
    132b
    functional assessment, 133
    nervous system, 133–134, 134b
    observation, 133
    planning, 131–132
    reassessment, 133
    testing positions, 133
  posteroanterior vertebral pressure,
    unilateral, 152b–153b, 152f
  PPIVMs, 153–155
  pre-treatment screening, 150–155
    cervical arterial dysfunction, 150,
      150b
    craniovertebral instability, 150,
      151f

  mobilization, 152–155,
    152b–153b
    rotation, 153b–155b, 153f–154f,
      156f
  rotation, 153b–155b, 153f–154f,
    156f
  self-management, 163f
  shoulder symptoms, 117
  spondylitic, 425–427
  subjective examination, 131, 131b
  traction, 164b–170b
  treatment, 155–160
    case study, 164b–170b
    central sensitization, 159
    context change, 159
    graded exposure, 163, 163b
    information/communication,
      155–156
    manual therapy, 159
    massage, 162
    neural mobilization, 160–162,
      160f
    neurodynamics, 160–163
    pain education, 156–157
    self-treatment, 162, 162f–163f
    testing position, 158–159
  see also lumbar spine; thoracic spine;
    and specific disorders
cervicogenic headache, 117, 185
Chartered Society of Physiotherapy,
    84–85
chest pain, 175f
  functional demonstration of
    symptoms, 191–192
  left-sided, 176, 177f, 180f
  radiating, 176, 181f
chin, poking, 189
Chronic Disease Self-efficacy Scales,
    24t
chronic regional pain syndrome
    (CRPS), 176, 179
circular model see mature organism
    model
clarification
  for accuracy, 30
  for completeness, 30
  for precision, 29
  for relevance, 30
clinical evidence, 2–5, 4f
clinical patterns, 249–250
  diaries of, 49
clinical practice, 27–31
clinical prediction rules, 253
  low back pain, 243b
  lumbar spine, 254t
clinical reasoning, 14–52
  biopsychosocial paradigm, 15, 18–19
  'brick wall' model see 'brick wall'
    model
  cervical spine, 118–119, 118f, 119b
  and cognition/metacognition, 26–27
  as collaborative process, 23–25
  complexity of, 44, 44f
  and critical thinking, 16–17
  definition, 15
  errors of, 44–46

and evidence-based practice, 15–16
and expert practice, 17–18
facilitation of, 48–49
hypothesis-oriented processes, 19–25
and knowledge, 25–26
learning through, 46–52
low back pain, 244–255
pelvic girdle pain, 337–341, 338t–340t
strategies, 32–33
theory, 48
see also specific types
clinical reasoning reflection form, 53f–71f
Clinical Standards Advisory Group, 234
clonus, 134b
closed questions, 90
cognition, 26–27, 51
cognitive behavioural therapy, 237–238, 270b–271b, 380
cognitive reinforcement, 98
collaborative goal setting, 94–95, 105–107
collaborative reasoning, 19–25, 20f, 32
  health perspectives, 21–23
  patients, 20–21
  physiotherapists, 19–20
combined movement tests, 430, 430f–431f
  thoracic spine, 194–195, 194f–195f
commitment to patient, 2
communication, 2, 83–114
  clarification, 29
  components of, 87–89
  during treatment interventions, 110–111
  eye contact, 87
  feedback loop, 88f
  immediate-response questions, 92, 99
  key words/phrases, 92
  listening, 2, 89–90
  movement diagram as, 407–408
  non-verbal, 87–89
  techniques, 90–93
  verbal, 87–89
  verbatim examples, 98–113
  see also therapeutic relationship; and specific conditions
communication errors, 86, 87f–88f
  bias, 92–93
communication styles, 389t
  directive, 111, 389t
  mirroring, 91, 111–112, 389t
  paralleling, 91–92
  questioning see questioning
compensation issues, 392b
completeness of examination, 30
compliance, 398–400
  barriers to, 398
    see also barriers to recovery
  enhancement, 398–399
    actions and decisions, 399
  motivational phase, 398

short-term, 398
soft tissue, 408
compliance diagrams, 412f
compression movement tests, thoracic spine, 195–196, 196f
compression test for pain provocation, 354, 354f
concern for patients, 2
conditional reasoning, 341
confidence, 2
  in own capabilities, 393
consultation
  ending, 97
  evaluation and reflection, 97–98
  examination see examination
  initial, 41t, 96–97, 99–103
  welcoming patient, 96, 99
contact points, 428–430, 429f
context change in cervical spine, 128b, 153–155, 159
contraindications
  manipulation, 215–216
  physical examination, 39–40
  sacroiliac region, 338t–340t
  treatment procedures, 39–40
contributing factors, 38–39
coping strategies, 263b, 392
  pelvic girdle pain, 343
costovertebral joint sprain, 178f–180f
costovertebral mobilization, 210, 211f
counselling, 84
craniovertebral instability, 150, 151f
creative thinking, 50–52
crepitus, 414f
critical phases, 95–98, 96f
  welcoming and information, 96, 99
  see also communication; examination
critical thinking, 16–17
  questioning, 27

D

D-plus-1 response, 197
Dallas Pain Questionnaire, 232
deformity
  cervical spine, 153b–155b
  disease-induced, 182
  protective, 191b, 272
demedicalization of low back pain, 229–230
dermatomes, nerve root pain, 35
descending modulatory pathways, 130–131
  strategies affecting, 131b
diagnosis, 4f, 32
  age of patient see age of patient
  blocking of joint movements, 306b, 414
  premature, 45
  problems, 3t, 52
    'brick wall', 4t, 14–15
  special questions, 344
  symptoms and signs, 3t
  see also clinical reasoning
diagnostic reasoning, 32

diagnostic titles, problems with, 3, 3t
diaphragm muscles, 363
  assessment, 364–365
differentiation tests, 7
  cervical spine, 164b–170b
  lumbar spine, 276b, 276f–277f
  thoracic spine, 197–198
directive communication, 111, 389t
directive interaction, 107
disability model of low back pain, 242t
discogenic disorders, 263
  clinical features, 265t–268t
discs, intervertebral see intervertebral discs
disinhibition, 130
disorders see specific conditions and areas
distraction test for pain provocation, 354, 354f
dizziness, 90
  cervical spine disorders, 117, 131b
  gravitational, 150b
  and rotational movements, 153b–155b
  vertebrobasilar insufficiency, 265

E

ectopic impulses, 124, 128–129
education
  about pain see pain education
  bodily awareness, 111–112
  movement diagrams as teaching aid, 407–408
  of patients, 400–401
  principles, 400–401
  therapeutic relationship in, 85–86
elbow
  flexion, slider technique using, 161f
  pain, 185
emotions, 51, 392b
empathy, 1–2, 83
empowerment, 84
end-of-range pain, 6, 408
  thoracic spine, 191, 198
endocrine system, 129
erector spinae, 335
errors
  of clinical reasoning, 44–46
  in communication, 86, 87f–88f
ethical reasoning, 32
evaluation see assessment
evidence-based practice (EBP), 15–16, 47
  definition, 340
  pelvic girdle pain, 340–341
  see also clinical reasoning
evolutionary biology model, 118
examination see physical examination; subjective examination
exercises
  breathing, 129
  cervical spine, 125b, 162, 162f–163f
  compliance, 94, 107, 399–400

functional restoration programmes, 387–390
low back pain, 234, 241t
record-keeping, 441–442
thoracic spine, 187b
see also self-management strategies; and specific exercises
experiential knowledge, 249–250
expert practice, 17–18
extension (cervical spine), 150, 159f
extension (lumbar spine)
  mobilization technique, 281b–282b
  physical examination, 295f–296f
extension (thoracic spine)
  physical examination, 194
  PPIVMs, 198–202
external oblique muscles, 334
eye contact, 87

F

face, cutaneous nerve supply, 137f
facial pain, 116–117, 175f
failed treatment, 52
family, 392b
Fear-avoidance Beliefs Questionnaire, 24t
fear-avoidance model, 118, 119b, 258
femoral nerve
  PKB, 292b, 293f
  slump in sidelying, 293b, 293f
femur
  medial rotation, 346, 374
  transference of forces, 332f
fight or flight response, 129
final assessment, 12
flat back, 272
flexion (cervical spine), 142f–144f
  PPIVMs, 153–155
  rotatory test, 150
flexion (lumbar spine)
  accessory movement, 299f
  mobilization technique, 278b–279b, 301b
  physical examination, 295f–296f
  side flexion, 283b, 297b
flexion (thoracic spine), 193–194, 195f
  C7-T3 areas, 216
  C7-T4 areas, 198–199, 198f
  lateral, 194, 199–201
  PPIVMs, 198–202
  side, 187b
  T4-11 areas, 200–201
follow-up sessions, record-keeping, 442
force closure, 332–334
  excessive, 367–368
  reduced, 366–367
  testing, 363–365
force-displacement curve, 405f
forearm, passive supination, 7
form closure, 332–333
  testing, 362–363
forward reasoning, 43

frontal (supraorbital) nerve, palpation, 136f–137f
function corners, 383, 388
functional capacity, 380–401
functional demonstration tests
  chest pain, 191–192
  lumbar spine, 273t–274t, 274–277, 275f
  thoracic spine, 190–192
functional restoration programmes, 386–390
  barriers to recovery, 390–395
  purpose of, 387–390
  see also self-management strategies

G

Gaenslen's test, 354, 354f
gait analysis, 346
gall bladder disease, 177f
gapping manipulation of sacroiliac joint, 371–372, 372f
gender of patient, 18–19
genitofemoral nerve, 185–186
Gilmore's groin, 185–186
glial cells, 129–130
gluteus maximus, 334–335
gluteus medius, 335
gluteus minimus, 335
goal-setting, 383, 395–396
grades of movement, 404–406
gravitational dizziness, 150b
groin pain, 178f–180f, 185–186
  right-sided, 176
guided graded exposure to activity, 393
gut feelings, 51

H

habitual movement patterns, 388
half-open questions, 90
halter, thoracic traction, 184, 212f
hand
  passive supination, 7
  tingling, 188f
hands-on vs. hands-off therapy, 382
headache, 117, 175f
  central sensitization, 126b
  cervicogenic, 117, 185
  clinical signs, 136b
  epidemiology, 116–117
  neurodynamic response, 138b
Health Assessment Questionnaire, 232
Health Evidence Network, 230
health literacy, 155–156
health perspectives, 21–23
heart disease, pain simulating, 177f, 180f
herniated disc, 3, 3t
  cervical spine disorders, 116
high velocity thrust manipulation, 185
hip joint
  adductors, 334
  differentiation test, 276b, 276f–277f

hypomobility, 37
mobilization, 349f
  active movement, 348–349
  movement abnormalities, 331b
  see also sacroiliac region
histamine, 122
history taking, 102–103
  communication *see* communication
  initial visit, 41t, 96–97, 99–103
  lumbar spine disorders, 263–265
  questioning *see* questioning
  record-keeping, 437, 438f
  sacroiliac disorders, 343–344
  subjective examination, 41t, 96–97, 99–103
    cervical spine, 131, 131b
    lumbar spine, 255–265
    pelvic girdle, 341–344
    thoracic spine, 176–182, 184b
  see also physical examination; subjective examination
hospital traction, 323
hyperaesthesia, 186
hyperalgesia, 125, 186
  primary, 122–123
  secondary, 123, 125
hypermobility
  movement diagrams, 416f, 417, 420–421, 423–424
  treatment, 421, 423–424
hyperpathia, 125
hypersensitivity, 117
hypervigilance, 21
hypogastric pain, right-sided, 176
hypomobility
  hip joint, 37
  lumbar spine, 243b, 254t, 320–321
  sacroiliac joint, 330
hypothesis categories, 33–42, 34b
  activity capabilities, 34
  contributing factors, 38–39
  interpretation of information, 42
  management and treatment, 40–41
  participation capabilities, 34
  pathobiological mechanisms, 34–37
  patient perspectives, 34
  patient safety, 39–40
  physical impairments, 37–38
  prognosis, 41–42
hypothesis generation/testing, 245–249
hypothesis-oriented processes, 19–25
hypothetico-deductive reasoning, 19–20, 50–51

I

ICFDH *see* International Classification of Functioning, Disability and Health
ilio-inguinal nerve, 185–186
ilium
  anterior position of, 375
  mobilization, 376
illness behaviour, 395
illness scripts, 43

immediate-response questions, 92, 99
immune boosting behaviours, 130b
immune system, 129–130
implicit theories of illness, 21–22
'impostership', 52
inclination, 428–430, 429f
inflammatory nociception, 122–123
  neurogenic contributions, 123
inflammatory soup, 122
information, interpretation of, 42
information-seeking, 96
infracostal pain, right-sided, 176, 177f
initial consultation, 41t, 96–97,
    99–103
  see also history taking; physical
      examination; subjective
      examination
injury
  high velocity, 182
  peripheral nerves, 124
  stinger/burner, 117–118
  whiplash see whiplash-associated
      disorder
innominate
  oscillatory movements, 358–360,
      359f–360f
  passive mobilization, 357–358,
      357f–358f
  position of
    in prone, 356–357, 357f
    in supine, 356, 356f
  rotation, 357–358, 357f–358f
    anterior, 369–370, 369f–370f
    posterior, 370–371, 370f–371f
input dominant pain mechanisms,
    121–123
instability, craniovertebral, 150, 151f
interaction, 83–84, 86–94
  directive, 107
  end phase, 89
  initial phase, 89
  middle phase, 89
  shaping of, 89–90
  see also therapeutic relationship
interactive reasoning, 32, 341
interleukin-1β, 122, 130
internal oblique muscles, 334
International Classification of
      Functioning, Disability and
      Health (ICFDH), 15, 18–19,
      18f
  cervical spine, 118
  lumbar spine, 231, 232f, 239b–240b
International Federation of
      Orthopaedic Manipulative
      Physiotherapists, 236
interoception, 127–128
intervertebral discs
  degeneration, 124, 190t
  healing, 307
  herniation, 3
  see also discogenic disorders
intervertebral joints
  lumbar spine, rotation, 303f
  pain arising from, 197–198
  PPIVMs see PPIVMs

thoracic spine, 201–202, 205,
    209–212, 214f
  Grade V mobilization, 216–218
  lateral flexion, 216
  longitudinal movement, 217
  rotation, 201–202
intervertebral pressures
  posteroanterior unilateral see
      posteroanterior vertebral
      pressure, unilateral
  rotary posteroanterior, 204–205,
      204f
  transverse, 205–207, 206f
Iowa Gambling Task, 127, 127b
irritability, 270b–271b, 408
ischaemic nociception, 122
ischiococcygeus, 361, 363

J

joints
  blocking of movements, 306b, 414
  costochondral, manipulation,
      225–226, 226f
  costovertebral, sprain, 178f–180f
  facet, 265t–268t
  intervertebral see intervertebral
      joints
  sacroiliac see sacroiliac joint
  sternochondral, manipulation,
      225–226, 226f

K

Kessler Physiological Distress Scale, 24t
key words/phrases, 92
kinesophobia, 395
knowledge, 25–26
  experiential, 249–250
Kuhn, Thomas, 15–16
kypholordosis, 272

L

L4-5 (lumbar spine) see lumbar spine,
    L4-5 areas
L5/S1 (lumbar spine) see lumbar
    spine, L5/S1 areas
latent pain, 36
lateral flexion of thoracic spine, 194,
    199–201
lateral sling of pelvic girdle, 335
lateral thinking, 50–52
latissimus dorsi, 334
learning through clinical reasoning,
    46–52
Leeds Assessment of Neuropathic
      Symptoms and Signs
      (LANSS), 125
left/right discrimination task, 127b
legs
  pain in, 265t–268t
  stiffness in, 258

lifestyle, 381
ligaments
  alar ligament test, 151f
  intermittent stretching, 5
  long dorsal SI ligament test, 355,
      355f
  sprains, 44–45
limit of range, 412–413, 417f
listening, 2, 89–90
  active, 90
  passive, 90
load transfer tests, 349–352
  see also stork test; straight leg raising
load-displacement curve, 405f
local muscle system, pelvic girdle,
    333–336
long dorsal SI ligament test, 355, 355f
longitudinal movements, 438t–439t
  thoracic spine, 217
longitudinal sling of pelvic girdle, 335
low back pain, 175f, 228, 228b
  advice to patients, 233–234
  alternative model, 231b
  chronic, 265t–268t
  classifications, subgroups and
      models, 240–244, 242t
  clinical assessment, 231–233
  clinical prediction rule, 243b
  clinical presentation, 265t–268t
  clinical reasoning, 244–255
  conceptualization, 230–231
  demedicalization, 229–230
  facet joint involvement, 265t–268t
  hypothesis generation/testing,
      245–249
  ICF domains, 231, 232f, 239b–240b
  multifactorial, 265t–268t
  nociceptive mechanisms, 265t–268t
  Paris Task Force, 228–229, 232–234,
      238
  physiotherapist's role in, 234–244
  reassessment, 247b–248b
  referral, 234
  treatment, 230, 233–234
    by phase, 240, 241t
    guidelines, 235b
    lumbar stabilization, 254t
    manual therapy, 243b
  see also lumbar spine
lumbago see low back pain
lumbar spine, 228–320
  assessment, 257, 308b–309b
  case studies, 320
  clinical prediction rules, 254t
  clinical presentations, 265,
      265t–268t
  disc lesions, thoracic mobilization/
      manipulation, 188–189
  extension
    mobilization technique,
        281b–282b
    physical examination, 295f–296f
  flexion
    accessory movement, 299f
    mobilization technique, 278b–
        279b, 301b

physical examination, 295f–296f
side flexion, 283b, 297b
history taking, 263–265
integrated treatment, 307–309
L4-5 areas, 258, 261
rotation, 304b
L5/S1 areas
flexion-extension, 295b–296b
intervertebral movement, 295f
palpation, 273t–274t
rotation, 296b
side flexion, 297b
low back pain see low back pain
manipulation (Grade V), 254t, 300, 304b
mobilization, 300–309
accessory movements, 265t–268t, 299f
active movement, 273t–274t, 277–278
anteroposterior central vertebral pressure, 300f
arthrogenic impairment, 313f–318f
clinical evidence, 306–307
extension, 281b–282b
flexion, 278b–279b, 301b
myogenic impairment, 310f–312f, 318f
neurodynamic techniques, 305–307, 305b
neurogenic impairment, 310f–315f, 318f
PKB, 292b
posteroanterior central vertebral pressure, 298f–299f
posteroanterior movement, 298f
posteroanterior unilateral vertebral pressure, 298f
with protective muscle spasm, 319f
side flexion, 283b
SLR, 289b, 289f
transverse vertebral pressure, 299f
movement abnormalities, 331b
palpation, 273t–274t, 292–295, 293f–295f
differentiation test, 276b, 276f–277f
skin temperature, 292–294, 363
sweating, 251, 292–294
T1/11-S1 areas, 273t–274t
physical examination, 269–295, 273t–274t
extension, 295f–296f
flexion, 295f–296f
functional demonstration, 273t–274t, 274–277, 275f
motor impairment, 273t–274t, 300
neurodynamic testing, 273t–274t, 288–292, 288t
neurological conduction tests, 273t–274t, 278–288
observation, 272, 273t–274t
PAIVMS, 273t–274t, 297

planning, 269
PPIVMs, 273t–274t, 295, 295b–297b, 296f
precautions, 269
reassessment, 308b–309b
rotation
mobilization technique, 286b, 302b–303b
with neurodynamic emphasis, 305b, 305f
physical examination, 296b
with SLR, 305f
stability dysfunction, 265t–268t
stabilization, 254t
stenosis, 254t, 265t–268t
subjective examination, 255–265
body charts, 259f–260f
history taking, 263–265
main problem, 257–258
making features fit, 262–263
perceived disability, 258
screening questions, 265
symptom behaviour, 262
symptom localization/quality, 258–262
T10/11-S1 areas
flexion/extension, 295f–296f
PAIVMs, 273t–274t, 297
palpation, 273t–274t
PPIVMs, 273t–274t, 295
rotation, 296b, 303f
side flexion, 297b
tests
active tests, 273t–274t, 277–278
slump in sidelying, 293b, 293f
slump test, 290b, 290f–292f, 292
traction, 318–319, 318f
treatment planning, 256f
see also cervical spine; thoracic spine; and individual disorders
lumbopelvic stability, 333–336, 334f
lumbopelvic-hip complex, 331b, 345
failed load transfer, 346b
impairments of, 345b
see also sacroiliac region
lumbosacral multifidi, 333b

M

machine traction, 318f
Maitland Concept, 1–13, 15
thoracic spine, 174–176, 175f
making features fit principle, 262–263
management see treatment; and individual conditions
mandibular nerve, palpation, 136f–137f
manipulation, 1–13, 382
cervical spine, cervical spine, manipulation (Grade V)
high velocity thrust, 185
lumbar spine see lumbar spine, manipulation (Grade V)

sacroiliac joint, 369
gapping, 371–372, 372f
therapeutic process, 387f
thoracic spine see thoracic spine, manipulation (Grade V)
manual muscle testing, 134b
massage, cervical spine, 162
mature organism model, 118f, 119b, 120
cervical nerve root lesions, 121b
maxillary nerve, palpation, 136f–137f
meaning perspective, 25
Measure Yourself Medical Outcome Profile (MYMOP), 307
mechanical loading model of low back pain, 242t
mechanical nociception, 122
mechanosensitivity, 133
median nerve
palpation, 139f–140f
slider technique, 160–161, 160f
ULNT, 143f–146f
metabolic syndrome, and neck pain, 117
metacognition, 26–27, 31b
lack of, 46
migraine, 117, 135
slump test, 141
see also headache
mind maps, 49–50
mirror neurons, 127
mirroring, 91, 111–112, 389t
misinterpretation
of body sensations, 21
of non-contributory information, 44–45
see also communication errors
mobility criteria, 232–233
mobilization, 1–13
cervical spine see cervical spine, mobilization
grades of, 404–406
hip, 348–349
lumbar spine see lumbar spine, mobilization
neurodynamic techniques see neurodynamic mobilization
passive see passive movement
sacroiliac region see sacroiliac region, mobilization
slider techniques see slider techniques
thoracic spine see thoracic spine, mobilization
see also movement
Modified Somatic Perceptions Questionnaire, 24t
motor control model of low back pain, 242t
motor control retraining, 367
motor impairment, 273t–274t, 300
motor system, 130, 130b
movement abnormalities
hip joint, 331b
lumbar spine, 331b

one-component vs. multicomponent, 249
pathobiological mechanisms, 249
see also specific disorders
movement continuum theory, 380–401
movement diagrams, 6, 404–422
clinical examples, 423–427
hypermobility, 416f, 417, 420–421, 423–424
Scheuermann's disease, 424–425
spondylitic cervical spine, 425–427
compiling, 407, 407f, 415–419, 419t
completion, 408f
depiction of, 404–406
examination refinements, 428–432
force-displacement curve, 405f
load-displacement curve, 405f
margins of error, 406f
modified, 415, 416f, 419, 420f
muscle spasm, 405f, 407, 413–415, 414f–415f, 419f
pain, 408–411
pain behaviour, 87, 410–411, 410f–411f, 418, 418f
pain intensity, 409, 409f–410f, 417f
pain onset, 408–409, 409f
passive movement, 440f
patient with one disorder, 431–432, 431f–432f
range limited by 50 percent, 419–420, 420f
range of movement, 409, 409f
reliability, 406
resistance, 404–406, 405f
resistance behaviour, 413, 413f–414f, 418f
as teaching aid/means of communication, 407–408
movements
accessory *see* accessory movements
active *see* active movements
combined, tests of, 430, 430f–431f
thoracic spine, 194–195, 194f–195f
grades of, 404–406
habitual patterns, 388
intervertebral, 295f
of joints, blocking, 306b, 414
longitudinal, 438t–439t
thoracic spine, 217
mobility criteria, 232–233
optimization of capacity, 238
oscillatory, 5
innominate, 358–360, 359f–360f
sacrum, 358–360, 359f–360f
passive *see* passive movement
see also mobilization; and specific areas
multifidus, 363, 363b
assessment, 364
muscle spasm, 405f, 407, 413–415, 414f–415f, 419f
muscles *see individual muscles*
myogenic impairment

with arthrogenic impairment, 315f–318f
with neurogenic impairment, 310f–312f, 318f

N

narrative reasoning, 32, 341
errors in, 45–46
neck
cutaneous nerve supply, 137f
palpation, 135–139
passive flexion, 196
neck pain, 175f
epidemiology, 116–117
and metabolic syndrome, 117
thoracic manipulation, 185
thoracic spinal symptoms, 188f
whiplash-associated disorder *see* whiplash-associated disorder
nerve blocks, 292
nerve root lesion
cervical, 117–118, 121b
context change, 128b, 153–155
subjective examination, 131b
nerves *see* neurons; and individual nerves
nervous system, examination of, 133–134, 134b
neural containers, 160
neural mobilization of cervical spine, 160–162, 160f, 161b
neurodynamic mobilization
cervical spine, 160–163
lumbar spine, 305–307, 305b
neurodynamic testing, 138b, 139–141
cervical spine, 141, 141b
lumbar spine, 270b–271b, 273t–274t, 288–292
responses to, 140–141
start position, 141, 149f
structural differentiation, 141
upper limb see upper limb neurodynamic tests
see also specific nerves
neurogenic impairment
with arthrogenic impairment, 313f–315f, 318f
with myogenic impairment, 310f–312f, 318f
neurogenic inflammation, 123
neurological conduction tests, 273t–274t, 278–288
neuromatrix model, 119b, 126
neuromusculoskeletal pain, 182t
neurons
axoplasmic flow, 125, 125f
ectopic impulses, 124, 128–129
nociceptive, 121
sensitivity, 124
see also individual nerves
neuropathic pain, 123–125
axoplasmic flow, 125, 125f
blood flow, 124
clinical detection, 125

palpation, 135
peripheral nerve injury, 123–124
neurophysiological model of low back pain, 242t
neurosignature, 126–128
nociceptive neurons, 121, 122t
activation, 121
location, 121
second order, 122
nociceptive pain, 35, 121
clinical detection, 123
inflammatory, 122–123
ischaemic, 122
mechanical, 122
second order neurons, 122
speed of messaging, 121–122
spinal, 261t
whiplash-associated disorder *see* whiplash-associated disorder
nociceptors, 121–123
non-propositional knowledge, 25
non-specific low back pain (NSLBP) *see* low back pain
non-steroidal anti-inflammatory drugs *see* NSAIDs
non-verbal communication, 87–89
noradrenaline, 128
Nottingham Health Profile, 232
NSAIDs, 234
pelvic girdle pain, 338t

O

O-P (overpressure)
lumbar spine, 277, 278b–279b, 278f–279f, 281b–282b
thoracic spine, 193f–194f, 221f
occipital nerve, 137f
greater, 136
lesser, 136
neurodynamic testing, 143f
palpation, 136b
one leg weight bearing-hip flexion test, 333b
open questions, 90
open-mindedness, 47
ophthalmic nerve, 135
Orebro Musculoskeletal Pain Screening Questionnaire, 24t
oscillatory movements, 5
innominate, 358–360, 359f–360f
sacrum, 358–360, 359f–360f
osteomyelitis, 182
osteoporosis, 182
Oswestry criteria, 232
output dominant pain mechanisms, 127–131
over-pressure *see* O-P (over-pressure)

P

P4 test, 340, 353, 353f
pain, 93–94, 156b
abdominal, 181f
arm, 188f

attitudes and beliefs, 392b
behaviour, 87, 410–411, 410f–411f, 418, 418f
brain changes in, 127, 127b
brain's role in, 126–127, 126b
cardiac, 177f, 180f
central processing, 35–36
chest *see* chest pain
contributing factors, 38–39
coping strategies, 263b
definition, 119–120
elbow, 185
end-of-range *see* end-of-range pain
facial, 116–117, 175f
groin, 178f–180f, 185–186
hypogastric, 176
infracostal, 176, 177f
intensity, 409, 409f–410f, 417f
irritability, 270b–271b, 408
latent, 36
low back *see* low back pain
movement diagrams, 408–411
nature of, 408
neck *see* neck pain
neuromuscular, 182t
neuromusculoskeletal, 182t
neuropathic *see* neuropathic pain
nociceptive *see* nociceptive pain
onset, 408–409, 409f
patient perspective, 21, 36
pelvic girdle *see* sacroiliac region
peripheral neurogenic, 35
pleural, 181f
provocation tests *see* pain
    provocation tests
radicular, 261t, 265t–268t
referred, 6, 197
    sites of, 183f, 190t
    somatic, 261–262, 261t
sense of control, 236–238
somatic, 182t
spontaneous, 36
systemic, 182t
types of, 261t
    see also specific types
understanding of, 22
visceral, 182t
pain behaviour, 87
pain education, 36
    cervical spine, 156–157
    low back pain, 85–86
pain mechanisms, 35, 119b, 120
    central sensitization, 125–126
    input dominant, 121–123
    nociception *see* nociceptive pain
    output dominant, 127–131
    reasoning framework, 120
pain provocation tests, 352–355
    compression, 354, 354f
    distraction, 354, 354f
    Gaenslen's test, 354, 354f
    long dorsal SI ligament test, 355, 355f
    P4 test, 340, 353, 353f
    palpation of symphysis pubis, 355, 355f
    Patrick's Faber test, 355, 355f

posterior pelvic, 353, 353f
    sacral thrust test, 354, 355f
pain schemas, 22
Pain Self-efficacy Questionnaire, 24t
'pain through range' problems, 6–7
pain-free neural mobilization, 125b, 129b
PainDETECT questionnaire, 125
PAIVMs
    cervical spine, 152–153
    lumbar spine, 273t–274t, 297
    thoracic spine, 197
palpation, 7, 97, 105
    brachial plexus, 136–139
    cervical spine, 135–139
        differentiation test, 164b–170b
        nerve roots, 136–139
    differentiation tests by
        cervical spine, 164b–170b
        lumbar spine, 276b, 276f–277f
    frontal (supraorbital) nerve, 136f–137f
    head, neck and upper limb nerves, 135–139
        see also specific nerves
    inclination and contact points, 428–430, 429f
    lumbar spine, 273t–274t, 292–295, 293f–295f
        differentiation test, 276b, 276f–277f
        L5/S1 areas, 273t–274t
        skin temperature, 292–294, 363
        sweating, 251, 292–294
        T1/11-S1 areas, 273t–274t
    mandibular nerve, 136f–137f
    maxillary nerve, 136f–137f
    median nerve, 139f–140f
    neuropathic pain, 135
    occipital nerve, 136b
    peripheral nerves, 134–139
        neuropathic pain, 135
        response to, 135
    sacroiliac region, 363
    skin sweating/temperature, 196, 292–294, 363
    symphysis pubis, 355, 355f
    thoracic spine, 196–198
paracetamol, pelvic girdle pain, 338t
paradigmatic assumptions, 47–48
paradigms, 236
    see also specific paradigms
paraesthesia, 35
    T4 syndrome, 179, 183f
paralleling, 91–92, 255
parasympathetic nervous system, 129
Paris Task Force on Back Pain, 228–229, 232–234, 238
participation capabilities, 34, 395
passive accessory intervertebral
    movements *see* PAIVMs
passive listening, 90
passive movement, 1–13, 408
    cervical spine
        assessment, 152–153
        treatment, 157, 158b, 158f

lumbar spine, disc lesions, 189
PPIVMs *see* PPIVMs
    record-keeping, 440, 440f
    role of, 381–384
sacroiliac joint
    in AP plane, 360–361, 361f
    in craniocaudal plane, 361–362, 362f
    sacroiliac region, 357–358
        innominate, 357–358, 357f–358f
    SLR *see* straight leg raising
    slump test *see* slump test
    thoracic spine, 189–202
    underlying mechanisms, 384
passive neck flexion (PNF), 196
passive physiological intervertebral
    movements *see* PPIVMs
passive testing
    lumbar spine, 295
    sacroiliac region, 345b, 356
patho-anatomical model of low back
    pain, 242t
pathobiological mechanisms, 34–37, 249
patient-centred approach, 85–86
patient-therapist collaboration, 23–25
patients
    activity capabilities, 34
    belief in, 175
    compliance, 398–400
    confidence in own capabilities, 393
    education, 400–401
    effect of questioning, 31
    health literacy, 155–156
    participation capabilities, 34
    perspectives on experience, 23, 34
    presentation, 87
    psychosocial issues, 392b
    reasoning process, 20–21
    sense of control, 236–238
    social environment, 395
    therapist commitment to, 2
    written records, 443
Patrick's Faber test, 355, 355f
pattern recognition, 43–44
    clinical pattern diaries, 49
    errors in, 44–46
pelvic belt, 338t
pelvic floor muscles, 333b, 363, 363b
    assessment, 364
pelvic girdle, 332, 332f
    force closure, 332–334
    form closure, 332–333
    local muscle system, 333–336, 334f
        anterior oblique sling, 330, 335–336
        lateral sling, 335
        longitudinal sling, 335
        posterior oblique sling, 330, 335
    mobility, 332–333
    pain *see* sacroiliac region
pelvic shift correction, 275b, 275f
perceived disability, 391
    lumbar spine, 258
Perceived Health Confidence Scale, 24t

Perceived Stress Scale, 24t
performance, 380–401
peripheral nerves
    injury, 124
    palpation, 134–139
        neuropathic pain, 135
        response to, 135
peripheral neurogenic pain, 35
peripheral neurogenic syndrome,
        265t–268t
peripheral pain generator model of low
        back pain, 242t
peroneal muscles, 335
personal knowledge, 25
phases of change, 396, 397b
PHQ2, 24t
PHQ9, 24t
physical activity, 381
    passive movement in promotion of,
        381–384
physical examination, 6–7, 41t,
        104–105, 394b
    active movements see active
        movements
    carrying out, 97
    and movement diagrams, 428–432
    palpation see palpation
    planning, 97, 131–132, 269
    precautions/contraindications,
        39–40
    record-keeping, 437
    see also subjective examination;
        tests/testing; and specific
        regions
physical impairment, 37–38, 38f, 38t
    contributing factors, 38–39
physiological movements
    accessory see accessory movements
    active see active movements
    see also PPIVMs
physiotherapists/physiotherapy
    collaboration with patients, 23–25
    commitment to patients, 2
    psychosocial assessment by, 23
    reasoning process, 19–20
    role of, 380–381
        in low back pain, 234–244
        in therapeutic relationship, 84
    scope of practice, 235–244, 237b
    treatment objectives, 236–244
PKB see prone knee bend
placebo effect, 84
planning
    physical examination, 97, 131–132,
        269
    treatment, 97–98, 105–107, 256f
pleural pain, 181f
poking chin position, 124
positional testing
    sacroiliac region, 356–357
        innominates
            in prone, 356–357, 357f
            in supine, 356, 356f
        pubic tubercles, 356
        sacrum in prone, 357, 357f
    thoracic spine, 197

posterior oblique sling of pelvic girdle,
        334–335
posterior pelvic pain provocation test
        (P4 test), 340, 353, 353f
posteroanterior movement
    sagittal see sagittal posteroanterior
        movements
    vertebral, lumbar spine, 298f
posteroanterior unilateral
        costovertebral pressure,
        thoracic spine, 208–210,
        208f–209f
posteroanterior vertebral pressure
    central
        lumbar spine, 298f–299f
        thoracic spine, 202–204, 203f
    unilateral
        cervical spine, 152b–153b, 152f
        lumbar spine, 298f
        thoracic spine, 207–208, 207f
posture, 346, 347f
    antalgic, 123, 133, 140–141, 165,
        168, 272, 346
PPIVMs
    C7-T4
        flexion, 198, 198f
        flexion/extension, 198–199, 199f
        lateral flexion, 199, 199f
        rotation, 199–200, 200f
    cervical spine, 153–155
    lumbar spine, 273t–274t, 295
    T2-12, rotation to right, 210,
        210f–211f
    T4-11
        flexion/extension, 200
        lateral flexion, 200–201, 201f
        rotation, 201–202, 201f
    T10/11-S1, 273t–274t, 295b–296b,
        296f
        flexion/extension, 295f–296f
        rotation, 296b, 296f
        side flexion, 297b, 297f
    thoracic spine, 198–202
predictive reasoning, 32
pregnancy, pelvic girdle pain, 330, 344
prescriptive assumptions, 48
pretreatment assessment, 8–10
problem oriented medical records
        (POMR), 434
procedural reasoning, 32–33, 341
professional craft knowledge, 25–26
professional manner, 86
prognosis, 41–42, 250–253, 252t
progressive assessment, 11
prone knee bend (PKB), 196,
        224–225, 224f
    femoral nerve, 292b, 293f
propositional knowledge, 25
prospective assessment, 308b–309b
protective deformity, 272
    see also antalgic posture
psoas major, 363, 363b
psychology models, 119b
psychosocial issues, 392b
    assessment, 23
pubic tubercles, position of, 356

Q

quadrant test, lumbar spine, 283f
Quebec Back Pain Disability Scale,
        232
questioning, 93–94, 99–100, 111–112,
        389t
    alternative questions, 90
    clinical practice, 27–31
    closed questions, 90
    critical thinking/learning, 27
    effect on patient, 31
    half-open questions, 90
    immediate-response questions, 92,
        99
    open questions, 90
    purpose of, 93
    screening questions, 24t, 30–31, 45
    Socratic, 17, 27, 28b–29b, 31b
    special questions, 344
    suggestive questions, 91
questionnaires, 435

R

R2-12 (thoracic spine) see thoracic
        spine, R2-12 areas
radial nerve
    palpation, 140f
    slider technique, 162f
    ULNT, 147f
radial sensory nerve, palpation, 140f
radicular pain, 261t, 265t–268t
radiculopathy, 118, 261t
range of movement
    determination of, 409, 409f
    lumbar spine, 232
    sacroiliac joint, 347
reassessment, 45–46, 98, 107–109
    low back pain, 247b–248b
    physical examination tests,
        109–110
reassurance, 2
record-keeping, 433–443
    active movement, 440
    asterisks, 268, 277, 435, 435b
    body charts, 259f–260f, 324f, 436,
        437f
    clinical tips, 436
    conditions, 435
    follow-up sessions, 442
    history-taking, 437, 438f
    information, instructions, exercises
        and warnings, 441–442
    passive movements, 440, 440f
    patient's written records, 443
    physical examination, 437
    problem oriented medical records,
        434
    retrospective assessment, 442–443
    SOAP notes, 434
    subjective examination, 436–437
    symbols, 438t–439t
    symptom behaviour, 436–437
    treatment interventions, 441

red flags, 40, 390
  low back pain, 234
  thoracic spine, 182, 184b
referred pain, 6, 197
  sites of, 183f, 190t
  somatic, 261–262, 261t
reflection, 47
  clinical reasoning reflection form,
      53f–71f
reflection in action, 97–98, 269
reflection on action, 97–98, 269
reflective practice, 255
reflex testing, 134b
rehabilitation *see* functional restoration
      programmes; treatment; and
      individual areas/conditions
reification, 47
relevance, 30
research, and therapeutic relationship,
      84–85
resistance, 404–406, 405f
  behaviour, 413, 413f–414f, 418f
  redefinition of, 406
  soft vs. firm, 406f
  spasm-free, 407, 411–413, 413f,
      417f–418f
retrospective assessment, 11–12, 98,
      112–113
  lumbar spine, 308b–309b
  record-keeping, 442–443
ribs, mobilization of, 210, 211f
Roland Morris Questionnaire, 232,
      243
rotary posteroanterior intervertebral
      pressures, 204–205, 204f
rotation (cervical spine), 153b–155b,
      153f–154f, 156f
  self-management, 163f
rotation (lumbar spine)
  mobilization technique, 286b,
      302b–303b
  in flexion and lateral flexion and
      lateral position left from
      below upwards, 304f
  in flexion and lateral position left
      from above downwards, 304f
  in flexion and lateral position left
      from below downwards, 304f
  localized manipulation, 304b
  with neurodynamic emphasis, 305b,
      305f
  physical examination, 296b
  with SLR, 305f
rotation (sacroiliac region), 348
  innominate, 357–358, 357f–358f
  anterior, 369–370, 369f–370f
  posterior, 370–371, 370f–371f
rotation (thoracic spine), 192,
      192f–193f, 195f
  PPIVMs, 198–202

S

sacral thrust test, 354, 355f
sacroiliac belt, 367

sacroiliac joint, 331b
  accessory movements, 358–362,
      368–369
  force closure
    excessive, 367–368
    reduced, 366–367
  manipulation, 369
    gapping, 371–372, 372f
  passive mobility/stability
    in AP plane, 360–361, 361f
    in craniocaudal plane, 361–362,
        362f
  range of motion, 347
  see also sacroiliac region
sacroiliac region, 254t, 330–372
  assessment, 340
  case study, 372b–376b
  classification, 336, 336f
  clinical presentations, 366–372
  clinical reasoning, 337–341,
      338t–340t
  contributing factors, 337, 338t–340t
  coping strategies, 343
  definition, 330
  evidence-based practice, 340–341
  force closure testing, 363–365
  form closure testing, 362–363
  illness experience, 338t–340t
  load transfer tests, 349–352
    SLR, 351–352, 351f–352f
    stork test, 333b, 350–351,
        350f–351f
  mobilization, 347–348, 347f
    backward bending, 347–348, 348f
    forward bending, 347, 347f
    from below upwards, 348, 349f
    rotation, 348
    side-bending, 348, 348f
  musculature *see individual muscles*
  pain provocation tests, 352–355
    compression, 354, 354f
    distraction, 354, 354f
    Gaenslen's test, 354, 354f
    long dorsal SI ligament test, 355,
        355f
    palpation of symphysis pubis, 355,
        355f
    Patrick's Faber test, 355, 355f
    posterior pelvic, 353, 353f
    sacral thrust test, 354, 355f
  palpation, 363
  passive mobilization, 356–358
    innominate, 357–358, 357f–358f
  physical examination, 344–345,
      345b
    gait, 346
    observation, 346–365
    posture, 346, 347f
  position tests, 356–357
    innominates in prone, 356–357,
        357f
    innominates in supine, 356, 356f
    pubic tubercles, 356
    sacrum in prone, 357, 357f
  precautions and contraindications,
      338t–340t

prognosis, 338t–340t
  rotation, 348
    innominate, 357–358, 357f–358f
  subjective examination, 341–344
    history, 343–344
    information phase, 342
    main problem, 342
    objectives, 341–344
    special questions, 344
    symptom behaviour, 342–343,
        344t
    symptom location, 342, 343f
  treatment, 337, 337t–340t,
      365–366, 365b
    motor control retraining, 333b,
        367
sacrotuberous ligament, 335
sacrum, 332
  oscillatory movements, 358–360,
      359f–360f
  position of, in prone, 357, 357f
sagittal posteroanterior movements,
      429f
  in combined positions, 430,
      430f–431f
scalp, cutaneous nerve supply, 137f
scapula
  pain, 175f
  pseudowinging, 189
Scheuermann's disease, 182, 424–425
sciatic nerve
  slider technique, 306b
  SLR, 278b–279b, 289f
sciatic pain, 188–189
scoliosis, 182, 189
screening questions, 24t, 30–31, 45
  lumbar spine, 265
second opinions, 52
  as barrier to recovery, 393–394
self-awareness, 46
  see also metacognition
Self-Efficacy for Managing Chronic
      Disease 6 Item Scale, 24t
self-management strategies, 109,
      237–238, 386–390
  cervical spine, 162, 162f–163f
  thoracic spine, 187b
self-reflection worksheets, 49
Semmes-Weinstein monofilaments,
      134b
sense of control, 236–238
sensitive practice, 395
sensory testing, 134b
SF-36, 232
Sharp-Purser test, 150
shoulders
  lateral rotation, 143f–144f
  range of movement, 130b
  rounded, 189
  symptoms, 117
  upper limb neurodynamic tests, 141,
      141b, 166f
  see also cervical spine
Sickness Impact Profile, 232
signs and symptoms model of low back
      pain, 242t

slider techniques, 160
cradle position, 168f
elbow flexion, 161f
median nerve, 160–161, 160f
radial nerve, 162f
sciatic nerve, 306b
SLR *see* straight leg raising
SLSSE, 176
slump long sitting technique with
sympathetic emphasis *see*
SLSSE
slump test, 6
lumbar disc lesions, 189
lumbar spine, 290b, 290f–292f, 292
thoracic spine, 186, 196, 220–224
SNAGS, 159, 159f
SOAP notes, 434
social environment, 395
Socratic questioning, 17, 27, 28b–29b,
31b
soft tissue changes, 7
cervical spine, 166
palpation examination
lumbar spine, 292, 294, 295f
sacroiliac region, 363
thoracic spine, 196–197
soft tissue compliance, 408
somatic pain, 182t
referred, 261–262, 261t
spasm *see* muscle spasm
spasm-free resistance, 407, 411–413,
413f, 417f–418f
special questions, 344
spine
cervical *see* cervical spine
lumbar *see* lumbar spine
thoracic *see* thoracic spine
spinous processes, position changes,
197
spondylitis *see* ankylosing spondylitis
spontaneous pain, 36
Stacey agreement, 44, 44f
sternochondral/costochondral joint
mobilization, 225–226, 226f
stinger/burner injury, 117–118
stork test, 333b, 350–351, 350f–351f
straight leg raising (SLR), 6
lumbar spine, 278b–279b, 289f,
305f
sacroiliac region, 351–352,
351f–352f
thoracic spine, 188–189, 196, 225,
225f
stress incontinence, 335
stress response, 129, 129b
structural differentiation, 141
structured reflection, 344–345
subjective examination, 41t, 96–97,
99–103
cervical spine, 131, 131b
hypothesis categories, 33–42, 34b
lumbar spine, 255–265
pelvic girdle, 341–344
record-keeping, 436–437
special questions, 344
thoracic spine, 176–182, 184b

see also physical examination; and
specific regions
suggestive questions, 91
'surface stirring', 5
sustained natural apophyseal gliding
movements *see* SNAGS
sway back, 272
sweating, palpation, 196
symbols, 438t–439t
sympathectomy, 186
sympathetic nervous system, 128–129
sympathoneural axis, 128
symphysis pubis, 332
palpation, 355, 355f
symptoms, 3t
behaviour, 100–101
lumbar spine, 262
record-keeping, 436–437
sacroiliac region, 342–343, 344t
dizziness *see* dizziness
localization, 37–38, 38f, 38t
dermatomes, 35
low back pain, 242t
lumbar spine, 258–262
shoulder, 117
thoracic spine, 188f, 190–192
synthesis, 26
systemic pain, 182t

T

T1-12 (thoracic spine) *see* thoracic
spine, T1-12 areas
T2-12 (thoracic spine) *see* thoracic
spine, T2-12 areas
T3-10 (thoracic spine) *see* thoracic
spine, T3-10 areas
T4 syndrome, 179, 183f
T4-7 (thoracic spine) *see* thoracic
spine, T4-7 areas
T4-11 (thoracic spine) *see* thoracic
spine, T4-11 areas
T5-7 (thoracic spine) *see* thoracic
spine, T5-7 areas
T10/11-S1 (lumbar spine) *see* lumbar
spine, T10/11-S1 areas
Tampa Scale of Kinesiophobia, 24t
tap test, thoracic spine, 196
teaching, reasoning about, 32
techniques, 5–6
arthrogenic, 305
as 'brainchild of ingenuity', 6
Buteyko, 129
cervical lateral glide, 157, 158f, 168f
communication, 90–93
grades of movement, 404–406
management, 5–6
manipulation *see* manipulation
mobilization *see* mobilization
neurodynamic *see* neurodynamic
mobilization
records *see* record-keeping
slider, 160
cradle position, 168f
elbow flexion, 161f

median nerve, 160–161, 160f
radial nerve, 162f
sciatic nerve, 306b
value of, 10–11
see also treatment; and specific
regions
temperature
extremes of, 121
palpation, 196, 292, 363
tensioner techniques, 160
ulnar nerve, 161, 161f
tensor fascia latae, 335
tests/testing
accessory movements, 7, 105
alar ligament test, 151f
Babinski test, 134b
cervical spine, 133, 158–159
combined movement tests, 430,
430f–431f
thoracic spine, 194–195,
194f–195f
compression movements tests,
195–196, 196f
differentiation tests *see*
differentiation tests
distraction test for pain provocation,
354, 354f
force closure, 363–365
form closure, 362–363
functional demonstration tests *see*
functional demonstration
tests
load transfer tests, 349–352
long dorsal SI ligament test, 355,
355f
manual muscle testing, 134b
neurodynamic testing *see*
neurodynamic testing
neurological conduction tests,
273t–274t, 278–288
one leg weight bearing-hip flexion
test, 333b
pain provocation *see* pain
provocation tests
positional testing *see* positional
testing
quadrant test, 283f
reflexes, 134b
sacral thrust test, 354, 355f
sensory testing, 134b
Sharp-Purser test, 150
slump test *see* slump test
stork test, 333b, 350–351,
350f–351f
tap test, 196
therapeutic climate, 89–90
therapeutic process, 385f
therapeutic relationship, 83–86
critical phases *see* critical phases
education and practice, 85–86
goal-setting, 383, 395–396
physiotherapist's role, 84
positive effects of, 84
and research, 84–85
therapists *see* physiotherapists/
physiotherapy

thoracic girdle pain, 186f
thoracic spine, 174–226
  appraisal, 192
  C7-T3 areas, Grade V manipulation, 216
  C7-T4 areas
    flexion, 198, 198f
    flexion/extension, 198–199, 199f
    lateral flexion, 199, 199f
    rotation, 199–200, 200f
  case studies, 178–182, 182f
  chronic conditions, 178–182
  differential diagnosis, 182
  examination and treatment techniques
    anteroposterior sternochondral/ costochondral joint mobilization, 225–226, 226f
    cervical anteroposterior unilateral vertebral pressure, 218–220, 219f
    PKB/slump, 224–225, 224f
    SLR, 225, 225f
    slump test, 196, 220–224
    see also mobilization (below)
  extension
    physical examination, 194
    PPIVMs, 198–202
  flexion, 193–194, 195f
    C7-T3 areas, 216
    C7-T4 areas, 198–199, 198f
    lateral, 194, 199–201
    PPIVMS, 198–202
    side, 187b
    T4-11 areas, 200–201
  Maitland Concept applied to, 174–176, 175f
  manipulation (Grade V), 186–188, 214–216
    contraindications, 215–216
    guidelines, 216–218
    indications, 215
    intervertebral joints (C7-13), 216, 217f
    intervertebral joints (T3-10), 217–218, 218f
    lumbar disc lesions, 188–189
    mechanical response, 214–215
    precautions, 215
    therapist action, 214
    when to use, 189–202
  mobilization, 185–188, 202–210
    anteroposterior unilateral vertebral pressure, 218–220, 219f
    lumbar disc lesions, 188–189
    posteroanterior central vertebral pressure, 202–204, 203f
    posteroanterior unilateral costovertebral pressure, 208–210, 208f–209f
    posteroanterior unilateral vertebral pressure, 207–208, 207f
    rotary posteroanterior intervertebral pressures, 204–205, 204f
    self-mobilization exercises, 187b

transverse vertebral pressure, 205–207, 206f
    PAIVMs, 197
  palpation, 196–197
    areas of sweating and temperature changes, 196
    differentiation test, 197–198
    soft tissue changes, 196–197
  physical examination, 189–202, 191b
    bony changes and position tests, 197
    flexion-extension, 192–194, 195f
    functional demonstration of symptoms, 190–192
    observation, 189
    PAIVMs, 197
    rotation, 192, 192f–193f, 195f
  posterior rami, 179f
  PPIVMs, 198–202
  present pain, 190
  prevalence of disorders, 176
  R2-12 areas, mobilization of ribs, 210, 211f
  red flags, 182, 184b
  rotation, 192, 192f–193f, 195f
  subjective examination, 176–182, 184b
  T1-12 areas, 191
    posterior primary rami, 179f
  T2-12 areas, rotation to right, 210, 210f–211f
  T3-10 areas, Grade V manipulation, 216–218, 217f
  T4-7 areas, 178
  T4-11 areas
    flexion/extension, 200
    lateral flexion, 200–201, 201f
    rotation, 201–202, 201f
  T5-7 areas, 189
  tests, 194–195
    combined movement, 194–195, 194f–195f
    compression movement, 195–196, 196f
    slump test, 196
    tap test, 196
  traction, 211–214
    lower spine, 212–214, 212f
    upper spine, 211–212, 212f
    see also cervical spine; lumbar spine; and specific disorders
thoracodorsal fascia, 334–335
thoracolumbar fascia, 334
thorax, flat, 189
touch, 383
    see also manipulation; palpation; passive movement
traction
  cervical, 164b–170b
  hospital, 323
  lumbar, 318–319, 318f
  machine, 318f
  thoracic, 211–214, 212f
    lower spine, 178f, 212–214, 212f–213f
    upper spine, 211–212, 212f

transverse abdominis, 333b, 334, 363, 363b
  assessment, 364
  posteroanterior pressure, 309f
transverse vertebral pressure
  lumbar spine, 299f
  thoracic spine, 205–207, 206f
trauma see injury
treatment, 5–6, 32–33, 40–41
  assessment of effects, 9–10
  cognitive behavioural therapy, 237–238, 270b–271b, 380
  consultative, 86
  failure, 52
  one-dimensional approach to, 386f
  precautions/contraindications, 39–40
  record-keeping, 441
  self-management strategies see self-management strategies
  techniques see techniques
  see also specific areas and conditions
treatment examples
  case studies, 164b–170b
  cervical spine, 155–160, 164b–170b
  lumbar spine, 230, 233–234, 235b, 320
  sacroiliac region, 372b–376b
  thoracic spine, 178–182, 182f
treatment objectives, 236–244
  optimization of movement capacity, 238
  psychosocial aspects, 238–240
  sense of control, 236–238
treatment planning, 97–98, 105–107
treatment sessions see assessment; consultation; and specific areas and conditions
trigeminal nerve, 136f–137f
  neurodynamic testing, 142f
  palpation, 135–136
TRPV1 channel, 121–122
trunk
  active movement, 345b, 347–348
  list correction, 275f
tumour necrosis factor-α, 122, 130
tumours, 182
two-point discrimination, 127b, 134b

U

ulnar nerve
  palpation, 139f
  tensioner technique, 161, 161f
  ULNT, 148f
ULNT see upper limb neurodynamic tests
unconditional regard, 90
upper limb neural tests (ULNTs), 196
upper limb neurodynamic tests, 141, 141b, 166f
  median nerve, 143f–146f
  radial nerve, 147f
  start position, 141, 149f
  ulnar nerve, 148f
urinary incontinence, 335, 344

V

verbal communication, 87–89
vertebral arteries, 159
vertebral disease
  ankylosing spondylitis, 101, 254t
    excessive compression in,
      367–368
    intra-articular injections for, 337t
  nerve root lesion *see* nerve root
    lesion
  osteoporosis, 182
  posture *see* posture
vertebral pressure
  anterior bilateral, cervical spine,
    138f
  anteroposterior central, lumbar
    spine, 300f

anteroposterior unilateral
  cervical spine, 138f, 218–220,
    219f
  thoracic spine, 218–220, 219f
vertebrobasilar insufficiency, 265
vertigo *see* dizziness
visceral pain, 182t

W

weak links, 252, 325
welcoming phase, 96
whiplash-associated disorder,
    116–117
  context change, 128b
  graded exposure therapy, 163,
    163b

motor impairment, 130b
  nociceptive patterns, 123b
wording skills
  bias, 15–16, 92–93
  paralleling, 91–92, 255
  see also communication
work, and disability, 392b
World Confederation of Physical
    Therapy, 83–85, 380–381
World Health Organization, ICF *see*
    International Classification of
    Functioning, Disability and
    Health

Y

yellow flags, 95–96, 233, 391